Modern Chromatographic Analysis of Vitamins

CHROMATOGRAPHIC SCIENCE SERIES

A Series of Monographs

Editor: JACK CAZES
Sanki Laboratories, Inc.
Mount Laurel, New Jersey

Additional Volumes in Preparation

Modern Chromatographic Analysis of Vitamins

Second Edition

edited by
André P. De Leenheer
Willy E. Lambert
Hans J. Nelis

State University of Ghent
Ghent, Belgium

Marcel Dekker, Inc.   New York • Basel • Hong Kong

Library of Congress Cataloging-in-Publication Data

Modern chromatographic analysis of vitamins / edited by André P. De
  Leenheer, Willy E. Lambert, Hans J. Nelis. -- 2nd ed.
      p.   cm. -- (Chromatographic science : v. 60)
    Includes bibliographical references and index.
    ISBN 0-8247-8626-2 (alk. paper)
    1. Vitamins-Analysis.   2. Chromatographic analysis.
  I. Leenheer, A. P. De. II. Lambert, Willy E.
  III. Nelis, Hans J. IV. Series.
    [DNLM: 1. Chromatography--methods. 2. Vitamins--analysis.   W1
  CH943 v. 60]
  QP771.M63 1992
  547.7'4046--dc20
  DNLM/DLC
  for Library of Congress   92-9991
                                                                        CIP

This book is printed on acid-free paper.

MARCEL DEKKER, INC.
270 Madison Avenue, New York, New York 10016

Current printing (last digit):
10 9 8 7 6 5 4 3 2 1

PRINTED IN THE UNITED STATES OF AMERICA

Preface

The first edition of *Modern Chromatographic Analysis of the Vitamins* was published in 1985. The past years have witnessed an enormous proliferation of chromatographic procedures for the determination of vitamins in different matrices.

This second edition constitutes an update of the state of the art of vitamin analysis and highlights the new important chromatographic trends in this area.

The first part covers the fat-soluble vitamins A, D, E, and K; the second part covers the water-soluble vitamins and coenzyme forms of ascorbate, folate, nicotinate, thiamine, flavins, pyridoxin, cyanocobalamin, biotin, and pantothenate. This new edition contains one additional chapter on pantothenic acid. We chose new authors for eight of the remaining twelve chapters.

Again, detailed information is given on quantitative analysis for each vitamin or vitamin group. In addition, the information on metabolism and biochemical function of each vitamin is updated.

The book is designed primarily for those who have an acquaintance with the different chromatographic techniques (e.g., GC, GC-MS, HPLC, and TLC). However, useful information for a beginner in this field is also included or referred to.

This work could not have been presented without the cooperation of the numerous authors and we are very grateful for their efforts.

André P. De Leenheer

Willy E. Lambert

Hans J. Nelis

Contents

Contributors

Arun B. Barua Biochemistry and Biophysics Department, Iowa State University, Ames, Iowa

Jiří Davídek Department of Food Chemistry and Analysis, Institute of Chemical Technology, Prague, Czechoslovakia

Tomáš Davídek Department of Food Chemistry and Analysis, Institute of Chemical Technology, Prague, Czechoslovakia

André P. De Leenheer Laboratory for Medical Biochemistry and Clinical Analysis, State University of Ghent, Ghent, Belgium

David S. Duch Division of Cell Biology, Wellcome Research Laboratories, Research Triangle Park, North Carolina

Harold C. Furr* Department of Biochemistry and Biophysics, Iowa State University, Ames, Iowa

Michel Gaudry Laboratoire de Chimie Organique Biologique, Université Pierre et Marie Curie, Paris, France

---

*Present affiliation: Department of Nutritional Sciences, University of Connecticut, Storrs, Connecticut.

Bruce W. Hollis Department of Pediatrics and Department of Biochemistry and Molecular Biology, Medical University of South Carolina, Charleston, South Carolina

Brian Irvin Analytical Development, Liposome Technology, Inc., Menlo Park, California

Glenville Jones Department of Biochemistry, Queen's University, Kingston, Ontario, Canada

Takashi Kawasaki Department of Biochemistry, Hiroshima University School of Medicine, Hiroshima, Japan

Willy E. Lambert Laboratory for Medical Biochemistry and Clinical Analysis, State University of Ghent, Ghent, Belgium

Johanna K. Lang Analytical Development, Liposome Technology, Inc., Menlo Park, California

Jan Lindemans Department of Clinical Chemistry, University Hospital Rotterdam Dijkzigt and Sophia Children's Hospital, Rotterdam, The Netherlands

Hugh Llewellyn John Makin Department of Chemical Pathology, The London Hospital Medical College, London, England

Robert J. Mullin Wellcome Research Laboratories, Research Triangle Park, North Carolina

Peter Nielsen Abteilung Medizinische Biochemie, Physiologisch-Chemisches-Institut Universitätskrankenhaus Eppendorf, Hamburg, Germany

Kristiina Nyyssönen Department of Clinical Chemistry, University of Kuopio, Kuopio, Finland

James Allen Olson Biochemistry and Biophysics Department, Iowa State University, Ames, Iowa

Markku T. Parviainen Department of Clinical Chemistry, University of Kuopio and University Central Hospital, Kuopio, Finland

CONTRIBUTORS

Olivier Ploux   Laboratoire de Chimie Organique Biologique, Université Pierre et Marie Curie, Paris, France

Michael Schillaci   Analytical Development, Liposome Technology, Inc., Menlo Park, California

Katsumi Shibata   Department of Food Science and Nutrition, Teikoku Women's University, Moriguchi, Osaka, Japan

Tatsuhisa Shimono   Department of Food Science and Nutrition, Teikoku Women's University, Moriguchi, Osaka, Japan

David James Hamilton Trafford   Department of Chemical Pathology, The London Hospital Medical College, London, England

Johan B. Ubbink   Department of Chemical Pathology, University of Pretoria, Pretoria, South Africa

Jan Velíšek   Department of Food Chemistry and Analysis, Institute of Chemical Technology, Prague, Czechoslovakia

RETINOIDS AND CAROTENOIDS

Harold C. Furr*, Arun B. Barua,
and James Allen Olson

Iowa State University, Ames, Iowa

1. RETINOL AND RELATED COMPOUNDS

1.1 Introduction

Chemical Properties

The structures and the IUPAC-approved numbering system of some naturally occurring compounds in the vitamin A group are depicted in Fig. 1. A group of synthetic retinoids is shown in Fig. 2. Approximately 2500 retinoids have thus far been synthesized, characterized, and, in many cases, evaluated for biological activity and toxicity (1–3). Although some of the more recently sythesized retinoids, such as 2.i and 2.j, bear little chemical resemblance to retinol (1.a), they all possess a highly conjugated double bond system, roughly similar physical dimensions, and similar types of biological activities. Inasmuch as some naturally occurring compounds, such as 1.c and 1.d, are also used as therapeutic agents, the distinction between naturally occurring and synthetic retinoids is not helpful relative to their usage in society. Thus, the general term "retinoids" embraces a large number of sometimes distantly related chemical compounds.

The so-called parent compound, all-*trans*-retinol (1.a), is an isoprenoid with five conjugated double bonds, absorption maximum at 325 nm in hexane or ethanol, and a single oxygen function. In acid, retinol rapidly dehydrates to anhydroretinol (1.h). In the presence of

*Present affiliation: Department of Nutritional Sciences, University of Connecticut, Storrs, Connecticut

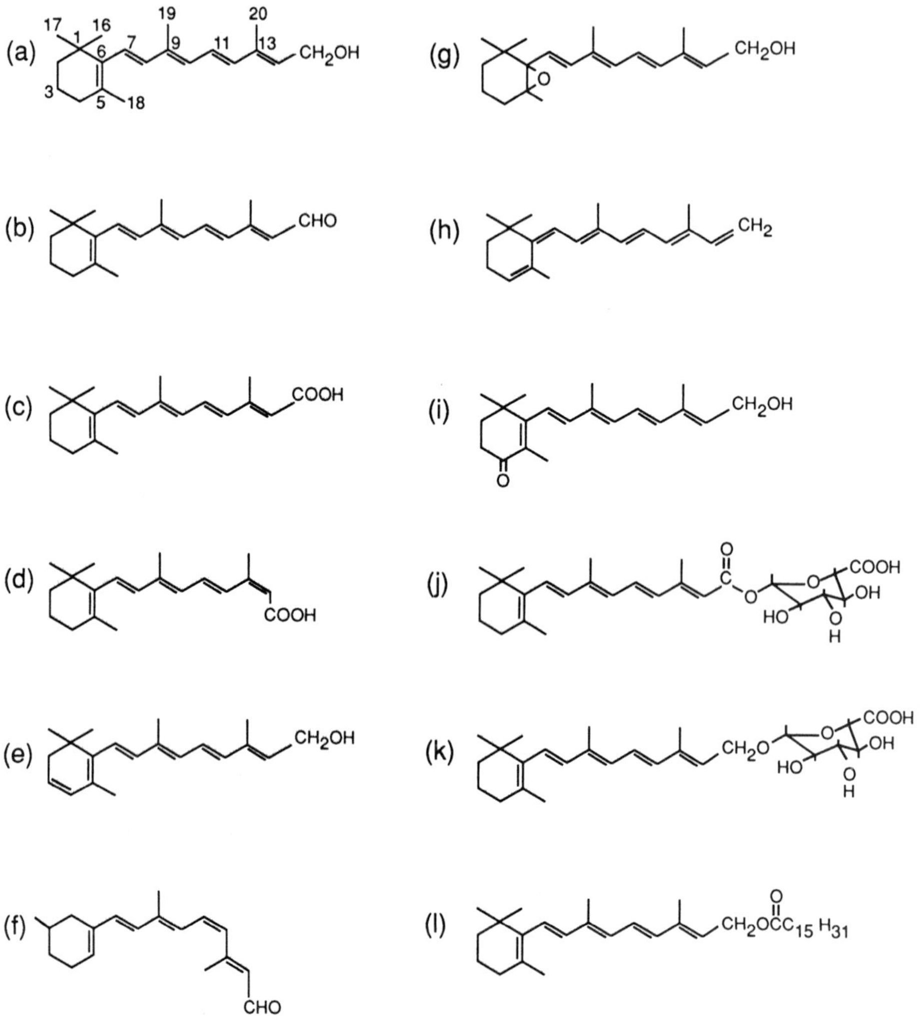

Figure 1 Some naturally occurring retinoids: (a) all-*trans*-retinol; (b) all-*trans*-retinal; (c) all-*trans*-retinoic acid; (d) 13-*cis*-retinoic acid; (e) all-*trans*-3,4-didehydroretinol; (f) 11-*cis*-retinal; (g) all-*trans*-5,6-epoxy retinol; (h) all-*trans*-anhydroretinol; (i) all-*trans*-4-oxoretinol; (j) all-*trans*-retinoyl β-glucuronide; (k) all-*trans*-retinyl β-glucuronid; (l) all-*trans*-retinyl palmitate.

light, retinol and its derivatives, such as 1.b, 1.c, and 1.l, isomerize to a mixture of isomers, primarily the 13-*cis* and 9-*cis* forms. Isomerization is much enhanced by iodine. The nature of the isomer mixture markedly depends on the solvent used.

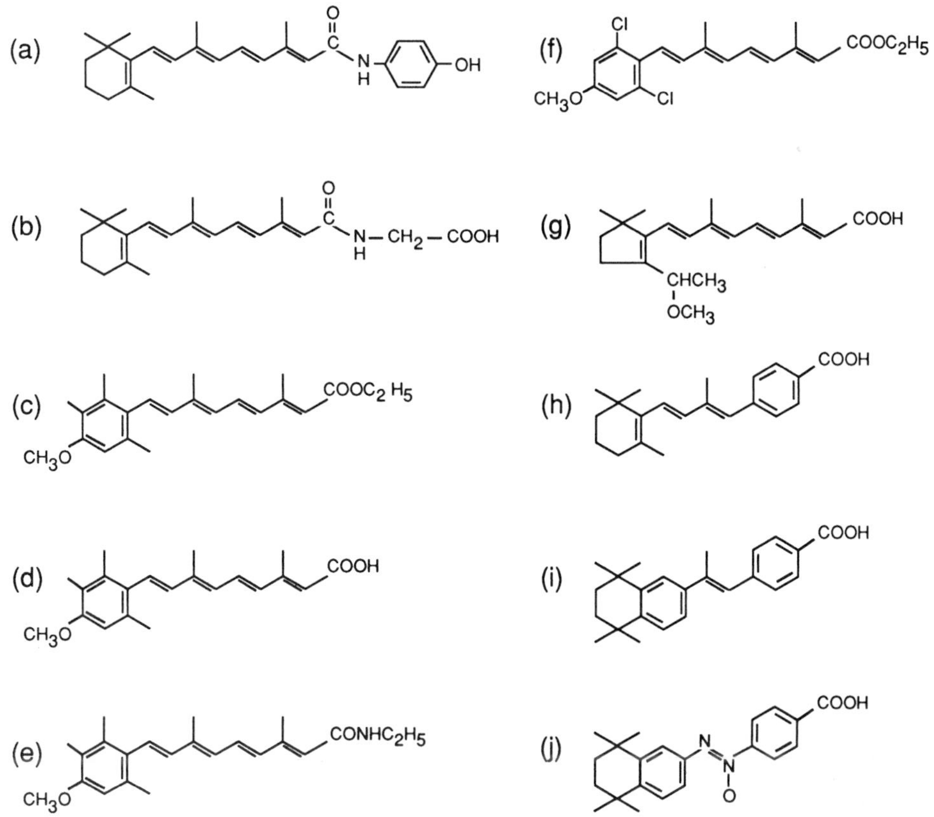

Figure 2 Some synthetic all-*trans* retinoids: (a) 4-hydroxyphenylretinamide (4-HPR), or *N*-retinoly-4-aminophenol; (b) *N*-retinoyl glycine; (c) the trimethyl-methoxyphenol analog of ethyl retinoate, also trivially called "etretinate"; (d) the trimethylmethoxyphenol analog of retinoic acid, also trivially called "acitretin"; (e) the trimethylmethoxyphenol analog of ethyl retinamide, also trivially called "motretinide"; (f) the methylmethoxydichlorophenol analog of ethyl retinamide, also trivially called "dichloroetretinate"; (g) the dimethylmethoxy-ethyl-cyclopentenyl analog of retinoic acid; (h) an aryl triene analog of retinoic acid; (i) tetrahydrotetramethylnaphthalenylpropenylbenzoic acid, abbreviated TTNPB and trivially termed an "arotinoid"; (j) tetrahydrotetramethylnaphthalenyl-azoxybenzoic acid, abbreviated TTNAOB and trivially called "Az90."

All retinoids are sensitive to oxidation and peroxidation, particularly in the presence of transition-group metals. A very large assortment of products results, including those with shortened carbon chains, ring oxidations, and hydroxymethyl groups.

Thus, to prevent the artefactual formation of such products, the following precautions are necessary: (a) the storage of biological samples at low temperature, preferably at $-70°C$, under argon in the dark, (b) the extraction with peroxide-free organic solvents, (c) the conduct of all analytical operations under yellow light, and (d) the analysis of reference compounds of high purity under identical sample conditions.

Because of its conjugated double bond system, vitamin A and other retinoids can be characterized and quantitated by their UV absorption spectra and often by their fluorescence. Proton and ^{13}C nuclear magnetic resonance (NMR) spectra are useful in characterizing *cis-trans* isomers, and mass spectrometry (MS) is valuable in assessing molecular weights and structures.

Formulas and molecular weights of some naturally occurring retinoids are: retinol ($C_{20}H_{30}O$, 286.44), retinal ($C_{20}H_{28}O$, 284.42), retinoic acid ($C_{20}H_{28}O_2$, 300.42), retinyl palmitate ($C_{30}H_{60}O_2$, 524.88), and retinoyl β-glucuronide ($C_{26}H_{36}O_8$, 476.54). At room temperature, retinol and its esters fluoresce strongly at 480–490 nm when excited at 325–345 nm, whereas retinal and retinoic acid do not. Fluorescence is enhanced in hexane and dioxane and depressed in ethanol and other alcohols. Because other polyenes, such as phytofluene, also fluoresce strongly under these conditions, care must be taken in differentiating between vitamin A fluorescence and that due to other compounds.

In addition to all-*trans*-vitamin A, all 15 of the other possible isomers have been characterized (4–6). In general, the introduction of increasing numbers of *cis* bonds lowers both the maximum wavelength and the molecular extinction coefficient relative to the all-*trans* isomer.

Biochemistry

Approximately 50 of the 600 known carotenoids can be oxidatively converted into retinal in mammals, primarily by central cleavage (7,8) but presumably also by eccentric cleavage (9,10). Retinyl esters, the major dietary form of vitamin A from animal products, are hydrolyzed in the intestinal lumen in the presence of pancreatic esterases and conjugated bile salts (11,12). Retinal produced from carotenoid cleavage is reduced to retinol, which is esterified and incorporated into chylomicra. Chylomicron remnants are taken up primarily by parenchymal cells of the liver but also by other tissues. Retinyl esters are hydrolyzed to retinol, which can (a) combine with the apo form of retinol-binding protein (RBP) to form holo-RBP, (b) be transferred to the stellate cells and be re-esterified, (c) be re-esterified in the parenchymal cell, (d) be oxidized through retinal to retinoic acid, (e) be conjugated with UDP-glucuronic acid to form retinyl β-glucuronide. In a similar way, retinoic acid forms retinoyl β-glucuronide. Although the mode of transferring retinol between parenchymal and stellate cells is still not clear, RBP has been suggested as a possible intercellular carrier within liver (13).

Vitamin A is inactivated biologically by either oxidation at the C-4 position to yield hydroxy and oxoderivatives or by oxidative shortening of the conjugated carbon chain. Hydroxylation of methyl groups also takes place.

Within cells, vitamin A is largely bound to specific carrier proteins, termed cellular retinoid-binding proteins. At least two such proteins bind retinol, another two bind retinoic acid, and another, uniquely in the eye, binds retinal. An additional binding protein for retinol and retinal, termed interphotoreceptor (interstitial) retinoid binding protein (IRBP), is found in the interphotoreceptor matrix between the retinal pigment epithelium and the outer segments of rod cells. In addition to the all-*trans* form, specific *cis* isomers are bound by some of these cellular binding proteins, but not by others. The binding proteins serve as transport and protective agents for retinoids and, in some cases, enhance their enzymatic transformations.

Another set of binding proteins, specific for retinoic acid, is found in the nucleus of cells. Because they influence genome expression, they have been called retinoic acid receptors (RAR). These RAR belong to a super-family of receptors, which also includes those for some steroids, tri-iodothyronine, and 1,25-hydroxycholecalciferol (14).

In the plasma, vitamin A is transported from its major depots in the liver to tissues in several forms, primarily as a 1:1 molar complex of all-*trans*-retinol with RBP, but also as all-*trans*- and 13-*cis*-retinoic acid, probably bound to albumin, and as retinyl and retinoyl β-glucuronides. Holo-RBP also interacts strongly with transthyretin in the plasma. All of these forms of vitamin A can be taken up by various tissue cells. Several tissues besides the parenchymal cells of the liver can also synthesize RBP, as evidenced by the presence of mRNA for RBP within such cells (15). Thus, the extensive recycling of retinol between the liver and peripheral tissue cells may well occur in both directions as complexes with RBP. Another possibility is that retinyl ester synthesized in essentially all cells of the body might be carried back to the liver in lipoproteins.

Vitamin A functions in vision and in cellular differentiation. In the visual process, holo-RBP of the plasma is taken up by the retinal pigment epithelium (RPE) by a receptor-mediated process. All-*trans*-retinol is isomerized to the 11-*cis* form in the RPE by a concerted reaction involving ester formation and hydrolysis (16,17). The 11-*cis* isomer, like the all-*trans* form, can be esterified by transacylation from endogenous membrane phospholipids or can be ferried to the rod outer segment on IRBP (18,19).

Within the RPE or outer segment, 11-*cis*-retinol is oxidized to 11-*cis*-retinal, which combines in the outer segment with opsin to yield rhodopsin. Light destabilizes rhodopsin by isomerizing the 11-*cis* chromophore through a transoid state to the all-*trans* isomer. Concomitantly, the protein passes through several conformational states to metarhodopsin II, which interacts with transducin, a G-protein with three subunits. A series of molecular events follow, including GTP binding, phosphodiesterase activation, a decrease in the cystosolic concentration of cGMP, a blocking of sodium ion uptake, and resultant hyperpolarization of the rod cell membrane (12,20). Needless to say, these events can be reversed. The three types of cone cells presumably have similar mechanisms for transducting impulses of light into membrane potentials.

In vitamin A deficiency, mucus-secreting epithelial cells in many tissues are replaced by squamous cells. Although this process of "keratinization" is the most prominent cellular manifestation of vitamin A deficiency, more subtle changes occur in most cells of the body. In the absence of vitamin A, keratinocytes produce a different pattern of keratins. Low concentrations of retinoic acid rapidly induce transglutaminase in macrophages (21), granulocytic differentiation in promyelocytic leukemia (HL-60) cells (22), and the differentiation of embryonic teratocarcinoma (F-9) cells (23). Retinoic acid, and, to a lesser extent, other naturally occurring retinoids produce a variety of cellular effects in other cell lines as well (24). Many synthetic retinoids show similar actions. Although these effects cannot readily be placed in a cohesive, all-embracing pattern, retinoids clearly influence gene expression in many cells.

The current leading hypothesis is that the nuclear RAR play a direct role in this process. Of the three known RAR, the γ form predominates in the skin. Because the K_a of RAR for retinoic acid is high (10^{10} mol/liter), RAR may be activated by physicochemical binding to free retinoic acid. Alternatively, covalent forms, that is, retinoyl derivatives of RAR, might also exist. Interestingly, retinyl and retinoyl β-glucuronide stimulate the differentiations of HL-60 cells well without evident conversion to retinol and retinoic acid, respectively (25). Retinoic acid has also been implicated as a morphogen in embryonic development (26). The adverse effects of vitamin A deficiency on reproduction, growth, and the immune response, in all likelihood, are an expression of perturbations in the process of cellular differentiation.

High doses of vitamin A and of other retinoids also cause serious toxic manifestations: namely, teratogenicity, chronic toxicity, and acute hypervitaminosis (11,12). Some individuals may also show a genetic sensitivity to vitamin A—termed vitamin A intolerance—at intakes not much above those normally ingested (27).

Sample Extraction and Handling

The retinoids are generally much more soluble in organic solvents than in aqueous systems, and hence must be extracted from biological or pharmaceutical matrices with lipophilic solvents. In the most favorable cases, the biological tissue can simply be ground with anhydrous sodium sulfate in a mortar (to facilitate tissue rupture and to remove water) under an appropriate solvent (e.g., dicholoromethane, dichloromethane:methanol, diethyl ether, or hexane: 2-propanol), and the resulting suspension filtered (28,29). Alternatively, the tissue may be homogenized before solvent extraction (30). Ito et al. have described a procedure for lyophilizing tissue homogenates before solvent extraction (31). The lyophilized homogenate may be extracted with dichloromethane:methanol and methanol (31), diethyl ether (32,33), or methanol and hexane (34).

In the most frequently used methods, blood plasma or serum samples are conveniently extracted with hexane or ethyl acetate (two or three extractions) after denaturing proteins with an equal volume of methanol or ethanol; the precipitating alcohol can be conveniently used as a carrier both for an internal standard and for an antioxidant. Alternatively, Peng et al. (35) have used 1/10 volume 5% perchloric acid to denature proteins and ethyl acetate for extraction of retinol. McClean et al. (36) and Nierenberg and Lester (37) used acetonitrile (including retinyl acetate, the internal standard) to denature serum proteins and then extracted retinol with ethyl acetate:1-butanol (1:1); an aliquot of the extract, without reduction in volume, was injected directly onto reversed-phase high-performance liquid chromatography (HPLC). The choice of denaturing solvent is a matter of personal preference; acetonitrile gives a more rubbery pellet of precipitated protein than does methanol, more difficult to resuspend for subsequent extraction.

Ionizable retinoids (such as retinoic acid or retinoid glucuronides) are more efficiently extracted with ethyl acetate after acidification of the aqueous medium, with, for example, dilute acetic acid (38,39). Alternatively, Wyss and Bucheli (40) have described a column-switching technique for HPLC of polar retinoids (retinoic acid, 13-*cis*-retinoic acid, and their 4-oxo metabolites) in serum that requires no separate solvent extraction: a plasma sample (diluted with acetonitrile solution containing internal standard and centrifuged after precipitation of plasma proteins) is injected onto a reversed-phase column, onto which the retinoids partition. Polar plasma components are washed out, and then the retained retinoids are back-flushed onto an analytical column and separated by gradient reversed-phase HPLC. A similar procedure could be useful for analysis of plasma retinol, but a similar method for analysis of retinol has not been reported.

More efficient breakup of tissues and extraction of retinol can be achieved by saponification of tissue or tissue homogenate. Conventionally, 1–4 parts aqueous 60% potassium hydroxide is used for low-fat samples, whereas ethanolic potassium hydroxide (5 g potassium hydroxide dissolved in 5 ml water and then diluted to 50 ml with 95% ethanol) is used for high-fat samples. The mixtures are heated at 60–100°C for 15–45 min; after cooling, retinol is extracted by addition of 1 part water and 3–5 parts hexane or ether (41). This approach is useful for determination of total vitamin A (as retinol), but provides no information on amount or composition of retinyl derivatives (e.g., esters, glucuronides) in the sample.

Open-column partition chromatography of tissue extracts on Sephadex LH-20 has been used to remove nonretinoid lipids and/or to resolve retinoids partially (31,42,43). Ion-exchange chromatography has been used for preliminary purification of ionic retinoids (44,45).

Ground animal feedstuffs can be extracted with isooctane:dioxane (80:20) with extensive shaking; the extract is filtered and concentrated for analysis of retinol and retinyl esters (46). For measuring total vitamin A in feedstuffs, saponification in the presence of sodium ascorbate or pyrogallol as antioxidant has been recommended (47–50). Disposable Kieselguhr columns (eluted with isooctane) may be used for preliminary purification of fatty samples after saponification (51).

For almost any chromatographic analysis it will be necessary to concentrate the original sample extract. For small extract volumes (<5 ml), it is convenient to evaporate volatile solvents (ether, dicholoromethane, hexane) under a gentle stream of inert gas. Argon is preferable to nitrogen, as commercial nitrogen may contain traces of oxygen, which can destroy retinoids in the trace quantities frequently present in tissue extracts. The residual lipid is then redissolved in a known amount of suitable solvent. Ideally this solvent should be of low volatility (to minimize volume changes by evaporation), capable of dissolving large amounts of lipid, and fully compatible with the chromatographic technique to be used (miscible and of similar polarity).

Driskell et al. (52,53) found that retinol is stable in frozen serum for at least 8 years, but that it was essential to add an antioxidant during extraction to prevent destruction of retinol. In contrast, Craft et al. (54) found that retinol and α-tocopherol were stable in frozen serum but that serum carotenoids were less stable, and that addition of antioxidant (ascorbic acid or butylated hydroxytoluene) had no effect on stability of the extracted compounds. Peng et al. (35) found retinol to be stable in their extraction solvent (ethyl acetate) for 24 h at $-20°C$; Barreto-Lins et al. (55) found that extracted retinol decomposed rapidly at ice temperatures. Clearly, each laboratory must establish its own optimum extraction and analysis conditions; the effect of climatic conditions (ambient temperature, light intensity, and relative humidity) on retinol stability has not been studied thoroughly. Since retinoids are labile to oxygen and light, especially when removed from the protection of their biological matrices, sample extracts should be analyzed as promptly as possible. Antioxidants (such as butylated hydroxytoluene) may be added at any stage of sample preparation to protect against oxidation, if it is confirmed that the antioxidant will not interfere with subsequent analysis. In this regard, it should be noted that pyrogallol (and presumably ascorbic acid) are poorly soluble in organic solvents; butylated hydroxyanisole (BHA) and butylated hydroxytoluene (BHT) are more soluble in organic solvents, but BHA's light absorption maximum (290 nm in methanol) approaches that of retinol, while BHT (absorption maximum 275 nm in methanol) is less well separated from retinol chromatographically (H. C. Furr, unpublished observations).

To prevent geometric isomerization of retinoids by white light, it is convenient to outfit the laboratory with yellow fluorescent lights ("F40 Gold" or equivalent) (56). Working in subdued lighting and keeping all retinoid and carotenoid solutions in amber glassware is helpful but provides less certain protection.

1.2. Thin-Layer Chromatography

Thin-layer chromatography (TLC) has traditionally been a method of choice for analysis of lipophilic compounds and was described extensively in the previous edition of this work, to which the interested reader is referred (57). TLC can be used for quantitative analysis, for example, for retinol (58). Recently TLC has been used less and less for analysis of retinoids and carotenoids because of the lability of these compounds to oxygen (particularly when adsorbed onto silica or alumina coatings in the presence of air), the expense of densitometers for quantitation of TLC plates, and the increasing availability of high-pressure liquid chromatographic equipment, which offers high resolution, lower limits of detection, and ready quantitation. TLC is still quite useful, however, for rapid analysis of reaction products when carrying out synthetic modification of retinoids and carotenoids, and for preliminary development of high-pressure liquid chromatographic separation techniques. Thus, short (7.5–8 cm) commercially available reversed-phase (C_8 and C_{18}) and adsorption (silica and alumina) TLC plates allow more rapid comparisons of chromatographic conditions (stationary and mobile phase) than do HPLC columns, which must be connected and equilibrated with various mobile phases before analysis.

Thin-layer chromatography is also useful for confirming the purity of concentrated solutions of retinoids and carotenoids, where impurities that do not absorb markedly at the wavelength of detection or that elute slowly from HPLC might not be detected by that technique. Similarly, TLC is preferable for analysis of radiochemical purity, since in other methods impurities may not be eluted and detected. Detection of radioactivity may be accomplished (after visualization of the retinoids by methods such as are described below) by autoradiography (exposure of the TLC plate to a sheet of x-ray film) (59), or by cutting the TLC plate into short sections, which are then counted individually in vials by liquid scintillation.

For initial "scouting" analysis by adsorption TLC (on silica or alumina plates), mobile phases of hexane:ether or hexane:acetone (4:1, v:v) frequently give adequate resolution. By altering the mobile-phase composition, R_f values (relative mobility) of desired components can be suitably adjusted. Tables of R_f values of representative retinoids on silica and alumina are given by John et al. (60), by Varma et al. (61), and by Fung and Rahwan (62). On reversed-phase TLC plates, methanol or acetonitrile gives adequate mobility and resolution for retinol and retinyl acetate; mixtures of less polar solvents (such as dichloroethane) with acetonitrile give good resolution of long-chain retinyl esters, and methanol:water or acetonitrile:water mixtures are suitable for polar retinoids.

Retinol and retinyl esters may be readily identified on TLC plates by their yellow-green fluorescence under a long-wave (366-nm) mercury lamp. Other retinoids (except anhydroretinol, which fluoresces with a red color), are not fluorescent under such conditions, and must be identified by nonspecific techniques, such as absorption of iodine vapor to form brown spots when placed in a chamber containing iodine crystals, quenching of the background fluorescence of fluorescent TLC plates (illuminated by a mercury lamp at 254 nm), or destructive tests such as charring with sulfuric acid.

1.3. High-Performance Liquid Chromatography

Introduction

Within the past 15 years, high-performance liquid chromatography (HPLC; also known as high-pressure liquid chromatography) has become the predominant method for separation and quantitation of retinoids. Of course, a number of factors are responsible for this popularity: ready availability of sturdy commercial equipment, with considerable standardization of equipment and techniques; appropriate lower limits of detection and facile quantitation; easily attained separation of most retinoids of interest within a reasonable length of time; and adaptability to crude biological tissue extracts or pure pharmaceutical preparations. The flood of vitamin A research in the past 20 years has depended heavily on HPLC. Several excellent reviews of the HPLC of retinoids may be cited, including those of Taylor (63), Lambert et al. (57), Bhat and Sundaresan (64), and De Leenheer et al. (65). Because the present review can not be exhaustive, the reader is referred to previous reviews for earlier information.

The two major, distinct methods of HPLC separation are referred to as normal-phase (adsorption) chromatography and reversed-phase (partition) chromatography. Polar bonded phases (cyano, amino), eluted with nonpolar mobile phases, also have been used in retinoid analyses. Historically, adsorption chromatography is the older technique, having been used for open-column separations since its introduction by Tswett (66), and so is often referred to as "normal-phase" or "straight-phase" chromatography. In this method, the sample is preferentially adsorbed onto a polar stationary phase, usually silica (sometimes alumina) in contemporary HPLC, and displaced from its adsorption sites by mobile phase, typically hexane containing low amounts of polar modifiers (67). Hence less polar sample components elute before more polar components. In traditional open-column adsorption chromatography, it was usual to adjust adsorption affinity both by adjusting the water content of the stationary phase and by adjusting polarity of the mobile phase with polar modifiers; in HPLC the water content of the stationary phase is adjusted only indirectly (deliberately or accidently), by adjusting water content of the mobile phase, and most adjustments of affinity and selectivity are made by modifying the mobile phase.

Reversed-phase HPLC is characterized by partitioning of the sample between a hydrophobic stationary phase (typically C_2, C_8, C_{18}, or phenyl chains covalently bonded to silica particles) and a more polar mobile phase, typically methanol or acetonitrile with small amounts of water added (68). Octadecylsilane (ODS, C_{18}) stationary phases have been most popular for retinoid analyses. In contrast to adsorption chromatography, polar sample components are eluted before less polar components in reversed-phase HPLC. Nonaqueous reversed-phase HPLC (mobile phases based on methanol or acetonitrile, with less polar solvent modifiers) has proven useful for separation of some nonpolar retinoids. To generalize, reversed-phase HPLC is frequently preferred for analysis of biological samples because the columns are more easily rinsed of impurities and because the sample separations are usually less sensitive to slight changes in mobile-phase composition; reversed-phase columns equilibrate with changing mobile phases much more rapidly than do adsorption stationary phases and hence are preferred for gradient elution. Adsorption HPLC, however, is capable of resolution of compounds (e.g., geometric isomers of retinoids) that are difficult or impossible to separate by reversed-phase HPLC.

Chromatographic analyses, whether adsorption or reversed-phase HPLC, should be designed so that the analytes of interest elute within the range $1 < k' < 10$, where the "capacity factor" $k' = (t_R - t_M)/t_M$ (t_R = retention time of sample component of interest, t_M = chromatographic dead time of the system). Chromatographic dead times may be determined by several methods (69,70), but can be approximated by the appearance of the well-known "solvent front" peak of the chromatogram. Large amounts of interfering substances in biological samples or excipients in pharmaceutical preparations may contribute to a large "solvent front," thus rendering difficult the quantitation of very early eluting peaks. On the other hand, late-eluting peaks are broadened and flattened, also making quantitation less certain; any chromatographic procedure that results in excessive values of k' also results in wasted time and wasted mobile phase. Separation of two adjacent peaks may be conveniently expressed by the "separation factor" $\alpha = k_2'/k_1'$ where k_2' and k_1' are the capacity factors of the two peaks. (More precise definitions of resolution also take into account the width of each peak.) The chromatographer must also note that merely increasing retention times of two peaks (by reducing mobile-phase flow or by adjusting mobile-phase composition) does not necessarily mean that their resolution is increased. For chromatography of a single component, the stationary phase and the composition of the mobile phase can be readily adjusted to give a capacity factor between 1 and 10. However, for analysis of several compounds differing significantly in polarity (for example, retinol and retinyl esters), it may be difficult or impossible to achieve this criterion with an isocratic (single) mobile phase, and gradient elution is required.

Quantitation of components separated by HPLC is achieved by comparison of peak areas or peak heights with those of standards. With the commercial availability of electronic reporting integrators, determination of peak area has become popular because peak areas tend to change less than heights when chromatographic conditions vary. Not every electronic integrator explicitly shows its baseline, however, and the chromatographer must beware that peak areas (or heights) are not erroneously increased because the integrator is drawing its baseline from a low point of the chromatogram (for example, a sharp depression associated with the solvent front). Gradient HPLC can be particularly troublesome, as some detectors respond to the varying refractive index of the mobile phase with dramatic changes of chromatogram baseline.

Standard curves are prepared by determination of the detector response (peak height or peak area) to known amounts of standards analyzed under identical conditions. Peak area is less susceptible to fluctuations in flow than is peak height. The standard curve should, of course, bracket the mass of sample analyzed, as detector responses may be nonlinear at the extremes. Despite the earlier use of international units (IU) or mass units (μg retinol equivalents), it is recommended that molar units be used for quantitation.

An appropriate internal standard is particularly important for correcting for losses during extraction and analysis. The internal standard, while being well resolved by chromatography, should be chemically and physically very similar to the analyte (i.e., itself a retinoid, preferably in the same chemical form) and should possess similar characteristics for extraction, chromatography, and detection. If the sample is not to be saponified subsequently or if the internal standard is not saponifiable, the internal standard may be added as a solution in the precipitating or extracting solvents. Retinyl acetate and propionate have been used as internal standards for retinol analysis (71), as have the hydrocarbons axerophthene (32) and anhydroretinol (72). Retinyl heptanoate and pentadecanoate have been used as internal standards for analysis of retinyl esters (73). Synthetic retinoids have been used as internal standards for quantitation of retinoic acid and other polar retinoids (40,74–76). Internal standards and external standardization using radioactive retinoids have been discussed by Cullum and Zile (34).

Concentrations of retinoid standards are conveniently determined by absorption spectroscopy of their solutions (Table 1). It must be emphasized, however, that purity of the standard solutions must be confirmed regularly (daily in some instances); retinoids are very labile to light, oxygen, and heat. Purity of a retinoid standard can be confirmed by comparison of its light absorption spectrum (not just absorbance at one wavelength) with that of a known standard and by demonstration of a single peak on chromatography (neither of these criteria is sufficient by itself). Commercially available all-*trans*-retinyl acetate, all-*trans*-retinyl palmitate, all-*trans*-retinal, and all-*trans*-retinoic acid are stable if stored appropriately (at $-20°C$ under inert gas such as argon), but should be checked before use and should be purified chromatographically if necessary. Commercial retinol is particularly unstable, in our experience; it is preferable to prepare retinol fresh by saponification of retinyl acetate or by reduction of retinal with sodium borohydride. [In the latter instance, a small quantity of retinal is dissolved in methanol and reduced by addition of solid sodium borohydride; after addition of water, the retinol is

Table 1 Light Absorbances of Selected Retinoids[a]

Compound	Solvent	λ_{max}	ϵ	$E_{1\,cm}^{1\%}$	Reference
All-*trans*-retinol	Ethanol	325	[52,770]	1845	77
	Hexane	325	[51,770]	1810	77
13-*cis*-Retinol	Ethanol	328	[48,305]	1689	77
11-*cis*-Retinol	Ethanol	319	[34,890]	1220	77
	Hexane	318	[34,320]	1200	77
All-*trans*-retinyl acetate	Ethanol	325	51,180	1560	12
	Hexane	325	[52,150]	1590	335
All-*trans*-retinyl palmitate	Ethanol	325	[49,260][b]	940	335
All-*trans*-retinal	Ethanol	383	[42,880]	1510	77
	Hexane	368	[48,000]	1690	77
13-*cis*-Retinal	Ethanol	375	[35,500]	1250	77
	Hexane	363	[38,770]	1365	77
11-*cis*-Retinal	Ethanol	380	[24,935]	878	77
	Hexane	365	[26,360]	928	77
All-*trans*-retinal oxime (*syn*)	Hexane	357	55,600	[1850]	147
(*anti*)	Hexane	361	51,700	[1723]	147
11-*cis*-Retinal oxime (*syn*)	Hexane	347	35,900	[1197]	147
(*anti*)	Hexane	351	30,000	[1000]	147
All-*trans*-retinoic acid	Ethanol	350	[45,300]	1510	335
All-*trans*-retinoic acid methyl ester	Ethanol	354	[44,340]	1415	335
13-*cis*-Retinoic acid	Ethanol	354	[39,750]	1325	335
13-*cis*-Retinoic acid methyl ester	Ethanol	359	[38,310]	1220	335
All-*trans*-retinoyl β-glucuronide	Methanol	360	50,700	[1065]	39
All-*trans*-retinyl β-glucuronide	Methanol	325	[44,950]	973	39
All-*trans*-3,4-didehydroretinol	Ethanol	350	[41,320]	1455	335
All-*trans*-3,4-didehydroretinal	Ethanol	401	[41,450]	1470	335
Anhydroretinol	Ethanol	371	[97,820]	3650	335
Axerophthene	Hexane	326	[49,950]	1850	335

[a] Values in brackets are calculated from corresponding ϵ or $E_{1\,cm}^{1\%}$ values.

[b] Medium- and long-chain fatty acyl esters of retinol have identical molar extinction coefficients (79).

extracted with hexane (77). If necessary, the hexane can be evaporated under a gentle stream of argon, and the retinol immediately dissolved in another solvent such as methanol or acetonitrile. Purity of the retinol is assessed by chromatography and its purity and concentration by absorption spectroscopy.] Other retinyl esters can be prepared by trans-esterification between retinyl acetate and the appropriate fatty acid methyl ester (78), or by condensation of retinol with either fatty acid anhydrides (79) or fatty acyl chlorides (80).

Retinoids tend to isomerize in solution, particularly when exposed to white light. Since the geometric isomers have lower extinction coefficients than do the all-*trans* forms, quantitation can be compromised if inappropriate standards are used. Reversed-phase HPLC frequently does not separate geometric isomers of retinoids well, so isomerization of standards and samples may be overlooked.

The most common mode of detection of retinoids in HPLC is by absorbance of ultraviolet light; because of their conjugated polyene chains, retinoids characteristically have high molar absorbances (molar extinction coefficients of 25,000–52,500) at wavelengths of 325–370 nm (Table 1), where few other compounds exhibit appreciable light absorbance. Thus the absorbance detectors currently popular for HPLC provide very good lower limits of detection and specificity for retinoids, with linear detector response over the range of most interest (typically up to 3.5 nmol, 1 μg retinoid). Values for lower limits of detection depend of course on electronic stability of the detector and the relative elution time of the peak of interest; late-eluting peaks are broader and more difficult to quantitate. Typical lower limits of detection are 3.5–35 pmol (1–10 ng) retinol at signal:noise ratios of 5:1 with absorbance detectors.

Detection of different retinoids with different absorption maxima (e.g., retinol and retinal) or of retinol and α-tocopherol or retinol and carotenoids necessitates either using a compromise wavelength (and sacrificing lower limits of detection) or switching wavelengths when a single-wavelength detector is used. These problems are obviated by use of a multiwavelength photodiode-array detector, which can monitor two to four wavelengths simultaneously (81–84). As these detectors are refined and made more sensitive it is expected that they will become increasingly popular, both because they provide the capability of monitoring several wavelengths at once and because they can provide complete absorption spectra for qualitative identification and for confirmation of peak purity.

Refractive index detectors are little used in retinoid research outside of preparative chromatography because they provide much poorer lower limits of detection and are not specific for retinoids. Refractive index detectors can not be used with gradient elution unless special steps are taken to eliminate changes of refractive index as the composition of the mobile phase varies.

Because retinol and its esters are highly fluorescent (excitation at 325 nm, emission about 480 nm), fluorescence detectors have been used to provide even lower limits of detection. For example, levels of 0.07 pmol (20 pg) retinol have been claimed to be measured in analysis of plasma (85–88) and in tear fluid (89) at a signal:noise ratio of 3:1, and 0.3 pmol (86 pg RE) retinyl palmitate at a signal:noise ratio of 6:1 (90,91) using fluorescence detection with adsorption HPLC. The fluorescence intensity of retinol and retinyl esters is dependent on solvent, being greater in non-polar solvents such as hexane; thus fluorescence detection offers greater advantages over light absorption detection in adsorption HPLC, where hexane-based mobile phases are used. This detection method provides specificity for retinol and its esters, but cannot be used for other retinoids because they are not fluorescent under ambient conditions.

Electrochemical detection of retinol has been demonstrated in reversed-phase HPLC by MacCrehan and Schonberger (92,93) and by Wring et al. (94), with a limit of detection of 0.29 pmol (82 pg) claimed at a signal:noise ratio of 2:1 (Fig. 3). Because water must be present for electrochemical detection, this method will find most application in reversed-phase HPLC, not in adsorption HPLC.

It is important to confirm identity and purity of chromatographic sample peaks. Probucol, an anticholesterolemic drug, has been reported to coelute with retinol and to interfere with its quantitation on reversed-phase HPLC (95); ubiquinones and beta-carotene coelute with retinyl esters in many HPLC systems (96). These interferences can be important, especially in samples with low retinoid content. Chromatographic peaks can be qualitatively identified by absorption spectroscopy (on-line, with photodiode-array absorbance detectors, or by off-line scanning of collected fractions), and identity confirmed by coelution with the appropriate standard in a completely different chromatographic system (e.g., adsorption chromatography after reversed-phase HPLC).

Retinol

All-*trans*-retinol is particularly easy to analyze by HPLC, whether it be from serum extracts or from saponified samples. Most published procedures for HPLC analysis of retinol differ in detail, not in concept. Hence the much-cited procedures of DeLeenheer et al. (97) and of Catignani and Bieri (98,99) for reversed-phase HPLC of retinol, which use methanol:water (95:5) with octadecylsilane (10-μm particle size) columns, are still appropriate as a beginning point for development of an assay in a new laboratory (Fig. 4). Reversed-phase columns using smaller particle size (5 or 3 μm) will offer sharper peaks (hence lower limits of

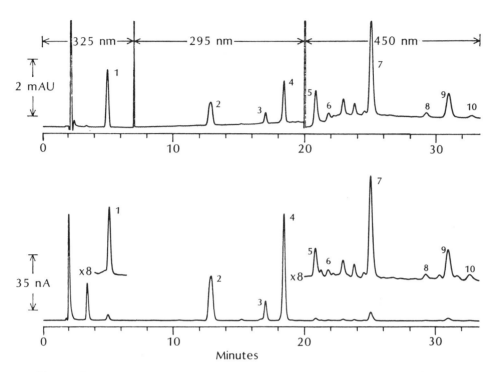

Figure 3 Gradient reversed-phase HPLC separation of retinol, tocopherols, and carotenoids in a serum extract with electrochemical and absorbance detection. Peak identification: 1, all-*trans*-retinol; 2, tocol (internal standard); 3, gamma-tocopherol; 4, alpha-tocopherol; 5, lutein; 6, zeaxanthin; 7, crypto-xanthin; 8, alpha-carotene; 9, all-*trans*-beta-carotene; 10, *cis*-beta-carotene. Chromatographic conditions: Vydac 5-μm TP 201 C_{18} column (4.6 × 250 mm), eluted with a linear gradient from methanol:water:1-butanol (75:15:10) (held 3 min initially) to methanol:water:1-butanol (88:2:10) over a 15-min period at 1.5 ml/min; both mobile phases contained ammonium hydroxide:acetic acid buffer at 0.02 M, pH 3.5. Detection: (lower trace) electrochemical detection at +900 mV with a glassy carbon electrode; (upper trace) absorbance at the indicated wavelength (93). Reprinted with permission from *Clinical Chemistry*.

detection). Of course, mobile-phase composition must be adjusted for the particular reversed-phase column in use to obtain retention times in the optimum range ($1 < k' < 10$, as discussed above); mobile phases of methanol:water or acetonitrile:water are appropriate for reversed-phase HPLC.

The challenges in analysis of retinol are to decrease lower limits of detection (thereby allowing use of smaller sample sizes) and to resolve

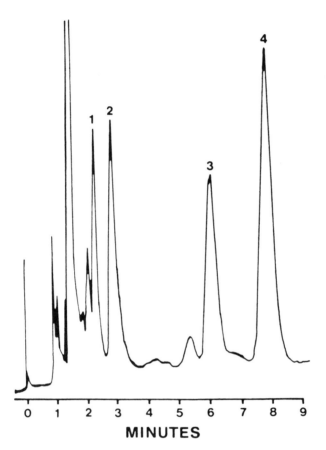

Figure 4 Chromatogram of retinol and α-tocopherol from normal plasma extract with internal standards added: Peak 1, retinol; 2, retinyl acetate (internal standard); 3, α-tocopherol; 4, α-tocopheryl acetate (internal standard). Chromatographic conditions: reversed-phase 10-μm μBondapak C_{18} column, eluted with methanol:water (95:5) at 2.5 ml/min; detection at 280 nm (98). Reprinted with permission from *Clinical Chemistry*.

geometric isomers. Many investigators are also interested in simultaneously determining either serum vitamin E and retinol levels, and/or serum carotenoids and retinol simultaneously. To improve limits of detection, narrow-bore adsorption HPLC (10 cm × 2.1 mm ID Spheri-5 Silica; mobile phase hexane:2-propanol, 99.5:0.5) has been used for analysis of retinol and retinyl palmitate (82,83). Unfortunately, lower limits of detection were not provided by the authors of those studies. Narrow-bore HPLC is not yet common in laboratories analyzing vitamin A, because more stringent demands are placed on equipment than are needed for conventional HPLC (e.g., accurate pumping at low flow, low-dispersion fittings and detector cells). Its application to the analysis of retinoids, particularly if coupled with sensitive fluorescence detection for retinol and retinyl esters, is highly promising.

Mansourian et al. (100) have used Lichrosorb-diol bonded-phase columns (mobile phase hexane:ethanol, 95:5) for analysis of serum retinol. The advantage claimed over adsorption HPLC is that irreversible adsorption of contaminants is much less, and the advantage over reversed-phase HPLC is that hexane extracts of samples can be injected directly onto the column, without evaporation and reconstitution. Palmer et al. (101) separated retinol from other liver components with hexane:2-propanol on a cyano-bonded phase column. Ohmacht et al. (102) have used amino- and cyano-bonded phases with gradient elution for determination of serum carotenoids and retinol.

Adsorption HPLC with fluorescence detection was used by Speek et al. (87,89) for analysis of retinol with lower limits of detection of 0.07 pmol (20 pg) retinol in 50 μl tear fluid. Biesalski et al. (103) have determined serum retinol and α-tocopherol simultaneously by isocratic adsorption HPLC with short retention times (< 10 min), and Van Haard et al. (104) have determined α-tocopherol, retinol, carotenes, and vitamin K_1 and 25-hydroxyvitamin D_3. Badcock and O'Reilly (88) determined retinol in human buccal mucosal cells by adsorption HPLC with fluorescence detection; 1-naphthol was used as internal standard, although it is not truly appropriate as it is not chemically similar to retinol.

Serum retinol and α-tocopherol were analyzed by reversed-phase HPLC by Nierenberg and Lester (37) and by Chow and Omaye (105). Serum retinol was analyzed with absorbance detection, and α-tocopherol simultaneously detected with amperometric detection by Huang et al. (106). Serum retinol, α-tocopherol, and carotenoids were analyzed by reversed-phase HPLC by Vuilleumier et al. (107), by Miller et al. (108), by Miller and Yang (81), by Nierenberg and Stukel (109), and by Hayes et al. (110). Retinol, α-tocopherol, and carotenoids also were analyzed in serum by Kaplan et al. (111) and by Brown et al. (112).

Bilic and Sieber (113) analyzed retinol (using retinyl acetate as internal standard) and α-tocopherol in milk and dairy products by reversed-phase HPLC after saponification. Similarly, Ciappellano et al. (114) also used saponification before HPLC analysis of retinol and carotenoids.

Nonaqueous reversed-phase HPLC was used by Nelis et al. (71) for determination of serum retinol, with retinyl propionate as internal standard.

Extraction is not necessarily required for the quantitation of plasma retinol. Retinol bound to plasma retinol-binding protein (RBP) can be directly detected by fluorescence in size-exclusion chromatography (115,116). With the size-exclusion columns used in the two reports to date (Toyo Soda TSK-SW and TSK-PW columns), retinol-RBP elutes in two peaks, namely, as the teritary retinol-RBP-transthyretin complex and as holo-retinol-RBP (115,116). Because fluorescence of retinol bound to RBP is enhanced to 10- to 14-fold over that of free retinol in solution (117), this method gives good limits of detection (3 pmol, 1 ng at a signal:noise ratio of 5:1) and requires as little as 20 μl serum sample at 0.17 μM retinol (5 μg retinol/dl). This method has the advantages of allowing direct injection of serum or plasma (with no extraction step) and of requiring only small samples (potentially, fingerprick blood samples). Its disadvantages are the requirements for fluorescence detection, a very different type of HPLC column and of mobile phase (albeit compatible with most HPLC equipment), and the need for secondary standardization with serum analyzed by conventional extraction techniques.

Retinyl Esters

Retinyl palmitate is both the most common retinyl ester found in most biological tissues and the most frequently available commercial form of vitamin A. Nonetheless, other long-chain fatty acid esters of retinol are also present in biological tissues. Because retinol and retinyl esters have the same molar absorptivity in a given solvent (79), retinyl palmitate may be used as a quantitative standard for all retinyl esters if peak area (not peak height) is used. The major problems in analyzing retinol and its esters from biological tissues are that (a) the difference in polarity between retinol and the common long-chain retinyl esters is too great to permit facile isocratic HPLC of both the alcohol and the esters, (b) it is equally difficult to elute all the esters as a single peak, and to resolve fully all the esters, and (c) the geometric isomers of individual retinyl esters in a mixture of retinyl esters cannot readily be resolved.

Retinyl ester composition varies from one biological tissue to another, but retinyl palmitate, stearate, and oleate usually predominate, with lesser amounts of shorter and unsaturated fatty acids present (79,118–120). Early attempts at isocratic reversed-phase HPLC of retinyl esters resulted in long retention times and sometimes in poor resolution of retinyl oleate from retinyl palmitate (79,118,121). DeRuyter and DeLeenheeer (122) cleverly effected the rapid separation of retinyl oleate from retinyl palmitate by argentation chromatography, that is, by incorporating silver nitrate in the mobile phase. Nonaqueous reversed-phase HPLC, however, proved effective for the rapid analysis of retinyl palmitate (123–126). Separation of the "critical pair" retinyl oleate and retinyl palmitate, as well as separation of most of the other naturally occurring vitamin A esters, was achieved by use of mobile phases containing chlorinated hydrocarbons (dichloroethane, dichloromethane, chloroform) in acetonitrile with short analysis times, k′ < 10 for all esters (96,127). This approach has subsequently been applied to analysis of retinyl esters in bovine retinal pigment epithelium (128), rabbit lacrimal gland (129), and milks and milk products (130) (Fig. 5). These methods were also used to determine the effects of dietary fatty acid composition on rat liver retinyl ester composition (120). In our experience, reversed-phase

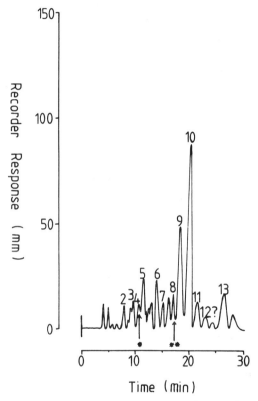

Figure 5 Nonaqueous reversed-phase HPLC of retinyl esters from bovine milk. Peak identification: 1, retinol; 2, retinyl caprylate; 3, retinyl caprate; 4, retinyl linolenate; 5, retinyl laurate + arachidonate; 6, retinyl linoleate; 7, retinyl myristate + palmitoleate; 8, retinyl pentadecanoate; 9, retinyl oleate; 10, retinyl palmitate; 11, retinyl eicosenoate; 12, retinyl heptadecanoate; 13, retinyl stearate; *, elution position of lycopene; **, elution position of β-carotene. Chromatographic conditions: two radially compressed NovaPak C_{18} columns in series, eluted with acetonitrile:dichloromethane (80:20) at 2 ml/min; detection at 325 nm (130). Reprinted with permission from *Journal of Micronutrient Analysis*.

mobile phases based on methanol (with tetrahydrofuran, toluene, or dichloromethane modifiers) provide resolution of retinyl esters by fatty acid chain length, but resolve retinyl oleate from retinyl palmitate poorly or not at all; only acetonitrile-based mobile phases modified with chlorinated hydrocarbons have provided good resolution of retinyl oleate from palmitate, as well as providing adequate resolution of most of the minor retinyl esters, with appropriately short retention times.

May and Koo (131) studied the effect of adding water to methanol-based mobile phases on the capacity factors (k') of a variety of retinyl esters on reversed-phase HPLC; essentially linear, parallel plots of log (k') versus percent water were found. For a given mobile-phase composition, linear relationships were found between log (k') and fatty acyl carbon number for saturated fatty acid retinyl esters, as has also been seen for mobile phases containing acetonitrile:dichloromethane (96). These relationships, and the retention time relative to retinyl palmitate, can be useful in tentative identification of retinyl esters on reversed-phase HPLC (127,131). Such studies of chromatographic behavior should facilitate optimization of conditions for retinoid separations.

High-pressure gel permeation chromatography (μStyragel columns eluted with dichloromethane or tetrahydrofuran) has been used for preliminary purification of retinyl palmitate (124,132,133).

The difference in polarity between retinol and its esters renders it difficult to obtain acceptable k' values for both using isocratic HPLC (either retinol elutes at an appropriate time after the solvent front and retinyl esters are eluted very late, or retinol is not well resolved from the solvent front). Lakshman et al. (134) found that a trimethylsilyl column (Zorbax TMS, 4.6 × 15 cm) eluted with acetonitrile:water (85:15) gave rapid elution of both retinol and retinyl palmitate standards; capacity factors and other details, however, were not given. A Whatman ODS-2 (C_{18}) column provided good retention of retinol (k' 2.5) with reasonably short retention times for retinyl palmitate (k' approximately 12) under conditions where other columns did not retain retinol adequately for confident quantitation (96). "Uncapped" reversed-phase columns could potentially retain retinol by hydrogen bonding, thereby bringing its k' closer to those of retinyl esters.

Adsorption HPLC in general is not as effective as reversed-phase HPLC at separating retinyl esters by fatty acyl chain length (135), but is particularly good at separating geometric isomers of retinoids. As in reversed-phase HPLC, it is difficult to obtain useful retention times for both retinyl esters and retinol under isocratic conditions. Biesalski and Weiser (91) have demonstrated the separation of all-*trans*, 13-*cis*, 11-*cis*, and 9-*cis*-retinyl palmitate, stearate, oleate, palmitoleate and linoleate (less than 14 min analysis time) on a 3-μm Spherisorb column, with lower limits of detection of 0.3 pmol by fluorescence detection and 0.8 pmol retinyl palmitate by UV detection. Full utilization of this method, however, requires careful control of mobile phase composition and moisture content, achieved by mobile-phase recycling (91).

Analysis of retinoids over a range of polarities is best achieved by gradient chromatography. Although gradient adsorption HPLC has been used to facilitate separation of geometric isomers of a range of retinoids (135, 136), the long times required for re-equilibration of adsorption stationary phases discourage their use for gradient chromatography. Reversed-phase HPLC is much more popular for gradient elution because the stationary phases reequilibrate rapidly with changes in mobile phase. Roberts et al. (32) used a single step gradient from 70:30 to 98:2 acetonitrile:water to elute retinoids from retinol to retinyl palmitate within 28 min. Neutral retinoids were separated on radial-compression C_{18} columns by use of methanol:water gradients, with partial resolution of retinyl esters (137). Cullum and Zile (34) have described a step-gradient system, using mobile phases of methanol:water (with ammonium acetate), methanol, and methanol: chloroform on an octadecylsilane column, which they used to elute compounds from the polar 4-oxo-retinoic acid and retinoyl β-glucuronide through retinoic acid, N-(4-hydroxyphenyl)retinamide, retinol, and retinyl acetate to the nonpolar retinyl palmitate and retinyl stearate. Van Kuijk et al. (138) used a step gradient from methanol (containing ammonium acetate) to 2-propanol to analyze retinoic acid, retinol, retinyl acetate (internal standard), retinal O-ethyl oxime, and retinyl esters in extracts of eye cups. Chaudhary and Nelson (139) analyzed retinoic acid, retinol, retinal, retinyl acetate, and retinyl palmitate by linear gradient elution from acetonitrile:water (with ammonium acetate), 70:30 to 98:2 on a C_{18} column; resolution of geometric isomers or retinyl esters was not attempted but separation of retinol and retinal was exceptionally good. Gradient reversed-phase HPLC on C_{18} columns has also been carried out with linear methanol:water to methanol:tetrahydrofuran gradients (140); depending on the composition of the final mobile phase, retinyl esters could be eluted as a single peak, or resolved by chain length. Methanol:water to methanol:dichloromethane gradients have been used to separate polar retinoids, retinol, and to achieve partial resolution of retinyl esters (38,39). Whereas methanol:tetrahydrofuran or methanol:dichloromethane mobile phases do not resolve retinyl oleate from retinyl palmitate, acetonitrile:water to acetonitrile:dichloroethane gradients can accomplish this separation (see discussion above and Ref. 127). In all of these gradient procedures, ammonium acetate is incorporated in the initial mobile phase to repress ionization of retinoic acid and other ionizable retinoids, thereby giving better peak shapes and more reproducible retention times (141,142). Reversed-phase gradient elution is flexible, in that mobile-phase composition can be adjusted to give convenient retention times for the particular column in use and the analytes of interest; if the most-polar retinoids (4-oxo-retinoic acid, retinoid glucuronides) are not to be analyzed, the proportion of water in the mobile phase may be reduced, and the analysis time correspondingly reduced. The disadvantages of gradient elution are that (a) a second pump (or single pump capable of gradient elution) must be available, (b) time for re-equilibration of the column with mobile phase (usually 5–10 min) must be allowed for reproducible retention times, and (c) changes in detector baseline due to the changing refractive index of the mobile phase may complicate quantitation by either peak area or peak height procedures.

Geometric Isomers of Retinal

Retinal is not used in pharmaceutical preparations or food supplements and occurs in significant quantities only in ocular tissues. Hence most analyses for retinal are concerned with its profile of geometric isomers as well as its quantitation. Isomerization of all retinoids can occur during food processing or saponification of samples for extraction and analysis, and knowledge of the extent of this isomerization may be important for estimating vitamin A value of foods (143).

Retinal is not well resolved from retinol in all reversed-phase HPLC systems. Curley et al. (144) compared chromatography of retinoids on a fully end-capped C_{18} column (Ultrasphere-ODS) and a non-end-capped column (Ultrasil-ODS). With a methanol:water mobile phase, retinol and retinal were baseline resolved on the end-capped column but not on the non-end-capped column; with an acetonitrile-water mobile phase, the opposite results were obtained. We have observed that on a given C_{18} column, effective resolution (separation factor $\alpha = k_2'/k_1'$) of retinol and retinal is not affected by the water content in methanol:water mobile phases (log k' for each compound increases proportionately as water content increases), but plots of log k' versus water content for retinol and retinal are not parallel for acetonitrile:water mobile phases (S. Cottingham and H. C. Furr, unpublished observations). Similarly, for reversed-phase HPLC of apo-retinoids and apo-carotenoid analogs, plots of log k' versus carbon chain length are parallel for alcohols and aldehydes/ketones in a given methanol:water mobile phase, but are not parallel for acetonitrile:water mobile phases (H. C. Furr, unpublished observations). Thus, separation of retinol and retinal on reversed-phase HPLC depends on the particular column and mobile phase, more so than most other retinoid separations. Van Kuijk et al. (138) prepared the O-ethyl oxime of retinal to improve retinal separation from retinol on reversed-phase HPLC, but without separation of geometric isomers.

MacCrehan and Schonberger (92) found that methanol:water mobile phases were superior to acetonitrile:water mobile phases for reversed-phase separation of geometric isomers of retinol (Vydac 201 TP or Zorbax ODS columns); the order of elution was di-*cis* < 11-*cis* < 9-*cis* < 13-*cis* < 7-*cis* < all-*trans*; separation factors ($\alpha = k_2'/k_1'$) were dependent on the column and mobile-phase composition. Replacement of part of the methanol in the mobile phase with *n*-butanol maintained the same separation factors but reduced total retention time to less than 30 min for complete isomer separation.

Resolution of geometric isomers of retinoids is generally better on adsorption HPLC than on reversed-phase HPLC (145). For separation of retinals, Zonta and Stancher (146) found that 2-propanol as a modifier in hexane separates all mono-*cis* isomers on a 5-μm Si-60 silica column, but does not separate di-*cis* isomers, whereas dioxane in hexane separates the di-*cis* isomers of retinal. Elution order is 11,13-di-*cis* < 13-*cis* < 9,13-di-*cis* < 11-*cis* < 9,11-di-*cis* < 9-*cis* < 7-*cis* < all-*trans*. For separation of retinols, 1-octanol is a more effective modifier of hexane than is 2-propanol; elution order is 11,13-di-*cis* < 11-*cis* < 9,13-di-*cis* < 13-*cis* < 9,11 di-*cis* < 9-*cis* < 7-*cis* < all-*trans*. In a comprehensive review of preparation and analysis of vitamin A isomers, Groenendijk et al. (147) demonstrated separations of isomers of retinyl esters, retinal, retinal oxime, and retinol by mobile phases of diethyl ether or dioxane in hexane.

Retinal oximes are conveniently prepared and are useful for the quantitative extraction of retinal from ocular tissue, where much of the retinal is held in Schiff-base linkage to the protein rhodopsin; the disadvantage to analyzing the oximes is that two conformers, *syn* and *anti*, are formed for each geometric isomer of retinal. Tsukida et al. (148) achieved resolution of the 10 isomers (*syn* and *anti* conformers) of 7-*cis*, 9-*cis*, 11-*cis*, 13-*cis*, and all-*trans*-retinal oxime using 0.2% 2-propanol in diethyl ether:benzene (3:97) on a Lichrosorb silica column. Landers and Olson (149) performed solvent optimization of separation of retinol and retinal oxime isomers on μPorasil and Excalibur silica columns; varying the ratios of isopropyl ether, dichloromethane, and chloroform in hexane had little effect on resolution of retinal oxime isomers, but isopropyl ether optimized separation of 9-*cis*- from all-*trans*-retinol, and dichloromethane plus chloroform optimized resolution of 11-*cis* from 13-*cis*-retinol. In further studies (150), these authors found that all the 9-*cis*, 11-*cis*, 13-*cis*, and all-*trans* isomers of retinal, retinal oxime, and retinol could be resolved from one another by use of ethyl acetate, dioxane, and 1-octanol as modifiers in hexane, on Lichrosorb Si-60 columns (Fig. 6). The elution order is retinyl esters (unresolved) < 13-*cis*-retinal < 11-*cis*-retinal < 9-*cis*-retinal < 7-*cis*-retinal < all-*trans*-retinal < *syn*-11-*cis*-retinal oxime < *syn*-all-*trans*-retinal oxime < *syn*-9-*cis*-retinal oxime +

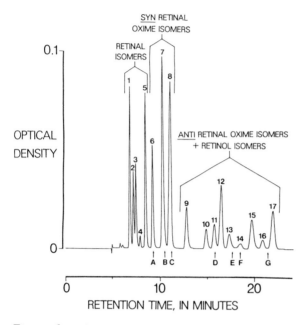

Figure 6 Adsorption HPLC separation of retinol, retinal, and retinal oxime isomer standards. Peak identification: 1, 13-*cis*-retinal; 2, 11-*cis*-retinal; 3, 9-*cis*-retinal; 4, 7-*cis*-retinal; 5, all-*trans*-retinal; 6, *syn*-11-*cis*-retinal oxime; 7, *syn*-all-*trans*-retinal oxime; 8, *syn*-9-*cis*-retinal oxime + *syn*-13-*cis*-retinal oxime; 9, *anti*-13-*cis*-retinal oxime; 10, *anti*-11-*cis*-retinal oxime; 11, 11-*cis*-retinol; 12, 13-*cis*-retinol; 13, *anti*-9-*cis*-retinal oxime; 14, 9,11-*cis*-retinol + 9,13-*cis*-retinol; 15, *anti*-all-*trans*-retinal oxime; 16, 9-*cis*-retinol; 17, all-*trans*-retinol; A, *syn*-9,11-*cis*-retinal oxime; B, *syn*-7-*cis*-retinal oxime; C, *syn*-9,13-*cis*-retinal oxime; D, *anti*-9,13-*cis*-retinal oxime; E, *anti*-9,11-*cis*-retinal oxime; F, *anti*-7-*cis*-retinal oxime; G, 7-*cis*-retinol. Chromatographic conditions: two 5-μm Lichrosorb Si-60 columns (4 × 250 mm) in series, mobile phase 11.2% ethyl acetate, 2% dioxane and 1.4% 1-octanol in hexane, flow 1 ml/min, detection at 325 nm (150). Reprinted with permission from *Journal of Chromatography*.

syn-13-*cis*-retinal oxime < *anti*-13-*cis*-retinal oxime < *anti*-11-cis-retinal oxime < 11-*cis*-retinol < 13-*cis*-retinol < *anti*-9-*cis*-retinal oxime < 9,11-*cis*-retinol + 9,13-*cis*-retinol < *anti*-all-*trans*-retinal oxime < 9-*cis*-retinol < all-*trans*-retinol < *syn*-9,11-*cis*-retinal oxime < *syn*-7-*cis*-retinal oxime < *syn*-9,13-*cis*-retinal oxime < *anti*-9,13-*cis*-retinal oxime < *anti*-9,11-*cis*-retinal oxime < *anti*-7-*cis*-retinal oxime < 7-*cis*-retinol for 11.2% ethyl acetate, 2% dioxane, and 1.4% 1-octanol in hexane. Retention of retinols relative to retinals and retinal oximes could be shifted by varying the proportion of 1-octanol.

Bridges et al. (136,151) used step gradients of ethyl ether in hexane or dioxane in hexane to separate retinyl esters (*cis* and *trans* isomers), retinal isomers, retinal oxime, retinol isomers, and 3-dehydroretinol (and its esters) on Lichrosorb, μPorasil, or Ultrasphere silica columns. As mentioned above, Biesalski and Weiser (91) have separated all-*trans*-, 13-*cis*-, 11-*cis*-, and 9-*cis*-retinyl palmitate, stearate, oleate, palmitoleate, and linoleate by isocratic adsorption HPLC (Fig. 7).

Bhat et al. (152,153) have used nonaqueous partition chromatography to separate isomers of retinol (dioxane in hexane or 2-octanol in hex-

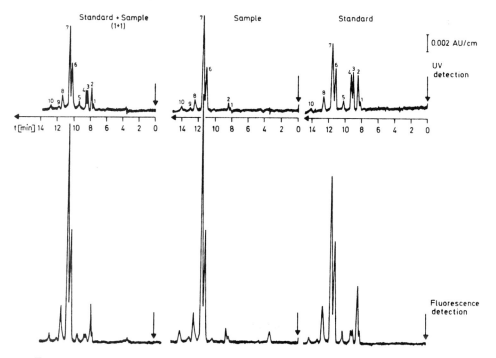

Figure 7 Isocratic adsorption HPLC of retinyl esters, with fluorescence and light absorbance detection. Peak identification: 1, 13-*cis*-retinyl stearate; 2, 13-*cis*-retinyl palmitate; 3, 11-*cis*-retinyl stearate; 4, 11-*cis*-retinyl palmitate; 5, 9-*cis*-retinyl palmitate; 6, all-*trans*-retinyl stearate; 7, all-*trans*-retinyl palmitate; 8, all-*trans*-retinyl oleate; 9, all-*trans*-retinyl palmitoleate; 10, all-*trans*-retinyl linoleate. Chromatographic conditions: 3-μm Spherisorb silica column (4.6 × 250 mm), mobile phase *n*-hexane:diisopropylether (98.5:1.5) at 2 ml/min; (lower trace) fluorescence detection (excitation at 332 nm, emission at 472 nm), (upper trace) absorbance detection at 325 nm. Note differences in sensitivity of fluorescence and absorbance detection for *cis* and all-*trans* isomers (91). Reprinted with permission from *Journal of Clinical Chemistry and Clinical Biochemistry*.

ane, on cyano- and octadecylsilane columns in series) or isomers of
retinoic acid (acetonitrile:dichloromethane:acetic acid, on a Zorbax
amino column); retention times were 25–50 min.

Extremely reproducible retention times for adsorption HPLC of
retinoid isomers are attainable if great care is taken in mobile-phase
preparation (including control of water content) and column equilibration.

Retinoic Acid and Other Polar Retinoids

HPLC has proven the method of choice for analysis of retinoic acid (tret-
inoin) and more polar retinoids. Since most of these compounds are not
fluorescent, absorbance detection is invariably used. Electrochemical
detection has not yet been reported with these compounds. Extraction of
acidic compounds from samples requires acidification, and HPLC
analysis requires addition of acid and/or a salt such as ammonium acetate to the mobile phase (39,154).

Adsorption HPLC can be used for analysis of retinoic acid if the
mobile phase is acidic; otherwise the polar compound adsorbs too tightly
to the stationary phase. Retinoic acid, 5,8-epoxyretinoic acid, 4-
oxoretinoic acid, and 4-hydroxyretinoic acid were separated on a silica
column (Partisil 10/50) with hexane:tetrahydrofuran:formic acid as
mobile phase (155); their methyl esters could be chromatographed on the
same column with a similar mobile phase (hexane:tetrahydrofuran)
without formic acid. DeRuyter et al. (154) and Thaller and Eichele (156)
used a mobile phase of acetonitrile and acetic acid in hexane on a silica
column. Methyl retinoate was also chromatographed with this column
and mobile-phase combination (154).

On a bonded-phase diol column, with a mobile phase of dichloromethane, 2-propanol, and acetic acid in hexane, DeRuyter et al. (154)
found that the capacity factor (k') of retinoic acid had a nonlinear
dependence on acetic acid concentration. The elution order on this
bonded phase column was retinal < retinoic acid < retinol.

Retinoic acid has been chromatographed on reversed-phase HPLC
with a methanol:water:acetic acid mobile phase on a C_8 column (154).
Frolik et al. (141) used acetonitrile:water mobile phases (with
ammonium acetate to repress broadening of the retinoic acid peak), and
showed clearly that the differences in retention on different reversed-
phase columns were due, at least in part, to differences in carbon load
(hydrocarbon coating of the stationary phase). Those authors (141) also
demonstrated the separation of 13-*cis*- from all-*trans*-retinoic acid by
reversed-phase HPLC. McCormick et al. (142,155) obtained separation
of 13-*cis*- from all-*trans*-retinoic acid, and separation of 4-oxo-, 4-
hydroxy-, 5,6-epoxy-, and 5,8-epoxyretinoic acids from retinoic acid,

using mobile phases of methanol:water with ammonium acetate on octa-decylsilane columns. The methyl esters of 4-oxo- and 4-hydroxyretinoic acid were not well resolved by reversed-phase HPLC (μBondapak C_{18} column), but could be resolved by adsorption HPLC (μPorasil column, hexane: tetrahydrofuran mobile phase) (142,155).

More recent analyses with newer columns (smaller particle size, higher carbon loading) can result in improved resolution, lower limits of detection, and better capacity factors (with adjustment of mobile phase). Thus, Barua et al. (38,39) quantitated retinoyl β-glucuronide, retinyl β-glucuronide, and retinoic acid from human plasma, using methanol:water (with ammonium acetate) on a Resolve 5-μm C_{18} column (Fig. 8), and Satre et al. (157) analyzed all-*trans*-4-oxoretinoic

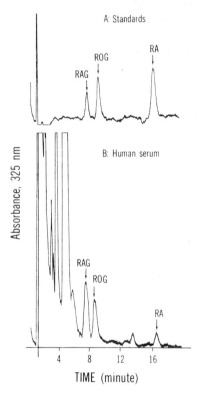

Figure 8 Isocratic reversed-phase HPLC of all-*trans*-retinoyl β-glucuronide (RAG), all-*trans*-retinyl β-glucuronide (ROG), and all-*trans*-retinoic acid (RA); A, standards; B, extract of human serum. Chromatographic conditions: Resolve 5-μm C_{18} column (3.9 × 150 mm); mobile phase methanol:water (68:32) containing 10 mM ammonium acetate, at 1.5 ml/min; detection at 325 nm (39). Reprinted with permission from *Methods in Enzymology*.

acid and 13-*cis*-4-oxoretinoic acid from mouse embryos with methanol:acetonitrile:water (with ammonium acetate) on a Partisil 5-μm ODS-3 column. Nonetheless, the principles of reversed-phase HPLC of retinoic acid have remained the same: mobile phases of methanol:water or acetonitrile:water, with incorporation of ammonium acetate at 0.1 to 1%.

Linear methanol:water mobile-phase gradients (with ammonium acetate) have been used with reversed-phase HPLC to separate all-*trans*-4-oxo-, all-*trans*-4-hydroxy-, and all-*trans*-5,6-epoxy-retinoic acid, 13-*cis*- and all-*trans*-retinoyl β-glucuronide, 13-*cis*- and all-*trans*-retinoic acid, all-*trans*-retinol, and methyl retinoate (43,158,159). Methanol:water gradients with acetic acid were used by Chaudhary and Nelson (160) for similar analyses. Cullum and Zile (34) used step gradients of methanol:water (also with ammonium acetate) to methanol:chloroform to resolve all-*trans*-4-oxo-, all-*trans*-5, 6-epoxy-, 13-*cis*-, and all-*trans*-retinoic acids, as well as 13-*cis*- and all-*trans*-retinoyl β-D-glucuronide, retinamides, and retinyl esters. A facile and more rapid resolution of a mixture of retinoids, including retinoyl β-glucuronide and retinyl β-glucuronide, retinoic acid, retinol, and retinyl esters, has been obtained with mobile phase gradients of methanol:water (with ammonium acetate) to methanol:dichloromethane on a Waters Resolve 5-μm C_{18} column (38,39) (Fig. 9). Swanson et al. (161) used gradients of acetonitrile:water (with ammonium acetate) on a Spherisorb 5-μm ODS column to separate retinoyl β-glucuronide and other metabolites of retinoic acid.

Because several analogs of retinoic acid have been used for dermatologic treatments in humans, monitoring their levels in plasma is important clinically. All-*trans*- and 13-*cis*-retinoic acid and several aromatic retinoid analogs were analyzed by adsorption HPLC on Partisil silica, with mobile phases of dichloromethane:glacial acetic acid or dichloromethane:methanol:glacial acetic acid (162). A number of isomers of retinoic acid (11,13-di-*cis*, 9,13-di-*cis*, 13-*cis*, 9-*cis*, and all-*trans*), 4-oxoretinoic acid (13-*cis* and all-*trans*), 4-hydroxyretinoic acid (13-*cis* and all-*trans*), and 5,6-epoxyretinoic acid (13-*cis* and all-*trans*) in whole human blood were analyzed by gradient reversed-phase HPLC (Whatman Partisil ODS, 10-μm particle size) using mobile phases of methanol:water:acetic acid (with ammonium acetate); an aromatic retinoic acid analog was used as internal standard (75). The lower limit of quantitation was about 0.03 nmol/ml (10 ng/ml).

Huselton et al. (163) used microbore adsorption HPLC on a diol column (1 mm × 25 cm; mobile phase 15% toluene in hexane) to chromatograph the pentafluorobenzyl ester derivatives of all-*trans*- and 13-*cis*-retinoic acid extracted from plasma, with direct-inlet negative-ion

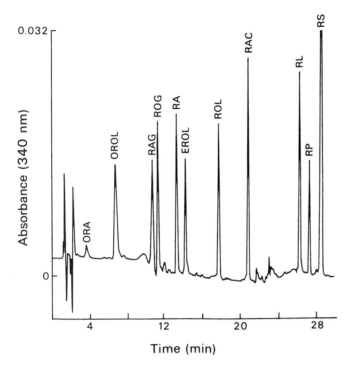

Figure 9 Gradient reversed-phase HPLC of retinoid standards. Peak identification: ORA, all-*trans*-4-oxoretinoic acid; OROL, all-*trans*-4-oxoretinol; RAG, all-*trans*-retinoyl β-glucuronide; ROG, all-*trans*-retinyl β-glucuronide; RA, all-*trans*-retinoic acid; EROL, all-*trans*-5,6-epoxyretinol; ROL, all-*trans*-retinol; RAC, all-*trans*-retinyl acetate; RL, all-*trans*-retinyl linoleate; RP, all-*trans*-retinyl palmitate; RS, all-*trans*-retinyl stearate. Chromatographic conditions: Resolve 5-μm C_{18} column (3.9 × 150 mm); 20-min linear gradient from methanol:water (68:32, containing 10 m*M* ammonium acetate) to methanol:dichloromethane (80:20) at 1 ml/min; detection at 340 nm (39). Reprinted with permission from *Methods in Enzymology*.

mass spectrometry for detection. Full-scan mass spectra could be obtained for standards; with selected ion monitoring at m/z 299, response was linear over the range 1.5–5 pmol. Tetradeuterated 13-*cis*-retinoic acid was used as internal standard.

To avoid extraction of plasma samples for analysis of all-*trans*- and 13-*cis*-retinoic acid and their 4-oxo metabolites, Wyss and Bucheli (40) employed column switching. Plasma proteins were precipitated by addition of 2-propanol (containing internal standard) and centrifugation. A large volume of the supernatant was injected onto a precolumn of C_{18} Corasil; polar components were flushed off, and then the retinoids were eluted from the precolumn and separated on an analytical column (5-μm Spherisorb ODS-1) with a gradient of acetonitrile:water:acetic acid (plus ammonium acetate). The limit of quantitation was 6 pmol/ml plasma (2 ng/ml).

Etretinate is the ethyl ester of an aromatic analog of retinoic acid (Fig. 2.c). An isocratic acetonitrile:water:acetic acid mobile phase was used on a Partisil ODS-2 reversed-phase column for quantitation of 13-*cis*-retinoic acid (isotretinoin), etretinate, and retinol, with retinyl acetate as internal standard; lower limits of detection were approximately 0.07 μmol/l (0.03 mg/l) serum (36). Use of a 5-μm Supelcosil LC-18 column allowed limits of detection of about 0.03 nmol (8 ng) etretinate (164). Bugge et al. (76) used a linear gradient of acetonitrile:water:acetic acid (with ammonium acetate) to analyze etretinate (and its 13-*cis* and all-*trans* free acids) and 13-*cis*-retinoic acid (and its 4-oxo and 4-hydroxy forms) in serum; other synthetic aromatic retinoids were used as internal standards. A Zorbax ODS column was used; the authors felt that the presence of exposed silanol groups (column not "end-capped") is important for resolution of *cis-trans* isomers of these compounds on reversed-phase HPLC. A similar chromatographic system was used to analyze metabolites of etretinate (mostly the all-*trans* and 13-*cis*- free acids, and chain-shortened acids) from human bile and plasma (165).

Retinyl phosphate and mannosylretinyl phosphate (MRP) were separated by anion exchange on Mono-Q columns, eluted with gradients of ammonium acetate or sodium chloride in methanol:water (166,167). These compounds were also separated on a Partisil-10 ODS column with acetonitrile: water; additional of ammonium acetate reduced "tailing" of the MRP peak (168). Several amide derivatives of retinoic acid have shown therapeutic promise. Hultin et al. (169) used a gradient of methanol:water to methanol on a Partisil-10 ODS-2 column to analyze the 13-*cis* and all-*trans* isomers of N-(4-hydroxyphenyl) retinamide (4-HPR) and its methoxy and ethoxy metabolites. An isocratic reversed-phase procedure was developed for analysis of 4-HPR in pharmaceutical products (170).

Retinoyl-coenzyme A has been chromatographed on a Spherisorb C_8 column using a methanol:water gradient (with ammonium acetate) (171). Ethyl retinoate, a metabolite formed from retinoic acid by rat liver microsomes, was analyzed by a similar gradient on a Zorbax ODS column (172). 4-Hydroxyretinol, a metabolite of retinol formed by rat liver microsomes, was analyzed by an acetonitrile:water:acetic acid gradient (with ammonium acetate) (173).

3-Hydroxyretinal (eye pigments of *Drosophila*) and 2-hydroxyretinal isomers and their oximes were separated by adsorption HPLC on silica columns (LiChrosorb Si60 or YMC-Pack A-012-3 S-3 SIL), using mobile phases of methanol and tetrahydrofuran in hexane or methyl t-butyl ether and methanol in benzene (174). 3-Hydroxyretinol and 3-hydroxyretinal oxime isomers were separated on a silica column (Lithosorb, 5-μm) using hexane:dioxane mobile phases (175). By the use of this procedure, the presence of all-*trans* and 11-*cis* isomers of 3-hydroxyretinol and 3-hydroxyretinal in several species of *Diptera* and *Lepidoptera* were demonstrated by Goldsmith et al. (175). A step gradient of t-butylmethyl ether and ethanol in benzene was used by Seki et al. (176) to resolve isomers of retinol, retinal oxime, 3-hydroxyretinol, and 3-hydroxyretinal oxime on a silica column; limits of detection of 1.2–2.1 pmol are claimed, with detection at 350 nm. Oximes of 11-*cis* and all-*trans* isomers of retinal, 3-hydroxyretinal, and 4-hydroxyretinal from extracts of squid eyes were separated by a step gradient of ethyl acetate and ethanol in hexane (177).

3,4-Didehydroretinoids

3,4-Didehydroretinol (3-dehydroretinol, vitamin A$_2$) has been demonstrated in some mammalian tissues (178,179), is a visual pigment in some fish and amphibia (180,181), and has been used in an indirect assessment of human vitamin A status (182). 3,4-Didehydroretinol, being more polar than retinol, elutes earlier on reversed-phase HPLC using methanol:water mobile phases (Resolve 5-μm C$_{18}$ column) (183) (Fig. 10) or acetonitrile:water mobile phases (Nucleosil 5-μm PEAB-ODS column) (178); 3,4-dehydroretinyl palmitate can be separated from retinyl palmitate by nonaqueous reversed-phase HPLC (183), although some vitamin A$_2$ and A$_1$ esters overlap. All-*trans* esters, aldehydes, and alcohols of retinol and 3,4-didehydroretinol were separated by step-gradient absorption HPLC, using dioxane in hexane as mobile phase; in every case the vitamin A$_2$ elutes after the vitamin A$_1$ form on adsorption chromatography (151). Geometric isomers of 3,4-didehydroretinal and retinal resolved by adsorption HPLC using mobile phases of dioxane and 2-propanol in hexane (146), and isomers of 3,4-didehydroretinol and retinol were separated using mobile phases of 2-propanol in hexane (184) or 1-octanol in hexane (146) on silica columns. Oximes of retinal and 3,4-didehydroretinal 11-*cis*, 13-*cis*, and all-*trans* isomers were separated by adsorption HPLC on a silica column (YMC-PAC A-012-3 S-3 SIL, 3-μm particle size) using diethyl ether and ethanol in hexane as mobile phase (181). Fatty acyl esters of 11-*cis*-, 3,4-didehydroretinol, all-*trans*-3,4-didehydroretinol, and all-*trans*-retinol were separated using diethyl ether in hexane (185). Since 3,4-didehydroretinol is much less fluorescent than is retinol (186), absorbance detection (usually at 340 nm) is used.

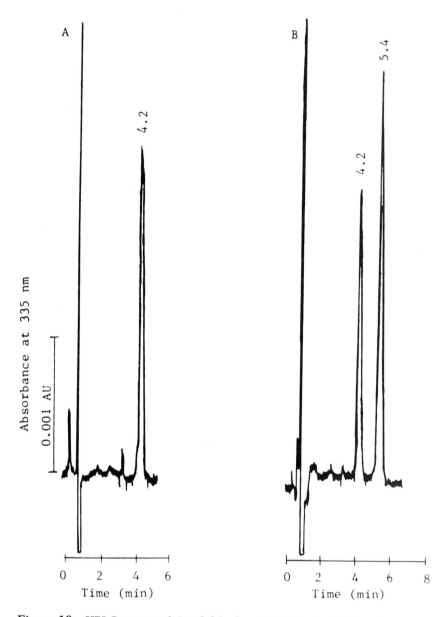

Figure 10 HPLC traces of 3,4-didehydroretinol standard (A) and a serum extract analyzed for 3,4-didehydroretinol and retinol (B). Retention times for 3,4-didehydroretinol and retinol were 4.2 and 5.4 min, respectively. Chromatographic conditions: Waters Resolve 5-μm C_{18} column (3.9 × 150 mm); methanol:water (85:15) at 1.5 ml/min, detection at 335 nm (S. Tanumihardjo and J. A. Olson, unpublished data).

1.4. Gas Chromatography

The lability of retinoids, particularly retinol and its esters, to heat and to incompletely inactivated column packings hindered early attempts at packed-column gas chromatography (GC). Dunagin and Olson (187) treated SE-30 packed columns by injecting β-carotene before successful chromatography of retinol and retinyl acetate; anhydroretinol, methyl retinyl ether, retinal, and methyl retinoate could be chromatographed without column pretreatment. Ninomiya et al. (188) earlier had described dehydration of retinol, retinyl acetate, and retinyl palmitate to anhydroretinol on GC packed columns. Cullum et al. (189) took advantage of the on-column dehydration of retinol to anhydroretinol for gas chromatographic-mass spectrometric analysis of deuterated retinol. Vecchi et al. (190) prepared the trimethylsilyl derivative of retinol for chromatography on QF-1 (fluorosilicone) packed columns. The *syn* and *anti* conformers of retinal methoxime were separated on a short QF-1 packed column (191). Taylor and Ikewa (192) have summarized the gas chromatography of catalytically hydrogenated carotenoids on packed columns.

Methyl retinoate, which can be prepared readily without apparent isomerization by treatment of retinoic acid in diazomethane, is stable to GC analysis on packed columns (154,193). Napoli et al. (45,194) analyzed methyl retinoate by GC-MS, using either positive-ion or negative-ion chemical ionization; the methyl-d_3 esters of all-*trans* and 13-*cis* retinoic acid were used as internal standards, and as little as 0.25 pmol (75 pg) could be detected. A short (1-m) packed column of 3% SP2100-DOH on Supelcoport was used, with methane as both carrier gas and reagent gas for chemical ionization-MS. The pentafluorobenzyl ester of an aromatic retinoic acid analog Ro 13–7410 was analyzed by capillary GC with column switching (194a): the peak of interest from a SE54 column was cut to an OV240 column, helium was used as carrier gas and ammonia as reagent gas for negative ion chemical ionization MS. The tetradeuterated analog was used as internal standard; as little as 0.07 pmol (25 pg) could be quantitated.

Bonded-phase capillary columns are inherently much more inert than packed columns, and provide much sharper peaks (i.e., better resolution and improved lower limits of detection.) The usefulness of on-column injection on capillary columns was demonstrated when Smidt et al. (195) showed that retinol could be chromatographed without derivatization on bonded-phase capillary columns without decomposition, with quantitation to 12 pmol (3.5 ng). Subsequently, this study was extended to capillary GC of underivatized apo-retinoids and retinoids on methylsilicone wall-coated open-tubular columns (DB-1; 15 m × 0.25 mm ID; 0.25 μm film thickness) with helium as carrier gas (196) (Fig. 11). Kovats

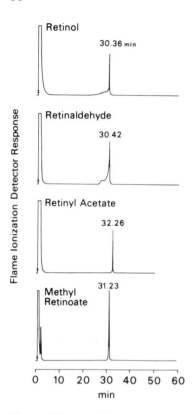

Figure 11 Capillary gas chromatography of retinoid standards. Chromatographic conditions: room-temperature on-column injection, bonded-phase methylsilicone wall-coated open-tubular capillary column (15 m × 0.25 mm ID, 0.25 μm film thickness); helium carrier gas at 34 kPa (5 psi) inlet pressure (2.5 ml/min), temperature gradient from 100 to 300°C at 5°C/min; flame-ionization detection. (H. C. Furr and J. A. Olson, unpublished data).

indices of these compounds were determined, and were found to be linear with increasing chain length for each class of compound (hydrocarbon, alcohol, acetate, aldehyde/ketone); by linear extrapolation, it was estimated that β-carotene should have a Kovats index of approximately 5000. By use of a short, thin-film DB-1 column (5 m × 0.25 mm ID; 0.1 μm film thickness) retinyl esters from retinyl acetate to retinyl dodecanoate as well as the apo-carotenoid β-apo-12'-carotenal were chromatographed without apparent decomposition; application of the technique to longer-chain compounds was limited by the upper temperature limit of the chromatograph. It is not yet known at what operating temperature the thermal isomerization of these polyene compounds will limit the usefulness of this technique. Separation of *cis-trans* isomers has not yet been studied. Kovats indices were also determined for anhydroretinol and methyl retinoate on a cyanopropyl-phenyl-methylsilicone capillary (DB-225) column (196).

Direct interfacing with mass spectrometers is an advantage of capillary GC over packed-column GC and HPLC (197). Capillary GC with on-column injection will probably not supplant HPLC for most types of retinoid analysis; nonetheless, the universal nature and low limits of detection of the flame-ionization detector and of mass spectrometric detection offer advantages over the more specific detectors used for liquid chromatography.

1.5. Other Methods

A wide variety of chemical and physical methods has been employed in the characterization, separation, and measurement of retinoids in addition to the methods discussed in the previous sections.

In characterizing retinoids, Raman spectra, infrared spectra, and x-ray analysis have been used in addition to UV/visible spectra, NMR spectra, and mass spectrometry (1). Retinoids can be separated on "open" columns (i.e., under atmospheric pressure) on alumina, silicic acid, ion-exchange resins, calcium phosphate, magnesium hydroxide, and Sephadex LH-20, as well as other, more or less inert solid supports, by the use of solvents of varying polarity (41). Usually, increasing concentrations of acetone or ethyl ether in hexane are used in adsorption chromatography, and mixtures of methanol and acetone are employed for hydrophobic (Sephadex LH-20) chromatography. The activity of the adsorbent can be increased by heating in an oven at 120–150°C to drive off water or reduced by adding water.

In addition to UV/visible absorbancy and fluorescence, vitamin A and its analogs can be measured colorimetrically by use of trifluoroacetic acid, trichloroacetic acid, antimony trichloride, ferric chloride in acetyl chloride, 4-toluene sulfonic acid, or sulfuric acid (41,198). In general, an intense blue color transiently appears that can be measured at 500–700 nm, depending on the given retinoid and conditions of analysis. Alternately, retinol extracted from plasma can be destroyed by exposure to intense light of 300–350 nm; the change in absorbancy at 325 nm before and after irradiation provides a good measure of retinol concentration (41,198).

Because most retinol in plasma is bound to the retinol-binding protein (RBP), the intense fluoresence of retinol on holo-RBP after size-exclusion chromatography (115,116) or after polyacrylamide gel electrophoresis (117,198) can be quantitatively measured. By use of antibodies, total RBP can be measured by radial immunodiffusion, by electroimmunoassay (198), or by enzyme-linked immunosorbent assay (ELISA)

(199,200). By a combination of fluorometry and electroimmunoassay, both holo-RBP and total RBP can be deteremined (198). Because apo-RBP is present in significant amounts in plasma even in severe vitamin A deficiency and because RBP levels are markedly affected by several nonspecific factors such as protein-energy malnutrition, the measurement of plasma retinol is usually preferred to that of RBP. A radio-immunoassay has also been developed for vitamin A (201). Although the procedure is quite sensitive, it is not highly specific for retinol.

1.6. Overview of Retinoid Analysis

Reversed-phase HPLC is the most popular mode of retinoid analysis, because the columns are not easily irreversibly fouled by extraneous lipids and because separations are usually not disturbed by slight changes in mobile-phase composition. However, exacting separations of geometric isomers of retinoids usually require adsorption chromatography. Although retinol itself is easily analyzed by isocratic chromatography, analyses of sample retinoids having a range of polarities (e.g., retinol plus retinyl esters; retinoyl β-glucuronides plus retinoic acid plus retinol) usually require gradient chromatography, and gradient elution is much more easily carried out in the reversed-phase mode. Absorbance detection is most popular for analysis of retinoids, because it is selective enough to ignore many possible interferences; lower limits of detection are on the order of 5 pmol (1.5 ng) for a retinoid eluting with an appropriate capacity factor $(1 < k' < 10)$, and detector responses are linear over an adequately wide range. However, fluorescence detection, especially when used with hexane-based mobile phases (i.e., adsorption chromatography), offers much better lower limits of detection for those retinoids that fluoresce appreciably. Appropriate internal standards increase the validity of quantitation.

We can wish for several developments in chromatographic analysis of retinoids and carotenoids. Better understanding of the separation mechanisms of reversed-phase chromatography of retinoids and carotenoids should rationalize the differences in elution behavior observed between acetonitrile-based and methanol-based mobile phases, and should also allow more rational choice of end-capped columns versus columns with free silanol groups. Effects of mobile-phase composition on column plate count may be more important than selectivity (202). Similarly, better understanding of chromatographic processes may lead to rapid isocratic analyses of retinol and retinyl esters (with acceptable capacity factors and resolution for both), with or without separation of geometric isomers. Analysis of serum retinoids without solvent extraction should be feasible, perhaps by column-switching techniques. Application of microbore HPLC techniques to analysis of retinoids may lead to lower limits of detection (smaller sample requirements) without major changes in detector technology. Development of detectors that are less sensitive to changes in mobile phase will facilitate quantitation in gradient liquid chromatography; improvements in photodiode array detectors will improve qualitative analysis.

Capillary gas chromatography should be explored further, both as an inlet method for mass spectrometry and as an analytical tool in itself. Supercritical fluid chromatography, which has features overlapping liquid and gas chromatography, has not yet been fully exploited as a separation technique for retinoids and carotenoids. Improved chromatograph-mass spectrometer interfaces for liquid chromatography and supercritical fluid chromatography, and new applications of fast-atom-bombardment mass spectrometry may well open new avenues for study of retinoid and carotenoid metabolism.

2. CAROTENOIDS

2.1. Introduction

Chemical Properties

Although the highly colored plant pigments, the carotenoids, have been of interest to biologists and chemists since the early 1800s, their chemical characteristics as a class were first well defined by Palmer (203) and then by Karrer and Jucker (204). A major treatise on carotenoids was edited by Otto Isler in 1971 (205).

All-*trans*-β-carotene (Fig. 12.5) is generally considered as a class prototype (206). β-Carotene is a symmetrical molecule of 40 carbon atoms, consists of 8 isoprene units, has 11 conjugated double bonds, and possesses two β-ionone rings at the ends of the molecule. Other common carotenoids possess hydroxy, aldehydic, oxo, or epoxy substituents, may be acyclic or contain different ring systems, and may contain variable numbers of conjugated and isolated double bonds (Fig. 12). The numbering system is similar to that for retinoids, in that the gem-dimethyl carbon in the ring is denoted C-1, the first carbon atom in the central chain C-7, and the two carbons at the point of symmetry C-15 and C-15′. Thus, violaxanthain (Fig. 12.10) is 3,3′-dihydroxy-5,6:5′, 6′-diepoxy-β-carotene. Carotenoids can also contain additional isoprene chains (homocarotenoids), less than 40 carbon atoms (apocarotenoids), and allenic and acetylenic bonds. Hydroxycarotenoids (xanthophylls) can form ester linkages with fatty acids and glycosidic linkages with sugars.

Karrer and Jucker (204) in 1948 identified 70–80 carotenoids. Straub, in an appendix to Isler's treatise (205), identified a total of 273

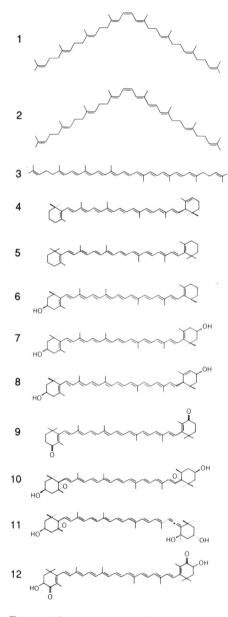

Figure 12 Some naturally occurring carotenoids: 1, phytoene; 2, phytofluene; 3, lycopene; 4, α-carotene; 5, β-carotene; 6, β-cryptoxanthin; 7, zeaxanthin; 8, lutein; 9, canthaxanthin; 10, violaxanthin; 11, neoxanthin; 12, astaxanthin (206). Reprinted with permission from *FASEB Journal.*

carotenoids in 1971, and then, in a 1987 update, 563 distinct compounds (207). Many *cis* isomers of each carotenoid are possible, and many have been specifically characterized. Carotenoids are very widely distributed in nature (208); indeed, it is rare to find a genus without some carotenoid-containing species.

Because of their highly conjugated double bond system, carotenoids show characteristic ultraviolet and visible absorption spectra. For most carotenoids, three peaks, or two peaks and a shoulder, absorb in the range of 400–500 nm. Absorption maxima, values of $E_{1\,cm}^{1\%}$, and molecular extinction values for common carotenoids in petroleum ether (209) are given in Table 2. Both the wavelength maximum and $E_{1\,cm}^{1\%}$ are significantly affected by the solvent used. Thus, for all-*trans*-β-carotene, the wavelength maximum and $E_{1\,cm}^{1\%}$ are 453 nm and 2592 in petroleum ether, 453 nm and 2620 in ethanol, 465 nm and 2337 in benzene, 465 nm and 2396 in chloroform, and 484 nm and 2008 in carbon disulfide (210). The *cis* isomers not only absorb less strongly than the all-*trans* isomer, but also show a so-called "cis-peak" of absorbance at 330–340 nm.

Carotenoids have also been characterized by nuclear magnetic resonance (NMR), infrared (IR), and Raman spectroscopy as well as by x-ray analysis and mass spectrometry (205). Because of their low volatility and

Table 2 Absorbances of Some Common Carotenoids in Petroleum Ether[a,b]

Fig. no.	Compound	Formula	Mol. wt.	Absorption maxima	$E_{1\,cm}^{1\%}$	$\epsilon \times 10^{-3}$
12.1	Phytoene	$C_{40}H_{64}$	544.95	275,$\underline{285}$,296	1250	68.1
12.2	Phytofluene	$C_{40}H_{62}$	542.93	331,$\underline{348}$,367	1350	73.3
12.3	Lycopene	$C_{40}H_{56}$	536.88	444,$\underline{472}$,502	3450	185.
12.4	α-Carotene	$C_{40}H_{56}$	536.88	422,$\underline{444}$,474	2800	150.
12.5	β-Carotene	$C_{40}H_{56}$	536.88	425,$\underline{453}$,479	2592	139.
12.6	β-Cryptoxanthin	$C_{40}H_{56}O$	552.88	425,$\underline{452}$,479	2386	132.
12.7	Zeaxanthin	$C_{40}H_{56}O_2$	568.88	426,$\underline{452}$,479	2348	134.
12.8	Lutein	$C_{40}H_{56}O_2$	568.88	421,$\underline{445}$,475	2550[c]	145.
12.9	Canthaxanthin	$C_{40}H_{52}O_2$	564.85	$\underline{466}$	2200	124.
12.10	Violaxanthin	$C_{40}H_{56}O_4$	600.88	420,$\underline{443}$,470	2550[c]	153.
12.11	Neoxanthin	$C_{40}H_{56}O_4$	600.88	416,$\underline{439}$,467	2243[c]	135.
12.12	Astaxanthin	$C_{40}H_{52}O_4$	580.85	$\underline{472}$	2135	124.

[a] $E_{1\,cm}^{1\%}$ and ϵ values are given for the major, underlined wavelength.

[b] From Ref. 209, except for astaxanthin (336).

[c] In ethanol.

relatively high molecular weight, the C-40 carotenoids have not as yet been separated by gas chromatography (196). Thus, carotenoids are primarily isolated by liquid chromatography on solid supports.

Carotenoids are unstable in the presence of light and oxygen (211). The central chain of conjugated double bonds is oxidatively cleaved at various points, giving rise to a family of apocarotenals (211,212). Most carotenoids, but not vitamin A, also serve as singlet oxygen quenchers (213). In essence, singlet oxygen, which is an electronically excited and highly reactive form of oxygen, interacts with the highly conjugated, ground-state carotenoid to give triplet states of both molecules. The triplet state of oxygen is its less active ground state, whereas the triplet carotenoid returns to the ground state by the emission of thermal energy (213). Carotenoids can also serve as antioxidants and free-radical quenching agents (213–215). Carotenoids interact rapidly with free radicals, or with oxygen, thereby inhibiting the propagation step of lipid peroxidation. Carotenoids serve this function best at low oxygen tensions (214); indeed, carotenoids can be pro-oxidants in 100% oxygen (214). These chemical properties of carotenoids, as noted below, are inherently related to their biological functions and actions.

Biochemistry

Carotenoids are primarily synthesized in plants and microorganisms. A major function of carotenoids clearly relates to the absorbance of light in the process of photosynthesis (216). Carotenoids serve as ancillary pigments in the antenna systems of photosynthetic organisms. Thus, the energy in the excited states of the carotenoids is ultimately transferred to the chlorophyll molecule at the reaction center of the antenna system (216).

A related function of carotenoids in photosynthetic organisms is photoprotection (217). Mutant photosynthetic organisms lacking carotenoids are killed by exposure to light and oxygen (217). Similarly, added carotenoids protect organisms from mutations induced by photooxidation (213,217).

As cis-trans isomerization is directly involved in the visual function of vitamin A in animals (11,12) and in energy transduction in bacteria via the bacteriorhodopsin system (12), so also might the cis-trans isomerization of carotenoids play physiological roles in microorganisms. For example, Nelis and DeLeenheer (218) found a high concentration of cis-canthaxanthin in the female reproductive system of the brine shrimp Artemia and a progressive decrease in the cis/trans ratio during nauplii development. Thus, the relation between isomeric forms of carotenoids and their biological actions deserves further attention.

In mammals, a small group of carotenoids, approximately 50 of the 600 known compounds, serve as precursors of vitamin A (11,12). Carotenoids in vertebrates seem to be oxidatively cleaved primarily at the central 15,15' double bond to yield two molecules of retinal (8), but eccentric cleavage to yield β-apo-carotenals also seems to occur (9,10). Fish and birds can also form vitamin A from hydroxy- and oxocarotenoids (206,219,220). In plants and microorganisms, eccentric cleavage is common (8).

Carotenoid cleavage products with physiologic roles in plants and microorganisms include abscisic acid, β-ionone, trisporic acid, and crocetin (221–223). Carotenoids undergo a variety of other biological transformations, including epoxidation (primarily at the 5,6 and 5',6' positions but also elsewhere in the molecule), reduction of oxo to hydroxy analogs and of epoxy to dihydrohydroxy compounds, esterification of hydroxy carotenoids, glycosylation of both hydroxy and carboxy compounds, and oxidation of methyl groups. Some of these metabolic reactions relate to physiological functions and others seem to be degradative in nature (221–223).

In mammals, carotenoids, freed from foodstuffs by proteolytic digestion of proteins in the stomach and small intestine, are solubilized by conjugated bile salts in the small intestine and are absorbed with other lipids (11,12). Carotenoids are primarily converted into vitamin A in the intestinal mucosa. A significant portion of absorbed carotenoids in humans, chickens, and cows, but not in rodents, is also incorporated per se into chylomicra, whose remnants are cleared from the plasma primarily by the liver.

Besides chylomicra, carotenoids are mainly associated in plasma with low-density lipoproteins (LDL) and high-density lipoproteins (HDL). The pattern of carotenoids in the plasma carotenoids includes lutein, zeaxanthin, lycopene, β-cryptoxanthin, α-carotene, and β-carotene. β-Carotene usually comprises 10–25% of the total plasma carotenoids (11,12).

Carotenoid patterns in the tissues of humans and monkeys are similar to those in plasma (224,225). Of various tissues, adipose tissue and liver seem to be major depositories of carotenoids in humans. Presumably carotenoids are both deposited in tissues and released from them into the plasma. Outside of the cleavage of several carotenoids into vitamin A, little is known of the manner in which other carotenoids, and particularly those that are nutritionally inactive, are metabolized.

Carotenoids also play a role in the coloration of living things, the most dramatic and pleasing example being the plumage of birds. Specific coloration may well serve as an attractant in sexual processes as well as providing protection from predators. In many cases, specific carotenoproteins are formed at given sites in these organisms (226). The ligands in such complexes are usually oxocarotenoids. Hydrocarbon carotenoids are usually loosely associated with lipoproteins in the plasma and tissues of animals, although a β-carotene binding protein of rat liver has recently been reported (227).

Apart from defined physiological functions, carotenoids have several biological actions. Whereas functions can be considered as essential physiological roles, actions can be defined as physiological or pharmacological responses, either beneficial or adverse, to treatment of an organism with carotenoids (206). In some cases, very little carotenoid is needed to invoke a response, in other cases, very large amounts are required.

Biological actions of carotenoids include enhancement of the immune response, a reduction of photoinduced or chemically induced neoplasm, decreased mutagenesis and sister-chromatid exchange, reduced cellular transformation, inhibited micronuclei formation in epithelial cells, and photoprotection of patients with erythropoietic protoporphyria (206,213).

Finally, carotenoids have been associated with a reduced incidence of some chronic diseases. These associations, although not inferring a cause-effect relationship, have nonetheless been seriously considered in a public health context (206,213,228). For example, the dietary intake of carotenoids, but not of vitamin A, is inversely associated in epidemiological surveys with the risk of lung cancer (228). Together with many other singlet oxygen- and free radical-quenching compounds found in fruits and vegetables, carotenoids may thereby be contributing to a reduced oxidative stress on cells of the lung.

Sample Extraction and Handling

Liaaen-Jensen (229) and Britton (230) have described in detail the extraction of carotenoids from plant and animal tissues. In brief, oxygen, light, and heat are the most destructive factors, and should be carefully avoided. The presence of oxygen during extraction may result in the formation of oxidative artifacts, or the disappearance of compounds (e.g., phytoene and phytofluene) due to complete oxidative breakdown. Furthermore, light and heat may cause isomerization. Peroxide-free solvents and an antioxidant such as butylated hydroxytoluene (BHT) should always be used during extraction of carotenoids. If possible, exposure to acid and alkali (except for saponification) should also be avoided. Carotenoids should be analyzed as rapidly as possible in fresh samples, inasmuch as rapid enzymatic destruction occurs. If immediate analysis is not possible, the samples should be freeze-dried, or stored in a freezer.

Because fresh plant and animal tissues contain a large percentage of water, carotenoids cannot be efficiently extracted into organic solvents unless water is removed. This can be done in two ways: (a) the sample can first be homogenized in a blender with water-miscible solvents such as acetone, methanol, or ethanol, and then the carotenoids can be extracted with hexane, peroxide-free diethyl ether, or ethyl acetate; or (b) the sample can be treated with anhydrous sodium sulfate and then extracted with hexane, dichloromethane, diethyl ether, or ethyl acetate. If the sample is dry, it is advantageous first to moisten the sample with water, then to extract with acetone, methanol, or ethanol, and then with hexane, ethyl acetate, or dichloromethane. Hard samples (e.g., shells of crustaceae) should first be ground to a powder, and then extracted.

Alkaline hydrolysis or saponification is carried out on carotenoid extracts almost as a matter of routine (230). Saponification is useful in destroying large amounts of chlorophylls (which can mask some carotenoids), or neutral lipids (oils and fats), which can make chromatography difficult. Saponification, however, will result in the conversion of carotenoid fatty acid esters to free alcohols. Thus, if the ester pattern is desired, saponification must be avoided. After saponification the organic extract should be washed with water carefully to remove traces of alkali, and the extract should be analyzed immediately. Extreme care should be taken during saponification, as up to 80% destruction of carotenoids can occur (231). On the other hand, saponification resulted in improved recovery of hydrocarbon carotenoids from serum (232), and no appreciable loss of carotenoids in vegetables and fruits (233).

The extraction of carotenoids from blood serum or plasma is essentially the same as described in section 1.1.3 for the extraction of retinoids. By using a mixture of ethyl acetate and hexane, the recovery of hydrocarbon carotenoids from serum can be improved (234). After removal of the extracting solvent, the residue should be dissolved in the required volume of a suitable solvent for analysis by HPLC. Because hydrocarbon carotenoids are poorly soluble in methanol and ethanol and xanthophylls are not soluble in hexane, a solvent mixture of dichloromethane, methanol, hexane, and acetonitrile is best used to dissolve the residue for HPLC analysis. An internal standard should be used in quantitation (235), inasmuch as the preparation of carotenoid samples for HPLC analysis can be accompanied by various analytical errors, such as sample loss during evaporation, partitioning, and redissolving. An internal standard is also useful in monitoring HPLC performance (column performance and detector response). In one case, a detector malfunction was observed from the internal standard response before the electronic diagnostics of the detector identified the problem (G. R.

Beecher, personal communication). The selection of a suitable internal standard is a major consideration, one that has been carefully dealt with in a previous review (65).

2.2. High-Performance Liquid Chromatography

In earlier spectrophotometric methods, the total hydrocarbon carotenoids ("carotenes") were estimated in plasma and foods by measuring the absorbancy of an extract at 450 nm. Various carotenoids in the extract clearly were not distinguished by this procedure. Currently much attention is being given to the individual carotenoids in blood and other tissues of animal origin, and also in fruits and vegetables. Since the early work on liquid chromatography of carotenoids by Stewart and Wheaton (236), a tremendous amount of progress has been made. Excellent recent reviews include those by DeLeenheer et al. (57,65), Taylor (63), Ruedi (237), Bushway (238), and Ruddat and Will (239). Consequently, this review will deal primarily with recent developments.

In the HPLC of carotenoids, it is now possible to analyze a whole range of very polar carotenoids like neoxanthin and violaxanthin to hydrocarbon carotenoids like α-carotene and β-carotene in a matter of minutes. Apart from speed, other advantages of HPLC over other methods of analysis, such as open-column chromatography and thin-layer chromatography, are (a) only a very small amount (nanograms to micrograms) of the compound in tissue extracts and a small volume of the solvent mixture are required; (b) exposure of the carotenoids to light and oxygen is avoided, thereby minimizing isomerization and decomposition; and (c) a single HPLC column, if properly maintained, can be used repeatedly over a long period of time. Depending on the type of the column and the applied solvent mixture, the resolution can remain good to excellent upon repeated usage.

HPLC can be either normal (or straight) phase or reversed-phase in nature. A single eluting solvent is used in isocratic HPLC, whereas a solvent of changing polarity is employed in gradient HPLC. The distinction between these two types of liquid chromatography has been discussed in detail in the section on the HPLC of retinoids.

Normal- (Straight-) Phase HPLC

Normal-phase HPLC (np-LC) is similar in nature to open-column chromatography. The most commonly used adsorbents are silica and alumina. The active sites in silica columns (such as Lichrosorb, Spherisorb, Zorbax etc.) are silanol groups, which are hydroxyl functions on silicon atoms. Because silica is acidic, basic substances are adsorbed very strongly. As in open-column chromatography, the least polar carotenoids (hydrocarbon carotenoids) elute first, followed in turn by carotenoids of increasing polarity. By using a silica column (Spheri 5) and an isocratic mobile phase of specially treated hexane:acetonitrile, Rhodes et al. (240) separated phytoene, phytofluene, zeta-carotene, neurosporene, lycopene, γ-carotene, and β-carotene. The advantage of np-LC is that *cis-trans* isomers (241,242) and diastereoisomers (243) can be resolved. However, *cis* isomers may be converted to the more stable *trans* isomer on silica columns (244). Tyczkowski et al. (245) were able to separate lutein esters and oxolutein esters from lutein on a silica gel (5 μm) cartridge using isooctane:acetone:methanol.

Although a complex mixture of geometric isomers of carotenoids can be resolved on alumina columns (246,247), the analysis time is much longer. Other adsorbents such as magnesia, zinc carbonate, and calcium carbonate are not sufficiently stable to be packed in a HPLC column. However, calcium hydroxide seems to be a good adsorbent (248). On a slurry-packed calcium hydroxide column using a mixture of hexane:acetone, *cis-trans* isomers of α- and β-carotene extracted from several fruits and vegetables were resolved (249).

When one class of polar or nonpolar carotenoids is resolved very efficiently by np-LC, the other classes of carotenoids are held very strongly on the column. Unless they are removed by extensive and time-consuming washing procedures, they may well interfere with the analysis after several runs. This problem is an inherent disadvantage of np-LC.

Reversed-Phase HPLC

Reversed-phase HPLC (rp-LC) differs from np-LC in two important aspects. In rp-HPLC, the retention behavior of solutes is reversed from np-LC; thus, the most polar compounds elute first and the least polar ones last. Second, rp-LC is not as sensitive as np-LC either to the presence of water in the solvent and extract or to slight differences in solvent composition. While np-LC resolves compounds of similar polarity well, including isomers, rp-LC is being widely used to resolve a wide range of carotenoids of different polarity. In recent years, rp-LC has also been used for separation of some isomers. In the analysis of carotenoids, rp-LC has been used much more extensively than has np-LC.

For carotenoid analysis, rp-LC columns generally contain octyl (C_8) or octadecyl (C_{18}) derived residues bonded to silica gel (e.g., Partisil ODS, μ-Bondapak C_{18}, Zorbax ODS, Lichrosorb RP), although other supports containing phenyl, amino, or cyano groups (250) can also be used. Khachik et al. (251) compared the efficacy of a low-carbon loading (Vydac C_{18}) and a high-carbon loading (Rainin Microsorb) column for the separation of the major carotenoids in fruits. Carotenoids were found to have a much higher adsorption affinity (longer retention time) for the Microsorb column with the smaller pore size than the Vydac column with larger pore size (251). Geometric isomers of hydrocarbon carotenoids were separated much better on a Vydac column than on a Microsorb column, whereas oxygenated carotenoids and their geometric isomers were better resolved on a Microsorb column (251).

Although most of the earlier available columns contained 10-μm particles, the use of columns with 5-μm particles results in sharper peaks and better resolution of carotenoids. More recently 3-μm columns have also been used (252–254). Column length also plays an important role in the resolution of a carotenoid mixture. Serum carotenoids, which are poorly resolved on a 15-cm column, separated very well on a 30-cm column of identical make (A. B. Barua, unpublished observations). Although most publications describe the use of 25-cm columns, the use of 15-cm columns is becoming popular.

It is wise to use a guard column preceding the main column. The guard column helps prevent clogging of the main column from unwanted materials, thereby increasing the life of the main column. An increase of column pressure is often associated with deposition of insoluble particles present in the extract on the frit in the guard column. The latter can be readily changed or cleaned. The main column sometimes may become clogged due to deposition of particles on the inner frits at both ends of the column. If replacement with new or cleaned frits will not solve the problem, the column must either be repacked, which is not a trivial process, or discarded. In the authors' laboratory, the final concentrated extract is routinely centrifuged briefly for about 10 s just before injection to get rid of undissolved material. The supernatant is then injected.

Because pure organic solvents rarely possess just the right elutropic properties for resolving a mixture of carotenoids within a reasonable period of time, mixtures of solvents are used. The most typical solvent mixtures consist of acetonitrile as a base solvent together with chloroform, dichloromethane, or dichloroethane as a modifier to control the eluotropic strength. Selectivity is often affected by methanol. Thus Nelis and DeLeenheer's (126) rp-isocratic solvent, namely, acetonitrile:dichloromethane:methanol (70:20:10), has also been found effective by other investigators (255,256). Addition of hexane to the above solvent mixture helps separate cis- and trans-neoxanthin, violaxanthin, neochrome, neolutein, β-carotene, and cis-β-carotene (231,257). Tetrahydrofuran (THF) has also been used in rp solvents (252,258–261). THF, however, often contains peroxides that can destroy up to 50% of the carotenoids during analysis (262); this problem can be overcome by using THF stabilized by BHT (262).

Lauren et al. (263) reported that the addition of n-decanol as a modifier to a mobile phase of ethyl acetate:acetonitrile rapidly conditioned new columns and avoided problems with trace solvent impurities. In the absence of n-decanol, activation of residual silanol groups in the rp packing can cause drastic deterioration in the column behavior (263). The best material for rapid isocratic separation of all major carotenoids is a high-carbon-loaded, non-end-capped material with ODS functionality. One end-capped C_8 material, however, gave similar results (264). Although the analysis of carotenoids by rp-isocratic HPLC seems to be preferred, rp-gradient HPLC has also been used (232,233,254,258,265–267). A combination of isocratic and gradient analysis often results in very good separation of carotenoids of closely related structures (257,268). For simultaneous determination of retinol, tocopherols, and carotenoids, rp gradients may be quite useful, inasmuch as retinol elutes at the solvent front in most of the isocratic systems used for carotenoid analysis.

The disadvantages of rp-gradient LC are twofold. First, it may be difficult to obtain a good baseline, especially when detection is done at low attenuation. By using appropriate conditions, however, baseline stability can sometimes be improved. Second, the column needs to be equilibrated after each run, which results in a significant period of time between runs.

The detection of carotenoids usually involves the absorption of visible light. Most carotenoids, due to the presence of a large number of conjugated double bonds, absorb light very strongly in the 400–500 nm region. A wavelength of 450 nm, which is the absorption maximum of β-carotene and of many other carotenoids, is usually selected. In general, interference by other biological compounds in this region is very little. Some carotenoids, however, absorb light maximally at higher wavelengths (e.g., lycopene at 470 nm) and some others at lower wavelengths (e.g., phytoene at 286 nm and phytofluene at 347 nm). If the detector is set at 450 nm, such carotenoids may well escape detection.

It is therefore preferable either to use two detectors set at appropriate wavelengths, or to monitor the chromatograms at different wavelengths by using a rapid-scanning ultraviolet/visible photodiode array detector. Using such a detector, Khachik et al. (251) simultaneously monitored the analysis of carotenoids at 470, 460, 450, 400, 350, and 286 nm, and were able to record 12 spectra/min. Milne and Botnen (253) programmed the photodiode array detector to detect retinol at 325 nm (0–1.6 min), tocopherols at 290 nm (1.6–2.5 min), and carotenoids at 460 nm (2.5–9 min). Online recording of absorption spectra often provides useful information about the compound eluting in a particular peak. For example, cis-carotenoids display a characteristic "cis peak" of absorbancy in the long-wavelength ultraviolet region. As one example, 15,15'-cis-β-carotene shows an almost identical spectrum with all-trans-β-carotene in the 400–500 nm region, but also shows an additional strong peak at 335 nm. The 5, 6-epoxycarotenoids show hypsochromic shifts of the main maximum by about 20 nm for each epoxy group after acid (HCl) treatment. Analysis of human serum extracted by ethyl acetate containing a trace of acetic acid showed a peak having the retention time of violaxanthin, but examination of the absorption spectrum revealed that the compound was actually bilirubin, which shows a single peak at 445–450 nm (234).

2.3. Applications

Human Blood

Stimulated by the inverse association shown in epidemiological surveys between dietary carotenoid intake and the risk of lung cancer (269–271), many investigators have analyzed human blood for carotenoids. While only the hydrocarbon carotenoids, namely, lycopene and α- and β-carotenes, have been analyzed in some studies, a whole range of carotenoids has been studied in others. So far, lutein, zeaxanthin, β-cryptoxanthin, lycopene, α-carotene, and β-carotene have been characterized in human blood. At least three major unidentified carotenoids are present in human blood; one of them is designated as "pre-cryptoxanthin" (as it elutes just before β-cryptoxanthin), and the other two elute in rp-HPLC between zeaxanthin and pre-cryptoxanthin (234,255). In addition, several minor carotenoid peaks are observed. Some of the HPLC systems used for the analysis of carotenoids in human plasma or serum from 1983 to 1989 are cited in Table 3 (54,81, 111,126,232,234,250,252,253,255,258,262,272–275).

Following the method of Vuillemier et al. (107), Wald et al. (276) analyzed serum levels of β-carotene in subjects who later developed breast cancer. Serum-level changes of β-carotene after administration of a pharmacological dose were studied by Costantino et al. (277) by Nierenberg's procedure (262). Using Craft's method (54), Brown et al. (278) studied the plasma response to the ingestion of vegetables or a dose of β-carotene. Similar studies (279–281) were conducted with the use of different HPLC procedures. Yet a different method (271) was used in analyzing the relation of plasma carotenoid level to the dietary intake of green vegetables (282) and carrot juice (283). Concentrations of β-carotene and retinol in plasma have also been correlated with age, smoking, and the use of cardiovascular drugs (262,284). A nonaqueous rp-isocratic HPLC procedure for the simultaneous analysis of carotenoids, retinol, retinyl esters, and tocopherols present in as little as 10 μl of human serum has been developed (A. B. Barua, H. C. Furr, D. Janick-Buckner, and J. A. Olson, unpublished results) (Fig. 13); baseline separation of α- and β-carotenes and of pre- and β-cryptoxanthins was achieved.

Other Human Tissues

Less information is available on the presence of carotenoids in other human tissues. By use of an acetonitrile:chloroform:water gradient on a C-18 rp column and a variable-wavelength detector, Parker (285) analyzed the composition of carotenoids and tocopherol in adipose tissues. Retinyl ester and carotenoid composition of human liver samples was analyzed by gradient elution (acetonitrile:water to acetonitrile:dichloroethane gradients) on a Waters Resolve 5-μm C_{18} column (286). The amounts of β-carotene in exfoliated buccal mucosal cells were measured by HPLC on a Vydac column using methanol containing 0.1% phosphoric acid and dichloromethane (287–289). β-Carotene in human skin has been analyzed by rp-LC on a BioSil C-18 column using acetonitrile:tetrahydrofuran:methanol containing ammonium acetate and butylated hydroxytoluene (259). Carotenoids of human colostrum have been analyzed by HPLC on a C-18 Ultrasphere column with acetonitrile:THF as the mobile phase (290).

Fruits and Vegetables

Of the very large number of recent publications in which HPLC has been used for the analysis of carotenoids in fruits, only a few will be selected in this review. Because detection by HPLC is very sensitive and a small quantity of the extract is sufficient, many carotenoids have now been identified that would have escaped detection by column or thin-layer chromatography. An excellent review of the carotenoid composition of plant foods has recently appeared (290).

Following the rp-LC procedure of Broich et al. (125), α-carotene and β-carotene in raw and cooked lettuce, spinach, beans, and carrot roots have been analyzed on a Supelcosil ODS column using methanol:acetonitrile:chloroform (291). Cooking enhanced the extractability of carotenoids from these vegetables (291). Nonaqueous rp-isocratic HPLC was used to optimize the separation of *cis-trans* isomers of α- and β-carotenes present in dried carrots (292). Using a photodiode array detector and Microsorb ODS column, Tan (293) identified phytofluene, β-carotene, phytoene, and lycopene in increasing order as the major carotenoids, and α-carotene, lycoxanthin, and *cis*-mutatoxanthin as minor carotenoids in tomato paste. The carotenoids of alfalfa products have been analyzed by isocratic-rp LC by using ethyl acetate:acetonitrile containing *n*-decanol on a Zorbax ODS column (294). Polar and nonpolar carotenoids and chlorophylls present in green spinach leaves have

Table 3 HPLC Systems Recently Used in the Analysis of Carotenoids in Human Plasma or Serum

Compounds	Stationary phase	Mobile phase	Internal standard	Reference
A,B,C,Ly,L,Z	Zorbax ODS 5 μm	MeCN:CH$_2$Cl$_2$:MeOH	RAc	(126)
A,B,Ly	Supelcosil LC-18 3 μm	MeCN:THF:MeOH	ACEE	(252)
A,B,Ly,R,T,Z	Radial Pak C$_{18}$ 5 μm	MeCN:CHCl$_3$:MeOH	TAc	(81)
A,B,C,L Ly,P,U,Z	Supelco LC-18	MeCN:CH$_2$Cl$_2$:MeOH	E	(255)
A,B,C,L, Ly,R,Z	Brownlee Spheri-5 RP18	MeCN:MeOH:H$_2$O/ BuOH (gradient)	None	(232)
A,B,C,L, Ly,Z	Chromsil-CN Chromsil-NH$_2$	Benzene:hexane (gradient) Benzene:hexane/MeOH (gradient)	None	(250)
A,B,Ly,R,T	Hypersil ODS 3 μm	MeOH	RAc	(253)
A,B,Ly	Biophase ODS 5 μm	MeCN/CHCl$_3$:2-PrOH:H$_2$O	RAc, TAc	(111)

A,B,Ly	NovaPak C18 4 μm	MeCN:MeOH:CH$_2$Cl$_2$:H$_2$O	None	(272,273)
A,B,Ly	Spherisorb ODS-2 3 μm	MeOH:MeCN:CH$_2$Cl$_2$	None	(254)
C,Ly,L,P U,Z	Ultrasphere C$_{18}$ 5 μm	MeCN:CH$_2$Cl$_2$:MeOH	E, TAc	(54)
A,B,C,L,Ly, R,T,Z	Spherisorb ODS-2	MeOH:hexane	TAc	(274)
A,B,Ly	Ultrasphere ODS	MeCN:CHCl$_3$:H$_2$O	Unknown structure	(275)
A,B,BR,C,L, Ly,P,U,Z	Resolve C$_{18}$ 5 μm	MeCN:CH$_2$Cl$_2$:MeOH/ H$_2$O:1-octanol	None	(234)
A,B,C,L,Ly, P,R,T,U,Z	Resolve C$_{18}$ 5 μm	MeCN:CH$_2$Cl$_2$:MeOH: 1-octanol	Retinyl hexanoate	(Unpublished)[a]
A,B,C,L,Ly	Ultrasphere ODS 5 μm	MeCN:MeOH:THF:H$_2$O	None	(258)

Abbreviations: A: α-carotene; ACEE: β-apo-8′-carotenoic acid ethyl ester; B: β-carotene; BR: bilirubin; C: β-cryptoxanthin; E: eichenone; L: lutein; Ly: lycopene; P: precryptoxanthin; R: retinol; RAc: retinyl acetate; T: α-tocopherol; TAc: α-tocopheryl acetate; U: structure unknown; Z: zeaxanthin; BuOH: 1-butanol; MeCN: acetonitrile; MeOH: methanol; 2-PrOH: 2-propanol; THF: tetrahydrofuran.

[a] A. B. Barua, H. C. Furr, D. Janick-Buckner, and J. A. Olson, unpublished observations.

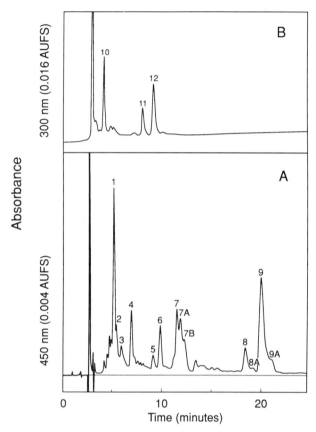

Figure 13 Separation of retinol, tocopherols, and carotenoids present in 10 μl of human serum. Column, 5 μm Waters Resolve C_{18} (30 cm × 3.9 mm ID); eluent, acetonitrile:dichloromethane:methanol:1-octanol (90:15:10:0.1, v/v/v/v), flow 1 ml/min. Lower panel (A): detection at 450 nm (carotenoids); upper panel (B); detection at 300 nm (retinol and tocopherols); two detectors (ISCO V4) in series; integrator, Shimadzu CR4A. Peaks: 1, lutein; 2, zeaxanthin; 3, carotenoid "X"; 4, carotenoid "Y"; 5, pre-cryptoxanthin; 6, β-cryptoxanthin; 7, all-*trans*-lycopene; 7A, 7B, *cis*-lycopenes; 8, all-*trans*-α-carotene; 8A, *cis*-α-carotene; 9, all-*trans*-β-carotene; 9A, *cis*-β-carotene; 10, retinol; 11, γ-tocopherol; 12, α-tocopherol. Identification of *cis*-carotenoids was based on Ref. 292 (A. B. Barua, H. C. Furr, D. Janick-Buckner, and J. A. Olson, unpublished observations).

been analyzed in approximately an hour by isocratic-rp LC on a Chromosil C-18 spherical column by use of acetonitrile:methanol:ethyl acetate (295). Bushway et al. (261,296) compared the carotenoid levels in 11 vegetables and one fruit collected from roadside stands and from supermarkets. Significant variations were found in the levels of β-carotene, but not of α-carotene, in produce from various sources. The differences in the β-carotene content in lettuce produced by various cultivation methods were analyzed by HPLC on a μ-Bondapak C_{18} column using acetonitrile:methanol:dichloromethane (297). By using rp-LC on a Whatman Partisil ODS column with acetonitrile:dichloromethane: methanol, Simon and Wolf (298) analyzed α-, β-, γ-, and ζ-carotenes, β-zeacarotene, and lycopene in carrots of diverse genetic background. Many carotenoids and carotenoid mono and di-fatty acid esters in several varieties of squash were separated on a Microsorb C-18 column using a combination of isocratic and gradient elution (257). By using a Spheri-5 column, solvent mixtures of methanol:acetonitrile:dichloromethane/hex-ane of varying compositions, and elution by isocratic, gradient or a com-bination of both methods, Khachik and Beecher (299) separated a number of straight-chain fatty acid esters of violaxanthin, auroxanthin, lutein, zeaxanthin, isozeaxanthin, and β-cryptoxanthin. The carotenoid and chlorophyll contents in extracts of raw and cooked broccoli, cab-bage, spinach, brussels sprouts, and kale have been separated by isocratic as well as by a combination of isocratic and gradient HPLC on a Micro-sorb C-18 column using several solvent systems (231). Nonapreno-β-caro-tene, a C-45 analog of β-carotene, has been used as an internal standard in the quantitation of *cis* and *trans* forms of lycopene, zeta-carotene, α-carotene, β-carotene, and $15,15'$-cis-β-carotene from extracts of carrots, sweet potato, pumpkin, and red palm oil (235). In these separations, a Brownlee C-18 cartridge and acetonitrile:dichloromethane:methanol mixture have been used (235). Zonta et al. (265) analyzed carotenoids and carotenoid esters by rp-LC on Lichrosorb and Supelcosil columns using a solvent gradient of dichloroethane:2-propanol:acetonitrile mix-ture. As in the case of 4-oxoretinoic acid and 4-hydroxyretinoic acid (300), the elution order of the oxocarotenoids (e.g., canthaxanthin) and the hydroxycarotenoids (e.g., zeaxanthin) was reversed when methanol was used in the mobile phase (265). These authors (265) also found that byproduct formation occurred when the carotenoids were kept in dichloroethane solution, but not when kept in carbon disulfide solution.

Philip and Chen (301) described a method for estimating the provi-tamin A carotenoids, β-carotene, β-cryptoxanthin, and cryptoxanthin esters, in a number of fruits (apricot, cantaloupe, grapefruit, mango, orange, pineapple, papaya, peaches, tangelo, watermelon, tomato, and red and yellow bell peppers) by HPLC on a Waters Resolve C_{18} column using a solvent gradient of methanol and ethyl acetate. The major fatty acid esters of carotenoids in persimmon and papaya were also analyzed (301). α-Carotene, β-carotene, and β-cryptoxanthin in orange juice have been analyzed by several HPLC procedures (126,302). By using a Vydac rp column with a mobile phase of acetonitrile:methanol:THF, Bushway (303) separated the carotenoids in 12 raw fruits and vegetables, namely, α- and β-carotene, 9- and 15-*cis* isomers of β-carotene, γ-carotene, canthaxanthin, β-cryptoxanthin, and 5, 6-epoxy-β-carotene.

Quackenbush (304) separated iodine-catalyzed isomers of α- and β-carotenes, lutein, and lycopene on a Vydac column with a mobile phase of methanol:chloroform. By this procedure, the occurrence of 9- and 13-*cis* isomers of carotenoids in raw carrot and canned peaches was demonstrated (304). Ben-Amotz et al. (305) separated the isomers of carotene and phytoene on a Vydac column using an acetonitrile:methanol mixture. Using a standard method (126), Heinonen et al. (233) separated and quantified the levels of α-, β- and γ-carotenes, lycopene, cryptoxanthin, and lutein in Finnish foods, which included 69 vegetables, fruits, berries, and mushrooms. The α- and β-carotene levels in some foods of East Africa were determined by HPLC on a Brownlee C-18 column with acetonitrile:methanol:hexane:dichloromethane (306). In the separation, identification, and quantitation of the major carotenoids in the extracts of apricots, peaches, cantaloupes, and pink grapefruit, a combination of isocratic and gradient methods involving both low (Vydac C-18) and high (Rainin Microsorb) carbon-loading columns were employed (251).

Chandler and Schwartz (249) identified *cis-trans* isomers of α- and β-carotenes in fresh and canned fruits and vegetables, and showed that canning resulted in increases of 9- and 13-*cis* isomers. Carotenoids in carrots, capsicum, orange, parsley, and tomato have been resolved both by rp-isocratic and rp-gradient LC procedures (267). Gradient LC gave better resolution but took more time (over 250 min for one run).

Scalia and Francis (307) described a method for preparative HPLC of carotenoids and carotenoid esters in paprika fruit, rose hips, and marigold flowers by use of a self-packing, axially compressed RP-18 column with a mobile phase of petroleum ether:acetonitrile:methanol:THF.

Milk and Other Animal Tissues

Due to high lipid levels, carotenoids in milk cannot be analyzed directly, but must be saponified prior to LC (308). Using an Alltech 5-μm C_{18} column with a mobile phase of acetonitrile:dichloromethane:methanol:2-octanol, Indyk (308) separated the saponified carotenoids from bovine milk. Carotenoids and retinoids in dairy products have been analyzed by HPLC (309). α-Carotene and β-carotene in cattle serum and liver have been separated on an Altex 5-μm column with a mobile phase of acetonitrile:chloroform (310). In another study, only β-carotene was identified in bovine serum (311). Alam et al. (312) analyzed plasma carotenoid levels as a function of dietary lipid intake in rats. By using a Radial Pak 5-μm cartridge with a mobile phase of isooctane: acetone:methanol, 3'-oxolutein, along with lutein, lutein esters, and zeaxanthin, were identified in tissues and egg yolks of chickens (244,245). Matsuno et al. (313) isolated carotenoids from hen's egg yolk and characterized three new ketocarotenoids by HPLC on a chiral resolution column Sumipax OA-2000. The distribution of β-carotene, along with retinol and tocopherols, in chick liver was studied by HPLC on a Lichrocart RP-18 column with a mobile phase of acetonitrile:chloroform:water or acetonitrile:THF:methanol containing ammonium acetate (314). Carotenoids and retinoids were analyzed by HPLC to study the conversion of astaxanthin to 3,4-didehydroretinol in fish (315). β-Carotene, retinal, and retinol were analyzed by HPLC to determine the carotene cleavage activity in bovine ovarian follicles (316). Vecchi et al. (317) separated astacene, semi-astacene, astaxanthin, and their *cis* isomers on Lichrosorb and Spherisorb (silica gel) columns coated with *ortho*-phosphoric acid.

Other Sources

By using standard rp-LC procedures (126), olive oil (256) and palm oil (318) carotenoids have been studied.

Kester and Thompson (319) used HPLC for the analysis of microbial carotenoids. Nam et al. (260) identified torulene, torularhodin, β-carotene, and γ-carotene in the yeast *Rhodotorula glutinis* by use of a Z-module C_{18} column with acetonitrile:THF:water.

Chen and Bailey (320) quantified neoxanthin, violaxanthin, lutein, and β-carotene in Bermuda grasses by rp-LC on an IBM-C_{18} column with acetonitrile:chloroform:water. Bailey and Chen (321) later showed that if saponification is not done prior to LC, lutein ester as well as chlorophylls can also be estimated in Bermuda grass.

The diastereomeric carotenoids, 2-hydroxy-β-carotene, 2, 2'-dihydroxy-β-carotene, and 2-hydroxy-echinenone, in the stick insect *Neohirosea japonica* and the sea louse *Ligia exotica* have been resolved (322) by using the chiral column, Sumipax OA-2000. By use of the same column, diastereomeric isomers of carotenoids with a 3-hydroxy-β end group (zeaxanthin) (323), a 3-hydroxy-4-oxo-β end group (astaxanthin and phoenicoxanthin) (324), and 3-oxo-ϵ end group (ϵ,ϵ-carotene-3, 3'-dione) (325) have been separated. By using a Chiralcel OD chiral column, the separation of carotenoids with a 4-hydroxy-β end group has been reported (326). Thirty-four carotenoids were isolated from two species of starfish, and five new acetylenic carotenoids have been identified by HPLC on a Sumipax OA-2000 column with a mobile phase of n-hexane:dichloromethane:ethanol (327).

2.4. Supercritical Fluid Chromatography

Supercritical fluid chromotography (SFC) has emerged as a new promising technique for the separation of carotenoids of closely related structures, including geometric isomers (328–330). In principle, SFC is very
similar to HPLC, but uses supercritical carbon dioxide, with or without
modifiers such as ethanol, as the mobile phase. The stationary phases for
SFC columns are the cyanopropylpolysiloxanes and polyethylene glycols.
In SFC analysis, both UV-visible and flame-ionization detectors can be
used. SFC can be combined with mass spectrometry to separate and to
identify unstable carotenoids such as fucoxanthin (329). SFC has been
used in separating α- and β-carotenes present in carrots and tomatoes
(330).

2.5. Other Methods

Using standard spectrophotometric methods, which involve recording
the absorption at 450 nm, total carotenoids in human plasma (331,332)
have been determined. Open-column chromatography (229), in combination with spectrophotometry, was widely used in the past for the
separation and quantitation of carotenoids. With the availability of
preparative and semipreparative HPLC, however, the use of open-
column chromatography has considerably declined. Nonetheless, open-
column chromatography is very useful for removing particulate matter
and substances of very different properties prior to HPLC analysis. Some
of the commonly used adsorbents in open-column chromatography are
alumina, silica, calcium hydroxide, calcium carbonate, magnesium carbonate, and magnesium oxide mixed with Hyflo Super Cel. Because
some of these adsorbents have high surface activity, carotenoids can be
isomerized and degraded during the relatively long period of chromatography. Nonetheless, mytitoxanthin and isomytitoxanthin have been
separated on a silica-gel column by use of a mixture of acetone and benzene (333).

Reversed-phase "flash" column chromatography has been used for
preparative scale analysis of carotenoids (334). By use of a glass column
packed with 50-μm C_{18} particles, and a solvent mixture of aceto-
nitrile:methanol:chloroform, provitamin A carotenoids present in a
number of fruits and vegetables have been separated (334). Because the
column is pressurized under nitrogen, the analysis time is short (10–15
min), thereby minimizing the chances of on-column degradation of the
carotenoids.

Thin-layer chromatography (TLC) (229) has also lost popularity
with the advancement of HPLC for the analysis of carotenoids (57).
Nonetheless, straight- and reversed-phase TLC can be used for sample

"cleanup," for checking the purity of standards, for determining the approximate composition of suitable solvent mixtures for HPLC analysis, and for rapidly following the rate of either biological or chemical reactions. By use of magnesia-Kieselguhr plates, good separation of α- and β-carotenes present in human colostrum has been reported (290).

3. SUMMARY

In the first edition of *Modern Chromatographic Analysis of the Vitamins*, published in 1985, high-performance liquid chromatography (HPLC) had already become the method of choice for the separation and quantitation of retinoids and carotenoids (57). Its dominance in this area of separation science has increased since that time. With improved adsorbents and hydrophobic supports of uniform, smaller particle sizes and with new solvent mixtures, the resolving power of HPLC systems has markedly improved. The development of new gradient systems and the combination of isocratic and gradient procedures has also given a new dimension of flexibility to HPLC separations. Furthermore, detectors of absorbance and fluorescence have improved in sensitivity and stability, and automatic sampling devices, gradient selection programs, and improved integrators have simplified the task of the analyst. Obviously, HPLC will remain as a major analytical tool for retinoids and carotenoids for the foreseeable future.

But new and improved techniques of other kinds also aid in the analysis of these polyenes. Gas chromatography on capillary columns is very promising, particularly with "cold" on-column injection of the sample. Supercritical fluid chromatography (SFC), now only in its inception, has been fruitfully applied to carotenoid analysis, and improvements in mass spectrometer design and in computerized data analysis have been of great value both in characterizing and in quantitating these substances. In a public health context, the interesting inverse association between the dietary intake of carotenoids and the incidence of some cancers has stimulated much interest. Similarly, the clinical effectiveness of many retinoids and some carotenoids in the treatment of certain skin disorders and of some types of cancer has fostered studies of their metabolism. As a result of these interests and concerns, better, highly specific analytical methods are increasingly needed. Significant further progress in these methodologies is anticipated in the next few years.

ACKNOWLEDGMENTS

The authors gratefully acknowledge support of their research studies on retinoids and carotenoids by the National Institutes of Health U.S. Public Health Service (CA-46406, DK-32793, DK-39733, EY-03677), the

U.S. Department of Agriculture (CRGO 87-CRCR-1-2320), and the
Trasher Research Fund (2800-8).

REFERENCES

1. F. Frickel, in *The Retinoids* (M.B. Sporn, A. B. Roberts, and D. S. Goodman, eds.), vol. 1, Academic Press, Orlando, FL, p. 7 (1984).
2. H. Kagechika, T. Himi, K. Namikawa, E. Kawachi, Y. Hashimoto, and K. Shudo, *J. Med. Chem.*, *32*:1098 (1989).
3. K. Teelman and W. Bollag, *Dermatologica*, *180:* 30 (1990).
4. A. E. Asato, A. Kim, M. Denny, and R. S. H. Liu, *J. Am. Chem. Soc.*, *105*: 2923 (1983).
5. R. S. H. Liu and A. E. Asato, *Tetrahedron*, *40*: 1931 (1984).
6. C. G. Knudsen, S. C. Carey, and W. H. Okamura, *J. Am. Chem. Soc.*, *102*: 6355 (1980).
7. M. R. Lakshman, I. Mychovsky, and M. Attlesey, *Proc. Natl. Acad. Sci. (USA)*, *86*:9124 (1989).
8. J. A. Olson, *J. Nutr.*, *119*:105 (1989).
9. G. W. Tang, J. D. Ribaya-Mercado, N. I. Krinsky, and R. M. Russell, *FASEB J.*, *4*:A924 (1990).
10. X. D. Wang, G. W. Tang, N. I. Krinsky, and R. M. Russell, *FASEB J.*, *4*:A1054 (1990).
11. J. A. Olson, in *Modern Nutrition in Health and Disease* (M. E. Shils and V. R. Young, eds.), 7th ed., Lea and Febiger, Philadelphia, p. 292 (1988).
12. J. A. Olson, in *Handbook of Vitamins* (L. J. Machlin, ed.), Marcel Dekker, New York, p. 1 (1990).
13. R. Blomhoff, T. Berg, and K. R. Norum, *Proc. Natl. Acad. Sci. (USA)*, *85*:3455 (1988).
14. R. M. Evans, *Science*, *240*:889 (1988).
15. D. R. Soprano, K. J. Soprano, and D. S. Goodman, *J. Lipid Res.*, *27*:166 (1986).
16. P. S. Deignor, W. C. Low, F. J. Canada, and R. R. Rando, *Science*, *244*:968 (1988).
17. H. Shi and J. A. Olson, *Biochim. Biophys. Acta*, *1035*:1 (1990).
18. S. L. Fong, W. B. Fong, T. A. Morris, K. M. Kedzie, and C. D. B. Bridges, *J. Biol. Chem.*, *265*:3648 (1990).
19. G. J. Chader, *Invest. Ophthalmol. Visual Sci.*, *30*:7 (1989).
20. L. Stryer, *Textbook of Biochemistry* 3rd Ed., W. H. Freeman, New York, p. 1027 (1988).
21. E. A. Chiocca, P. J. Davies, and J. P. Stein, *J. Cell Biochem.*, *39*:293 (1989).
22. N. Takahashi and T. R. Breitman, *J. Biol. Chem.*, *264*:5159 (1989).
23. G. J. LaRosa and L. J. Gudas, *Proc. Natl. Acad. Sci. (USA)*, *85*:329 (1988).

24. A. B. Roberts and M. B. Sporn, in *The Retinoids* (M. B. Sporn, A. B. Roberts, and D. S. Goodman, eds.), vol. 2, Academic Press, Orlando, FL p. 209 (1984).
25. J. M. Gallup, A. B. Barua, H. C. Furr, and J. A. Olson, *Proc. Soc. Exp. Biol. Med.*, *186*:269 (1987).
26. M. Maden, D. E. Ong, D. Summerbell, F. Chytil, and E. A. Hearst, *Dev. Biol.*, *135*:124 (1989).
27. J. A. Olson, *J. Nutr.*, *119*:1820 (1989).
28. S. R. Ames, H. A. Risley, and P. L. Harris, *Anal. Chem.*, *26*:1378 (1954).
29. J. A. Olson, *Arch. Latinam. Nutr.*, *29*:521 (1979).
30. E. G. Bligh and W. J. Dyer, *Can. J. Biochem. Physiol.*, *37*:911 (1959).
31. Y. L. Ito, M. H. Zile, H. M. Ahrens, and H. F. DeLuca, *J. Lipid Res.*, *15*:517 (1974).
32. A. B. Roberts, M. D. Nichols, C. A. Frolik, D. L. Newton, and M. B. Sporn, *Cancer Res.*, *38*:3327 (1978).
33. A. Frolik, T. E. Tavela, G. L. Peck, and M. B. Sporn, *Anal. Biochem.*, *86*:743 (1978).
34. M. E. Cullum and M. H. Zile, *Anal. Biochem.*, *153*:23 (1986).
35. Y. -M. Peng, M. -J. Xu, and D. S. Alberts, *J. Natl. Cancer Inst.*, *78*:95 (1987).
36. S. W. McClean, M. E. Ruddel, E. G. Gross, J. J. DiGiovanna, and G. L. Peck, *Clin. Chem.*, *28*:693 (1982).
37. D. W. Nierenberg and D. L. Lester, *J. Chromatogr.*, *345*:275 (1985).
38. A. B. Barua, R. O. Batres, and J. A. Olson, *Am. J. Clin. Nutr.*, *50*:370 (1989).
39. A. B. Barua, *Methods Enzymol.*, *189*:136 (1991).
40. R. Wyss and F. Bucheli, *J. Chromatogr.*, *424*:303 (1988).
41. C. A. Frolik and J. A. Olson, in *The Retinoids*, vol. 1 (M. B. Sporn, A. B. Roberts, and D. S. Goodman, eds.), Academic Press, New York, p. 181 (1984).
42. M. Holasova and J. Blattna, *J. Chromatogr.*, *123*:225 (1976).
43. M. H. Zile, R. C. Inhorn, and H. F. DeLuca, *J. Biol. Chem.*, *257*:3537 (1982).
44. K. Lippel and J. A. Olson, *J. Lipid Res.*, *9*:580 (1968).
45. J. L. Napoli, B. C. Pramanik, J. B. Williams, M. I. Dawson, and P. D. Hobbs, *J. Lipid Res.*, *26*:387 (1985).
46. H. Cohen and M. Lapointe, *J. Agric. Food Chem.*, *26*:1210 (1978).
47. D. B. Parrish, *CRC Crit. Rev. Food Sci. Nutr.*, *9*:375 (1977).
48. H. Egan, R. S. Kirk, and R. Sawyer, *Pearson's Chemical Analysis of Foods*, 8th ed., Churchville Livingstone, Edinburgh, p. 539 (1981).
49. Analytical Methods Committee, Royal Society of Chemistry, *Analyst*, *110*:1019 (1985).
50. A. Bognar, Z. *Lebensm. Unters. Forsch.*, *182*:492 (1986).
51. C. F. Bourgeois and N. Ciba, *J. Assoc. Off. Anal. Chem.*, *71*:12 (1988).
52. W. J. Driskell, M. M. Bashor, and J. W. Neese, *Clin. Chim. Acta.*, *147*:25 (1985).

53. W. J. Driskell, A. D. Lackey, J. S. Hewett, and M. M. Bashor, *Clin. Chem.*, *31*:871 (1985).

54. N. E. Craft, E. D. Brown, and J. C. Smith, Jr., *Clin. Chem.*, *34*:44 (1988).

55. M. H. Barreto-Lins, F. A. C. S. Campos, M. C. N. A. Azevdo, and H. Flores, *Clin. Chem.*, *34*:2308 (1988).

56. G. M. Landers and J. A. Olson, *J. Assoc. Off. Anal. Chem.*, *69*:50 (1986).

57. W. E. Lambert, H. J. Nelis, M. G. M. DeRuyter, and A. P. DeLeenheer, in *Modern Chromatographic Analysis of the Vitamins* (A. P. DeLeenheer, W. E. Lambert, and M. G. M. DeRuyter, eds.), Marcel Dekker, New York, p. 1 (1985).

58. F. Tataruch, *Mikrochim. Acta*, *1*:235 (1984).

59. R. M. McKenzie, M. L. McGregor, and E. C. Nelson, *J. Label. Compounds Radiopharm.*, *15*:265 (1977).

60. K. V. John, H. R. Lakshmanan, F. B. Jungwala, and H. R. Cama, *J. Chromatogr.*, *18*:53 (1965).

61. T. N. R. Varma, T. Panalaks, and T. K. Murray, *Anal. Chem.*, *36*:1864 (1964).

62. Y. K. Fung and R. G. Rahwan, *J. Chromatogr.*, *147*:528 (1978).

63. R. F. Taylor, *Adv. Chromatogr.*, *22*:157 (1983).

64. P. V. Bhat and P. R. Sundaresan, *CRC Crit. Rev. Anal. Chem.*, *20*:197 (1988).

65. A. P. DeLeenheer, H. J. Nelis, W. E. Lambert, and R. M. Bauwens, *J. Chromatogr.*, *429*:3 (1988).

66. M. Tswett, *Deutsche Bot. Ges.*, *24*:316, 384 (1906).

67. D. L. Saunders, *J. Chrom. Sci.*, *15*:372 (1979).

68. C. Horvath and W. Melander, *J. Chrom. Sci.*, *15*:393 (1977).

69. R. J. Smith, J. K. Haken, and M. S. Wainwright, *J. Chromatogr.*, *334*:95 (1985).

70. H. C. Furr, *J. Chrom. Sci.*, *27*:216 (1989).

71. H. J. Nelis, J. DeRoose, H. Vandenbaviere, and A. P. DeLeenheer, *Clin. Chem.*, *29*:1431 (1983).

72. J. C. Wallingford and B. A. Underwood, *J. Chromatogr.*, *381*:158 (1986).

73. A. C. Ross, *Methods Enzymol.*, *123*:68 (1986).

74. A. P. DeLeenheer, W. E. Lambert, and I. Claeys, *J. Lipid Res.*, *23*:1362 (1982).

75. F. M. Vane, J. K. Stollenborg, and C. J. L. Bugge, *J. Chromatogr.*, *227*:471 (1982).

76. C. J. L. Bugge, L. C. Rodriquez, and F. M. Vane, *J. Pharm. Biomed. Anal.*, *3*:269 (1985).

77. R. Hubbard, P. K. Brown, and D. Bownds, *Methods Enzymol.*, *18C*:615 (1971).

78. S. Futterman and J. S. Andrews, *J. Biol. Chem.*, *239*:81 (1964).

79. A. C. Ross, *Anal. Biochem.*, *115*:324 (1981).

80. H. S. Huang and D. S. Goodman, *J. Biol. Chem.*, *240*:2839 (1965).

81. K. W. Miller and C. S. Yang, *Anal. Biochem.*, *145*:21 (1985).

82. M. Mulholland and R. J. Dolphin, *J. Chromatogr.*, *350*:285 (1985).

83. M. Mulholland, *Analyst*, *111*:601 (1986).
84. M. D. Greenspan, C. -Y. L. Lo, D. P. Hanf, and J. B. Yudkovitz, *J. Lipid Res.*, *29*:971 (1988).
85. R. Schindler, A. Klopp, C. Gorny, and W. Feldheim, *Int. J. Vit. Nutr. Res.*, *55*:25 (1985).
86. A. T. Rhys Williams, *J. Chromatogr.*, *341*:198 (1985).
87. A. J. Speek, C. Wongkham, N. Limratana, W. Saowakontha, and W. H. Schreurs, *J. Chromatogr.*, *382*:284 (1986).
88. N. R. Badcock and D. A. O'Reilly, *J. Chromatogr.*, *382*:290 (1986).
89. A. J. Speek, E. J. van Agtmaal, S. Saowakontha, W. H. Schreurs, and N. J. van Haeringen, *Curr. Eye Res.*, *5*:841 (1986).
90. C. A. Collins and C. K. Chow, *J. Chromatogr.*, *317*:349 (1984).
91. H. K. Biesalski and H. Weiser, *J. Clin. Chem. Clin. Biochem.*, *27*:65 (1989).
92. W. A. MacCrehan and E. Schonberger, *J. Chromatogr.*, *417*:65 (1987).
93. W. A. MacCrehan and E. Schonberger, *Clin. Chem.*, *33*:1585 (1987).
94. S. A. Wring, J. P. Hart, and D. W. Knight, *Analyst*, *113*:1785 (1988).
95. G. S. Shephard, B. J. Hough, M. E. van Stuijvenberg, and D. Labadarios, *Clin. Chim. Acta*, *153*:249 (1985).
96. H. C. Furr, D. A. Cooper, and J. A. Olson, *J. Chromatogr.*, *378*:45 (1986).
97. A. P. DeLeenheer, V. O. R. C. DeBevere, M. G. M. DeRuyter, and A. E. Claeys, *J. Chromatogr.*, *162*:408 (1979).
98. G. L. Catignani and J. G. Bieri, *Clin. Chem.*, *29*:708 (1983).
99. G. Catignani, *Methods Enzymol.*, *123*:215 (1986).
100. R. Mansourian, E. Shepherd, and H. Dirren, *Int. J. Vit. Nutr. Res.*, *52*:227 (1982).
101. D. N. Palmer, M. A. Anderson, and R. D. Jolly, *Anal. Biochem.*, *140*:315 (1984).
102. R. Ohmacht, G. Toth, and G. Voigt, *J. Chromatogr.*, *395*:609 (1987).
103. H. Biesalski, H. Grieff, K. Brodda, G. Hafner, and K. H. Bassler, *Int. J. Vit. Nutr. Res.*, *56*:319 (1986).
104. P. M. Van Haard, R. Engel, and T. Postma, *Biomed. Chromatogr.*, *2*:79 (1987).
105. F. I. Chow and S. T. Omaye, *Lipids*, *18*:837 (1983).
106. M. L. Huang, G. J. Burckart, and R. Venkataramanan, *J. Chromatogr.*, *380*:331 (1986).
107. J. P. Vuilleumier, H. E. Keller, D. Gysel, and F. Hunziker, *Int. J. Vit. Nutr. Res.*, *53*:265 (1983).
108. K. W. Miller, N. A. Lorr, and C. S. Yang, *Anal. Biochem.*, *138*:340 (1984).
109. D. W. Nierenberg and T. Stukel, *Am. J. Med. Sci.*, *294*:187 (1987).
110. R. B. Hayes, J. F. Bogdanovicz, F. H. Schroeder, A. De Bruijn et al., *Cancer*, *62*:2021 (1988).
111. L. A. Kaplan, J. A. Miller, and E. A. Stein, *J. Clin. Lab. Invest.*, *1*:147 (1987).
112. E. D. Brown, A. Rose, N. Craft, K. E. Seidel, and J. C. Smith, Jr., *Clin. Chem.*, *35*:310 (1989)

113. N. Bilic and R. Sieber, Z. *Lebensm. Unters. Forsch.*, *186*:514 (1988).
114. S. Ciappellano, F. Brighenti, M. Porrini, and G. Testolini, *Acta Vitaminol. Enzymol.*, *7*:223 (1985).
115. H. C. Furr and J. A. Olson, *Anal. Biochem.*, *171*:360 (1988).
116. B. J. Burri and M. A. Kutnink, *Clin. Chem.*, *35*:582 (1989).
117. J. Glover, *Methods Enzymol.*, *67F*:282 (1980).
118. P. V. Bhat and A. Lacroix, *J. Chromatogr.*, *272*:269 (1983).
119. R. Schindler, M. Scholz, and W. Feldheim, Z. *Lebensm. Unters. Forsch.*, *185*:208 (1987).
120. H. C. Furr, A. J. Clifford, L. M. Smith, and J. A. Olson, *J. Nutr.*, *119*:581 (1989).
121. M. G. M. DeRuyter and A. P. DeLeenheer, *Clin. Chem.*, *24*:1920 (1978).
122. M. G. M. DeRuyter and A. P. DeLeenheer, *Anal. Chem.*, *51*:43 (1979).
123. N. A. Parris, *J. Chromatogr.*, *157*:161 (1978).
124. W. O. Landen, *J. Assoc. Off. Anal. Chem.*, *65*:810 (1982).
125. C. R. Broich, L. E. Gerber, and J. W. Erdman, Jr., *Lipids*, *18*:253 (1983).
126. H. J. C. F. Nelis and A. P. DeLeenheer, *Anal. Chem.*, *55*:270 (1983).
127. H. C. Furr, *Methods Enzymol.*, *189*:85 (1991).
128. J. C. Saari and D. L. Bredberg, *J. Biol. Chem.*, *263*:8084 (1988).
129. J. L. Ubels, T. B. Osgood, and K. M. Foley, *Curr. Eye Res.*, *7*:1009 (1988).
130. D. C. Woollard and H. Indyk, *J. Micronutr. Anal.*, *5*:35 (1989).
131. H. E. May and S. I. Koo, *J. Liq. Chromatogr.*, *12*:1261 (1989).
132. W. O. Landen, *J. Assoc. Off. Anal. Chem.*, *63*:131 (1980).
133. B. A. Bidlingmeyer and F. V. Warren, *LC-GC*, *6*:780 (1988).
134. M. R. Lakshman, P. R. Sundaresan, L. L. Chambers, and P. K. Shoff, *Lipids*, *23*: 144 (1988).
135. D. D. Bankson, R. M. Russell, and J. A. Sadowski, *Clin. Chem.*, *32*:35 (1986).
136. C. D. B. Bridges, S.-L. Fong, and R. A. Alvarez, *Vision Res.*, *20*:355 (1980).
137. J. B. Williams, B. C. Pramanik, and J. L. Napoli, *J. Lipid Res.*, *25*:638 (1984).
138. F. J. G. M. Van Kuijk, G. M. Handelman, and E. A. Dratz, *J. Chromatogr.*, *348*:241 (1985).
139. L. R. Chaudhary and E. C. Nelson, *J. Chromatogr.*, *294*:466 (1984).
140. H. C. Furr, O. Amedee-Manesme, and J. A. Olson, *J. Chromatogr.*, *309*:299 (1984).
141. C. A. Frolik, T. E. Tavela, and M. B. Sporn, *J. Lipid Res.*, *19*:32 (1978).
142. A. M. McCormick, J. L. Napoli, and H. F. DeLuca, *Anal. Biochem.*, *86*:25 (1978).
143. H. Steuerle, Z. *Lebensm. Unters. Forsch.*, *181*:400 (1985).
144. R. W. Curley, D. L. Carson, and C. N. Ryzewski, *J. Chromatogr.*, *370*:188 (1986).
145. B. Stancher and F. Zonta, *J. Chromatogr.*, *234*:244 (1982).
146. F. Zonta and B. Stancher, *J. Chromatogr.*, *301*:65 (1984).

147. G. W. T. Groenendijk, P. A. A. Jensen, S. L. Bonting, and F. J. M. Daemen, *Methods Enzymol.*, *67F*:203 (1980).
148. K. Tsukida, M. Ito, T. Tanaka, and I. Yagi, *J. Chromatogr.*, *331*:265 (1985).
149. G. M. Landers and J. A. Olson, *J. Chromatogr.*, *291*:51 (1984).
150. G. M. Landers and J. A. Olson, *J. Chromatogr.*, *438*:383 (1988).
151. A. T. C. Tsin, R. A. Alvarez, S.-L. Fong, and C. D. B. Bridges, *Vision Res.*, *24*:1835 (1984).
152. P. V. Bhat, H. T. Co, and A. Lacroix, *J. Chromatogr.*, *260*:129 (1983).
153. P. V. Bhat and A. Lacroix, *Methods Enzymol.*, *123*:75 (1986).
154. M. G. DeRuyter, W. E. Lambert, and A. P. DeLeenheer, *Anal. Biochem.*, *98*:402 (1979).
155. A. M. McCormick, J. L. Napoli, and H. F. DeLuca, *Methods Enzymol.*, *67F*:220 (1980).
156. C. Thaller and G. Eichele, *Nature*, *327*:625 (1987).
157. M. A. Satre, J. D. Penner, and D. M. Kochhar, *Teratology*, *39*:341 (1989).
158. D. P. Silva and H. F. DeLuca, *Biochem. J.*, *206*:33 (1982).
159. D. A. Miller and H. F. DeLuca, *Arch. Biochem. Biophys.*, *244*:179 (1986).
160. L. R. Chaudhary and E. C. Nelson, *Int. J. Vit. Nutr. Res.*, *55*:17 (1985).
161. B. N. Swanson, C. A. Frolik, D. W. Saharevitz, P. P. Roller, and M. B. Sporn, *Biochem. Pharmacol.*, *30*:107 (1981).
162. C. V. Puglisi and J. A. F. DeSilva, *J. Chromatogr.*, *152*:421 (1978).
163. C. A. Huselton, B. E. Fayer, W. A. Garland, and D. J. Liberato, in *Liquid Chromatography/Mass Spectrometry* (M. A. Brown, ed.), American Chemical Society, Washington, D. C., p. 166 (1990).
164. P. Thongnopnua and C. L. Zimmerman, *J. Chromatogr.*, *433*:345 (1988).
165. F. M. Vane, C. J. L. Bugge, and L. C. Rodriguez, *Drug Metab. Dispos.*, *17*:275, 280 (1989).
166. K. E. Creek, D. Rimoldi, C. S. Silverman-Jones, and L. M. DeLuca, *Biochem. J.*, *227*:695 (1985).
167. K. E. Creek, D. Rimoldi, M. Brugh-Collins, and L. M. DeLuca, *Methods Enzymol.*, *123*:61 (1986)
168. P. V. Bhat, L. M. De Luca, and M. L. Wind, *Anal. Biochem.*, *102*:243 (1980).
169. T. A. Hultin, R. G. Mehta, and R. C. Moon, *J. Chromatogr.*, *341*:187 (1985).
170. W. R. Sisco, P. A. Schrader, A. M. McLaughlin, and B. H. Clark, *J. Chromatogr.*, *368*:184 (1986).
171. A. Kutner, B. Renstrom, H. K. Schnoes, and H. F. DeLuca, *Proc. Natl. Acad. Sci. (USA)*, *83*:6781 (1986).
172. D. A. Miller and H. F. DeLuca, *Proc. Natl. Acad. Sci. (USA)*, *82*:6419 (1985).
173. M. A. Leo and C. S. Lieber, *J. Biol. Chem.*, *260*:5228 (1985).
174. M. Ito, N. Matsuoka, K. Tsukida, and T. Seki, *Chem. Pharm. Bull.*, *36*:78 (1988).

175. T. H. Goldsmith, B. C. Marks, and G. C. Bernard, *Vision Res.*, 26:1763 (1986).
176. T. Seki, S. Fujishita, M. Ito, N. Matsuoka, and K. Tsukida, *Exp. Biol.*, 47:95 (1987).
177. S. Matsui, M. Seidou, I. Uchiyama, N. Sekiya, K. Hiraki, K. Yoshihara, and Y. Kito, *Biochim. Biophys. Acta*, 966:370 (1988).
178. H. Torma and A. Vahlquist, *J. Invest. Dermatol.*, 85:498 (1985)
179. H. Torma and A. Vahlquist, *Biochim. Biophys. Acta*, 961:177 (1988).
180. A. T. C. Tsin, S. T. Morales, and J. M. Flores, *Can. J. Zool.*, 64:2066 (1986).
181. T. Seki, S. Fujishita, M. Azuma, and T. Suzuki, *Zool. Sci.*, 4:475 (1987).
182. S. A. Tanumihardjo, H. C. Furr, J. W. Erdman, and J. A. Olson, *Eur. J. Clin. Nutr.*, 44:219 (1990).
183. S. A. Tanumihardjo and J. A. Olson, *J. Nutri.*, 118:598 (1988).
184. B. Stancher and F. Zonta, *J. Chromatogr.*, 287:353 (1984).
185. M. Azuma, T. Seki, and S. Fujishita, *Vision Res.*, 28:959 (1988).
186. A. T. Tsin, H. A. Pedrozo-Fernandez, J. M. Gallas, and J. P. Chambers, *Life Sci.*, 43:1379 (1988).
187. P. E. Dunagin and J. A. Olson, *Methods Enzymol.*, 15:289 (1969).
188. T. Ninomiya, K. Kidokoro, M. Horiguchi, and N. Higosaki, *Bitamin*, 27:349 (1963).
189. M. E. Cullum, J. A. Olson, and S. W. Veysey, *Int. J. Vit. Nutr. Res.*, 53:3 (1983).
190. M. Vecchi, W. Vetter, W. Walther, S. F. Jermstad, and G. W. Schutt, *Helv. Chim. Acta.*, 50:1243 (1967).
191. A. P. DeLeenheer and M. G. M. DeRuyter, *Anal. Biochem.*, 63:169 (1975).
192. R. F. Taylor and M. Ikawa, *Methods Enzymol.*, 67:233 (1980).
193. T. C. Chiang, *J. Chromatogr.*, 185:335 (1980).
194. J. L. Napoli, *Methods Enzymol.*, 123:112. (1986).
194a. H. J. Egger, U. B. Ranalder, E. U. Koelle and M. Klaus, *Biomed. Environ. Mass Spec.*, 18:453 (1989).
195. C. R. Smidt, A. D. Jones, and A. J. Clifford, *J. Chromatogr.*, 434:21 (1988).
196. H. C. Furr, S. Zeng, A. J. Clifford, and J. A. Olson, *J. Chromatogr.*, 527:406 (1990).
197. A. J. Clifford, A. D. Jones, and H. C. Furr, *Methods Enzymol.*, 189:94 (1991).
198. G. Arroyave, C. O. Chichester, H. Flores, J. Glover, L. A. Mejia, J. A. Olson, K. L. Simpson, and B. A. Underwood, *Biochemical Methodology for the Assessment of Vitamin A Status*, International Vitamin A Consultative Group, ILSI-NF, Washington, DC, 1982.
199. N. Monji and E. Bosin, *Methods Enzymol.*, 123:85 (1986).
200. D. Topping, H. W. Forster, C. Dolman, C. M. Luczynska, and A. M. Bernard, *Clin. Chem.*, 32:1863 (1986).
201. G. H. Wirtz and S. S. Westfall, *J. Lipid Res.*, 22:869 (1981).
202. R. E. Pauls and R. W. McCoy, *J. Chromatogr. Sci.*, 23:181 (1985).

203. L. S. Palmer, *Carotenoids and Related Pigments*, American Chemical Society Monograph Series, Chemical Catalog Co., New York (1922).
204. P. Karrer and E. Jucker, *Carotenoids*, Elsevier, New York (1950).
205. O. Isler (ed.), *Carotenoids*, Birkhauser Verlag, Basel (1971).
206. A. Bendich and J. A. Olson, *FASEB J.*, 3:1927 (1989).
207. H. Pfander (ed.), *Key to Carotenoids by Otto Straub*, 2nd ed., Birkhauser Verlag, Basel (1987).
208. T. W. Goodwin, *The Biochemistry of the Carotenoids*, 2nd ed., vols. I and II, Chapman and Hall, London (1980, 1984).
209. E. DeRitter and A. E. Purcell, in *Carotenoids as Colorants and Vitamin A Precursors* (J. C. Bauernfeind, ed.), Academic Press, Orlando, FL, p. 883 (1981).
210. O. Isler, H. Lindlar, M. Montavon, P. Ruegg, and P. Zeller, *Helv. Chim. Acta*, 39:249 (1956).
211. A. H. El-Tinay and C. O. Chichester, *J. Org. Chem.*, 35:2290 (1970).
212. G. J. Handelman and N. I. Krinsky, *FASEB J.*, 4:A923 (1990).
213. N. I. Krinsky, *Prev. Med.*, 18:592 (1989).
214. G. W. Burton, *J. Nutr.*, 119:109 (1989).
215. J. E. Packer, J. S. Mahood, V. O. Mora-Arellano, T. F. Slater, R. L. Willson, and B. S. Wolfenden, *Biochim. Biophys. Res. Commun.*, 98:901 (1981).
216. R. J. Cogdell and H. A. Frank, *Biochim. Biophys. Acta*, 895:63 (1987).
217. N. I. Krinsky, *Pure Appl. Chem.*, 51:649 (1979).
218. H. J. Nelis, P. Lavens, M. M. Van Steenberge, G. R. Criel, and A. P. DeLeenheer, *J. Lipid Res.*, 29:491 (1988).
219. A. B. Barua, *World Rev. Nutr. Diet.*, 31:89 (1978).
220. T. W. Goodwin, *Annu. Rev. Nutr.*, 6:273 (1986).
221. J. A. Olson, in *Biosythesis of Isoprenoid Compounds* (J. W. Porter and S. L. Spurgeon, eds.), vol. 2, John Wiley, New York, p. 371 (1983).
222. B. V. Milborrow, in *Biosynthesis of Isoprenoid Compounds* (J. W. Porter and S. L. Spurgeon, eds.), vol. 2, John Wiley, New York, p. 413 (1983).
223. J. D. Bu'Lock in *Biosynthesis of Isoprenoid Compounds* (J. W. Porter and S. L. Spurgeon, eds.), vol. 2, John Wiley, New York, p. 437 (1982).
224. H. H. Schmitz, C. L. Poor, R. B. Wellman, and J. W. Erdman, Jr., *FASEB J.*, 4:A1055 (1990).
225. N. I. Krinsky, M. M. Mathews-Roth, S. Welankiwar, P. K. Sehgal, N. C. G. Lausen, and M. Russett, *J. Nutr.* 120:81 (1990).
226. P. F. Zagalsky, *Methods Enzymol.*, 111:216 (1985).
227. C. Okoh and M. R. Lakshman, *FASEB J.*, 4:A1056 (1990).
228. R. G. Ziegler, *J. Nutr.*, 119:116 (1989).
229. S. Liaaen-Jensen, in *The Carotenoids* (O. Isler, ed.), Birkhauser Verlag, Basel, p. 61 (1971).
230. G. Britton, *Methods Enzymol.*, 111:113 (1985).
231. F. Khachik, G. R. Beecher, and N. F. Whittaker, *J. Agric. Food Chem.*, 34:603 (1986).
232. J. N. Thompson, S. Duval, and P. Verdier, *J. Micronutr. Anal.*, 1:81 (1985).

233. M. I. Heinonen, V. Ollilainen, E. K. Linkola, P. T. Varo, and P. E. Koivistoinen, *J. Agric. Food Chem.*, 37:655 (1989).

234. A. B. Barua, R. O. Batres, H. C. Furr, and J. A. Olson, *J. Micronutr. Anal.*, 5:291 (1989).

235. F. Khackik and G. R. Beecher, *J. Agric. Food. Chem.*, 35:732 (1987).

236. I. Stewart and T. A. Wheaton, *J. Chromatogr.*, 55:325 (1971).

237. P. Ruedi, *Pure Appl. Chem.*, 57:793 (1985).

238. R. J. Bushway, *J. Liquid Chromatogr.*, 8:1527 (1985).

239. M. Ruddat and O. H. Will, *Methods Enzymol.*, 111:189 (1985).

240. S. H. Rhodes, A. G. Netting and B. V. Milborrow, *J. Chromatogr.*, 442:412 (1988).

241. A. Fiksdahl, J. T. Mortensen, and S. Liaaen-Jensen, *J. Chromatogr.*, 157:111 (1978).

242. G. Englert and M. Vecchi, *Helv. Chim. Acta.*, 63:1711 (1980).

243. M. Vecchi, G. Englert, and H. Mayer, *Helv. Chim. Acta*, 65:1050 (1982).

244. J. Tyczkowski, J. L. Schaeffer, C. Parkhurst, and P. B. Hamilton, *Poult. Sci.*, 65:2135 (1986).

245. J. Tyczkowski and P. B. Hamilton, *Poult. Sci.*, 65:1526 (1986).

246. S. K. Reeder and G. L. Park, *J. Assoc. Off. Anal. Chem.*, 55:595 (1975).

247. M. Vecchi, G. Englert, R. Maurer, and V. Meduna, *Helv. Chim. Acta*, 64:2746 (1981).

248. K. Tsukida, K. Saiki, T. Takii, and Y. Koyama, *J. Chromatogr.*, 245:359 (1982).

249. L. A. Chandler and S. J. Schwartz, *J. Food Sci.*, 52:669 (1987).

250. R. Ohmacht, G. Toth, and G. Voigt, *Chromatographia*, 22:189 (1986).

251. F. Khachik, G. R. Beecher, and W. R. Lusby, *J. Agric. Food Chem.*, 37:1465 (1989).

252. C. C. Tangey, *J. Liquid Chromatogr.*, 7:2611 (1984).

253. D. B. Milne and J. Botnen, *Clin. Chem.*, 32:874. (1986).

254. V. J. Gatautis and K. H. Pearson, *Clin. Chim. Acta*, 166:195 (1987).

255. J. G. Bieri, E. D. Brown, and J. C. Smith, Jr., *J. Liquid Chromatogr.*, 8:473 (1985).

256. B. Stancher, F. Zonta, and P. Bogoni, *J. Micronutr. Anal.*, 3:97 (1986).

257. F. Khachik, G. R. Beecher, and W. R. Lusby, *J. Agric. Food Chem.*, 36:938 (1988).

258. R. S. Parker, *J. Nutr.*, 119:101 (1989).

259. A. J. Culling-Berglund, S. A. Newcomb, M. Gagne, W. S. Morfitt, and T. P. Davis, *J. Micronutr. Anal.*, 5:139 (1989).

260. H. S. Nam, S. Y. Cho, and J. S. Rhee, *J. Chromatogr.*, 448:445 (1988).

261. R. J. Bushway, *J. Agric. Food Chem.*, 34:409 (1986).

262. D. W. Nierenberg, *J. Chromatogr.*, 339:273 (1985).

263. D. R. Lauren, M. P. Agnew, and D. E. McNaughton, *J. Liquid Chromatogr.*, 9:1997 (1986).

264. D. R. Lauren and D. E. McNaughton, *J. Liquid Chromatogr.*, 9:2013 (1986).

265. F. Zonta, B. Stancher, and G. P. Marletta, *J. Chromatogr.*, 403:207 (1987).

266. T. Philip and T. Chen, *J. Food Sci.*, *53*:1720 (1988).
267. R. B. H. Wills, H. Nurdin, and M. Wootton, *J. Micronutr. Anal.*, *4*:87 (1988).
268. F. Khachik and G. R. Beecher, *J. Agric. Food Chem.*, *36*:929 (1988).
269. R. Peto, R. Doll, J. D. Buckley, and M. B. Sporn, *Nature (Lond.)*, *290*:201 (1981).
270. W. C. Willet, *Nutr. Rev.*, *48*:201 (1990).
271. M. S. Menkes, G. W. Comstock, J. P. Vuilleumier, K. J. Helsing, A. A. Rider, and R. Brookmeyer, *N. Engl. J. Med.*, *315*:1250 (1986).
272. Y. Ito, R. Sasaki, M. Minohara, M. Otani, and K. Aoki, *Clin. Chim. Acta.*, *169*:197 (1987).
273. Y. Ito, M. Minohara, N. Ogitsu, Y. Kusuhara, R. Sasaki, M. Otani, M. Ito, and K. Aoki, *Japn. J. Clin. Chem.*, *16*:18, (1987).
274. G. Cavina, B. Gallinella, R. Porra, P. Pecora, and C. Suraci, *J. Pharm. Biomed. Anal.*, *6*:259 (1988).
275. G. Wang, M. R. Root, X. Ye, J. Chen, and T. C. Campbell, *J. Micronutr. Anal.*, *5*:3 (1989).
276. N. J. Wald, J. Boreham, J. L. Hayward, and R. D. Bulbrook, *Br. J. Cancer*, *49*:321 (1984).
277. J. P. Costantino, L. H. Kuller, L. Begg, C. K. Redmond, and M. W. Bates, *Am. J. Clin. Nutr.*, *48*:1277 (1988).
278. E. D. Brown, M. S. Micozzi, N. E. Craft, J. G. Bieri, G. Beecher, B. K. Edwards, A. Rose, P. R. Taylor, and J. C. Smith, Jr., *Am. J. Clin. Nutr.* *49*:1258 (1989).
279. M. Stacewicz-Sapuntzakis, P. E. Bowen, J. W. Kikendall, and M. Burgess, *J. Micronutr. Anal.*, *3*:27 (1987).
280. N. V. Dimitrov, C. Meyer, D. E. Ullrey, W. Chenoweth, A. Michelakis, W. Malone, C. Boone, and G. Fink, *Am. J. Clin. Nutr.* *48*:298 (1988).
281. C. T. Henderson, S. Mobarhan, P. Bowen, M. Stacewicz-Sapuntzakis, P. Langenberg, R. Kiani, D. Lucchesi, and S. Sugerman, *J. Am. Coll. Nutr.*, *8*:625 (1989).
282. A. Shibata, R. Sasaki, Y. Ito, N. Hamajima, S. Suzuki, M. Ohtani, and K. Aoki, *Int. J. Cancer*, *44*:48 (1989).
283. H. Kim, K. L. Simpson, and L. E. Garber, *Nutr. Res.*, *8*:1119 (1988).
284. D. W. Nierenberg, T. A. Stukel, J. A. Baron, B. J. Dain, E. R. Greenberg, and Skin Cancer Prevention Study Group, *Am J. Epidemiol.*, *130*:511 (1989).
285. R. S. Parker, *Am. J. Clin. Nutr.*, *47*:33 (1988).
286. S. A. Tanumihardjo, H. C. Furr, O. Amedee-Manesme, and J. A. Olson, *Int. J. Vit. Nutr. Res.* *60*:307 (1990).
287. H. F. Stitch and M. P. Rosin, *Int. J. Cancer*, *37*:389 (1986).
288. H. F. Stitch, A. P. Hornby, and B. P. Dunn, *Cancer Lett.*, *30*:133 (1986).
289. L. M. Cameron, M. P. Rosin, and H. F. Stitch, *Cancer Ltt.*, *45*:203 (1989).
290. D. B. Rodriguez-Amaya, *J. Micronutr. Anal.*, *5*:191 (1989).
291. J. M. Dietz, S. S. Kantha, and J. W. Erdman, Jr., *Plant Foods Hum. Nutr.*, *38*:333 (1988).

292. E. Lesellier, C. Marty, C. Berset, and A. Tchapla, *J. High Resolution Chromatogr.*, *12*:447 (1989).
293. B. Tan, *J. Food Sci.*, *53*:954 (1988).
294. D. R. Lauren, D. E. McNaughton, and M. P. Agnew, *J. Assoc. Off. Anal. Chem.*, *70*:428 (1987).
295. H. G. Daood, B. Czinkotai, A. Hoschke, and P. Biacs, *J. Chromatogr.*, *472*:296 (1989).
296. R. J. Bushway, A. Yang, and A. M. Yamani, *J. Food Qual.*, *9*:437 (1986).
297. K. Kobayaski, A. Tsurumizu, M. Toyoda, and Y. Saito, *Nippon Shokuhin Kogyo Gakkaishi*, *36*:676 (1989).
298. P. W. Simon and X. Y. Wolff, *J. Agric. Food Chem.*, *35*:1017 (1987) and *36*:938 (1988).
299. F. Khachik and G. R. Beecher, *J. Chromatogr.*, *449*:119 (1988).
300. A. B. Barua and J. A. Olson, *Biochem. J.*, *263*:403 (1989).
301. T. Philip and T. Chen, *J. Food Sci.*, *53*:1703 (1988).
302. J. F. Fisher and R. L. Rouseff, *J. Agric. Food Chem.*, *34*:985 (1986).
303. R. J. Bushway, *J. Agric. Food Chem.*, *34*:985 (1986).
304. F. W. Quackenbush, *J. Liquid Chromatogr.* *10*:643 (1987).
305. A. Ben-Amotz, A. Lers, and M. Avron, *Plant Physiol.*, *86*:1286 (1988).
306. F. Pepping, C. M. J. Vencken, and C. E. West, *J. Sci. Food Agric.*, *45*:359 (1988).
307. S. Scalia and G. W. Francis, *Chromatographia*, *28*:87129. (1989).
308. H. Indyk, *J. Micronutr. Anal.*, *3*:169 (1987).
309. V. Ollilainen, M. Heinonen, E. Linkola, P. Vero, and P. Koivistoinen, *J. Dairy Sci.*, *72*:2257 (1989).
310. N. Hidiroglou, L. R. McDowell, and A. Boning, *Int. J. Vit. Nutr. Res.*, *56*:339 (1986).
311. H. Boyd, N. S. Ritchier, B. C. Cooke, and J. F. Roche, *Irish Vet. J.*, *38*:95 (1984).
312. B. S. Alam, S. Q. Alam, A. Bendich, and S. S. Shapiro, *Nutr. Cancer*, *12*:57 (1989).
313. T. Matsuno, T. Hirono, Y. Ikuno, T. Maoka, M. Shimizu, and T. Komori, *Comp. Biochem. Physiol.*, *84B*:447 (1986).
314. S. T. Mayne and R. S. Parker, *Lipids*, *21*:164 (1986).
315. A. Gillou, G. Choubert, T. Storebakken, J. d. L. Noue, and S. Kaushik, *Comp. Biochem. Physiol.*, *94B*:481 (1989).
316. F. J. Schweigert, M. Wierich, W. A. Rambeck, and H. Zucker, *Theriogenology*, *30*:923 (1988).
317. M. Vecchi, E. Glinz, V. Meduna, and K. Schiedt, *J. High Resolution Chromatogr.*, *10*:349 (1987).
318. J. H. Ng and B. Tan, *J. Chromatogr. Sci.*, *26*:463 (1988).
319. A. S. Kester and R. E. Thompson, *J. Chromatogr.*, *310*:372 (1984).
320. H. Chen and C. A. Bailey, *J. Chromatogr.*, *393*:297 (1987).
321. C. A. Bailey and B. H. Chen, *J. Chromatogr.*, *455*:396 (1988).
322. T. Maoka and T. Matsuno, *J. Chromatogr.*, *478*:379 (1989).
323. T. Maoka, A. Arai, M. Shimizu, and T. Matsuno, *Comp. Biochem. Physiol.*, *83B*:121 (1986).

324. T. Maoka, K. Komori, and T. Matsuno, *J. Chromatogr.*, *318*:122 (1985).
325. Y. Ikuno, T. Maoka, M. Shimizu, T. Komori, and T. Matsuno, *J. Chromatogr.*, *328*:387 (1989).
326. T. Maoka and T. Matsuno, *J. Chromatogr.*, *482*:189 (1989).
327. T. Maoka and T. Matsuno, *Comp. Biochem. Physiol.*, *93B*:829 (1989).
328. J. C. Giddings, L. McLaren, and M. N. Meyers, *Science, 159*:197 (1968).
329. N. M. Frew, C. G. Johnson, and R. H. Bromund, *ACS Symp. Ser.*, *366*:208 (1987).
330. H. H. Schmitz, W. E. Artz, C. L. Poor, J. M. Dietz, and J. W. Erdman, Jr., *J. Chromatogr.*, *479*:261 (1989).
331. S. Krasinski, R. M. Russel, C. L. Ostradovec, J. A. Sadowski, S. C. Hartz, R. A. Jacob, and R. B. McGandy, *Am. J. Clin. Nutr.*, *49*:112 (1989).
332. L. Hussein and M. El-Tohamy, *Int. J. Vit. Nutr. Res.*, *59*:229 (1989).
333. A. K. Chopra, A. Khare, G. P. Moss, and B. C. L. Weedon, *J. Chem. Soc. Perkins Trans.*, *I*:1371 (1988).
334. S. Tsai, S. C. S. Tsou, and K. L. Simpson, *J. Micronutr. Anal.*, *5*:171 (1989).
335. U. Schwieter and O. Isler, in *The Vitamins*, 2nd ed. (W. H. Sebrell, Jr., and R. S. Harris, eds.), Academic Press, New York, vol. 1, p. 5 (1967).
336. M. Buchwald and W. P. Jencks, *Biochemistry*, 7:834 (1968).

2

VITAMIN D: CHOLECALCIFEROL, ERGOCALCIFEROL, AND HYDROXYLATED METABOLITES

Glenville Jones

Queen's University, Kingston, Ontario, Canada

David James Hamilton Trafford
and Hugh Lewellyn John Makin

The London Hospital Medical College, London, England

Bruce W. Hollis

Medical University of South Carolina, Charleston, South Carolina

1. INTRODUCTION

The demonstration over two decades ago (1) of the conversion of vitamin D_3 into 25-hydroxyvitamin D_3 (25-OH-D_3) triggered a dramatic surge of interest in the basic biochemistry and physiology of vitamin D. The resultant elucidation of the metabolism and role of vitamin D in calcium homeostasis (1–5) has led to a change of emphasis from the study of the parent vitamin itself to the study of its metabolites. Older methods of bioassay, colorimetric and ultraviolet (UV) absorption assay, have been replaced by newer techniques based upon chromatography, radioligand procedures, and mass spectrometry (reviewed in Ref. 6). Present methods separate and specifically measure a wide variety of metabolites and chemical analogs instead of a heterogeneous "vitamin D" group. The increased sensitivity and specificity offered by modern assays have enabled the measurement of picogram quantities of vitamin D metabolites, thereby permitting these techniques to be applied to the analysis of vitamin D and its metabolites in physiological fluids. Chemical synthesis of vitamin D metabolites for clinical trials has led to improvements in the separation and analysis of the vitamin D family of compounds, which has also been beneficial to analytical chemists in the pharmaceutical and food industries.

1.1   Basic Formulas

Vitamin D and its metabolites are a group of 9,10-seco-steroids with the basic structure shown in Fig. 1. The A ring of the steroid nucleus is rotated about the C6 position. The conjugated *cis*-triene system gives rise to the characteristic UV-absorption spectrum of vitamin D (molar extinction coefficient = 18,300; λ_{max} = 264 nm; λ_{min} = 228 nm). The D_3 series has a side chain derived from cholesterol; the D_2 series has a side chain derived from ergosterol containing an additional C22(23) double bond and a C24 methyl group.

1.2   Chemistry

Vitamin D_2 and vitamin D_3 are derived by photoirradiation from their respective 5,7-diene sterol precursors: 7-dehydrocholesterol or ergosterol. The intact sterol precursor, known as a provitamin, undergoes photolysis when exposed to UV light of wavelength 280–320 nm to yield a variety of photoirradiation products, the principal ones being pre-vitamin D, tachysterol, and lumisterol, the structures of which are illustrated in Fig. 2. The previtamin D undergoes spontaneous thermal rearrangements to

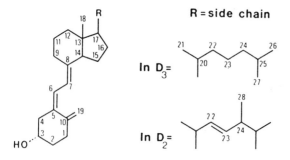

Figure 1   Basic formula of vitamin D compounds.

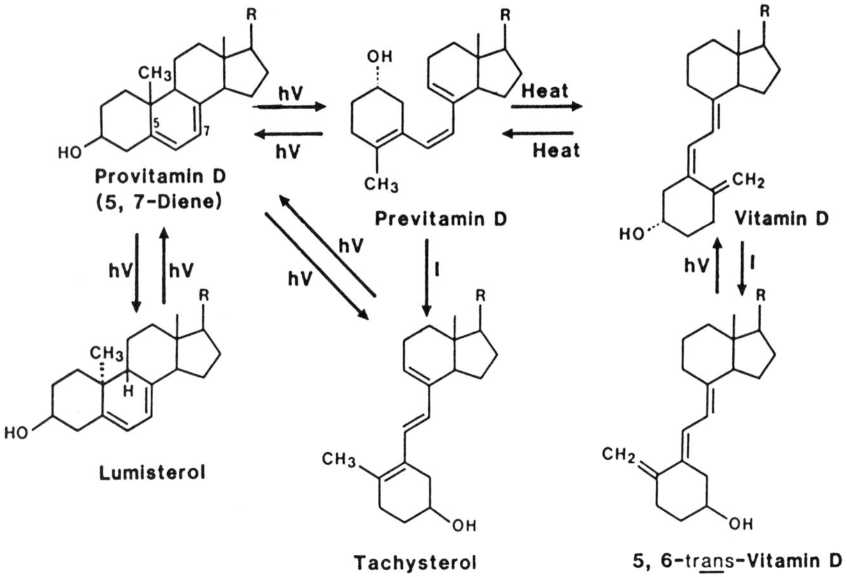

Figure 2 Irradiation products of provitamin D.

vitamin D (7). Vitamin D has a number of other closely related isomers and derivatives that have little biological activity but can be formed during synthesis, derivatization, or handling.

The isolation and identification of the metabolites of vitamin D have been followed by a keen interest in the chemical synthesis of the D vitamins. Clinical use of these new compounds has led to more efficient synthesis (8). A popular approach to the synthesis of vitamin D metabolites, involves the preparation of a suitably hydroxylated or substituted provitamin, conversion of this to the equivalent previtamin, followed by thermal isomerization to the vitamin D, but other more sophisticated procedures have been used where the molecule is synthesized in two halves (9–12). Besides the natural hydroxylated metabolites described below, chemists have synthesized a series of fluorinated vitamin D compounds [e.g., 24-difluoro-25-OH-D_3 (10) and 26,26,26,27,27,27-hexafluoro-1, 25-$(OH)_2$-D_3 (11)], a series of vitamin D analogs containing a 25,26,27-cyclopropane ring [e.g., MC969 (12):1α-OH-D_3 with a C25,26,27 ring], and a series of side-chain oxa-compounds [e.g., 22-oxa-1,25-$(OH)_2$-D_3] where specific carbon atoms of the side chain are replaced by an oxygen atom. A further series of compounds arises from modification of the A-ring by reduction of the irradiation intermediate, tachysterol, to give dihydrotachysterol (with a 19-methyl group and a 180° rotated A-ring).

Many of these drugs are now in clinical trial because of their potential therapeutic use in hypocalcemia, malignancies, and psoriasis.

1.3 Biochemistry

Vitamin D_3 is synthesized in the skin from 7-dehydrocholesterol by a process closely resembling the photochemical process in the test tube (13). Previtamin D_3 made by UV light exposure undergoes thermal isomerization to vitamin D_3, which is selectively removed by the vitamin D-binding globulin (DBP) of the blood (13). Alternatively, preformed vitamin D_3 or D_2 in the diet is absorbed from the intestine into lymph, enters the circulation, and is rapidly taken up by the liver (14). Vitamin D_3 is converted in the liver to 25-OH-D_3 (1) (see Fig. 3). Two enzymes are present in the liver to carry out 25-hydroxylation and are located in the endoplasmic reticulum and mitochondrion, respectively (14a,15). The former appears to be the specific 25-hydroxylase enzyme with an apparent K_m for 25-OH-D_3 of $5.6 \times 10^{-8}M$ (16), a limited binding capacity, and tight regulation (15). The mitochondrial enzyme, on the other hand, appears to be nonspecific and unregulated but with a high

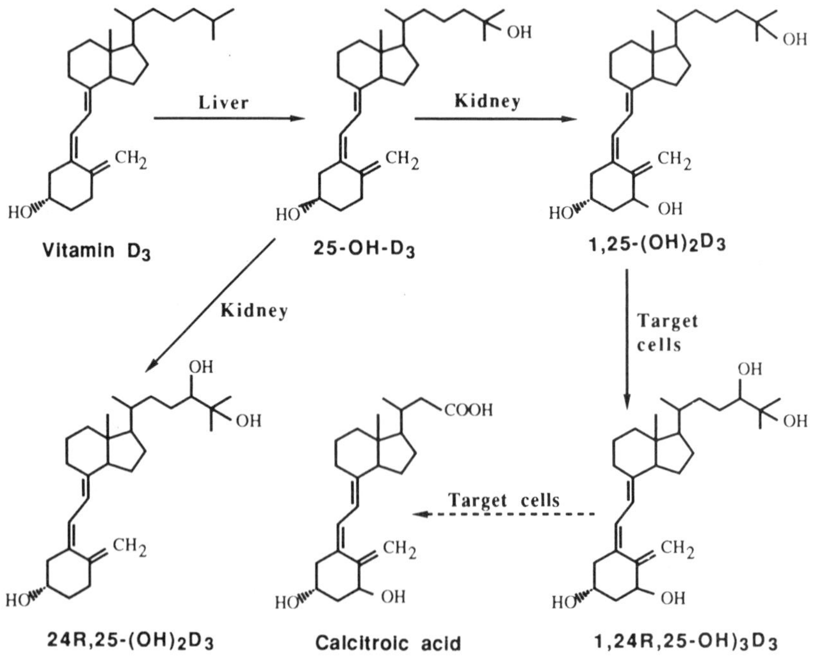

Figure 3 Metabolism of vitamin D_3.

capacity (16), perhaps utilizing bile acid precursors as its normal substrate (17). In vivo regulation of the level of 25-OH-D_3 is thus incomplete and 25-OH-D_3 is the circulating vitamin D metabolite in highest concentration.

25-Hydroxyvitamin D_3 is metabolized by the kidney (see Fig. 3) into a series of dihydroxylated compounds, the important ones being $1\alpha,25$-dihydroxyvitamin D_3 [$1\alpha,25$-$(OH)_2$-D_3] (18,19) and $24R,25$-dihydroxyvitamin D_3 [24 (R), 25-$(OH)_2$-D_3] (20,21). $1\alpha,25$-Dihydroxyvitamin D_3 is believed to be the active form of vitamin D necessary for the repletion of calcium and phosphate homeostasis (2) and is at least 10 times more biologically active in this respect than vitamin D_3. $1\alpha,25$-Dihydroxyvitamin D_3 raises serum calcium and phosphate by stimulating intestinal calcium and phosphate absorption (22–24) and, together with parathyroid hormone (PTH), by stimulating bone resorption (25). It may also play a role in calcium and phosphate reabsorption by the kidney. All of these functions of 1,25-$(OH)_2$-D_3 are mediated by a specific vitamin D receptor protein (VDR) (3), which interacts directly with vitamin D-responsive genes at a transcriptional level. Recent work by Suda's group (26–28) suggests that 1,25-$(OH)_2$-D_3 may play an additional receptor-mediated role in bone cell differentation by inducing maturation of monocyte-like cells into preosteoclasts and stimulating fusion of preosteoclasts to produce multinucleated cells, bone-resorbing osteoclasts. Since $1\alpha,25$-$(OH)_2$-D_3 is such a potent hormone, it is not surprising to find that its synthesis is tightly controlled. The kidney 1-hydroxylase (29) is stimulated by low concentrations of calcium (30), phosphate (31), or parathyroid hormone (32) and inhibited by $1\alpha,25$-$(OH)_2$-D_3 (33). Thus, the circulating level of $1\alpha,25$-$(OH)_2$-D_3 in the plasma rarely exceeds 100 pg/ml in any mammalian species (3). The synthesis of $24(R),25$-$(OH)_2$-D_3 is a detoxication pathway of vitamin D_3 (2,3). The synthesis of $24(R),25$-$(OH)_2$-D_3 is stimulated by $1\alpha,25$-$(OH)_2$-D_3 administration (34), and $24(R),25$-$(OH)_2$-D_3 is the major dihydroxylated metabolite in the plasma of normocalcemic mammals. A role for $24(R),25$-$(OH)_2$-D_3 in the bone mineralization has been suggested by some authors (35,36), but is now largely discredited (37). The metabolism of vitamin D_2 in general parallels that of vitamin D_3 in most mammalian species with the synthesis of 25-OH-D_2 (38), 1,25-$(OH)_2$-D_2 (39) (Fig. 4), and $24(R),25$-$(OH)_2$-D_2 (40), although there may be quantitative differences in 25-hydroxylation (41,42). In addition, a "unique" metabolite of vitamin D_2, $24,26$-$(OH)_2$-D_2, has been described (43).

1,24(R),25-Trihydroxyvitamin D_3 was originally isolated as the product of the administration of $1\alpha,25$-$(OH)_2$-D_3 to a normocalcemic animal (44). More recently it has been recognized as the initial product of a catabolic pathway commonly referred to as 24-oxidation, present in a

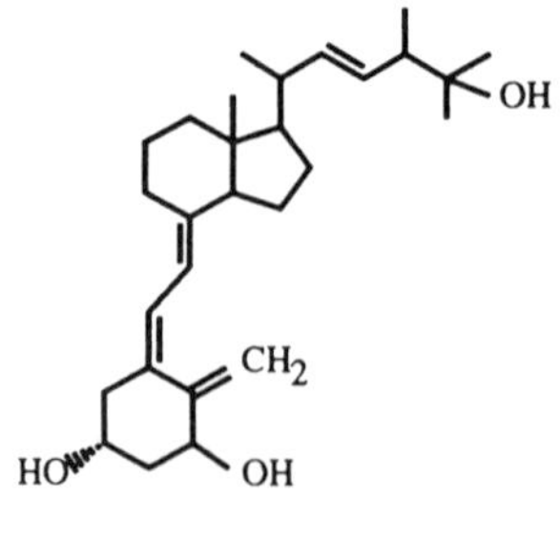

1,25-(OH)₂D₂   **25S,26-(OH)₂D₃**

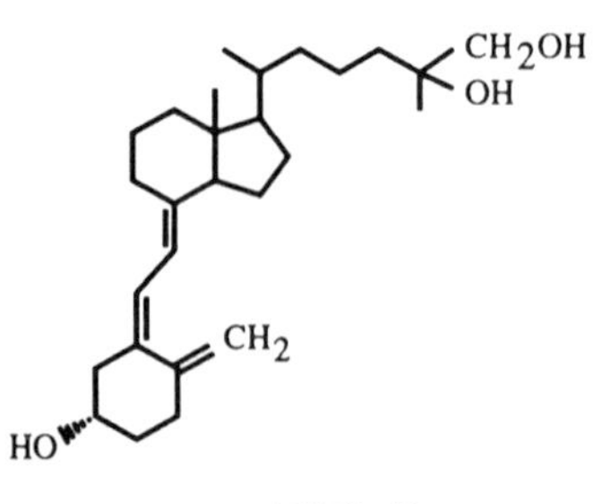

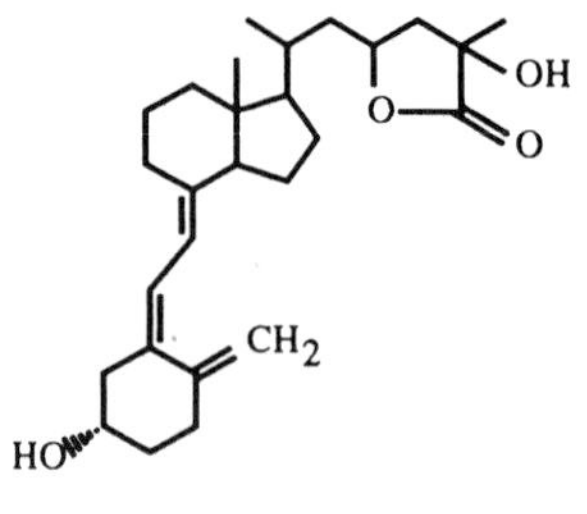

25-OH-D₃-26,23-lactone 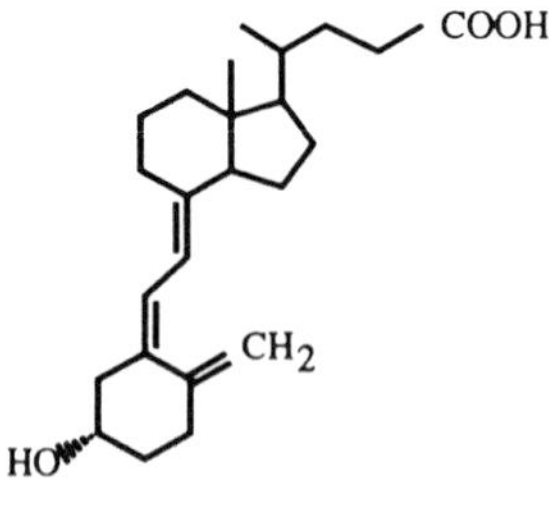   **Cholecalcioic acid**

Figure 4   Other biological metabolites of vitamin D₃.

variety of 1,25-(OH)₂-D₃ target cells (45–47). The enzymes in this pathway are induced by 1,25-(OH)₂-D₃ and seem tightly coupled to vitamin
D receptor occupation. 1α,25-(OH)₂-D₃ is 24-hydroxylated to give
1,24(R),25-(OH)₃-D₃ and then is 24-oxidized and 23-hydroxylated
before it undergoes side-chain cleavage (48) to calcitroic acid (49) (Fig.
3). 24(R),25-(OH)₂-D₃ is probably converted to cholecalcioic acid (50)
(Fig. 4). The kidney is the likely site of the formation of two other vitamin D metabolites, 25-OH-D₃-26,23-lactone (51) and 25(S),26-
(OH)₂-D₃ (52), shown in Fig. 4.

Many other minor metabolites are being reported, but little is known
beyond their structure. These include 1,25(S),26-(OH)₃-D₃, 1α,25-
(OH)₂-D₃-26-lactone, 24-OH-D₂, 25, 26-(OH)₂-D₂, vitamin D₃ sulfate,
and 5,6-trans-25-OH-D₃ (53–58).

1.4   Application

The analysis of vitamin D and its metabolites is worthy of attention for
many reasons. The measurement of the level of vitamin D metabolites

provides important knowledge about the etiology, pathogenesis, and treatment of diseases involving disturbances of calcium and phosphorus metabolism. The analysis of vitamin D compounds in drug formulations, such as multivitamin tablets, injectable solutions, and new metabolite preparations, is required to ensure the purity, stability, and potency of the compounds.

There is at present tremendous interest in elucidating the full details of the metabolism and mode of action of vitamin D. The need for unequivocal identification of increasing numbers of metabolites in animal studies in vivo and in vitro is placing increased demands on the resolving capabilities of modern chromatographic techniques and the sensitivity of detection and measurement.

Part of the interest in the study of the vitamin D stems from the availability of pure radioisotope-labeled derivatives of vitamin D and its metabolites and chemically synthesized metabolites. Present techniques of quality control can accurately determine purity and specific activity in radioactively labeled vitamin D, and chemical synthesis has been greatly aided by chromatographic techniques able to resolve stereoisomers.

Last but not least, the food industry has now introduced liquid chromatographic (LC) and gas chromatographic-mass spectrometry (GC-MS) methods for vitamin D analysis of the traditional vitamin D-supplemented human foods. Infant milk formulas and margarine provide the analyst with the task of measuring nanogram quantities of vitamin D in a matrix containing milligram or gram quantities of fat. Animal feeds also contain added vitamin D. It is likely that if vitamin D metabolites are used in the beef and dairy science industry on any major scale, there will be a need for accurate methods for the analysis of vitamin D and its metabolites in tissues and milk.

Attempts will be made in this chapter to describe examples of the methods used to solve the many problems of analysis of vitamin D and its metabolites.

2. LIQUID CHROMATOGRAPHIC ANALYSIS

2.1 Preparation of Samples

The need for sample preparation, extraction, concentration, and partial purification prior to final analysis naturally depends upon the nature of the sample matrix and the methods of quantitation used. Minimal prepurification is required for concentrated samples of synthetic vitamin D compounds during chemical synthesis. At the other extreme, the analysis of vitamins D_2 and D_3 in foodstuffs involves saponification, extraction, and concentration prior to quantitation. The analysis of trace quantities of vitamin D metabolites, such as $1,25\text{-}(OH)_2\text{-}D_3$, in human plasma requires the extraction of picogram quantities, purification by column chromatography, and finally, radioligand assay. Much attention has been paid to sample preparation, as a significant reduction in analysis time can be achieved by optimizing purification procedures.

Saponification

Where samples contain significant quantities of lipid, such as in the analysis of such foodstuffs as infant formulas, fortified milk, and margarine, a saponification step using ethanolic KOH is usually included to eliminate the bulk of the neutral lipid (e.g., triglyceride and phospholipid) prior to extraction. A typical saponification will include equal volumes of a foodstuff and a solution of 5M ethanolic KOH. The saponification takes place in a closed vessel at 60°C for 20 min after which the solution is cooled and extracted with hexane. It is very important to note that an internal standard or radiolabeled tracer should be added to the solution prior to saponification to correct for losses of endogenous compound that occur throughout the quantitation processes. There is also the possibility that conjugates or esters of vitamin D might be released by saponification.

Extraction

Since vitamin D and its metabolites are fat-soluble sterols, partition into organic solvents provides significant purification by removal of water-soluble contaminants. Solvent systems for extraction fall into two basic categories (Table 1).

Table 1 Extraction Procedures for Vitamin D Compounds

Solvent	Metabolite	Reference
Methanol-chloroform (2:1)	General	59
Methanol-methylene chloride (2:1)	General	60
Ethyl acetate-cyclohexane (1:1)	General	61
Hexane-isopropanol (1:2)	General	62
Ethanol	D, 25-OH-D	63
Hexane (after saponification)	D	64
Ether	25-OH-D	65
Methanol:water (Sep-Pak)	25-OH-D	66
Dichloromethane	$24,25\text{-}(OH)_2\text{-}D_3$ $1,25\text{-}(OH)_2\text{-}D_3$	67
Dichloromethane on Extrelut	$24,25\text{-}(OH)_2\text{-}D_3$ $1,25\text{-}(OH)_2\text{-}D_3$	68

1. Total lipid extraction, for example, methanol-chloroform-water (2:1:0.8) (59) or ethanol-water (9:1) (69).
2. Selective lipid extraction, for example, ether, ethylacetate-cyclohexane (1:1), hexane, dichloromethane, or hexane-isopropanol (1:2).

Clearly, though solvents in the second class are desirable to minimize contamination of vitamin D extracts, they pose problems in that they tend to provide efficient extraction for one particular metabolite or group of metabolites (e.g., the dihydroxylated metabolites) and poorly extract those of a different polarity. When simultaneous analysis of several vitamin D metabolites with a wide range of polarities is required, a total lipid extraction (59) may be necessary.

The high efficiency of the Bligh and Dyer technique (59) for total lipid extraction (i.e., methanol:chloroform 12:1, v/v) is probably due to the formation of a monophasic dispersion of sample in extracting solvent, followed by return to the classic two-phase system by addition of extra chloroform and saturated KCl. All hydroxylated nonacidic vitamin D metabolites can be extracted quantitatively by this technique. Substitution of methylene chloride for chloroform avoids the known carcinogenicity of chloroform and reduces evaporation times by taking advantage of the lower boiling point of methylene chloride. The use of ethanol is a rapid method for precipitation of protein and extraction of vitamin D metabolites but becomes increasingly impractical as sample volumes exceed 1 ml.

Two-phase liquid-liquid extraction of samples is the preferred choice of sample preparation in the majority of applications. Vitamin D and its photoisomers are relatively nonpolar and can be extracted with hexane or other low-polarity solvents, providing the matrix is broken down by saponification, etc. Acid hydrolysis must be avoided due to the tendency to dehydrate the 1-hydroxyl and to give rise to isomerization. In the biochemical areas of analysis, all types of saponification are avoided, chiefly because of concern about the stability of vitamin D metabolites but also because of lack of convenience. More polar solvents, such as modified hexane mixtures, cyclohexane-ethyl acetate (1:1) (61), hexane-isopropanol (1:2) (62), or hexane-isopropanol-n-butanol (93:3:4) (70), are employed for the extraction of metabolites of vitamin D and to break protein-bound vitamin D complexes. Horst et al. (56) use ether followed by methanol-methylene chloride (1:3) in a lengthy but ingenious attempt to analyze a series of vitamin D_2 and D_3 metabolites simultaneously. Care must be taken when using ether, since this solvent may contain peroxides that can react with the cis-triene of vitamin D.

Methylene chloride is frequently used for the extraction of 24(R),25-$(OH)_2$-D_3 and 1,25-$(OH)_2$-D_3 from plasma. Though the use of methylene chloride was originally as a two-phase system with plasma

(67), one modification is to adsorb the plasma onto Kieselguhr packed in a column (commercial version, Extrelut, Merck, Darmstadt, West Germany) and elute by passing methylene chloride through the column (68). A total of 80–90% extraction of both dihydroxylated metabolites is obtained, and the amount of lipid extracted is so small as to make additional cleanup steps unnecessary.

An additional postextraction prechromatographic step that can be used is to backwash the extract with a low-ionic-strength, weakly basic (ph 9–10) buffer, such as phosphate. This tends to remove any acidic lipid components poorly ionized at neutral pH levels.

Minicolumns and Prepacked Cartridges

The use of an inexpensive, disposable, gravity-flow minicolumn as a penultimate step prior to LC serves several useful purposes.

1. It protects the expensive LC column from lipid, particulate matter, etc.
2. It eliminates remaining neutral and highly polar lipid contaminants, further reducing the lipid load applied to the LC.
3. It can be used to fractionate the vitamin D metabolites into major classes for subsequent analysis using different solvent systems.
4. It can serve as a support for solid-phase extractions.

    Minicolumns have disadvantages, too.

1. Batch-to-batch and manufacturer-to-manufacturer variability, requiring frequent calibration checks.
2. The minicolumn sometimes provides unwanted resolution of D_2 and D_3 metabolites, particularly when using Sephadex-LH 20 and hydroxyalkoxypropyl Sephadex (HAPS), giving misleading results when using radioactive vitamin D metabolites as internal standards, unless larger fractions are collected to include both D_2 and D_3 metabolites.
3. Losses can occur without achieving any substantial purification of the sample.
4. Adsorbants used in the minicolumns can be dirty and introduce interference into subsequent analyses.

It is fair to say that many of these disadvantages of minicolumns have been overcome with the introduction of prepacked cartridges, particularly those based upon the syringe-type minicolumn. On balance then, the advantages of such cartridges outweigh the disadvantages and their introduction has revolutionized sample preparation, streamlining the procedures greatly and in some clinical assays eliminating the need for HPLC altogether (71). Cartridges have largely replaced the use of liquid-liquid extraction since they can act as a solid-phase extraction surface in the same way that Extrelut was used a decade ago. Cartridges can also be used as a separation tool to resolve vitamin D and its metabolites. Cartridges can be used for a combination of solid-phase extraction and separation procedures (72).

Cartridges are now available in a number of different chemistries ranging from straight-phase packings such as silica to exotic bonded-phase packings (e.g., C_{18} or octadecasilane). An increasing number of different packing materials is becoming available from the manufacturers (Analytchem and Waters), but the full use of these different packings has yet to be fully realized in the vitamin D field. Present-day procedures focus mainly on use of silica and C_{18} packings.

SILICIC ACID.   This material has been used for some time to resolve vitamin D and 25-OH-D fractions (63,65), and it has been incorporated into a method for LC assay of 25-OH-D (73,74). Recoveries with silicic acid can be low, and care must be taken to select the appropriate particle size to permit adquate flow and good performance. Koshy (75) recommends use of columns containing 2 g silica gel 60 (230–400 mesh, E. Merck, Darmstadt, West Germany). 25-Hydroxy-vitamin D can be eluted with ether-ethyl acetate (9:1).

Sep-Pak SIL cartridges (Waters Associates, Milford, MA) use high-efficiency silica particles and offer minimal variability. These cartridges have been used by Hollis and colleagues (76) to demonstrate the lack of vitamin D sulfate in human milk and by Adams et al. (77) to fractionate classes of vitamin D metabolites in human plasma. Evaluations of the use of Sep-Pak SIL as a means of preliminary fractionating vitamin D and its metabolites have been published (77,78). Hollis et al. (76) demonstrated the use of these cartridges for the rapid separation of vitamin D and vitamin D sulfate. The plastic coating of the Sep-Pak is made of virgin polyethylene with minimal or zero amounts of plasticizers. Early versions of the Sep-Pak SIL were not completely devoid of UV-absorbing impurities, and as a result numerous interfering peaks were introduced into the sample during "purification." Leaching may still occur from Sep-Paks with chlorinated hydrocarbons. Bond-Elut cartridges, on the other hand, are encased in surgical-grade polypropylene and leaching of plastics into the solvents has not been a problem. This issue becomes of great importance when using subsequent sensitive analytical techniques such as HPLC or GC-MS.

In our hands, the separation of vitamin D metabolites on a Waters silica Sep-Pak cartridge is inferior to that achieved using the higher-quality microsilica supplied by Analytichem International as Bond-Elut cartridges (Fig. 5).

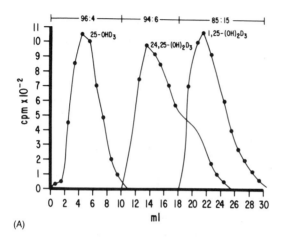

(A)

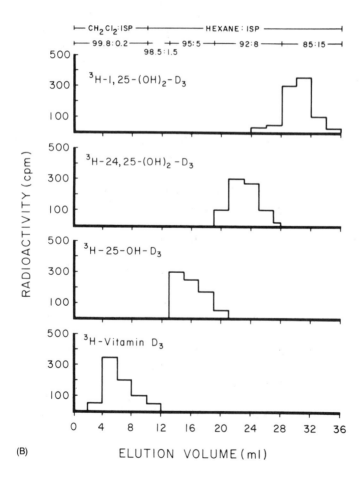

(B)   ELUTION VOLUME (ml)

C_{18} OR ODS-BONDED SILICA CARTRIDGES. Sep-Pak C_{18} is the reverse-phase analog of the silica cartridge and uses a bonded octadecasilane (C18) phase. It can also be used to fractionate plasma in the reverse manner to that described by Adams et al. (77). Dabek et al. (66), Turnbull et al. (80), and Fraher et al. (81) have developed methods for 25-OH-D_2 and 25-OH-D_3 using Sep-Pak C18 for both extraction (80,81) and preliminary purification (66) of the sample. The method of Dabek et al. (66) utilizes the properties of methanol as both an extraction solvent and as a mobile phase. However, these procedures did not extract the parent compound, vitamin D. Hollis and Frank (79) have recently described a technique that does remove vitamin D from serum or plasma using a modified solid-phase extraction technique.

Further investigation into the utility of ODS-bonded silica cartridges has led to a procedure that has been described as "phase-switching" (72). This procedure uses a concept by which solid-phase extraction and subsequent normal-phase separation of vitamin D metabolites can be performed on a single cartridge. This study by Hollis (72) demonstrated that the type of ODS-microsilica packing used greatly affects the resolution one achieves with respect to metabolites of vitamin D. This concept is displayed in Fig. 6. Using a fully end-capped ODS-silica cartridge results in little resolution between 24,25-$(OH)_2$-D_3 and 1,25$(OH)_2$-D_3 (Fig. 6A). However, using a partially end-capped ODS-silica material (ODS-OH) excellent resolution is achieved between these two important vitamin D_3 metabolites (Fig. 6B) (82), but it will be noted that using ODS-OH cartridges the resolution previously achieved between 25-OH-D_3 and 24,25-$(OH)_2$-D_3 is lost. However such a system has proved very useful in the purification of 1,25-$(OH)_2$-D_3 prior to radioligand assay (71) and is now available as part of a commercial assay (Incstar Corporation, Stillwater, MN). Other reverse-phase type silica cartridges ($-NO_2$) have been used to separate 25-OH-D_3 and 1,25-$(OH)_2$-D_3 (83).

SEPHADEX-LH20 (PHARMACIA, UPPSALA, SWEDEN). This gel was first used with the solvent systems hexane-chloroform (50:50-35:65) (84) for vitamin D and its metabolites. In fact, without Sephadex-LH 20,

Figure 5   Elution profiles of radiolabeled vitamin D_3 and its metabolites, (A) on silica SEP-PAK cartridges: the column was developed in 10ml hexane:isopropanol (96:4), which elutes 25-OH-D, followed by an 8-ml wash with hexane:isopropanol (94:6), which elutes the majority of 24,25-$(OH)_2$-D. Finally the 1,25-$(OH)_2$-D was eluted with 10 ml hexane:isopropanol (85:15) (from Ref. 71). (B) On a silica BOND-ELUT cartridge: each bar represents the amount of radioactivity in 2 ml of eluent during batch elution with various mixtures of isopropanol in methylene chloride or hexane (from Ref. 79).

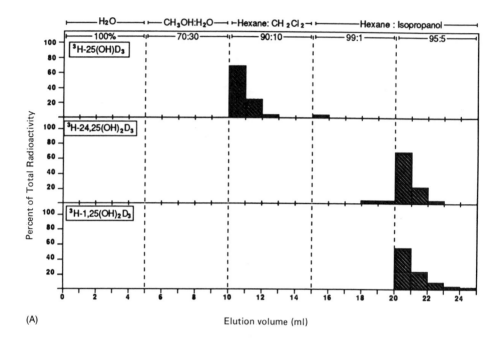

(A)   Elution volume (ml)

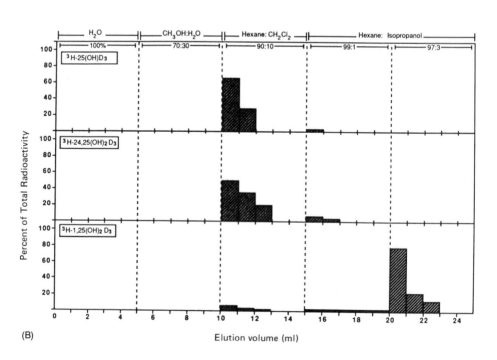

(B)   Elution volume (ml)

it is doubtful if the early metabolites would have been purified sufficiently for MS identification. Later solvent systems based upon hexane-methanol-chloroform (9:1:1) gave much sharper peaks and permitted reduction of column size to 15 × 0.6 cm bed dimension (67). A sample elution pattern for vitamin D metabolites in plasma is shown in Fig. 7 (56). Sephadex-LH 20, although widely used for preliminary purification of the hydroxylated metabolites of vitamin D, provides poor resolution of vitamin D and neutral lipid and is rarely used for analysis of vitamin D itself.

HYDROXYALKOXYPROPYL SEPHADEX-LH 20. Coupling of a C11-C14 or C15-C18 chain in the form of an olefin epoxide (Nedox 114 or 1518, Ashland Chemical Co., Peoria, IL) to Sephadex-LH 20 generates a gel, HAPS, that is far less polar than its precursor (85). This permits the use of solvents such as hexane, which swells the gel and increases the retention of nonpolar vitamin D metabolites, such as vitamin D itself and its photoisomers (39). Thompson et al. (86) used HAPS instead of alumina to purify vitamin D from unsaponifiable material of milk samples. HAPS is now commercially available under the name of Lipidex 5000 and has been used in place of LH20. Both Shepard et al. (87) and Horst et al. (56) have incorporated it into their schemes for simultaneous vitamin D metabolite assay. Jones et al. (39) used the solvent hexane-chloroform (95:5) to separate vitamin D_2 from its photoisomers on a HAPS column.

ALUMINA. This adsorbent is particularly suitable for the purification of vitamin D from the unsaponifiable lipid milk, margarine, and infant formulas.

TLC. This technique is mainly used for prepurification of saponified samples for gas-liquid chromatography (GLC) and has been used for the separation of vitamin D from cholesterol (88) and in combination with GLC for the estimation of 25-OH-D_3 in chick plasma (88). Care must be taken to avoid oxidation of vitamins on the TLC place during drying of the applied sample and during removal of the plate from the tank. Such oxidation can be minimized by running plates at $0°C$ in the atmosphere of nitrogen, in a similar fashion to the TLC procedure used for the removal of cholesterol prior to GC-MS (89). Thin-layer chromatography (TLC) is relatively inexpensive and yet offers high resolution and has the advantage that many samples can be purified using one TLC run. It is also valuable for use in countries where HPLC may not yet be readily available (90). Vieth et al. (91) used TLC to separate tritiated products

---

Figure 6 Elution of radiolabeled vitamin D_3 metabolites from (A) an ODS-BOND-ELUT cartridge and (B) an ODS-BOND-ELUT-OH cartridge (from Refs. 72 and 82).

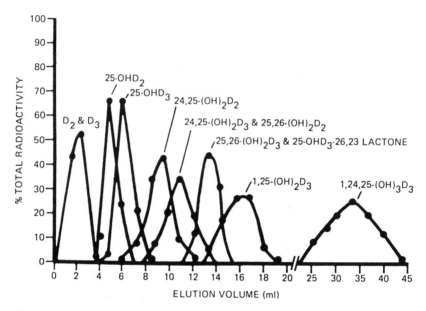

Figure 7 Elution pattern of vitamin D metabolites on a 0.6 × 15.5 cm
Sephadex-LH 20 column developed with hexane-chloroform-methanol (9:1:1).
(From Ref. 56.)

in biochemical studies of renal 25-OH-D hydroxylases. Several methods
for the measurement of vitamin D_3 and 25-OH-D_3 using mass spectrometry utilize TLC as a prepurification step sometimes after derivatisation (e.g., 89, 92, & 93). High-performance (HP) TLC has been described (94) for the separation of vitamin D metabolites using microparticulate silica in the stationary phase with a chloroform:ethyl acetate solvent.

Other Procedures

Estradiol has been extracted from human plasma prior to mass fragmentography (95) by the use of an affinity column where a specific antigen to
the compound of interest is covalently bound to the column support
material (Sepharose). The analyte binds to the antigen, and after washing the column the analyte can be removed from the column. It should
be possible to carry out a similar procedure by adding antigen bound to,
for example, magnetic particles, which could then be removed, washed,
and the analyte recovered. Unfortunately, antigens with high specific
affinity for vitamin D metabolites are not readily available. However,
such a procedure has been used for the isolation of vitamin D binding
protein from plasma (96).

Since vitamin D metabolites are bound to vitamin D binding protein (DBP), isolation of this protein from plasma could also be used as a method of extracting vitamin D metabolites as well. Indeed, precipitation of DBP from plasma with ammonium sulfate, centrifugation, and the examination of the washed pellet gave a recovery of $1,25\text{-}(OH)_2\text{-}D_3$ of 72% (97).

One of the most common problems with LC is the presence of particulate matter in the samples for injection. Unchecked, this ultimately leads to clogging of the injector or, worse, the inlet frit of the column. Changing the inlet frit of the column is a procedure to be avoided by the inexperienced chromatographer if at all possible, since, unless great care is taken, disturbance of the bed may occur, in which case column efficiency may be reduced. Thus, filtering of samples prior to injection is recommended. Such a procedure is described by Jones (98). Use of a relatively inexpensive guard column may also give greater protection to the main analytical column. Waters Associates (Milford, MA) markets a syringe fitted with a Swinney filter holder containing a Millipore 0.45-μm Teflon filter (called an organic sample clarification kit) but its use may lead to losses. Alternatively, samples for LC analysis can be transferred to a 5-ml conical screw-capped vial (Reactivial; Pierce Chemical Co., Rockford, IL) and centrifuged at low speed (around $500 \times$ g for 5 min), although this is not always a completely satisfactory procedure.

It is our experience that the principal determinant of the lifetime of an LC column used in the assay of plasma and kidney perfusate samples is not the lipid content of the sample but the mechanical and physical abuse the column takes. Thus, specific columns will withstand heavy lipid loads very well without major diminution in column efficiency provided the adsorbed lipids can subsequently be eluted. Columns that permit washing with highly polar solvents such as methanol, water, and even 0.1 N nitric acid (Zorbax-SIL, Dupont Instruments, Wilmington, DE) allow their use as preparative columns (without sample cleanup) prior to LC analysis on a second LC system (98). Washing the column at the end of each day of analysis is sufficient. Jones (98) used silica adsorption LC followed by reverse-phase LC on octadescasilane-bonded phase (Fig. 8). A similar technique, but reversing the order of the LC columns, C18-LC followed by silica LC, has been used successfully by Okano and colleagues (99). The use of reverse-phase Sep-Pak C18 cartridges followed by straight-phase LC on Zorbax-SIL (80) is a similar approach. The main advantage is the use of the resolving power of both types of LC (straight-phase and reverse-phase). Clearly, this is advantageous over a combination of open column and one LC step. It also permits greater automation of LC and overcomes the disadvantages of minicolumns

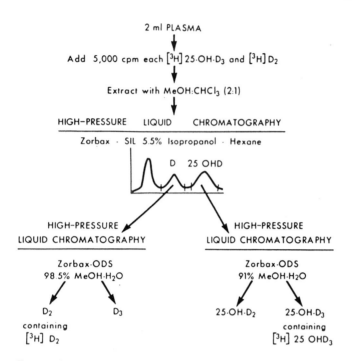

Figure 8 Scheme for the analysis of vitamins D_2 and D_3 and 25-OH-D_2 and 25-OH-D_3 in human plasma by LC with UV detection. (From Ref. 98, ©1978, Clinical Chemistry.)

alluded to in section 2.3 above. The disadvantages are the need for expensive instrumentation, that samples are run serially rather than in parallel, and that the LC column needs frequent washes. An alternative procedure (100) for plasma 25-OH-D used two separate straight-phase Zorbax-SIL columns but interpolated a simple specific chemical reaction [formation of isotachysterol isomers (101)] between the two LC separations.

2.2 Liquid Chromatography

General Considerations

LC analysis of vitamin D has only become practically feasible over the last 15 years with tremendous improvements in LC instrumentation. Major advances in detector sensitivity and column particle technology have made possible the detection of as little as 1 ng vitamin D under ideal conditions. Extra column peak broadening has been minimized by the design of eddy-free flow connectors and injectors and use of minimum dead-space tubing. The objective of all good LC analyses is to maximize resolution R, which is defined by the equation

$$R = \frac{1}{4} \underbrace{\left(\frac{\alpha - 1}{\alpha} \right)}_{\text{Selectivity}} \underbrace{\left(\sqrt{N} \right)}_{\text{Plates}} \underbrace{\left(\frac{k'}{1 + k'} \right)}_{\text{Retention}}$$

The value of N is determined by the size and nature of the particles used to make the column and by the quality of the packing procedure. Most vitamin D applications utilize particles in the 3–10 μm size range, and values of N in excess of 10,000 per column should be expected. The selectivity factor (α) and capacity factor (k') can be altered by changing the chemical characteristics and the strength of the solvent, respectively. Examples of the effect of increasing R by changing either α or k' are given below.

The nature of the type of analysis to be carried out and the design of the LC system may be important considerations in the selection of the type and size of the column to be used, since they may influence N. Some practical rules or considerations are given:

1. Use a column size appropriate to the volume of the injection, weight of solute, etc.
2. Use small-volume injections since these are theoretically best for sharp peaks (i.e., large N). However, practical considerations of sample handling may dictate a compromise to a larger injection volume.
3. Use mobile phase as the sample solvent to avoid peak artifacts.
4. Standardize injection volumes for more reproducible results, since change in injection volume will influence the retention time and hence peak height-area ratio. If peak areas are used for quantitation instead of peak heights, changes in injection volume have little effect.

Whereas a 25 × 0.21 cm microbore LC column may be ideal for analysis of repeated 2–5 μl injections containing microgram quantities of a synthetic vitamin D metabolite using UV detection, it is not ideal for the analysis of 25-OH-D$_3$ in human plasma. Here the samples may still contain considerable amounts of lipid and a column with excellent loading capacity is the choice. Some of the newer 3–μm particle columns (8 cm × 0.62 cm diameter e.g., Zorbax, Golden Series) are ideal for the HPLC of biological samples since they are very tolerant of large injection volumes (100–200 μl) and large lipid load (i.e., whole extract from 2–5 ml plasma), and yet give minimal sample losses and minimal effects of extracolumn band broadening. In addition, we recommend the use of an automatic injection system (Fig. 9; for example, WISP, Waters Associates, Milford, MA) that has the capability of injecting from minimum volume inserts. The WISP can be programmed to make 200-μl injections from a total volume of 210 μl, thus losing only 5% of the sample (the WISP has a 6-μl dead space). The chromatography of biological extracts also makes it preferable to have a precolumn filter (e.g., Rheodyne Inlet Filter) or a precolumn to protect the inlet end of the LC column, since direct injection of extracts from large volumes of sample increases the likelihood of column contamination. Though these devices help to prolong column life, they can also cause extracolumn band broadening, especially if they are poorly installed or badly packed. Larger columns (25 × 0.62 cm) are less affected by these protective devices. The mobile phase is a rich source of contaminants over the lifetime of a column, and a preinjector filter or precolumn is therefore again recommended for prolonging column life.

Columns and Solvents

SILICA. Several microparticulate (3–6 μm) spherical silicas are now available: Lichrospher, Zorbax-SIL, and Spherisil. The advantage of these packings is that they pack more uniformly than irregularly shaped particles, and have less tendency to settle with time and pressure.

Isopropanol-Hexane Mixtures. These mixtures provide a good solubility for the vitamins D and have been widely applied to the resolution of a variety of compounds ranging in polarity from photoirradiation mixtures of vitamin D to 1,24,25-$(OH)_3$-D_3. Isocratic mixtures of 2.5% isopropanol in hexane separate vitamins D_2 and D_3 from 24-OH-D_2, 24-OH-D_3, 25-OH-D_2, and 25-OH-D_3 (Fig. 10). Isopropanol-hexane (10:90) provides resolution of most of the known vitamin D_3 metabolites (102) in

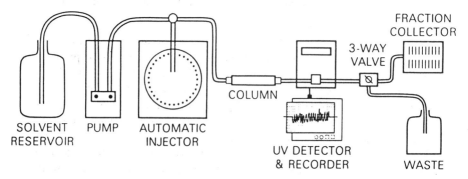

Figure 9 Typical LC apparatus used for the analysis of vitamin D and its metabolites in human plasma. (Modified from Ref. 61).

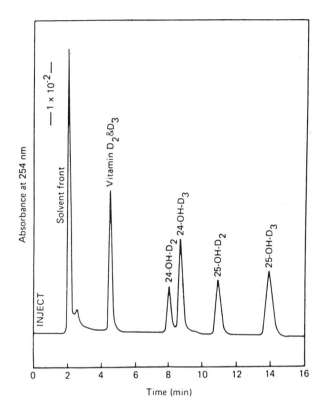

Figure 10 LC separation of vitamin D_2 and D_3, 24-OH-D_2, 24-OH-D_3, 25-OH-D_2, and 25-OH-D_3, using Zorbax-SIL and 2.5% isopropanol in hexane. (From Ref. 102)

a single chromatographic run (Fig. 11), and can also be useful for vitamin D_2 metabolites (Fig. 12). These early separations can now be achieved on a single 25 × 0.46 or 25 × 0.62 cm column using similar solvent systems. The use of ternary solvent systems, incorporating methanol into the standard isopropanol-hexane mixture (103), greatly minimizes peak tailing, particularly of 24(R),25-(OH)$_2$-D_3. Figure 13 shows the results of using a hexane-isopropanol-methanol (87:10:3) system solvent on the separation of 25-OH-D_3, 24(R),25-(OH)$_2$-D_3, and 1,25-(OH)$_2$-D_3. The polarity of the solvent can be reduced while keeping the proportion of isopropanol-methanol approximately the same.

Methanol-Methylene Chloride Mixtures. Ikekawa and Koizumi (104) have described a gradient solvent system of 0.02-6% methanol in methylene chloride to resolve a mixture of dihydroxy metabolites on

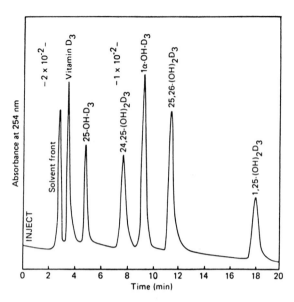

Figure 11 LC separation of vitamin D_3 and its metabolites on Zorbax-SIL using the solvent system 10 % isopropanol in hexane. (From Ref. 102).

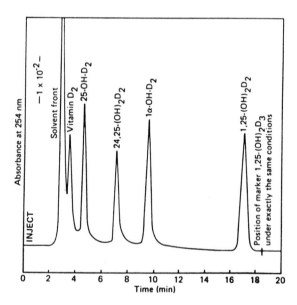

Figure 12 LC separation of vitamin D_2 and its metabolites on Zorbax-SIL using the solvent system 10 % isopropanol in hexane. (From Ref. 102).

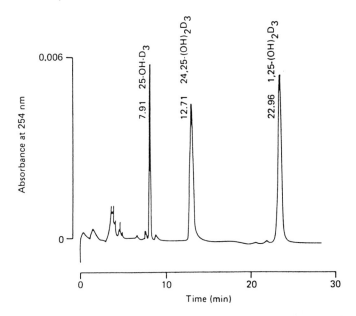

Figure 13 LC separation of 25-OH-D$_3$, 24(R), 25-(OD)$_2$-D$_3$, and 1,25-(OH)$_2$-D$_3$ on Zorbax-SIL (25 cm × 6.2 mm) using the solvent system hexane-isopropanol-methanol (87:10:3). (Redrawn after Ref. 103).

Zorbax-SIL (25 × 0.21 cm) (Fig. 14). This solvent system gives a higher theoretical plate count N than does the isopropanol-hexane-methanol mixture under otherwise identical conditions. However, the low viscosity of methylene chloride-methanol mixtures can lead to bubble problems with some solvent delivery systems. Replacing some of the methylene chloride with hexane and using a hexane-methylene chloride-methanol mixture (90:10:10) overcomes some of the viscosity problems, but poor miscibility and poor sample solubility develop. The hexane-methylene chloride-methanol (90:10:10) mixture beautifully separates D$_2$ and D$_3$ metabolites (Fig. 15), but not D$_2$ and D$_3$ themselves.

Figure 16 illustrates the influence of small changes in solvent composition (α) on the resolution of 1,25-(OH)$_2$-D$_2$ and 1,25-(OH)$_2$-D$_3$ using the same column (Zorbax-SIL, 25 × 0.62 cm) while keeping the retention time approximately the same.

One further solvent system that should be mentioned, which separates 25-OH-D$_3$-26,23-lactone and 24(R),25-(OH)$_2$-D$_3$, is a methylene chloride-isopropanol (96.5:3.5) mixture (105). The lactone

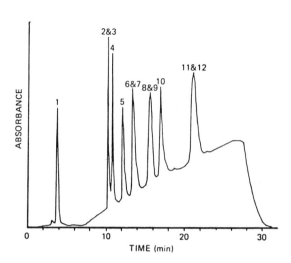

Figure 14 LC separation of vitamin D_3 metabolites on Zorbax-SIL using a gradient of 0.02-6% methanol in methylene chloride. Peaks: (1) vitamin D_3; (2,3) 24(R)-OH-D_3 and 24(S)-OH-D_3; (4) 25-OH-D_3; (5) 1α-OH-D_3; (6,7) 24(R),25-$(OH)_2$-D_3 and 24(S),25-$(OH)_2$-D_3; (8,9) 1α-24(R)-$(OH)_2$-D_3 and 1α,24(S)-$(OH)_2$-D_3; (10) 1α,25-$(OH)_2$-D_3; (11,12) 1α,24(R),25-$(OH)_3$-D_3 and 1α,24(S),25-$(OH)_3$-D_3. (Modified from Ref. 104).

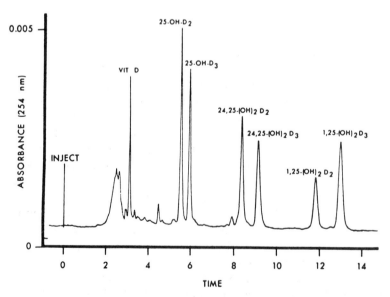

Figure 15 LC separation of vitamin D_2 and D_3 metabolites on Zorbax-SIL using the solvent system hexane-methanol-methylene choride (80:10:10). (From Ref. 103).

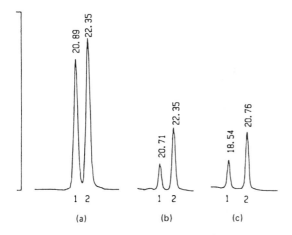

Figure 16   LC separation of $1,25\text{-}(OH)_2\text{-}D_2$ (peak 1) and $1,25\text{-}(OH)_2\text{-}D_3$ (peak 2) on Zorbax-SIL using (a) hexane-isopropanol (85:15); (b) hexane-isopropanol-methanol (87:10:3); and (c) hexane-ethanol-chloroform (80:10:10). Retention times in minutes are shown above peaks. Note the effect of changing solvent selectivity α on resolution. (Modified from Ref. 103).

runs with a retention time almost identical to $24,25\text{-}(OH)_2\text{-}D_3$ with isopropanol-hexane mixtures but elutes with $25\text{-}OH\text{-}D_3$ with a solvent mixture rich in methylene chloride.

OCTADECASILANE (ODS OR C18) BONDED PHASES.   Matthews et al. (106) were first to report LC of vitamin D metabolites using the pellicular packing ODS-Permaphase and a gradient of methanol and water. With the advent of the microparticulate bonded phases, such as μBondapack C18 and Zorbax-ODS, analysts have successfully used reverse-phase LC for many compounds. However, in the vitamin D field, their use has been sparing for all but the separation of vitamins D_2 and D_3 (Fig. 17). Mixtures of methanol-water or acetonitrile-methanol-water (105) are preferred for vitamin D and its metabolites. Acetonitrile greatly reduces the viscosity of the solvent mixture and results in lower back pressures. The limited use of reverse-phase packings stems from the aversion of vitamin D analysts to aqueous mobile phases, particularly when competitive binding assay of collected fractions is used for quantitation, since aqueous phases are difficult to evaporate, tend to dissolve support material, and, since they contain dissolved oxygen, may give rise to oxidation to the 5,7-diene system. Second, the resolution of the dihydroxylated compounds is not as good as that achieved using silica (see Fig. 18). Plate counts on bonded-phase columns are generally lower,

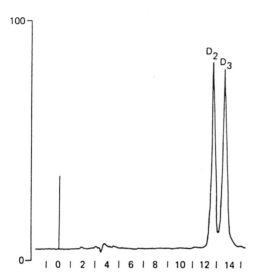

Figure 17   LC separation of vitamins D_2 and D_3 on Zorbax-ODS using the solvent system methanol-water (98.5:1.5). (From G. Jones, unpublished results).

pressures are higher, and column lifetimes are shorter than systems using straight-phase silica LC.

A recent application of ODS-cartridges and HPLC columns is in the purification of calcitroic acid from tissue extracts. Here, the ionization properties of the weak acid group can be minimized and the molecule retarded by its interaction with the C18 hydrophobic surface. An example of such an interaction during sample preparation and quantitation on HPLC has been described (47). Mobile phases for calcitroic acid are rich in water and contain a small percentage of acetic acid or other acid to lower pH (acetonitrile-water-GAA, 40:60:1) (Fig. 19).

CYANO AND OTHER PHASES.   There has been limited use of other packings. Straight-phase bonded packings offer excellent recoveries, but often the solvent strength has to be weakened significantly in comparison to that for silica in order to conserve adequate retention. μBondapak-CN and Zorbax-CN (107) have been used with some success for the separation of hydroxylated metabolites of vitamin D from those containing aldehyde or keto groups. One excellent example of this is the difficult separation of 25-OH-D_3-26,23-lactone and 24,25-(OH)$_2$-D_3 referred to earlier. Zorbax-CN can be used to provide baseline resolution, the 26,23-lactone being strongly retarded by this packing and emerging much after the 24,25-(OH)$_2$-D_3 (108). Contrast this with the other means of resolution: methylene chloride/isopropanol mixtures where the 26,23-lactone comigrates with 25-OH-D_3. The cyano packing has proven to be very useful in the recent identification of several oxo-compounds

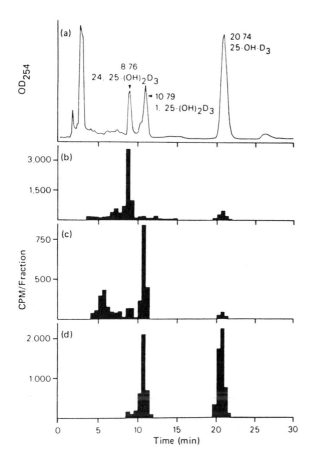

Figure 18 LC separation of in vitro generated metabolites of [^{3}H]-25-OH-D$_3$ on µBondapak-C$_{18}$ using the solvent system methanol-water (85:15). Fetal kidney tissue was homogenized and mitochondria prepared, and these were incubated with [^{3}H]-25-OH-D$_3$ to produce two major metabolites, [^{3}H]-1,25-(OH)$_2$-D$_3$ and [^{3}H]-24,25-(OH)$_2$-D$_3$. The extract was chromatographed initially on Zorbax-SIL, as in Fig. 12 and the metabolite regions isolated and rechromatographed as above. (a) nonradioactive standards; (b) [^{3}H]-24,25-(OH)$_2$-D$_3$ region; (c) [^{3}H]-1,25-(OH)$_2$-D$_3$ region; and (d) radioactive standards. (From M. Rawlins, S. W. Kooh, and G. Jones, unpublished results.)

found on the pathway from 1,25-(OH)$_2$-D$_3$ to calcitroic acid (46), and in the purification of metabolites of 25-hydroxydihydrotachysterol$_3$ (109).

Methods of Detection

ULTRAVIOLET ABSORBANCE (FIXED OR VARIABLE-WAVELENGTH). Variable-wavelength detectors are useful for distinguishing compounds in photoirradiation mixtures, where they take

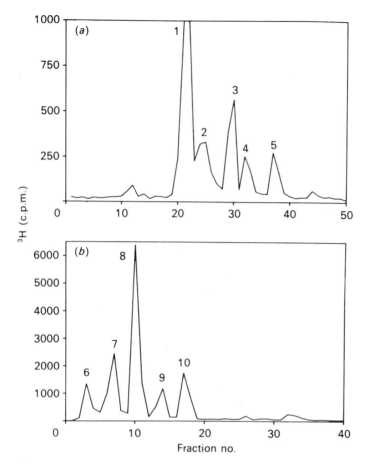

Figure 19 HPLC of extracts of bone cells incubated with [1β-^{3}H]-1,25 (OH)$_2$-D$_3$ (a) Methylene chloride layer on Zorbax-Sil, 3 μm particle size, hexane/propan-2-ol/methanol (91:7:2, by volume), flow rate 2 ml/min. (b) Aqueous layer on Zorbax-ODS, 3μm; acetonitrile/water/glacial acetic acid (40:60:1, by volume), 2 ml/min. Peaks numbers repesent tentative assignment based upon a single HPLC run by comparison with retention time of standards. 1, 1,25-(OH)$_2$-D$_3$; 2, 24-oxo-1,25-(OH)$_2$-D$_3$; 3, tetranor-1,23-(OH)$_2$-D$_3$; 4, 24-oxo-1,23,25-(OH)$_3$-D$_3$; 5, 1,24,25-(OH)$_3$-D$_3$; 6, unknown; 7, unknown; 8, cal-citroic acid; 9, tetranor-1,23-(OH)$_2$-D$_3$; 10, 1,24,25-(OH)$_3$-D$_3$. (From Ref. 47, with permission).

advantage of the differences in the UV spectra of the various photoiso-mers. Normally little is gained in the analysis of vitamin D metabolites, since ϵ254 is 90% of ϵ265 and usually variable-wavelength detectors are noisier at comparable sensitivity than fixed-wavelength detectors due to an inherently weaker lamp intensity. Similarly dihydrotachysterol

($\epsilon251 = 37,00$) metabolites with the 5,7-diene structure are best detected using a fixed wavelength detector because of the closeness of the 254-nm mercury line to the λ_{max}.

However, optimizing UV absorbance is not the only reason to switch detection from 254 to 265 nm. Many sample matrices, whether biological or artificial, contain UV interferences of an aromatic nature absorbing in the 254 nm region, such as ketones and benzene derivatives. Effects of these can be minimized by switching to 265 nm or an even higher wavelength. Unfortunately, estrogens and several other compounds (e.g., peptides and phenolics) often absorb in the 270–290 nm range so that variable-wavelength detectors offer no panacea.

But variable-wavelength detectors can have a considerable value when, for example, isotachysterol derivatives are used for LC, since these isomers at 290 nm give approximately twice the absorbance of unisomerized vitamin D metabolites at 264 nm (110). Isotachysterols have been used to improve the sensitivity and specificity of an LC system for plasma 25-OH-D$_2$ and 25-OH-D$_3$. A simple method for 25-OH-D$_2$ and 25-OH-D$_3$ in plasma has been described using LC of isotachysterols and monitoring at 301 nm, where absorbance of vitamin D metabolites is minimal but where isotachysterols still absorb significantly (80).

DIODE-ARRAY SCANNING SPECTROPHOTOMETRIC DETECTORS. UV detection has been hampered by its lack of specificity. In most cases the major criterion for peak identification has been on the basis of comparison of retention time with known standards. Recently, however, a new type of UV detector has been introduced based upon the diode-array scanning spectrophotometer (111). Such an instrument is able to make repeated 200–400 nm scans of chromatographic effluent passing through the detector flow cell in as little as 100 ms or less. Using a microcomputer and associated data storage devices, vast amounts of chromatographic data can be acquired in a single 20-min chromatographic run. Jones et al. (45) have applied this technique to the separation of vitamin D metabolites in extracts of kidney perfusates. As illustrated in Fig. 20 the diode-array scanning spectrophotometric detector adds another dimension, wavelength, to the conventional absorbance versus time plot. Vitamin D metabolite peaks can be recognized at 590, 700, 870, and 890 s from their $\lambda_{max} = 265$ nm, $\lambda_{min} = 228$ nm properties without the use of known standards. In fact, the technique allowed Jones et al. (45) to recognize the existence of two new metabolites: 24-oxo-23,25-(OH)$_2$-D$_3$ and 24,25,26,27-tetranor-23-(OH)-D$_3$ formed in the perfused kidney in vitro. It should be noted, however, that mass spectrometry and comparison to chemically synthesized material provided the means of identification of the metabolites in these studies (45,112). In

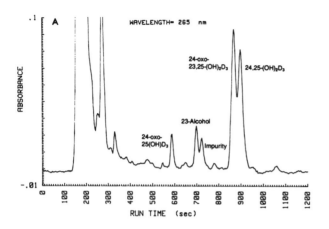

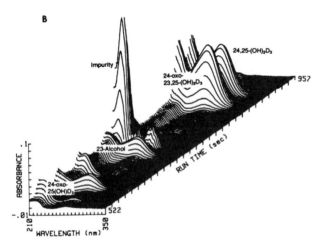

Figure 20 HPLC separation of metabolites of 24,25-$(OH)_2$-D_3 made in the perfused rat kidney. Extract of perfusate from kidneys perfused in the presence of 1250 nM 24,25-$(OH)_2$-D_3. (A) Absorbance at 265 vs. run time. (B) Absorbance vs. wavelength vs. run time. (A) and (B) represent the same chromatographic run. Note in (A) that the peak marked as an impurity appears minor because the wavelength used for monitoring is 265 nm. The impurity peak absorbs strongly at 225 nm and in the 275–280 nm region. Note also that all metabolite peaks have the classical vitamin D absorption spectrum. Conditions: Zorbax-SIL (6.2 mm × 25 cm); hexane-isopropanol-methanol (94/5/1); 1.5 ml/min. (From Ref. 112 with permission).

another example shown in Fig. 21 it has been used to study metabolites of the vitamin D analog, dihydrotachysterol$_3$ (DHT$_3$), generated *in vivo* (109). DHT$_3$ has a characteristic tricusped peak with maxima at 242, 251, and 260 nm, which make its metabolites stand out in the three-

102

dimensional (3-D) profile. Later generations of these detectors (e.g., Waters 990 diode array detector) offer excellent performance even at high sensitivity (0.01 AUFS) due to data bunching, smoothing, and noise reduction software. We have found diode-array detectors to be more than just a pretty picture.

Irrespective of the type of spectral representation we used, 3-D plot or isoabsorbance plot, the scanning spectrophotometry provides valuable information regarding the purity of vitamin D preparations. This is of tremendous value in predicting when, during a metabolite purification scheme, direct probe-MS will be feasible and will not be hampered by impurities.

Diode-array detection may move into the analytical field shortly as its price becomes more competitive. Consider the use of acid (80,101) which converts vitamin D metabolism into the isotachysterol isomer but where the complete spectrum of the isotachysterol isomer is observed. Such a procedure provides a degree of specificity unheard of with single-run HPLC with single-wavelength detection and derivatisation (Fig. 22).

RADIOACTIVITY DETECTOR.   One manufacturer (Berthold, West Germany) has developed an extremely sensitive radioactivity monitor to measure radiolabeled compounds flowing through a flow cell placed between two photomultiplier tubes. Early models were bulky and used a spirally arranged Teflon tube between two plates as the flow cell. A post-LC column mixer was used to mix effluent with scintillation fluid. The mixture flowed through the flow cell, where counting efficiencies for ^3H were high but residence time short. Results are shown in Fig. 23.

Later models (e.g., LB503HS) have reduced lead shielding and use highly sensitive electronics as before. The liquid scintillation fluid and mixer have been replaced by a flow cell of 300 μl volume containing a solid glass scintillator. Adsorption of lipids to the scintillator is minimal, but counting efficiency for ^3H is in the 2–5 % range. Nevertheless, peaks are much sharper than when liquid scintillator is used (Fig. 24). The detector provides excellent online counting efficiencies for $[^{14}C]$-25-OH-D_3 of around 80 % .

OFF-LINE RADIOLIGAND ASSAYS.   One of the most common uses of LC in the analysis of clinical samples, where UV sensitivity is at its limit, is in the preparation of purified extracts containing individual metabolites (or groups of metabolites) for competitive protein-binding assay or radioimmunoassay. Specific binding proteins, such as vitamin D-binding globulin (DBP; VDBG), the blood carrier protein (69), or target tissue receptors for 25-OH-D_3 or 1,25-$(OH)_2$-D_3, can be used in these systems (reviewed in Refs. 6 and 14). Antibodies have been raised in sheep and rabbits (61,115) and various radioimmunoassays described

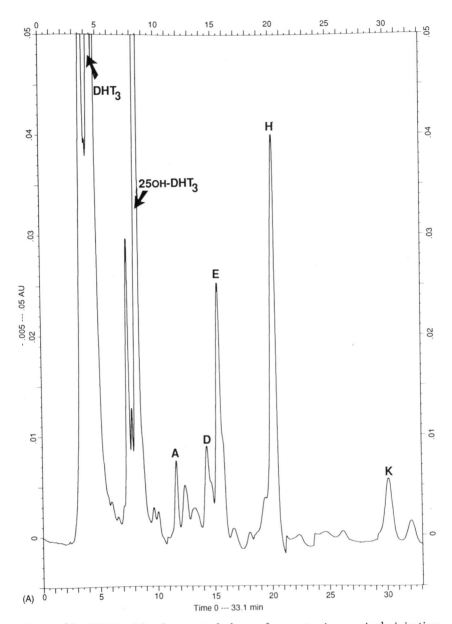

Figure 21 HPLC of lipid extract of plasma from rats given a single injection of DHT_3, 18 h previously. (A) Single-wavelength (251 nm) detection. (B) Diode array spectrophotometric detection. Conditions used were as follows: Zorbax-SIL (0.62 × 25 cm); hexane-2-propanol-methanol (91:7:2 v/v/v); 2 ml/min. Metabolites are labeled A-L. The metabolite peaks A, D, and E were given the same letter designations as metabolites observed in kidney perfusions on the basis of their retention on HPLC. In the case of peak E, subsequent identification by MS confirmed this letter designation. (From Ref. 109 with permission).

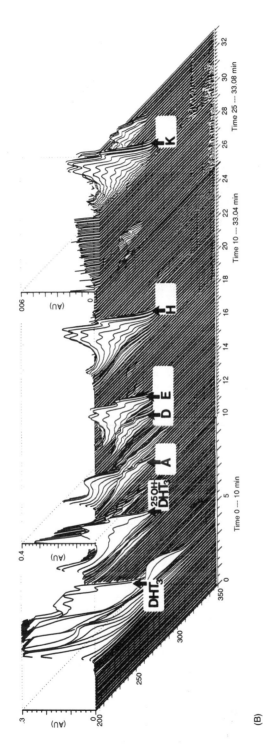

Figure 21

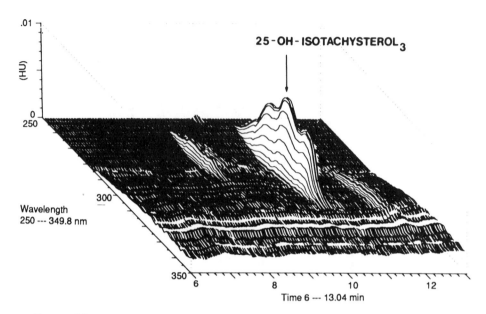

Figure 22 High-performance liquid chromatography of an extract of plasma after conversion to isotachysterol isomers. A plasma sample was extracted as illustrated in Fig. 3 and the 25-OH-D fraction from the Sep-Pak SIL was chromatographed on Zorbax SIL. The fraction corresponding to 25-OH-D$_3$ was collected, and isotachysterols formed (92). The isotachysterol isomer was rechromatographed on Zorbax SIL (25 cm × 6.2 mm ID) using the solvent hexane:isopropanol:methanol (94:5:1, by volume). The eluate was monitored using a Waters photodiode array assembly and a three-dimensional plot was produced. The 25-OH-isotachysterol$_3$ peak from the plasma extract had a retention time of 10.73 min (a standard run immediately afterward had a retention time of 10.75 min). The 3-D plot showed that the plasma peak had a typical isotachysterol UV spectrum in the range 250–350 nm and appeared to be uncontaminated with other UV-absorbing compounds. (From Ref. 113 with permission).

(114). Simple clinical assays for 25-OH-D and 1,25-(OH)$_2$-D now utilize sample preparation on cartridges, and improvements in the assay conditions have largely eliminated the need for HPLC (see Fig. 25).

Applications

VITAMIN D AND 25-OH-D MEASUREMENT IN PLASMA.   Vitamin D and 25-OH-D can be measured in plasma by LC with UV monitoring at 254 nm as described by Shepard et al. (87), Horst et al. (56), Jones (98), and Lambert et al. (60). Schemes shown in Figs. 8 and 26 illustrate two examples of different approaches used to purify the sample prior to LC. Examples of chromatograms from Ref. 98 are shown in Figs. 27 and 28.

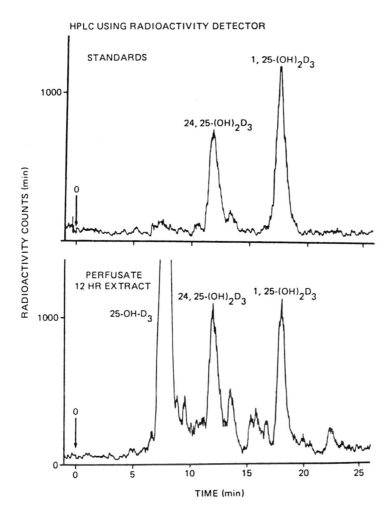

Figure 23 LC using an on-line liquid scintillation counter for detecting radioactive (^{3}H or ^{14}C) peaks of vitamin D. The example illustrates the metabolic picture obtained from the analysis of an incubation of [^{3}H]-25-OH-D_3 with an isolated perfused rat kidney. (From Ref. 107).

24,25-Dihydroxyvitamin D_3 can also be measured by LC with UV monitoring at 254 nm, but identification of the small peak is tentative. The potentially interfering 25-OH-D_3-26,23-lactone can be rapidly eluted with methylene chloride-isopropanol mixtures. An LC method for plasma 24,25-$(OH)_2$-D_3 has been described (116) using two Zorbax-SIL LC steps and UV absorption, but no proper evaluation of this method has been carried out and it has not been applied by subsequent workers for the measurement of this metabolite in plasma.

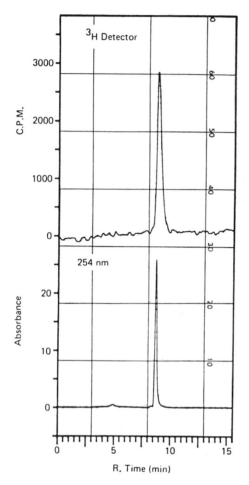

Figure 24   LC of [^{3}H]-25-OH-D (400,000 dpm) as in Fig. 13, using a radioactivity detector (Berthold). Upper panel: ^{3}H detector. Lower panel: Waters 440 UV detector at 254 nm. Note the slight peak broadening effect of the 300 μl flow cell.

ANALYSIS OF *IN VITRO* AND *IN VIVO* PRODUCED METABOLITES OF VITAMIN D.   This is a relatively straightforward application of the technique of LC to separate and identify radioactively labeled peaks by comigration with authentic standards. Examples have already been shown in Figs. 18, 20 and 23. Unfortunately, although this is one of the potentially useful applications of LC analysis, it is also one of the most abused. It is not valid to assume that because a radioactive compound (e.g., peak b of Fig. 18) comigrates with the standard in a single

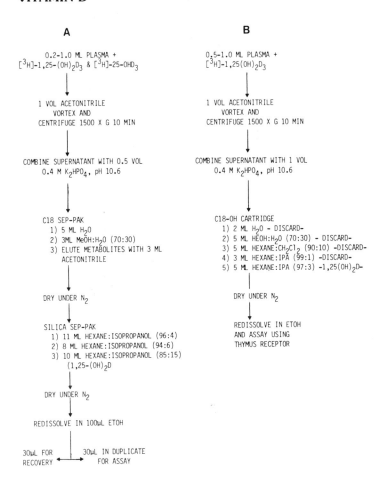

Figure 25 Flow charts of 1,25-(OH)$_2$-D radioreceptor assay based on (A) dual-cartridge and (B) single-cartridge technology.

LC system, it is unequivocally identified. Too often it is believed that liquid chromatography always produces "high-performance" results. Clearly, comigration depends on all factors in the R_s equation, and several solvent and column systems should be tested before firm identification of unknown peaks is made. Interpolation of specific chemical transformation (such as isotachysterol formation), changing the chromatographic properties of the peaks under investigation, also enhances specificity.

SEPARATION OF STEREOISOMERS. Cochromatography of chemically synthesized stereoisomeric mixtures with biologically generated me-

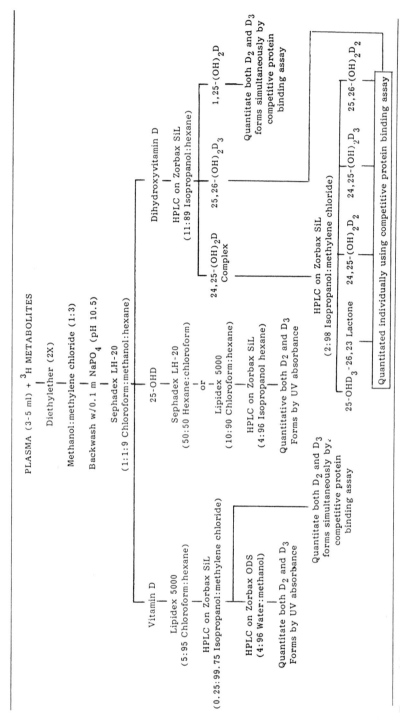

Figure 26 Schematic diagram of a comprehensive scheme for the analysis of vitamin D and its metabolites using a combination of HPLC and competitive-binding assay (from Ref. 56 with permission).

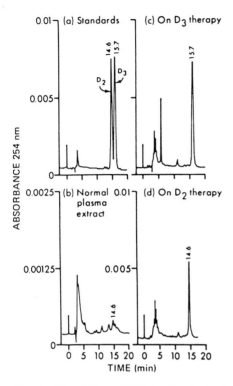

Figure 27 LC analysis of vitamin D fractions from human plasma using the scheme shown in Fig. 8. (a) Standards (D_2, 112 ng; D_3, 117 ng). (b) Plasma extract of normal adult. (c) Plasma extract of child treated with 50,000 IU vitamin D_3 daily. (d) Plasma extract of child treated with 100,000 IU vitamin D_2 daily. Fractions b, c, and d were purified by Zorbax-SIL LC before the reverse-phase LC shown here. Numbers above peaks represent retention times in minutes. Flow rate = 1.5 ml/min; solvent system, methanol-water (98.5:1.5); k_{D2} = 6.3; k_{D3} = 6.85; α = 1.087; N = 4720; R = 1.19. Column: Zorbax-ODS (6.2 mm × 25 cm). (From Ref. 98, 1978, Clinical Chemistry.)

tabolites has led to the identification of at least six naturally occurring compounds as: $24(R),25$-$(OH)_2$-D_3, $24(R),25$-$(OH)_2$-D_2, $23(S),25$-$(OH)_2$-D_3, $23(S),25(R)$-25-OH-D_3 26,23-lactone, $1,24(R),25$-$(OH)_3$-D_3, and $25(R),26$-$(OH)_2$-D_3. The separation of $24(R,S),25$-$(OH)_2$-D_2 is shown in Fig. 29.

PHARMACEUTICAL PREPARATIONS. Aside from the specially formulated vitamin D metabolite preparations now being produced by Leo (1α-OH-D_3), Phillips-Duphar (DHT$_2$, vitamin D_2 and D_3), Upjohn (25-OH-D_3), and Hoffman-La Roche [$1\alpha,25$-$(OH)_2$-D_3], the major type of

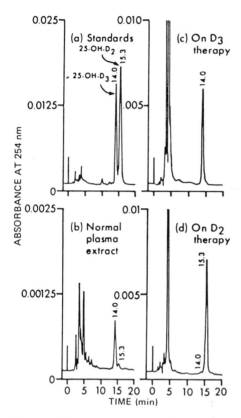

Figure 28 LC analysis of 25-OH-D fractions from human plasma using the scheme shown in Fig. 8. (a) Standards (25-OH-D$_3$, 250 ng; 25-OH-D$_2$, 345 ng). (b) Plasma extract of normal adult. (c) Plasma extract of child treated with 50,000 IU vitamin D$_3$ daily. (d) Plasma extract of child treated with 100,000 IU vitamin D$_2$ daily. Fractions b, c, and d were purified by Zorbax-SIL LC before the reverse-phase LC shown here. Numbers above peak represent retention times, in minutes. Flow rate = 1.5 ml/min; solvent system, methanol-water (91:9, v/v); $k'_{25\text{-OH-D3}}$ = 6.80; $k'_{25\text{-OH-D2}}$ = 6.05; α = 1.12; N = 4314; R = 1.51. Column: Zorbax ODS (6.2 mm × 25 cm). (From Ref. 98, 1978, Clinical Chemistry.)

vitamin D analysis in the pharmaceutical industry is measurement of vitamin D in multivitamin preparations and vitamin D resin-containing powders. Methodology involves a reverse-phase chromatographic step followed by separation of 4,6-cholestadienol (internal standard), vitamin D, and previtamin D. Concentrations of vitamin D represent the sum of previtamin D and vitamin D in the mixture (117). An example of

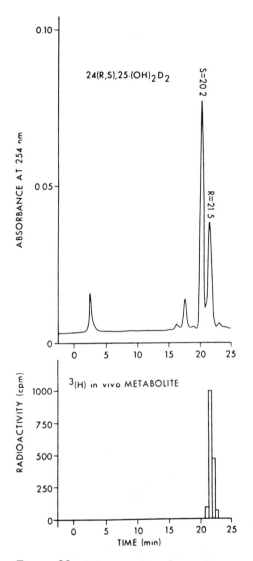

Figure 29   LC separation of stereoisomers of $24(R,S),25\text{-}(OH)_2\text{-}D_2$. (Reprinted with permission from Ref. 40, ©1979, American Chemical Society.)

analysis of dry multivitamin concentrates after saponification and extraction is shown in Fig. 30.

FOODSTUFFS.   As stated earlier, current methodology for margarine involves saponification, selective extraction, and alumina column chromatography followed by a combination of silica, 5 μm, and reverse-

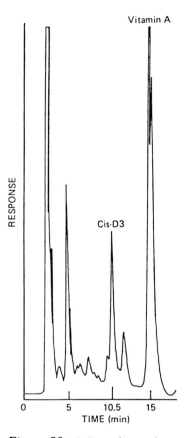

Figure 30   LC analysis of vitamin D_3 in a multivitamin concentrate after saponification and extraction. The concentrate contained 200,000 IU D_3 (5 mg) per gram. Note the good resolution of vitamins D and A. (From H. Hofsass, in Symposium Proceedings of the Association of Vitamin Chemists, Oak Brook, Illinois, March 30, 1979. Reproduced courtesy of Waters Associates.)

phase Radial Pak-C18 separation of vitamins D_2 and D_3. See Fig. 31 for the type of separation. Milk analysis can be achieved without the alumina step.

More recently, Hollis and Frank (118) have successfully utilized a combination of saponification, organic liquid/liquid extraction with hexane, preliminary chromatography on silica Bond-Elut cartridges (Fig. 5b), and nonaqueous reverse-phase HPLC to produce a reliable single-step HPLC assay for the direct UV determination of vitamins D_2 and/or D_3 in infant formula, fortified milk, or animal feeds (118). The advantage of this method is that it requires very little sample, for example,

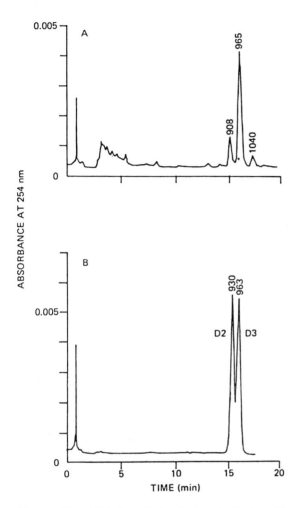

Figure 31 (A) LC analysis of vitamin D₃ in milk after saponification, extraction, and alumina chromatography. (B) LC of standards of D₂ and D₃ under identical conditions. Retention times are marked above the peaks in seconds. Spherisorb ODS (25 cm × 4.6 mm, 10 μm). Solvent system: methanol-acetonitrile (1:9). Flow rate: 1 ml/min. Detection: 254 nm. The milk sample contained 24 IU D₃ per 100 ml according to area under peak at 965 sec. (Modified from Ref. 64.)

0.5–1.0 ml liquid or 1–2 g feed, and is very rapid and cost-effective. Figure 32 demonstrates the resolution and subsequent quantitation of vitamins D₂ and D₃ in infant formula using this rapid one-step HPLC procedure.

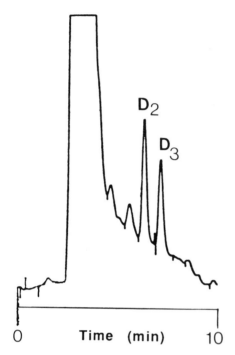

Figure 32 Actual HPLC profile of infant milk formula containing vitamins D_2 and D3 (elution times 6.16 and 7.0 min, respectively). One milliliter of infant formula was saponified in an equal volume of ethanolic KOH and then extracted with hexane. The extract was dried under nitrogen, chromatographed on a BOND-ELUT silica cartridge as already illustrated in Fig. 5b. The eluent containing vitamin D was collected, dried under nitrogen, and applied to a nonaqueous reverse-phase HPLC system for direct UV quantitation at 254 nm. The HPLC column (Vydac-ODS) was eluted with acetonitrile-methylene chloride (75:25) at a flow rate of 1.5 ml/min.

3. GAS CHROMATOGRAPHIC ANALYSIS

3.1 B-Ring Closure

A prerequisite for the use of gas-liquid chromatography is that the solute should be in the vapor phase during the process of partition between the mobile gas phase and the stationary liquid phase. For compounds of molecular mass in excess of around 200 D, this requires analysis to be carried out at elevated temperatures, usually in excess of 100°C. At these temperatures, vitamin D and its hydroxylated metabolites undergo thermal rearrangement involving B-ring closure. In the naturally occurring steroid, the 19-methyl attached to C10 is always β and is *trans* with

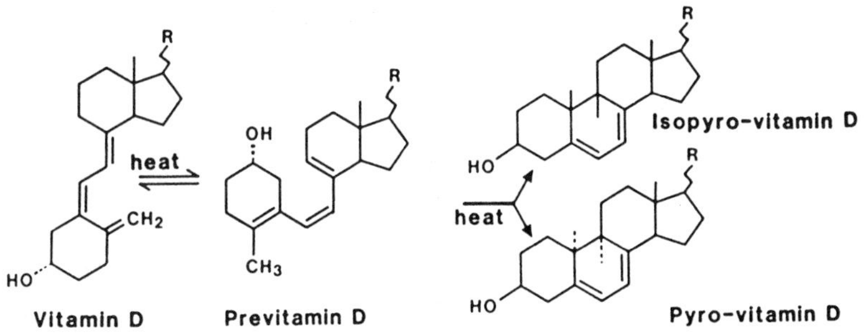

Figure 33 Thermal transformation of vitamin D to pyro and isopyro isomers.

respect to the 9α-hydrogen. When B-ring closure occurs in the vitamin D series, two isomers are formed, both of which are *cis* across the 9–10 carbon-carbon bond (i.e., C19β, 9β, isopyro; and C19α, 9α, pyro). The formation of these isomers was originally described in 1932 by Askew and his colleagues (119), who heated vitamin D in the test tube to around 190°C. Although isomerization took place rapidly at this temperature and was complete in about 4 h, ring closure has been shown to occur at all temperatures in excess of 125°C (120). It is irreversible and the ratio of pyro and isopyro remains at 2:1. This reaction occurs in the absence of oxygen, and it is now thought that the immediate precursor of these isomers is the previtamin (see Fig. 33).

At the temperatures at which GLC is carried out, therefore, vitamin D and its metabolites are all converted irreversibly and quantitatively to a 2:1 mixture of pyro and isopyro isomers that separate in all the GLC systems so far examined (88,101,121,122). The formation of these two isomers during GLC was first demonstrated by Ziffer et al. (123).

3.2 Derivatives for GLC

As with all GLC systems for steroid analysis, the stability and volatility of vitamin D and its metabolites can be increased by the formation of derivatives on the polar hydroxyl groups. Free underivatized hydroxyl groups may give rise to adsorption during chromatography (124) and nonlinearity of detector response. The 25-hydroxyl group in vitamin D is sterically hindered. If vitamin D and particularly its polyhydroxylated metabolites are injected into a GC without derivatization, broad peaks are obtained, indicating some degree of adsorption. In addition, dehydration of the 25-hydroxyl can occur, giving rise to two extra peaks in addition to the pyro and isopyro isomers. This dehydration is variable, but 100% conversion to the 25-dehydro derivative can sometimes be

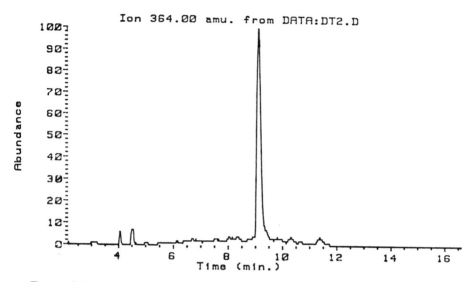

Figure 34 Mass chromatography of dehydrated 25-OH-D$_3$, monitoring the molecular ion, m/z 364.

achieved by introducing powdered glass at the top of the GC column, thus allowing use of the dehydro peaks for quantitation.

The use of powdered glass to achieve dehydration is not always effective, however, and more consistent results can be obtained if required using aluminium powder at 400°C. Although it would be expected that pyro and isopyro isomers would still be formed during chromatography, only one major peak is observed for each metabolite during GC-MS, probably because the isopyro isomer has only low-intensity ions (Fig. 34). Mass spectra obtained for each peak indicated that the expected dehydration had occurred (Fig. 35). Dehydration can occur in a number of ways; for example, loss of the 25-hydroxyl could lead to a double bond between C24 and C25 or C25 and C26. Use of a high-resolution capillary column indicates that two isomers are formed during dehydration of 25-OH-D, and use of stable isotope-labeled compounds has confirmed that both the expected dehydration products are formed. Dehydration of dihydroxylated vitamin D metabolites also occurs, and the products from 24,25-(OH)$_2$-D$_3$ and 25,26-(OH)$_2$-D$_3$ are easily resolved during GC because in 25,26-(OH)$_2$-D$_3$ both the 25- and 26-hydroxyls cannot be removed simultaneously and the remaining hydroxyl makes the product more polar than that from 24,25-(OH)$_2$-D$_3$ (see Fig. 36).

Formation of derivatives on the polar hydroxyl groups of vitamin D and metabolites, although it improves stability and volatility, does not

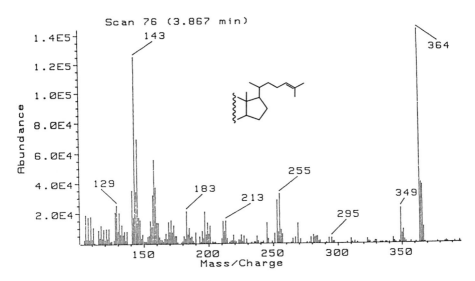

Figure 35 El(+) mass spectrum of dehydration product of 25-OH-D$_3$ illustrated in Fig. 34. There are two possible dehydration products but only one is illustrated. Note the relatively high intensity of the molecular ion.

overcome the problem of the B-ring closure and the formation of the two pyro and isopyro peaks. The formation of these isomers is quantitative, and either or both peaks can be used for measurement (125–129), but the separation of a number of metabolites in a single run can be complicated by the multiplicity of peaks. Figure 37a illustrates the separation of trimethylsilyl ether derivatives on a conventional packed column. In this separation, the 25-hydroxyl has been derivatized by the formation of a 25-trimethylsilyl ether. Because the 25-hydroxyl is sterically hindered, it is difficult to derivatize, and only two reagents have proved satisfactory for the low levels present in plasma trimethylsilylimidazole (TMSI) and a mixture of bis-trimethylsilytrifluoroacetamide (BSTFA): trimethylchlorosilane (TMCS) (3:1, v/v). Improvement in separation can be achieved by using capillary columns, and Fig. 37b shows the separation of a persilylated mixture, similar to that used in Fig. 37a, on a 25-cm wallcoated capillary column.

In attempts to simplify the chromatographic profile obtained, a considerable amount of study has been undertaken into the formation of derivatives of vitamin D that were thermally stable and did not isomerize during GLC. Nair and DeLeon (122), using trifluoroacetic anhydride, formed "acetate esters" and suggested that although pyro and isopyro derivatives were still formed during GLC, they did not separate as acetates. This is now known to be incorrect, and it is recognized that the

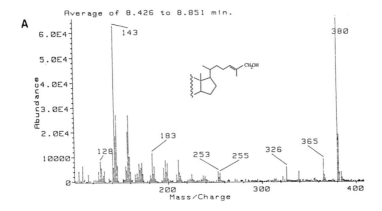

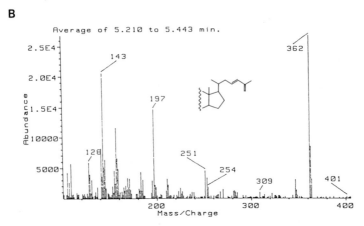

Figure 36 El(+) mass spectra of dehydration products from (B) 24,25-$(OH)_2$-D_3 and (A) 25,26-$(OH)_2$-D_3. Possible structures for the products are illustrated. Note the different molecular ion (m/z 362 in B and m/z 380 in A) indicating the loss of a different number of hydroxyls. The retention time of the product from 25,26-$(OH)_2$-D_3 is 3 min longer than that of the product from 24,25-$(OH)_2$-D_3.

use of trifluoroacetic anhydride gave rise to the acetate of the isotachysterol isomer of vitamin D, which because of the rearrangement of the A ring is resistant to thermal cyclization (see Fig. 38). Injection of isotachysterol isomers onto GLC columns gives rise, therefore, to single peaks. Adsorption and dehydration of the 25-hydroxyl group still occur, however, and the use of derivatives is still necessary. 1α-Hydroxylated derivatives of vitamin D do not undergo this isomerization, probably because the suggested reaction mechanism for this reaction (illustrated in Fig. 38) involves the intermediate formation of isovitamin D with a Δ^1

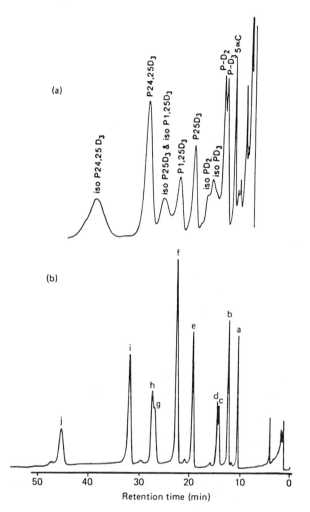

Figure 37 Gas chromatography of trimethylsilyl ether derivatives of vitamin D and various metabolites using (a) conventional packed column and (b) wall-coated glass capillary column. (a) Separation by GLC of the trimethysilyl ether derivatives of ergocalciferol, cholecalciferol, and some metabolites of chole-calciferol. P = pyro, isoP = isopyro, $5\alpha C$ = 5α=cholestane, D_2 = ergocalci-ferol, D_3 = cholecalciferol, $25D_3$ = 25-hydroxycholecalciferol, $1,25D_3$ = 24,25-dihydroxyvitamin D_3. Gas chromatography was carried out on OV1 at 230°C using total ion current detection. (From Ref. 101) (b) Total ion current chromatogram of a mixture of the TMS ethers of five cholecalciferols showing peaks corresponding to cyclized isomers: vitamin D_3 (pyro, a, and isopyro, c), 1α-hydroxyvitamin D_3 (peak I, b, and peak II, d), 25-hydroxyvitamin D_3 (peak I, e, and peak II, g), 1α-25-dihydroxyvitamin D_3 (peak I, f, and peak II, h), and 24(R), 25-dihydroxyvitamin D_3 (peak I, i, and peak II, j). (From Ref. 130.)

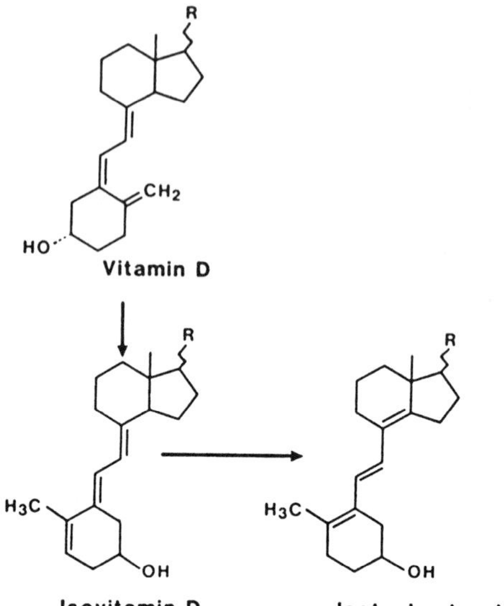

Figure 38 Formation of the isotachysterol isomers of vitamin D. (From Ref. 131).

double-bond (131). The presence of a 1α-hydroxyl may well inhibit the formation of this intermediate. Figure 39 shows the GLC separation of the same mixture as that illustrated in Fig. 37a after formation of isotachysterol isomers.

A wide variety of reagents has been used to affect this isomerization: acetyl chloride (122), trifluoroacetic anhydride (122), penta- and heptafluorobutyryl chlorides (122), and heptafluorobutyric anhydride (132,133). These reagents not only give rise to the formation of the isotachysterol isomer but at the same time form derivatives on the hydroxyl group. Acetyl chloride esterifies all groups, including the sterically hindered 25-hydroxyl, whereas anhydrides do not esterify the 25-hydroxyl.

Other reagents that have been used to form the isotachysterol isomers, without concomitant ester formation, include boron trifluoride (134), antimony trichloride (135), and a number of acidic reagents (136). None of these reagents were found to be of value when forming the isotachysterol isomers of the very small amounts of vitamin D and its metabolites present in human plasma. Seamark et al. (101) described a new procedure that gave quantitative conversion down to 1-ng levels using hydrochloric acid gas in chloroform or methylene chloride. At levels below 100 ng, carrier vitamin D_2 was added to protect against destruction. This simple HCl procedure, which takes only 54 min, allows iso-

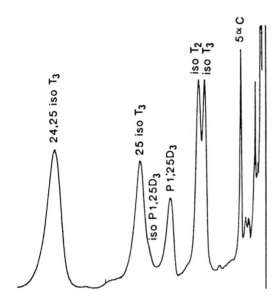

Figure 39 Gas chromatography of trimethylsilyl ether derivatives of isotachysterol isomers of vitamin D and various metabolites. Separation by GLC of the
trimethylsilyl ether derivatives of ergocalciferol, cholecalciferol, and some metabolites of cholecalciferol, after isomerization to isotachysterol derivatives. P =
pyro, isoP = isopyro, isoT$_2$-isotachysterol$_2$, isoT$_3$-isotachysterol$_3$, 5αC = 5α-
cholestane, D$_2$ = ergocalciferol, D$_3$ = cholecalciferol, 25D$_3$ = 25-hydroxy-
cholecalciferol, 1,25D$_3$ = 1α,25-dihydroxycholecalciferol. Gas chromatography
was carried out on OV1 at 230°C using total ion current detection. This is the
same mixture separated before isomerization in Fig. 37a. (From Ref. 101).

merization without formation of esters, thus allowing a choice of derivative without the interpolation of a hydrolysis step. A recent improvement
in this isomerization procedure, which does not require the addition of
carrier vitamin D at low levels and uses HCl in 2-butanol (137), has been
published.

Although these isomers give single peaks during GLC, formation of
derivatives improves linearity of detector response and prevents destruction and adsorption in the same way as for isomerized vitamins.
Underivatized 25-hydroxyisotachysterols still show dehydration. Figure
40 shows an example of this during the GLC separation of methoxy
derivatives of isotachysterol isomers using conventional packed columns.
It is not clear whether this dehydration occurs during GLC or, as sug-

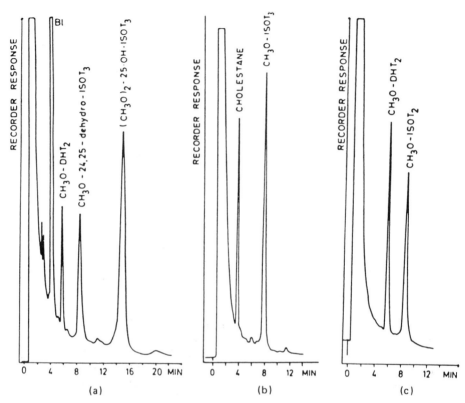

Figure 40 GLC of methoxy derivatives of isotachysterol isomers of vitamin D$_2$, vitamin D$_3$, and 25-OH-D$_3$. (a) Gas-liquid chromatography (FID) of 3β-methoxydihydrotachysterol$_2$ (CH$_3$O-DHT$_2$: 1 μg) and derivatized 25-hydroxy-vitamin D$_3$ (4 μg), i.e., 3β-methoxy-24,25-dehydroisotachysterol$_3$ (CH$_3$O-24, 25-dehydro-ISOT$_3$) and 3β,25-bismethosyisotachysterol$_3$ [(CH$_3$O)$_2$-25-OH-ISOT$_3$]. (b) GLC (FID) of cholestane (0.75 μg) and 3β-methoxyisotachysterol$_3$ (CH$_3$-ISOT$_3$,3μg). (c) GLC (FID) of 3β-methoxydihydrotachysterol$_2$ (CH$_3$O-DHT$_2$,4μg). and 3β-methoxyisotachysterol$_2$ (CH$_3$O-ISOT$_2$, 4 GLC conditions: A 2% QF-1 column is operated at an oven temperature of 225°C and at a linear velocity of nitrogen (carrier gas) of 6 cm/sec. (From Ref. 138).

gested by De Leenheer and Cruyl (139), during formation of the methoxy derivative or during the isomerization itself (140) using antimony trichloride. The quantitative formation of methoxy derivatives requires careful control and so far has only been examined using micro-gram amounts of vitamin D and 25-OH-D (139).

3.3 Removal of Cholesterol

Unlike LC, in which the presence of large amounts of cholesterol in biological extracts can largely be ignored since cholesterol does not absorb in the UV, the presence of unesterified cholesterol during GLC is a major problem. It is present in human plasma in very much larger concentrations (50 mg/100 ml) than vitamin D_3. (1 μg/100 ml) and has very similar GLC properties to vitamin D_3. The removal of cholesterol prior to quantitation by GLC is therefore essential, but it has unfortunately proved to be extremely difficult to find a completely satisfactory method, although a number of procedures, such as TLC (121), digitonin precipitation (132,133), and LC on silver nitrate-impregnated columns (125), have been described.

3.4 Flame Ionization and Electron-Capture Detectors

Although it is clear that vitamin D and its metabolites can be separated by GLC, their measurement in biological fluids has been hampered by the lack of a suitable detector with the required sensitivity and specificity. Two relevant column detectors for gas chromatography are in use today, the flame-ionization detector (FID) and the electron-capture detector (ECD), and a number of methods using FID have been described for the estimation of vitamin D in pharmaceutical preparations or animal foodstuffs (141–143). However, the FID is not sufficiently sensitive for the estimation of vitamin D metabolites in human plasma, although Sklan (144) briefly described some recovery experiments for 25-OH-D in plasma. The ECD, however, is sufficiently sensitive, and GLC methods have been described in which very low levels of vitamin D (5–10 ng/ml) (138,145) using pure standards and a 25-OH-D_3 (50 pg) (88) using chick plasma have been detected. However, the electron capture detector, although sufficiently sensitive, lacks specificity, and its use for the analysis of vitamin D in human plasma has so far not been described.

3.5 Mass Spectrometry

MS as a Detector

Linking the gas chromatograph to a mass spectrometer, which can be used for specific identification and as a quantitative detector, may give comparable sensitivity to the ECD but also provides greatly enhanced specificity. Low-resolution mass spectrometers are not as sensitive (defined as signal to noise ratio) as high-resolution machines but are at the moment much cheaper to purchase and operate. There are increasingly available cheap "benchtop" systems that are now within reach of any analytical laboratory. Such systems are usually based on quadrupole machine (i.e., Hewlett–Packard mass-selective detector HP 5970), although there is a different type involving the so-called "ion trap system" (Finnigan MAT). Such systems are linked to simple personal computer systems that allow the provision of sophisticated control of the GC-MS system acquisition and manipulation of data. Figure 41 illustrates in diagrammatic form how such a system is put together.

Conventional packed columns with carrier gas flow rates around 40 ml/min can be linked to some mass spectrometers via a separator system, which would be expected to be a source of destruction and/or loss of sen-

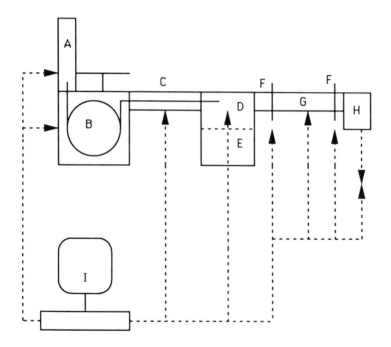

Figure 41 Schematic outline of a simple "bench-top" mass spectrometer linked to a gas chromatograph: (A) automated sample injection system, (B) oven and capillary GC column, (C) heated transfer line, (D) ion source of mass spectrometer, (E) vacuum generating system, (F) prefilters and slits for focussing, (G) mass filter (i.e., quadrupole), (H) electron or photon multiplier, amplifier and electronics, (I) computer for data handling and control. Control and/or information flow to and from the computer indicated · · ·

sitivity. However, modern mass spectrometers, including benchtop systems mentioned above, are usually designed to be used with capillary or megabore columns.

Such columns can be linked directly to the mass spectrometer since the carrier gas flow rate is low (1–2 ml/min), and the column can be inserted directly into the ion source of the spectrometer, thus eliminating the loss of analyte in the separator system. Apart from its use as a detector on the end of a gas chromatograph, the mass spectrometer has found considerable use in the vitamin D field as a means of establishing the identity of isolated metabolites (e.g., 146–150) and checking the purity of biological extracts prior to assay (see Fig. 42). For example, Jones (98)

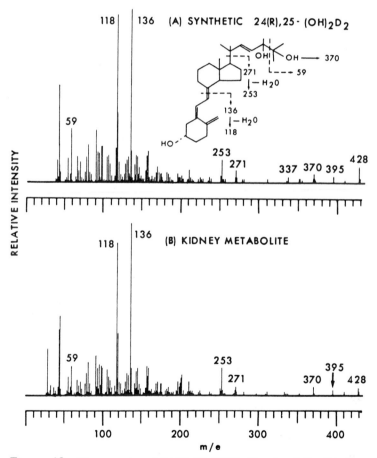

Figure 42   Mass spectra of 24(R),25-(OH)$_2$-D$_2$ after LC. (A) Chemically synthesized. (B) Biologically generated. (Reprinted with permission from Ref. 40, © 1979, American Chemical Society.)

has used mass spectrometry as a means of confirming the purity of a 25-OH-D$_3$ fraction isolated from plasma in an LC method for the measurement of 25-OH-D$_2$ and 25-OH-D$_3$ (see Fig. 28). At this point, however, a note of caution should be sounded, since the demonstration that an apparently homogeneous HPLC peak gives a mass spectrum that is consistent with that of the expected analyte may lead to a false assumption that the peak in question is indeed pure. This has been clearly demonstrated by Holmberg et al. (151) during a mass spectrometric study of an HPLC method for 25-OH-D. Apparently homogeneous HPLC peaks had the correct mass spectrum, but analytical results obtained by HPLC when compared to those obtained by GC-MS on the same plasma showed no correlation.

The mass spectrometer can be used as detector for gas chromatography in two ways. The most sensitive method relies on the ability of the MS to focus on specific ion fragments. There are numerous ways of arranging this that depend upon the type of mass spectrometer being used. The spectrometer can be focussed on a single ion fragment or on different ion fragments at different times. The dwell time on each fragment is of course directly related to sensitivity. In a single focusing magnetic sector machine the focusing on different fragments can be achieved by altering the accelerating voltage so that different ions are sequentially focused on the electron multiplier. Modern laminated magnets now allow rapid alteration of the magnetic field without associated hysteresis effects, and focusing can thus be achieved by altering the current through the magnet. Quadrupole mass spectrometers operate on a different principle and focus ions by altering radio frequency and direct current applied across four rods through the axis of which the ions travel. As mentioned previously, quadrupole mass spectrometers are assuming increasing importance in analytical laboratories. The process of mass fragmentography (MF) is the most sensitive mode of operation, but an alternative approach can be adopted. All modern mass spectrometers are now equipped with sophisticated data acquisition and manipulation computing systems and thus are capable of scanning the effluent gas from the GC at regular intervals (1–5 scans/s) and storing the complete mass spectrum obtained. At the end of the GC run data can be recalled and total ion or single ion chromatograms can be constructed. Such a system (mass chromatography) is not as sensitive as MF but provides a very valuable method of establishing the ion fragment to monitor for the best sensitivity and specificity.

Derivatives for MS

The use of the MS as a detector would appear to place an extra requirement of the derivatives of vitamin D used for such analyses. Not only must they have satisfactory GLC properties, but in addition they should fragment in the mass spectrometer to give a suitable ion of high m/z, preferably specific to the metabolite of interest. However, because of the much enhanced specificity of the mass spectrometer, selectivity during chromatography assumes less importance. However, little attention has been paid to the gas chromatographic characteristics of derivatives of vitamin D metabolites. Provided that symmetrical peaks are obtained and adsorption during GC is minimal, the GC system is regarded as satisfactory. No investigation of selective stationary phases has been carried out, and all methods so far published have used nonselective methylsilicone type phases for GC. Very few authors have used modern capillary WCOT columns, which might be expected to provide increased selectivity and sensitivity. In a recent survey of 14 published methods for the GC-MS of vitamin D metabolites, only five had used capillary GC columns. Interestingly, of those five, three were published more than 10 years ago (see Table 2).

There are various methods of producing ion fragments, but in the vitamin D field, electron impact (EI) has been most commonly used. Chemical ionization (CI) has been used, with ammonia as the reagent gas, in the GC-MS separation and identification of vitamin D_3 and previ-

Table 2 Publications Using Capillary Columns for GC-MS of Vitamin D and Its Metabolites in Human Plasma and Urine[a]

Analyte	Stationary phase	Details of WCOT column (ID × length)	Reference	Date of reference
25-OH-D_3, 24,25-$(OH)_2$-D_3, 1,25-$(OH)_2$-D_3	OV 101	0.35 mm × 25 m	127*	1978
D_2 and 25-OH-D_3	SE 30	0.29 mm × 25 mm	125*	1978
D_3, 25-OH-D_3, 1,25-$(OH)_2$-D_3	OV 101	0.32 mm × 25 m	140**	1978
Metabolites of ^{3}H-25-OH-D_3 in urine	SE 52	15 m long (no details on ID)	153***	1980
1,25-$(OH)_2$-D_3	Superox 4	0.25 mm × 4 m	152****	1988

[a] All methods used EI(+) and single-focusing magnetic sector mass spectrometers (*VG Micromass 16F, **LKB 9000, or ***Hitachi-M52) or quadrupole (****Finnigan 1020) systems.

tamin D_3 after irradiation of the skin of vitamin D-deficient rats by ultraviolet light (154).

The most extensive evaluation of the mass spectrometric properties of vitamin D and its metabolites has been carried out in Lisboa's laboratory using open tubular capillary column GLC and a conventional low-resolution mass spectrometer. Trimethylsilylated derivatives of D_3, 25-OH-D_3, their isotachysterol derivatives, and 1,25-$(OH)_2$-D_3 have been examined by mass chromatography (140). Increased intensity of the molecular ion in the mass spectrum of the isotachysterol$_3$ trimethylsilyl (TMS) ether compared with that obtained from either the pyro- or isopy-rovitamin D_3 trimethylsilyl ether was observed. This has also been described by Seamark et al. (89), and comparative values are given in Table 3. Thus, not only does the formation of isotachysterol derivatives give single peaks during GLC, but it also increases the sensitivity of mass fragmentography. Mass spectrometric data and retention times of these TMS ether derivatives on OV101-coated capillary columns have been obtained (130).

Although the use of isotachysterols during chromatography achieves the chromatographer's desire for single peaks, isotachysterols have not been used in more recent methods for GC-MS of vitamin D metabolites. We have not found it possible to form isotachysterol derivatives of the more polar vitamin D_2 metabolites without considerable destruction occurring, and the mass spectra obtained from the n-butylboronate-trimethylsilyl ether derivatives of isotachysterol isomers of 24,25-$(OH)_2$-D_3 have a major ion at m/z 253 and very low intensity high m/z ions. Since these methods (155,156) utilize stable isotope-labeled internal standards with the label on carbons 26 and 27, the m/z 253 ion is of little

Table 3 Comparison of the Peak Areas of ITS-TMS and Pyro-D_3-TMS + Isopyro-D_3-TMS Prepared from Equal Amounts of D_3 as a Measure of Relative Ion Intensity [a]

Compound	"Area"
ITS$_3$-TMS	0.924
Pyro-D_3-TMS	0.585
Isopyro-D_3-TMS	0.175
ITS/(pyro + isopyro)	1.22
ITS/pyro	1.58
ITS/isopyro	5.28

[a] ITS = isotachysterol$_3$, D_3 = vitamin D_3. The isotachysterol derivative was prepared by the method described in Ref. 101 and analyzed by mass spectrometry. The molecular ion (m/z 456) was analyzed in each case, as was the ion $(M-57)^+$ of cholesteryl-t-BDMS, used as an internal standard.

value for quantitation since it represents the ring structure after loss of the side chain.

An interesting derivative for 24,25-(OH)$_2$-D$_3$ has been described by Lisboa and Halket (130), who formed a cyclical boronate across the adjacent 24- and 25-hydroxyl groups as previously described for steriods (157–159). Halket et al. (160) obtained mass spectrometric and retention times for methyl- and n-butylboronate-3-trimethylsilyl ether derivatives of 24,25-(OH)-D$_3$ and found that the use of the cyclic boronate derivative stabilized the molecule and gave rise to considerably enhanced intensity of ions of high mass-charge ratio. Figure 43 compares the normalized mass spectra of 24,25-(OH)$_2$-D$_3$-TMS with that obtained from the methylboronate TMS derivative, showing the greatly increased mass

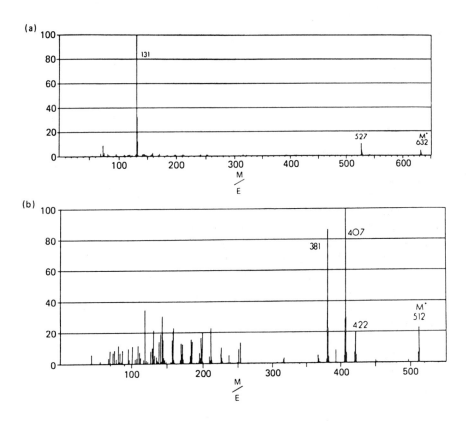

Figure 43 Normalized mass spectra of two derivatives of 24,25-(OH)$_2$-D$_3$ during GC-MS on a 50-m OV-17 capillary column at 260°C. In each case the pyro peak was scanned. (a) 24(R),25-Dihydroxycholecalciferol-tris-trimethysilyl ether. (b) 3-Trimethysilyl ether-24,25-methylboronate ester derivative of 24(R),25-dihydroxycholecalciferol. (From Ref. 160.)

fragments at m/z 381, $(M-131)^+$, the fragment probably obtained by A-ring cleavage containing C2, C4, and C3-O-TMS, and m/z 407, $(M-90+15)^+$.

The use of n-butylboronate-trimethylsilyl derivatives also has the advantage that these derivatives of 24,25-$(OH)_2$-D_3 and 25,26-$(OH)_2$-D_3 separate during GC on a nonselective stationary phase (155), and such derivatives have been used in the development of mass fragmentographic assays for both these vitamin D metabolites (156). Vicinal hydroxyls and 1,3-cis-diols can both form cyclic boronates, and n-butyl-, n-phenyl-, and n-methylboronates of 24,25-$(OH)_2$-D_3 can easily be formed. Interestingly only n-butyl- and n-phenylboronates can be formed with ease from 25,26-$(OH)_2$-D_3, whereas n-methylboronates appear not to be formed (156).

Trimethylsilyl ether derivatives have been widely used for GC-MS, but as can be seen from Fig. 43, they are not ideal derivatives for mass fragmentography in the vitamin D field, since intensities of ion fragments of high mass are very low. The mass spectra of TMS ethers of 25-hydroxylated vitamin D_3 metabolites all contain a base peak at m/z 131 (the fragment obtained by side-chain cleavage, between C24 and C25, containing C26, C27, and C25-O-TMS). 26-Hydroxylation increases the mass of this peak to m/z 219 because of the presence of the extra 26-trimethylsilanol group. Use of other derivatives, such as the cyclic boronates, can, as illustrated for 24,25-$(OH)_2$-D_3, greatly enhance the intensities of higher mass fragments more suitable for use in MF analysis. Both mass spectra in Fig. 43 were obtained using the pyro peak, since formation of these derivatives does not prevent the thermal cyclization of the B ring. Other derivatives have been used in attempts to improve the mass spectral characteristics, and studies have been carried out using t-butyldimethylsilyl (t-BDMS) ether derivatives (161), which have been shown to give greatly enhanced intensity of the $(M-57)^+$ ion fragment for steroids (162). Retention time data have been obtained for these derivatives and for mixed derivatives containing the 25-trimethylsilyl ether (130).

Figure 44 illustrates the EI(+) mass spectra obtained for a mixed t-BDMS/TMSi derivatives of 25-OH-D_3 in comparison to that obtained from 25-OH-D_3 per-TMSi. One further way of enhancing high mass ions can be applied to quadrupole mass spectrometers, because they show mass discrimination and have electronic means of changing the intensity of high mass ions. Figure 44 also shows the enhancement of high-mass ions that can be achieved using a single benchtop quadrupole system for 25-OH-D_3-per-TMSi.

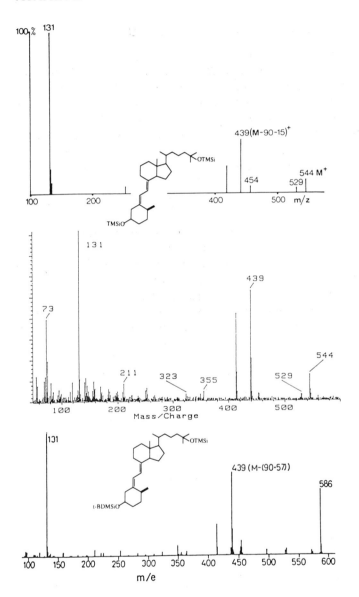

Figure 44 El(+) mass spectra obtained from 25-OH-D as (A) per-trimethylsilyl (TMS) ether on a single focusing magnetic sector GC-MS (LKB 2091), (B) per-TMS ether on a benchtop quadrupole system tuned to high mass, (C) mixed TMS ether/t-butyldimethylsilyl ether on a magnetic sector GC-MS (LKB 2091). (C) from Ref. 92.

3.6 Vitamin D Estimation in Plasma Using GC-MS

The first mass fragmentographic assay of a vitamin D metabolite in human plasma was described for 25-OH-D$_3$ using [26-^{2}H$_3$]-25-OH-D$_3$ as an internal standard (128). A brief communication (162a) did illustrate a mass fragmentograph of 25-OH-D$_3$-TMS extracted from plasma, but no quantitative data were given. Stable isotope-labeled 25-OH-D$_3$ was synthesized by the route shown in Fig. 45, and after purification a preparation containing 92% trideuterated molecules was obtained. Serum (2.5 ml) was extracted with chloroform-methanol, the 25-OH-D$_3$ fraction eluted from a LH 20 column, and the TMS derivative formed and analyzed by GC-MS using a conventional packed column (1% SE30). The ion fragments m/z 131 (for 25-OH-D$_3$) and 134 (for [^{2}H$_3$] 25-OH-D$_3$) were monitored. Because the mass fragments monitored were so low, interference was occasionally encountered, so that the m/z 131 channel was obscured and it was not possible to estimate 25-OH-D$_3$. In such cases, alternative ions could not be monitored since their intensities were too low. However, it was suggested that the 25-OH-D$_3$-TMS derivative could be resolved from the interfering substances by reducing the column temperature. A subsequent modification of this procedure was published in 1980 (92) in which the LH20 column was replaced with TLC and a mixed tBDMS/TMSi derivative was formed. This procedure has recently been used to evaluate an HPLC method for plasma

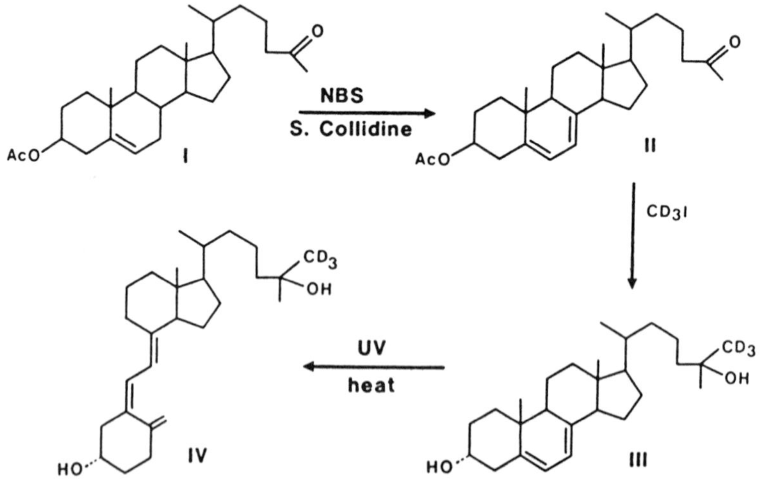

Figure 45 An outline of a typical synthetic route for the synthesis of 26-trideuterated 25-OH-D$_3$. (From Ref. 128).

25-OH-D_3 (151) and, as already mentioned, values obtained by both methods on the same plasma showed no correlation—the GC-MS values being substantially lower than those by HPLC.

De Leenheer and Cruyl (132,133) described a method for plasma D_3 in which the interfering cholesterol was removed by digitonin precipipation and D_3 was purified using Lipidex 5000. After formation of heptafluorobutyrate using heptafluorobutyric anhydride, mass fragmentography was carried out monitoring the molecular ion (M^+ = 580). Dihydrotachysterol$_2$ was used as the internal standard. A similar procedure for assaying plasma D_3 using added D_2 as an internal standard was described by Bjorkhem and Larsson (129). Cholesterol was removed by TLC and trimethylsilyl ether derivatives formed. Although the base peak was at m/z 351, $(M-90+15)^+$, it was considered better to monitor smaller peaks at m/z 325 (and m/z 337 for D_2). Again, pyro and isopyro peaks were formed during chromatography.

The first use of capillary columns in the GC-MS of vitamin D derivatives was by Zagalak et al. (125), who described a procedure for D_3 and 25-OH-D_3 in human serum. A number of deuteriated metabolites were synthesized and used as internal standards. TLC was followed by LC using different columns for 25-OH-D_3 and D_3. Trimethylsilyl ethers were formed and the pyro peaks monitored using the molecular ion (m/z 456). However, this method was not properly evaluated and no data on precision or accuracy was provided.

1,25-Dihydroxyvitamin D_3 has also been assayed (126) using GC-MS. After extraction, LH 20 chromatography, and straight-phase followed by reverse-phase LC, trimethylsilyl ethers were formed and analyzed on a packed column (1.5% SE30) monitoring the fragment m/z 131, derived from side-chain cleavage, in a similar fashion to that described previously for 25-OH-D_3 (128). This assay required 20 ml serum and used $[26\text{-}^2H_3]$-1,25-$(OH)_2$-D_3 as an internal standard. This assay, of course, requires too much plasma for use as a routine procedure. However, it does provide a valuable means of assessing other less rigorous methods of measuring what is one of the most important metabolites of vitamin D_3. Such an evaluation of the calf thymus assay (71) has been carried out (152) giving excellent correlation between the two methods and indicating that the calf thymus assay probably measures 1,25-$(OH)_2$-D reasonably accurately.

In an attempt to develop a mass fragmentographic "profile" for the major metabolites of vitamin D in plasma, a method was described (89) in which D_2, 25-OH-D_2, 25-OH-D_3, and 24,25-OH-D_3 were assayed. After extraction and Lipidex 5000 chromatography, isotachysterol isomers were formed using the HCl method of Seamark et al. (101).

Trimethylsilyl ethers were formed using TMSi and mass fragmentography was carried out, monitoring the molecular ions of each metabolite. More recent work in our laboratory has demonstrated that GC-MS can successfully be used for the measurement of all the major metabolites of vitamins D_2 and D_3. Recently, a method for measuring 25-OH-D_2, 25-OH-D_3, 24,25-$(OH)_2$-D_2, and 25,26-$(OH)_2$-D_2 in a single sample of plasma has been described by our laboratory (163), and this method has been used to measure these metabolites in people taking D_2 (164). Similar procedures for the measurement of metabolites of vitamin D_3 have also been described (155,156,165). These methods are all based on the scheme outlined in Fig. 46 and use trimethylsilyl ether derivatives for

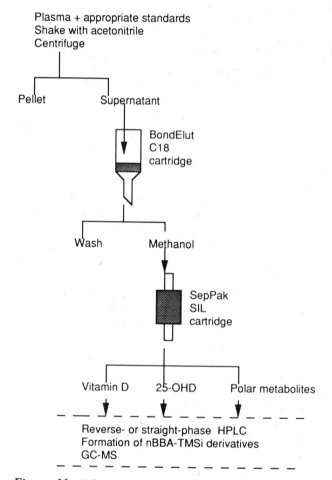

Figure 46 Scheme for extraction of vitamin D and its metabolites from plasma prior to GC-MS.

GC-MS or, in the case of metabolites with vicinal hydroxyl groups on the side chain, mixed trimethylsilyl ether-cyclic n-butyl boronate derivatives. Mass fragmentographic procedures require standard material both labeled, as internal standards, and unlabeled, for quantitation, and there is a dearth of such material available. It is sometimes possible to overcome the lack of a suitable internal standard by judicious use of another labeled metabolite. For example, in the method described above for metabolites of vitamin D_2, deuteriated 25-OH-D_3 was used as an internal standard for the measurement of both 25-OH-D_2 and 25-OH-D_3 and deuteriated 24,25-(OH)$_2D_3$ as an internal standard for the measurement of 24,25-(OH)$_2D_2$. Such procedures, while necessary, are not entirely satisfactory, particularly when labeled vitamin D_2 metabolites are used as standards for the measurement of metabolites of vitamin D_3 or vice versa. Vitamins D_2 and D_3 have very different chemical properties, the D_2 series being much more labile, and thus if inappropriate standards are used, analytical values may be over- or underestimated.

So far no satisfactory method for the measurement of 1,25-(OH)$_2$-D that uses reasonable volumes of plasma has been described. Indeed, only one fully evaluated method (126) has been described, which used 20 ml of plasma, a volume that makes this difficult to carry out. It may be possible using better mass spectrometers, particularly quadrupole systems tuned to high mass and capillary GC, to improve sensitivity and thus reduce the volume of plasma required for assay. Figure 47 illustrates the

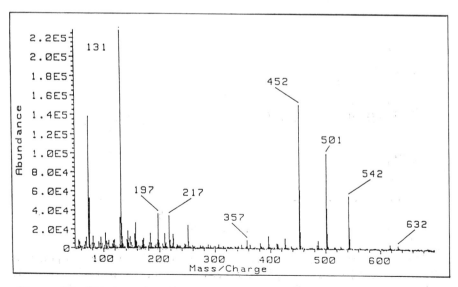

Figure 47   El(+) mass spectrum of the per-TMS ether derivative of 1,25-(OH)$_2$-D$_3$ on a benchtop quadrupole system, tuned to high mass.

mass spectrum of the per-trimethylsilyl ether derivative of $1\alpha,25$-$(OH)_2$-D_3 obtained by such a quadrupole system (Hewlett-Packard GC-MSD, model 5970). Even though the system is tuned to high mass, the intensity of the molecular ion (m/z 632) is still very low, and GC-MS methods that monitor this ion have low sensitivity and cannot be used to measure the concentration of this analyte in human plasma without the use of unacceptably large volumes of sample. However, monitoring the $(M$-90-$90)^+$ ion in the "high-tune" mode has given sufficient sensitivity to enable 15 pg of injected standard $1\alpha,25$-$(OH)_2$-D_3-TMSi to be seen easily (Fig. 48). However, the analysis of plasma/serum is more difficult, and nonspecific interference reduces the signal to noise ratio and the sensitivity achieved with standard material is not achieved with such biological samples. A further area that might prove fruitful in this regard is the use of chemical ionization mass spectrometry monitoring negative ions $[CI(-)]$. This requires the formation of suitable electron-capturing

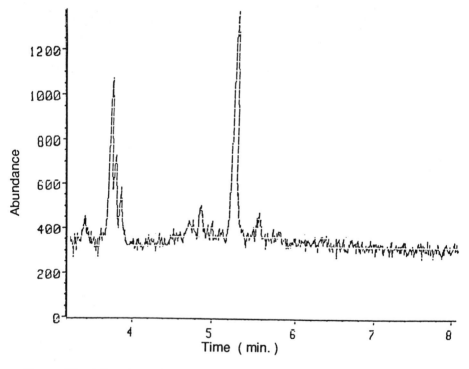

Figure 48   Selected ion monitoring of the $(M$-90-$90)^+$ ion (m/z 452) produced from 15 pg 1,25-$(OH)_2$-D_3 per-TMS derivative using a capillary GC and the Hewlett-Packard model 5970 mass selective detector (by courtesy of Dr. Ruth Coldwell).

derivatives with good GC properties, which retain the negative ion during mass spectrometry. So far no such procedure has been described, though as noted earlier CI(+) and CI(−) MS has been used for the identification of vitamin D metabolites formed *in vivo* (e.g., 166–168).

The mass fragmentographic assays so far developed are summarized in Table 4, which gives details of those methods already described above and the more recent ones developed by our laboratory. Normal values obtained using methods published since 1980 are given in Table 5. Details of values obtained prior to 1980 and more information than is given here can be obtained from a number of reviews (6,114,173–175).

3.7 *In Vitro* Studies Using GC-MS

Apart from the use of GC-MS for the analysis of plasma levels of vitamin D and its metabolites, Bjorkhem's group have made use of mass fragmentography in their numerous studies of *in vitro* metabolism. Early investigators examined the properties of mitochondrial (17,176,177) and microsomal (178,179,181,182) 25-hydroxylase enzyme systems. In these studies, previous published procedures were slightly modified and GC-MS methods were developed that used the mixed *t*-butyldimethylsilyl/trimethylsilyl derivatives discussed earlier in this chapter. Mass fragmentography of the trimethylsilyl ether of putative 23,25-dihydroxyvitamin D_3, formed *in vivo* in 1,25-$(OH)_2$-D_3-treated guinea pigs, proved to be of value in identification when a standard mass spectrum was not adequate (183). Further examples of the use of GC-MS in studies of vitamin D metabolizing enzymes *in vitro* are given in Table 6.

3.8 Synthesis of Deuteriated Standards

It is clear that the best mass fragmentographic methods utilize stable isotope-labeled analogues as internal standards (isotope dilution mass spectrometry, IDMS). Such internal standards dispense with the need for chemical analogues, which may not behave in the same way as the analyte in the purification procedures prior to GC-MS, and with tritiated standards and the attendant need for liquid scintillation counting. However, deuteriated standards are not widely available for most of the metabolites of vitamin D, and it may be necessary to use a deuteriated standard of one metabolite for the measurement of another (see 163). Table 7 summarizes some of the deuteriated standards of vitamin D metabolites that have been synthesized and used in mass fragmentographic analyses for vitamin D and its metabolites. However, it should not be assumed that stable isotope-labeled standards always behave the same way as unlabeled standards, since it is possible that labeled and unlabeled metabolites can separate in some chromatographic systems, and

Table 4   GC-MS Methods for the Analysis of Vitamin D and Its Metabolites in Human Plasma/Serum

Analyte	Derivative used for GC	Type of GC column[a]	Internal standard	Ion monitored	Reference
D_3	ITS-HFB	1% FFAP	DHT_2	M^+	133
	TMS	1.5% SE30	D_2	$(M-131)^+$	129,169
	TMS	2% OV1	D_2	M^+ and $(M-90)^+$	89
25-OH-D_3	TMS	1.5% SE30	$[26-^2H_3]$-25-OH-D_3	m/z 131, side-chain fragment	128
	TMS/tBDMS	1.5% SE30	$[26-^2H_3]$-25-OH-D_3	M^+	92
	TMS	2% OV1	D_2	M^+	89
	TMS	2% OV1	$[26,27-^2H_6]$-25-OH-D	$(M-90-15)^+$	163–165
25-OH-D_2	TMS	2% OV1	$[26,27-^2H_6]$-25-OH-D_3	$(M-90-15)^+$	163–165
	TMS	2% OV1	D_2	M^+	89
24,25-$(OH)_2$-D_3	TMS-nBBA	2% OV1	$[26,27-^2H_6]$-24,25-(OH)-D_3	$(M-90-15)^+$	155,164
24,25-$(OH)_2$-D_2	TMS-nBBA	2% OV1	$[28-^2H_5]$-24,25-$(OH)_2$-D_2	$(M-90-15)^+$	163–165
25,26-$(OH)_2$-D_3	TMS-nBBA	2% OV1	$[26,27-^2H_5]$-25,26-$(OH)_2$-D_3	$(M-90-15)^+$	156
1,25-$(OH)_2$-D_3	TMS	Superox 4[1]	$[26-^2H_3]$-1,25-$(OH)_2$-D_3	$(M-90)^+$	152
	TMS	SE30[2]	$[26-^2H_3]$-1,25-$(OH)_2$-D_3	$(M-90)^+$	126

[a] All methods use conventional packed columns (0.4 cm ID) except [1], which uses a WCOT capillary column (see Table 2), and [2], which used a conventional packed column but with smaller ID (0.2 cm). TMS = per-trimethylsilyl ether, tBDMS = tertiary-butyldimethylsilyl ether, nBBA = n-butylboronate.

injudicious selection of HPLC fractions can cause problems. Nonlabeled standards are of course a prerequisite for accurate GC-MS analyses, and many such standards are not readily available. Small quantities have been donated to us from several sources, for which we are extremely grateful. The continuing provision of both labeled and unlabeled

Table 5 Concentrations of Vitamin D Metabolites Measured by Mass
Fragmentography in Human Plasma/Serum and Urine (Published Since 1980) [a]

Analyte	Extraction and purification	Reference	Normal values
D_2	Methanol-methylene dichloride, hexane (esters), alumina, digitonin-celite-water	170	136 ng/ml in urine (268 ng/ml after enzyme hydrolysis)
D_3	column, and SP- and RP-HPLC		4.5 ± 5.3 ng/ml serum 120 ng/ml in urine after enzyme hydrolysis
25-OH-D_3			21.4 ± 5.3 ng/ml serum
24,25-$(OH)_2$-D_3	Acetonitrile, Sep-Pak C18, Sep-Pak SIL, SP-HPLC	155	1.6 ± 0.6 ng/ml plasma (in UK summer) 3.1 ± 1.3 ng/ml (Australian winter)
25,26-$(OH)_2$-D_3	Acetonitrile, Sep-Pak C18, Sep-Pak SIL, SP-HPLC	156	Mean: 0.39 ng/ml (UK) Range: 0.05–0.8 ng/ml Mean: 0.76 ng/ml (Australia) Range: 0.3–1.3 ng/ml
25-OH-D_2	Acetonitrile, Bond-Elut C18, Sep-Pak SIL,	163	0.12–6.6 ng/ml
25-OH-D_3	SP-HPLC		2.3–32.6 ng/ml
24,25-$(OH)_2$-D_2			ND (normals), 4.1–29.5 ng/ml (in patients on D_2)
25,26-$(OH)_2$-D_2			ND (normals), 0.85–2.11 (in patients on D_2)
25-OH-D_3	Sodium carbonate/ ethyl acetate, t-BMDS/ TMS formation, TLC	171 172	15.3 ± 1.6 (SD) ng/ml 19.2 ± 2.0 (SD) ng/ml (Sweden)

[a] Methods published prior to 1980 have been reviewed in Refs. 6, 114, and 173–175. ND = not detectable. TMS = per-trimethylsilyl ether. t-BDMS = t-butyldimethysilyl ether.

Table 6 Mass Fragmentographic Methodology used for *In Vitro* Studies of Vitamin D-Metabolizing Enzymes

Tissue used	Method[a]	Reference
D₃-25-hydroxylase		
Rat liver mitochondria	1	176.
Rat liver mitochondria and microsomes[b]	1 and 2	177
Reconstituted system from rat liver microsomes	1	179
Reconstituted system from rat liver mitochondria cytochrome p450	1	17
Uptake of vitamin D₃ and metabolism in isolated hepatocytes	1 and 3	180
Cytochrome P-450 from rat liver microsomes	1	178,181
Inhibition by a protein fraction from liver microsomes	1	182
Difference in hydroxylation of vitamins D₂ and D₃	1	184,185
25-OHD₃-24-hydroxylase		
In rat kidney mitochondria	4	186
25-OHD₃-1-hydroxylase		
Assay in pig kidney mitochondria	2	187
Assay and properties in guinea pig kidney	2	188
Variation during development and pregnancy in guinea pig kidney	2	189
Simulatory effect of testosterone in guinea pig kidney	2	190

[a] Methods:

1. As described in Ref. 92 using mixed t-butyldimethylsilyl/trimethylsilyl derivative of 25-OHD₃, monitoring the molecular ions of the analyte (m/z 586) and trideuteriated internal standard (m/z 589).
2. As described in Ref. 126 using trimethylsilyl ether derivative of 1,25-dihydroxyvitamin D₃ and monitoring $(M-90-90)^+$ ions using a trideuteriated internal standard.
3. As described in Ref. 169 using trimethylsilyl ether derivative of vitamin D₃ and monitoring $(M-131)^+$ but using a heptadeuteriated internal standard.
4. As described in Ref. 186 using trimethylsilyl ether derivative of 24,25-dihydroxyvitamin D₃ and monitoring m/z 131 and m/z 134 (for trideuteriated internal standard).

[b] Also studied 1α-hydroxyvitamin D₃-25-hydroxylase (method 2).

Table 7 Synthesis of Some Deuteriated Analogues of Various Vitamin D Metabolites for Use as Internal Standards during Mass Fragmentography

Metabolite	Carbon atom on which ^{2}H attached	Number of ^{2}H molecules per mole	Reference
D_3	3,4	2	125
D_3	2,3,4,6	6	125
D_3	26	3	191
D_3	26,27	6	192
25-OH-D_3^a	26	3	125,128,175,191
25-OH-D_3	26,27	6	192
1,25-$(OH)_2$-D_3	26	3	125,126,174,[a]187,191
24,25-$(OH)_2$-D_3	26	3	186,[a]191
24,25-$(OH)_2$-D_3	26,27	6	192
25,26-$(OH)_2$-D_3	26	3	191
25,26-$(OH)_2$-D_3	25,26	5	156
1,24,25-$(OH)_3$-D_3	26	3	191
24,25-$(OH)_2$-D_2	28	3	174

[a] Deuteriated 24,25-$(OH)_2$-D_3 and 1,25-$(OH)_2$-D_3 were generated from deuteriated 25-OH-D_3 by incubation with kidney preparation preparations in vitro (refs. 174 and 186). Synthesis and use of deuteriated vitamin D metabolites in mass fragmentography has been reviewed in Ref. 174.

material is essential to allow further development of GC-MS methodology. GC-MS methods for vitamin D metabolites provide definitive procedures against which the specificity of many of the commonly used competitive binding, radioreceptor, and radioimmunoassays can be assessed. Such assessments have been carried out by Bjorkhem's group, evaluating an HPLC method for 25-OH-D3 (193), the calf thymus receptor assay for 1,25-(OH)2-D3 (71), and two commercial kits and an HPLC method for 25-OH-D3 (152). Two other HPLC methods for 25-OH-D3 have also been evaluated with reference to GC-MS (194). Future quality assurance procedures for vitamin D metabolite assay methods will need GC-MS target values.

ACKNOWLEDGMENTS

Some of the work described in this chapter was supported by grants from the Medical Research Council of Canada (G.J.), the Medical Research Council (UK) (H.L.J.M. and D.J.H.T.), and the Wellcome Trust (H.L.J.M.).

REFERENCES

1. J. W. Blunt, H. F. DeLuca, and H. F. Schnoes, *Biochemistry*, 7:3317 (1968).
2. H. F. DeLuca, *FASEB J.*, 2:224 (1988).
3. M. R. Haussler, *Annu. Rev. Nutr.*, 6: 527 (1986).
4. A. W. Norman, J. Roth, and L. Orci, *Endocrinol. Rev.*, 3:331 (1982).
5. H. L. Henry and A. W. Norman, *Annu. Rev. Nutr.*, 4:493 (1984).
6. C. E. Porteous, R. D. Coldwell, D. J. H. Trafford, and H. L. J. Makin, *J. Steroid Biochem.*, 28:785 (1987).
7. E. Havinga, *Experientia*, 29:1181 (1973).
8. W. G. Salmond, in *Vitamin D: Basic Research and Its Clinical Application* (A. W. Norman, K. Schaefer, D. V. Herrath, H.-G. Grigoleit, J. W. Coburn, H. F. DeLuca, E. B. Mawer, and T. Suda, eds.), Walter de Gruyter, Berlin, p. 25. (1979).
9. S. J. Shiuey, J. J. Partridge, and M. R. Uskokovic, *J. Org. Chem.*, 53:1040 (1988).
10. S. Yamada, M. Ohmori, and H. Takayama, *Tetrahedron Lett.*, 21:1859 (1979).
11. Y. Kobayashi, T. Taguchi, N. Kanuma, N. Ikekawa, and J.-I. Oschide, *J. Chem. Soc. Chem. Commun.*, 10:459 (1980).
12. M. J. Calverley, *Tetrahedron*, 43:4609 (1987).
13. M. F. Holick, N. M., Richtand, S. C., McNeill, S. A. Holick, J. E. Frommer, J. W. Henley, and J. T. Potts, *Biochemistry*, 18:1003 (1979).
14. G. Ponchon and H. F. DeLuca, *J. Clin. Invest.*, 48:1273 (1969).
14A. M. Horsting and H. F. DeLuca, *Biochem. Biophys. Res. Commun.*, 36:251 (1969).
15. M. H. Bhattacharyya and H. F. DeLuca, *Arch. Biochem. Biophys.*, 160:58 (1974).
16. T. Suda, N. Horiuchi, M. Fukushima, Y. Nishii, and E. Ogata, in *Vitamin D: Biochemical, Chemical and Clinical Aspects Related to Calcium Metabolism* (A. W. Norman, K. Schaefer, J. W. Coburn, H. F. DeLuca, D. Fraser, H.-G. Grigoleit, and D. V. Herrath, eds.), Walter de Gruyter, Berlin, p. 201 (1977).
17. I. Bjorkhem, I. Holmberg, H. Oftebro, and J. I. Pedersen, *J. Biol. Chem.*, 255:5244 (1980).
18. D. E. M. Lawson, D. R. Fraser, E. Kodicek, H. R. Morris, and D. H. Williams, *Nature*, 230:228 (1971).
19. M. F. Holick, H. K. Schnoes, and H. F. DeLuca, *Proc. Natl. Acad. Sci. USA*, 68:803 (1971).
20. M. F. Holick, H. K. Schnoes, H. F. DeLuca, R. W. Gray, I. T. Boyle, and T. Suda, *Biochemistry*, 11:4251 (1973).
21. J. C. Knutson and H. F. DeLuca, *Biochemistry*, 13:1543 (1974).
22. J. F. Myrtle and A. W. Norman, *Science*, 171:79 (1971).
23. M. R. Haussler, D. W. Boyce, E. T. Littledike, and H. Rasmussen, *Proc. Natl. Acad. Sci. USA*, 68:177 (1971).
24. T. C. Chen, L. Castillo, M. Korycka-Dahl, and H. F. DeLuca, *J. Nutr.*, 104:1056 (1974).

25. Y. Tanaka and H. F. DeLuca, *Arch. Biochem. Biophys.*, *146*:574 (1971).
26. C. Miyaura, E. Abe, T. Kuribayaski, H. Tanaka, K. Konno, Y. Nishii, and T. Suda, *Biochem. Biophys. Res. Commun.*, *102*:937 (1981).
27. E. Abe, C. Miyaura, H. Sakagami, M., Takeda, K. Konno, T. Yamazaki, S. Yoshiki, and T. Suda, *Proc. Natl. Acad. Sci. USA*, *78*:4990 (1981).
28. E. Abe, C. Miyaura, H. Tanaka, Y. Shiina, T. Kuribayashi, T. Suda, Y. Nishii, H. F. DeLuca, and T. Suda, *Proc. Natl. Acad. Sci. USA*, *80*:5583 (1983).
29. D. R. Fraser and E. Kodicek, *Nature*, *228*:764 (1970).
30. U. Trechsel, J. A. Eisman, J. A. Fischer, J. P. Bonjour, and H. Fleisch, *Am. J. Physiol.*, *239*:E119 (1980).
31. Y. Tanaka and H. F. DeLuca, *Arch. Biochem. Biophys.*, *154*:566 (1973).
32. M. Garabedian, M. F. Holick, H. F. DeLuca, and I. T. Boyle, *Proc. Natl. Acad. Sci. USA*, *69*:1673 (1972).
33. R. W. Gray, J. L. Omdahl, J. G. Ghazarian, and H. F. DeLuca, *J. Biol. Chem.*, *247*:7528 (1972).
34. Y. Tanaka and H. F. DeLuca, *Science*, *183*:1198 (1974).
35. P. Bordier, H. Rasmussen, P. Marie, L. Miravet, J. Gueris, and A. Ryckwart, *J. Clin. Endocrinol. Metab.*, *46*:284 (1978).
36. D. Goodwin, D. Noff, and S. Edelstein, *Nature*, *276*:517 (1978).
37. R. Brommage, K. Jarnagin, H. F. DeLuca, S. Yamada, and H. Takayama, *Am. J. Physiol.* *244*:E298 (1983).
38. T. Suda, H. K. Schnoes, H. F. DeLuca, and J. W. Blunt, *Biochemistry*, *8*:3515 (1969).
39. G. Jones, H. K. Schnoes, and H. F. DeLuca, *Biochemistry*, *14*:1250 (1975).
40. G. Jones, A. Rosenthal, D. Segev, Y. Mazur, F. Frolow, Y. Halfon, D. Rabinovich, and Z. Shakked, *Biochemistry*, *18*:1094 (1979).
41. I. Holmberg, *Biochim. Biophys. Acta*, *800*:106 (1984).
42. I. Holmberg, T. Berlin, S. Ewerth, and I. Bjorkhem, *Scand. J. Clin. Lab. Invest.*, *46*:785 (1986).
43. N. J. Koszewski, T. A. Reinhardt, J. L. Napoli, D. C. Beitz, and R. L. Horst, *Biochemistry-USA*, *27*:5785 (1988).
44. M. F. Holick, A. Kleiner-Bossaller, H. K. Schnoes, P. M. Kasten, I. T. Boyle, and H. F. DeLuca, *J. Biol. Chem*, *248*:6691 (1973).
45. G. Jones, M. Kung, and K. Kano, *J. Biol. Chem.*, *258*:12920 (1983).
46. D. Lohnes and G. Jones, *J. Biol. Chem.*, *262*:14394 (1987).
47. G. Makin, D. Lohnes, V. Byford, R. Ray, and G. Jones, *Biochem. J.*, *262*:173 (1989).
48. D. Harnden, R. Kumar, M. F. Holick, and H. F. DeLuca, *Science*, *193*:493 (1976).
49. R. P. Esvelt, H. F. Schnoes, and H. F. DeLuca, *Biochemistry*, *18*:3977 (1979).
50. H. F. DeLuca, and H. K. Schnoes, in *Vitamin D: Basic Research and Its Clinical Application* (A. W. Norman, K. Schaefer, D. V. Herrath, H.-G. Grigoleit, J. W. Coburn, H. F. DeLuca, E. B. Mawer, and T. Suda, eds.), Walter de Gruyter, Berlin, p. 445, (1979).

51. J. K. Wichman, H. F. DeLuca, H. K. Schnoes, R. L. Horst, R. M. Shepard, and N. A. Jorgensen, *Biochemistry*, *18*:4775 (1979).
52. J. J. Partridge, S.-J. Shiney, N. K. Chadha, E. G. Baggiolini, J. F. Blount, and M. R. Uskokovic, *J. Am. Chem. Soc.*, *103*:1253 (1981).
53. Y. Tanaka, H. K. Schnoes, C. M. Smith, and H. F. DeLuca, *Arch. Biochem. Biophys.*, *210*:104, (1981).
54. N. Ohnuma, K. Bannai, H. Yamaguchi, Y. Hashimoto, and A. W. Norman, *Arch. Biochem. Biophys.*, *204*:387 (1980).
55. G. Jones, H. K. Schnoes, L. Levan, and H. F. DeLuca, *Arch. Biochem. Biophys.*, *202*:450 (1980).
56. R. L. Horst, E. T. Littledike, J. L. Riley, and J. L. Napoli, *Anal. Biochem. 116*:189 (1981).
57. N. LeBoulch, C. Gulat-Marney, and Y. Raoul, *J. Vitamin Nutr. Res.*, *44*:167 (1974).
58. R. Kumar, S. Nagubandi, I. Jardine, J. Landowski, and S. Bollman, *Am. Soc. Bone Mineral Res. Abstr.* 51A (1981).
59. E. G. Bligh and W. J. Dyer, *Can. J. Biochem.*, *37*:911 (1957).
60. P. W. Lambert, P. B. DeOreo, B. W. Hollis, I. Y. Fu, D. J. Grinsberg, and B. A. Roos, *J. Lab. Clin. Med.*, *98*:536 (1981).
61. R. Bouillon, P. DeMoor, E. G. Baggiolini, and M. R. Uskokovic, *Clin. Chem.*, *26*:562 (1980).
62. M. T. Parviainen, K. E. Savolainen, P. H. Korhonen, E. M. Alhava, and J. K. Visakorpi, *Clin. Chim. Acta*, *114*:233 (1981).
63. R. Belsey, H. F. DeLuca, and J. T. Potts, *J. Clin. Endocrinol. Metab.*, *33*:554 (1971).
64. J. N. Thompson, G. Hatina, W. B. Maxwell, and S. Duval, *J. Assoc. Off. Anal. Chem.*, *65*:624 (1982).
65. E. E. Delvin, M. Dussault, and F. H. Glorieux, *Clin. Biochem.*, *13*:106 (1980).
66. J. T. Dabek, M. Harkonen, O. Wahlroos, and H. Adlercreutz, *Clin. Chem.*, *27*:1346 (1981).
67. J. A. Eisman, A. J. Hamstra, B. E. Kream, and H. F. DeLuca, *Science*, *193*:1021 (1976).
68. R. S. Mason, D. Lissner, C. Reek, and S. Posen, in *Vitamin D: Basic Research and Its Clinical Application* (A. W. Norman, K. Schaefer, D. V. Herrath, H.-G. Grigoleit, J. W. Coburn, H. F. DeLuca, E. B. Mawer, and T. Suda, eds.), Walter de Gruyter, Berlin, p. 243 (1979).
69. R. E. Belsey, H. F. DeLuca, and J. T. Potts, *J. Clin. Endocrinol. Metab.* *38*:1046 (1974).
70. N. J. M. Jongen, W. J. F. Van der Vijgh, H. J. J. Willems, and J. C. Netelenbos, *Clin. Chem.*, *27*:444 (1981).
71. T. A. Reinhardt, R. L. Horst, J. W. Orf, and B. W. Hollis, *J. Clin. Endocrinol. Metab.*, *58*:91 (1984).
72. B. W. Hollis, *Clin. Chem.*, *32*:2060 (1986).
73. K. T. Koshy and A. L. Vanderslik, *Anal. Biochem.*, *74*:282 (1976).
74. T. J. Gilbertson and R. P. Stryd, *Clin. Chem.*, *23*:1700 (1977).
75. K. T. Koshy, *Methods Enzymol.*, *67*:357 (1980).

76. B. W. Hollis, and B. A. Roos, H. H. Draper, and P. W. Lambert, *J. Nutr.*, *111*:384 (1981).

77. J. S. Adams, T. Clemens, and M. F. Holick, *J. Chromatogr.*, *226*:198 (1981).

78. A. A. Rhedwi, D. C. Anderson, and G. N. Smith, *Steroids*, *39*:149 (1982).

79. B. W. Hollis, and N. E. Frank, *J. Chromatogr.*, *343*:43 (1985).

80. H. Turnbull, D. J. H. Trafford, and H. L. J. Makin, *Clin. Chim. Acta*, *120*:65 (1982).

81. L. J. Fraher, G. Jones, T. L. Clemens, S. Adami, and J. L. H. O'Riordan, *Acta Endocrinol.* 97(Suppl. 243), abstr. 8 (1981).

82. B. W. Hollis and T. Kilbo, in *Vitamin D: Molecular, Cellular and Clinical Endocrinology* (A. W. Norman and K. Schaffer, eds.), Walter de Gruyter, Berlin, p. 710, (1988).

83. M. J. M. Jongen, W. J. F. van der Vijgh, P. Lips, and S. C. Netelenbos, *Nephron*, *36*:230 (1984).

84. M. F. Holick and H. F. DeLuca, *J. Lipid Res.*, *12*:460 (1971).

85. J. N. Ellingboe, E. Nystrom, and J. Sjovall, *J. Lipid Res.*, *11*: 266 (1970).

86. J. N. Thompson, W. B. Maxwell, and M. L'Abbe, *J. Assoc. Off. Anal. Chem.*, *60*:998 (1977).

87. R. M. Shepard, R. L. Horst, A. J. Hamstra, and H. F. DeLuca, *Biochem. J.*, *182*:55 (1979).

88. D. Sklan, P. Budowski, and M. Katz, *Anal. Biochem.*, *56*:606 (1978).

89. D. A. Seamark, D. J. H. Trafford, and H. L. J. Makin, *Clin. Chim. Acta*, *106*:51 (1980).

90. V. Justova and L. Starka, *J. Chromatogr.*, *209*:337 (1981).

91. R. Vieth, D. Fraser, and G. Jones, *Anal. Chem.*, *50*:2150 (1978).

92. I. Bjorkhem and I. Holmberg, *Methods Enzymol.*, *67*:385 (1980).

93. S. Dueland, I. Holmberg, T. Berg, and J. I. Pedersen, *J. Biol. Chem.*, *256*:10430 (1981).

94. M. Thierry-Palmer and T. K. Gray, *J. Chromatogr.*, *262*:460 (1983).

95. S. J. Gaskell and B. G. Brownsey, *Clin. Chem.*, *29*:677 (1983).

96. R. Bouillon, E. van Herck, I. Jans, B. Keng Tan, H. van Baelan, P. DeMoor, *Clin. Chem.*, *30*:1731 (1984).

97. V. Justova, Z. Wildtova, and V. Pacovsky, *Endocrinol. Exp.* *18*:241 (1984).

98. G. Jones, *Clin. Chem.*, *24*:287 (1978).

99. T. Okano, N. Mizuno, S. Shida, N. Takahashi, T. Kobayashi, E. Kuroda, S. Kodama, and T. Matsuo, *J. Nutr. Sci. Vitaminol*, 27:43 (1981).

100. D. J. H. Trafford, D. A. Seamark, H. Turnbull, and H. L. J. Makin, *J. Chromatogr.*, *226*:351 (1981).

101. D. A. Seamark, D. J. H. Trafford, and H. L. J. Makin, *J. Steroid Biochem.*, *13*:1057 (1980).

102. G. Jones and H. F. DeLuca, *J. Lipid Res.*, *16*:448 (1975).

103. G. Jones, *J. Chromatogr. Biomed. Applic.*, *221*:27 (1980).

104. N. Ikekawa and N. Koizumi, *J. Chromatogr.*, *119*:227 (1976).

105. R. L. Horst, *Biochem. Biophys. Res. Commun.*, *89*:286 (1979).

106. E. W. Matthews, P. G. H. Byfield, K. W. Colston, I. M. A. Evans, L. S. Galante, and I. MacIntryre, *FEBS Lett.*, *48*:122 (1974).

107. A. M. Rosenthal, G. Jones, S. W. Kooh, and D. Fraser, *Am. J. Physiol.*, 239:E12 (1980).
108. J. Cunningham, R. D. Coldwell, G. Jones, H. S. Tenenhouse, D. J. H. Trafford, and H. L. J. Makin, *J. Bone Miner. Res.* 5:173 (1990).
109. G. Jones, N. Edwards, D. Vriezen, C. Porteous, D. J. H. Trafford, J. Cunningham, and H. L. J. Makin, *Biochemistry*, 27:7070 (1988).
110. D. A. Seamark, D. J. H. Trafford, P. G. Hiscocks, and H. L. J. Makin, *J. Chromatogr.*, 197:271 (1980).
111. J. C. Miller, S. A. George, and B. G. Willis, *Science*, 218:241 (1982).
112. G. Jones, K. Kano, S. Yamada, T. Furusawa, H. Takayama, and T. Suda, *Biochemistry*, 23:3749 (1984).
113. R. D. Coldwell, C. E. Porteous, D. J. H. Trafford, and H. L. J. Makin, *Steroids*, 49:155 (1987).
114. D. A. Seamark, D. J. H. Trafford, and H. L. J. Makin, *J. Steroid Biochem.*, 14:111 (1981).
115. T. L. Clemens, G. N. Hendry, R. F. Graham, E. G. Baggiolini, M. R. Uskokovia, and J. L. H. O'Riordan, *Clin. Sci. Mol. Med.*, 54:329 (1978).
116. B. E. Dreyer, and D. B. P. Goodman, *Anal. Biochem.*, 114:37 (1981).
117. E. deVries, F. J. Mulder, and B. Borsje, *J. Assoc. Off. Anal. Chem.*, 64:61 (1981).
118. B. W. Hollis and N. E. Frank, *Methods Enzymol.*, 123:167 (1986).
119. F. Askew, R. B. Bourdillon, H. M. Bruce, R. K. Callow, J. Philpot, and T. A. Webster, *Proc. R. Soc., Ser. B*, 107:76 (1932).
120. B. Pelc and D. H. Marshall, *Steroids*, 31:23 (1978).
121. P. P. Nair, C. Bucana, S. DeLeon, and D. A. Yruner, *Anal. Chem.*, 37:631 (1965)
122. P. P. Nair and S. DeLeon, *Arch. Biochem. Biophys.*, 128:663 (1968).
123. H. Ziffer, W. J. A. Vanden Heuvel, E. O. A. Haahti, and E. C. Horning, *J. Am. Chem. Soc.*, 82:6411 (1960).
124. H. L. J. Makin and D. J. H. Trafford, in *Methodological Surveys in Biochemistry*, vol. 7 (E. Reid, ed.), Ellis Horwood, Chichester, p. 312, (1978).
125. B. Zagalak, H. D. L. Curtius, R. Foschi, G. Wipf, V. Redweik, and M. J. Zagalak, *Experientia*, 34:1537 (1978).
126. I. Bjorkhem, I. Holmberg, T. Kristiansen, and J. L. Pedersen, *Clin. Chem.* 25:584 (1979).
127. J. M. Halket and B. P. Lisboa, *Acta Endocrinol. (Kbh.)*, 87 (Suppl. 251):120 (1978).
128. I. Bjorkhem and I. Holmberg, *Clin. Chim. Acta*, 68:215 (1976).
129. I. Bjorkhem and A. Larsson, *Clin. Chim. Acta*, 88:559 (1978).
130. B. P. Lisboa and J. M. Halket, in *Recent Developments in Chromatography and Electrophoresis* (A. Frigerio and L. Renoz, eds.), pp. 141–162 (1979).
131. T. Kobayashi and A. Adachi, *J. Nutr. Sci. Vitaminol. (Tokyo)*, 19:311 (1973).
132. A. P. DeLeenheer and A. A. M. Cruyl, in *Quantitative Mass Spectrometry in Life Sciences* (A. P. DeLeenheer and R. R. Roncucci, eds.), Elsevier, Amsterdam, p. 165 (1977).

133. A. P. DeLeenheer and A. A. M. Cruyl, *Anal. Biochem.*, 91:293 (1978).
134. H. H. Inhoffen, K. Bruckner, and R. Grundel, *Chem. Bericht.*, 87:1 (1954).
135. T. K. Murray, K. C. Day, and E. Kodicek, *Biochem. J.*, 98:293 (1966).
136. T. Kobayashi and A. Adachi, *J. Nutr. Sci. Vitaminol. (Tokyo)*, 19:303 (1973).
137. V. K. Argarwal, *J. Steroid Biochem.*, 35:149 (1990).
138. A. P. DeLeenheer and A. A. M. Cruyl, *Methods Enzymol.*, 67:335 (1980).
139. A. P. DeLeenheer and A. A. M. Cruyl, *J. Chromatogr. Sci.*, 14:434 (1976).
140. J. M. Halket and B. P. Lisboa, in *Recent Developments in Mass Spectrometry in Biochemistry and Medicine*, vol. 1 (A. Frigerio, ed.), Plenum Publishing, New York, p. 457 (1978).
141. T. K. Murray, P. Erdody, and T. Panalaks, *J. Assoc. Off. Anal. Chem.*, 51:839 (1968).
142. D. O. Edlund, *Methods Enzymol.*, 67:343 (1980).
143. T. Kobayashi, *Methods Enzymol.*, 67:347 (1980).
144. D. Sklan, *Methods Enzymol.*, 67:355 (1980).
145. P. W. Wilson, D. E. M. Lawson, and E. J. Kodicek, *J. Chromatogr.*, 39:75 (1969).
146. V. Trechsel, J. A. Eisman, J. A. Fischer, J. P. Bonjour, and H. Fleishch, *Am. J. Physiol.*, 239:E119 (1980).
147. N. Ohnuma, K. Bannai, H. Yamaguchi, Y. Hashimoto, and A. W. Norman, *Arch. Biochem. Biophys.*, 204:387 (1980).
148. L. W. LeVan, H. K. Schnoes, and H. F. DeLuca, *Biochemistry*, 20:222 (1981).
149. Y. Takasaki, T. Suda, S. Yamada, H. Takayama, and Y. Nishii, *Biochemistry*, 20:1681 (1981).
150. T. A. Reinhardt, J. L. Napoli, D. C. Beitz, E. T. Littledike, and R. L. Horst, *Biochem. Biophys. Res. Commun.*, 99:302 (1981).
151. I. Holmberg, T. Kristiansen, and M. Sturen, *Scand. J. Clin. Lab. Invest.*, 44:275 (1984).
152. H. Oftebrow, J. A. Falch, I. Holmberg, and E. Hang, *Clin. Chim. Acta*, 176:157 (1988).
153. C. H. L. Shackleton, E. Roitman, and J. J. Whitney, *J. Steroid Biochem.*, 12:521 (1980).
154. T. Okano, K. Mizuno, N. Matsuyama, N. Nobuhara, and T. Kobayashi, *Rec. Trav Chim. Pays-Bas*, 98:253 (1979).
155. R. D. Coldwell, D. J. H. Trafford, H. L. J. Makin, M. J. Varley, and D. N. Kirk, *Clin. Chem.*, 30:1193 (1984).
156. R. D. Coldwell, D. J. H. Trafford, H. L. J. Makin, M. J. Varley, and D. N. Kirk, *J. Chromatogr. Biomed. Appl.*, 338:289 (1984).
157. C. J. W. Brooks and B. S. Middleditch, *Clin. Chim. Acta*, 34:145 (1971).
158. C. J. W. Brooks and D. J. Harvey, *J. Chromatogr.*, 54:193 (1971).
159. T. A. Baillie, C. J. W. Brooks, and B. S. Middleditch, *Anal. Chem.*, 44:30 (1972).
160. J. M. Halket, I. Ganschow, and B. P. Lisboa, *J. Chromatogr.*, 192:434 (1980).

161. B. Lindback, T. Berlin, and I. Bjorkhem, *Clin. Chem.*, *33*:1226 (1987).
162. G. Phillipou, D. A. Bigham, and R. F. Seamark, *Steroids*, *26*:516 (1975).
162A. J. M. Halket and B. P. Lisboa, *Acta Endocrinol. (Kbh.)*, *87*(Suppl. 215):120 (1978).
163. R. D. Coldwell, D. J. H. Trafford, M. J. Varley, D. N. Kirk, and H. L. J. Makin, *Clin. Chim. Acta*, *180*:157 (1989).
164. R. D. Coldwell, R. D., D. J. H. Trafford, H. L. J. Makin, A. Trube, D. Lisner, R. S. Mason, and S. Posen, *J. Bone Mineral Res.*, *1*: (Suppl. 1): abstr. 376 (1986).
165. R. D. Coldwell, D. J. H. Trafford, M. J. Varley, D. N. Kirk, and H. L. J. Makin, *Biomed. Environ. Mass Spectrom.*, *16*:81 (1988).
166. J. K. Wichmann, H. K. Schnoes, and H. F. DeLuca, *Biochemistry*, *20*:7385 (1981).
167. R. L. Horst, T. A. Reinhardt, B. C. Pramanik, and J. L. Napoli, *Biochemistry*, *22*:245 (1983).
168. J. L. Napoli, B. C. Pramanik, P. M. Royal, T. A. Reinhardt, and R. L. Horst, *J. Biol. Chem.*, *258*:9100 (1983).
169. I. Holmberg and A. Larsson, *Clin. Chim. Acta*, *100*:173 (1980).
170. B. Zagalak, F. Neuheiser, M. J. Zagalak, T. Kuster, H. C. Curtius, G. U. Exner, S. Franconi, and A. Prader, in *Chromatography and Mass Spectrometry in Biomedical Sciences* (A. Frigerio, ed.), Elsevier, Amsterdam, vol. 2, p. 347 (1983).
171. T. Berlin, L. Emtestam, and I. Bjorkhem, *Scand. J. Clin. Lab. Invest.*, *46*:723 (1986).
172. T. Berlin, I. Holmberg, and I. Bjorkhem, *Scand. J. Clin. Lab. Invest.* *46*:367 (1986).
173. H. L. J. Makin and D. J. H. Trafford, in *Vitamin D* (R. Kumar, ed.), Martinus Nijhoff, Boston, p. 497 (1984).
174. R. D. Coldwell, D. J. H. Trafford, M. J. Varley, D. N. Kirk, and H. L. J. Makin, *Steroids*, *55*:418 (1990).
175. I. Bjorkhem, I. Holmberg, J. Kristiansen, A. Larsson, and J. I. Pedersen, in *Vitamin D: Basic Research and Its Clinical Application* (A. W. Norman, K. Schaefer, D. V. Herrath, H.-G. Grigoleit, J. W. Coburn, H. F. DeLuca, E. B. Mawer, and T. Suda, eds.), Walter de Gruyter, Berlin, p. 183, (1979).
176. I. Bjorkhem and I. Holmberg, *J. Biol. Chem.*, *253*:843 (1978).
177. I. Bjorkhem and I. Holmberg, *J. Biol. Chem.*, *254*:9518 (1979).
178. R. Hansson, I. Holmberg, and K. Wikvall, *J. Biol. Chem.*, *256*:4345 (1981).
179. I. Bjorkhem, R. Hansson, I. Holmberg, and K. Wikvall, *Biochem. Biophys. Res. Commun.*, *90*:615 (1979).
180. S. Dueland, I. Holmberg, T. Berg, and J. I. Pedersen, *J. Biol. Chem.*, *256*:10430 (1981).
181. S. Andersson, I. Holmberg, and K. Wikvall, *J. Biol. Chem.*, *258*:6777 (1983).
182. I. Holmberg, *Biochem. Biophys. Res. Commun.*, *123*:1209 (1984).
183. J. I. Pedersen, Y. Hagenfeldt, and I. Bjorkhem, *Biochem. J.*, *250*:527 (1988).

184. I. Holmberg, *Biochim. Biophys. Acta*, *800*:106 (1984).
185. I. Holmberg, T. Berlin, S. Ewerth, and I. Bjorkhem, *Scand. J. Clin. Lab. Invest.*, *46*:785 (1986).
186. J. I. Pedersen, H. H. Shobaki, I. Holmberg, S. Bergseth, and I. Bjorkhem, *J. Biol. Chem.*, *258*:742 (1983).
187. I. Holmberg, K. Saarem, J. I. Pedersen, and I. Bjorkhem, *Anal. Biochem.*, *159*:317 (1986).
188. Y. Hagenfeldt, J. I. Pedersen, and I. Bjorkhem, *Biochem. J.*, *250*:521 (1988).
189. Y. Hagenfeldt, H. Eriksson, and I. Bjorkhem, *Biochim. Biophys. Acta*, *1002*:84 (1989).
190. Y. Hagenfeldt, I. Bjorkhem, and H. Eriksson, *Biochim. Biophys. Acta*, *1042*:94 (1990).
191. J. O. Whitney, C. H. L. Shackleton, C. G. Edmonds, A. L. Burlingame, and C. F. Piel, in *Stable Isotopes*, Proceedings of the Third International Conference (E. R. Klein and P. D. Klein, eds.), Academic Press, New York (1979).
192. D. N. Kirk, M. J. Varley, H. L. J. Makin, and D. J. H. Trafford, *J. Chem. Soc. Perkin Trans.*, *1*:2563 (1983).
193. I. Holmberg, K. Kristiansen, and M. Sturem, *Scand. J. Clin. Lab. Invest.* *44*:275 (1984).
194. D. J. H. Trafford, D. A. Seamark, H. Turnbull, and H. L. J. Makin, *J. Chromatogr.*, *226*:351 (1981).

3

VITAMIN E

Johanna K. Lang, Michael Schillaci, and Brian Irvin

Liposome Technology, Inc., Menlo Park, California

1. INTRODUCTION

1.1 Discovery and Biological Function

Vitamin E was first discovered as a nutritional factor (factor X) that prevented the death and resorption of fetuses in pregnant rats (1). Compounds that exhibited vitamin E activity were also referred to as tocopherols, derived from Greek and meaning "to bear offspring." Other manifestations of vitamin E deficiency that were observed in animals reared on a vitamin-E-free diet were testicular atrophy in male rates, central nervous system (CNS) lesions in young chicks, muscular dystrophy, and exudative diathesis, a leakage of plasma into subcutaneous tissues (2). In humans, vitamin-E-deficient diets did not provoke a characteristic disease state or disorder. Recent research, however, has shown a strong link between vitamin E deficiency and atherosclerosis (3). In epidemiological studies, the mortalities from atherosclerosis-related heart attacks correlated well with low plasma vitamin E levels, and even better with plasma vitamin E/cholesterol ratios (4). Although the various biological manifestations of vitamin E activity are not fully understood, there is a broad consensus that the basis of its bioactivity is its ability to act as a lipid soluble antioxidant that protects vulnerable polyunsaturated fatty acids in cell membranes and plasma lipoproteins from harmful and potentially fatal lipidperoxidation processes (3,5).

153

1.2   Chemistry of Vitamin E

Since the first vague descriptions of vitamin E as an essential dietary component, chemists have identified the chemical equivalents of vitamin E activity and determined their molecular structures. In pure form vitamin E is a yellow viscous liquid that decomposes easily in the presence of light, oxygen, alkaline pH, or traces of transition metal ions. The structural element common to all vitamin E active compounds is tocol, a chroman ring system with a terpenoid side chain of three terpene units. Essential to its biological activity are the hydroxyl group in position 6 and the methyl group in position 2 of the chroman ring. The terpenoid side chain can exist in the saturated or unsaturated form. The saturated form is far more prevalent and constitutes the group of tocopherols, while the unsaturated tocols are referred to as tocotrienols (Fig. 1, Table 1). Within the tocopherols and tocotrienols, the alpha (α), beta (β), gamma (γ), and delta (δ) homologs differ in number and position of methyl substituents on the chroman ring. α-Tocopherol, the most abundant of vitamin E active compounds carries three methyl groups on carbons 5, 7, and 8 of the aromatic ring. In the isomeric beta and gamma species, two methyl groups are in positions 5 and 8 or 7 an 8, respectively, while delta-tocopherol has only one methyl group in position 8. Vitamin E active species can thus be classified into tocopherols (T) and tocotrienols (T-3) and their respective alpha, beta, gamma, and delta homologs (Table 1). Historically, α-, β-, and γ-tocotrienol series were referred to as epsilon-, eta-, and theta-tocopherols, but the classification into tocopherols and tocotrienols as adopted by IUPAC (6) clearly does better justice to their structural differences and similarities.

Table 1   Compounds of the Vitamin E Family

Trivial name	Abbreviation	Chemical name
α-Tocopherol	α-T	5,7,8-Trimethyltocol
β-Tocopherol	β-T	5,8-Dimethyltocol
γ-Tocopherol	γ-T	7,8-Dimethyltocol
δ-Tocopherol	δ-T	8-Methyltocol
α-Tocotrienol	α-T3	5,7,8-Trimethyltocotrienol
β-Tocotrienol	β-T3	5,8-Dimethyltocotrienol
γ-Tocotrienol	γ-T3	7,8-Dimethyltocotrienol
δ-Tocotrienol	δ-T3	8-Methyltocotrienol

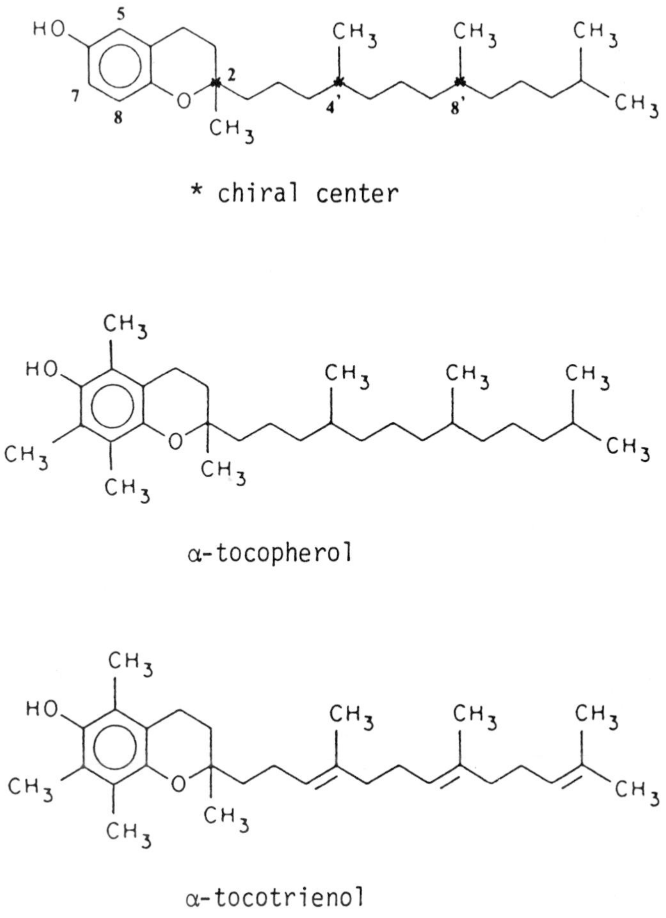

* chiral center

α-tocopherol

α-tocotrienol

Figure 1 Structure of tocopherols and tocotrienols. Top: General structure, numbers indicate positions of methyl grops (5, 7, 8) as referred to in Table 1 and location of chiral centers (2, 4′, 8′). Middle: Structure of α-tocopherol. Bottom: Structure of α-tocotrienol.

Due to the presence of chiral centers at position 2 of the chroman ring and the 4′ and 8′ carbons of the terpenoid side chain, tocopherols can exist in eight diastereomeric forms; moreover, tocotrienol double bonds can form cis and trans isomers. So far, only all-*trans*-tocotrienols have been found in nature. α-Tocopherol occurs naturally only as the 2R, 4′R, and 8′R isomer (RRR-tocopherol, d-α-tocopherol), whereas pharmaceutical tocopherol supplements often contain synthetic α-tocopherol racemates. Depending on the optical purity of the starting material, isophytol, synthetic α-tocopherol is composed of the C-2 enantiomers (2RS-α-tocopherol, d,l-α-tocopherol) or a racemic mixture of all possible stereomers (2RS-, 4'RS,- 8'RS-α-tocopherol, all-*rac*-α-tocopherol) (Table 2).

Commercial vitamin supplements often contain vitamin E esters such as tocopheryl acetate or tocopheryl succinate. These derivatives are more stable, as the reactive 6-hydroxy group is protected by the esterification, but this modification also renders them biologically inactive. In vivo, however, unspecific esterases rapidly cleave the ester bond and set free the active compound.

1.3 Biological Activity and Natural Abundance

The discovery and characterization of the members of the vitamin E family of compounds were possible when the early bioassays were complemented by more and more powerful chemical analyses. Chromatography made it feasible to separate the tocopherols and tocotrienol homologs and diastereomers and to isolate them in pure form. Biological activities or biopotencies of vitamin E active compounds as determined by the classical rat fetal resorption test (7) vary from less than 0.1 to 1.7 IU. The International Unit of activity (IU) was defined as the activity of 1 mg 2RS-α-tocopheryl acetate (d,l-α-tocopheryl acetate). Bioassays are notoriously difficult to standardize, and this is reflected in conflicting opinions as to the true bioactivity of the individual tocopherol and tocotrienol homologs and their stereomers (8). There is agreement, however, that RRR-α-tocopherol (d-α-tocopherol) is the most potent compound. Esters of RRR-α-tocopherol have similar potencies (compared on a molar

Table 2 α-Tocopherol Stereoisomers and Racemates

Chemical name	Trivial name	Other names
2R, 4'R, 8'R- 2R, 4'R, 8'S- 2R, 4'S, 8'S- 2R, 4'S, 8'R-	d-	RRR-
2S, 4'S, 8'S- 2S, 4'S, 8'R- 2S, 4'R, 8'S- 2S, 4'R, 8'R-		
2RS, 4'R,8'R-	d,1-	2RS-, RS-, 2-ambo-
2RS, 4'RS,8'RS	all-*rac*-	2-ambo-, 4'-ambo-, 8'-ambo-

basis); a value of 1.66 IU was suggested for 1 mg of RRR-α-tocopheryl acetate (9). The beta and gamma homologs are only half as active, and δ-tocopherol even less. A change in sterochemistry, especially at C-2, abolishes more than 50% of the bioactivity, as does the presence of double bonds in the side chain (tocotrienols). The bioactivities of the tocopherol homologs reflect their effectiveness to act as lipid-soluble antioxidants (5). The low bioactivities of "unnatural" stereomers have been attributed to impaired uptake and increased turnover (8). The wide variation in bioactivity among the tocopherols underscores the importance of differentiating between them when analyzing for vitamin E. In animal tissues, isomer distribution is influenced by diet, but RRR-α-tocopherol is by far the most abundant. Vegetable fats and oils are the best sources of vitamin E and may contain large amounts of β-, γ-, and δ-tocopherols as well as tocotrienols and tocopherylesters (10).

2. THIN-LAYER CHROMATOGRAPHY

2.1 General Considerations

Historically, thin-layer chromatography (TLC), and with it the ability to separate the tocopherol homologs, was a significant advancement from earlier colorimetric vitamin E assays such as the Emmerie-Engel method (11), where were nondiscriminating for tocopherols and were subject to interferences from other reducing substances, including antioxidants present for the protection of tocopherols (12). Today, TLC has value as a straightforward and inexpensive qualitative or semiquantitative assay method. For quantitative analyses, high-performance liquid chromatography (HPLC) or gas chromatography (GC) has surpassed TLC, as quantitative TLC assays lack precision, are labor intensive, and are difficult to automate. Given proper sample preparation TLC is suitable for all sample types. TLC systems are capable of separating tocopherol and tocotrienol homologs. One-dimensional systems are often satisfactory; additional resolution can be achieved by developing in a second dimension. Quantitation can be done in situ by densitometry (13,14) or by the more traditional approach of eluting the spots from the plate and performing colorimetric assays (15–18). TLC is also popular as a sample cleanup for other quantitative procedures, such as GC.

2.2 Separation Systems

For thin-layer chromatography of vitamin E silica gel plates have been widely used, either as silica gel G (18,19), silica gel 60 (16,17), or silica gel GF (14), or other commercially available precoated silica gel plates

(13,15,20). Alternatives are aluminum oxide plates, which have been used in the past with mixed results. Herting et al. reported that tocopherol spots originating from whole plasma lipids were less defined on aluminum oxide plates that when spotted on silica gel (15). With saponified blood lipids, however, alumnium oxide was superior to silica gel. The number of tocopherols, tocotrienols, or matrix-related compounds to be separated determines whether one- or two-dimensional techniques are necessary. The first successful separation of all four natural tocopherols was achieved on a silica gel G plate developed in one dimension with chloroform and in a second with hexane/isopropyl ether 80/20 (v/v) (18,21). This system also separates most of the tocotrienols and the naturally occurring tocopheryl esters. Another two-dimensional system, petroleum ether/isopropyl ether/acetone 85/12/4) after chloroform, is useful for the separation of the tocopherol homologs (19). A one-dimensional system developed by Mueller-Mulot (17) also separates all tocopherols and tocotrienols but cannot resolve γ-tocopherol from β-tocotrienol. It calls for three successive developments of a silica gel 60 plate with n-hexane/ethyl acetate 92.5/7.5 (v/v). See Table 3 for a summary of TLC separation systems.

2.3 Detection

The most common mode of detection is fluorescence quenching on supports impregnated with a fluorescent indicator, such as fluorescein. Fluorescent plates can be obtained from commercial sources (13,17), or made in-house with dichlorofluorescein (18), or sodium fluorescein (16), 0.002-0.003% by volume added to the silica slurry. Illuminated under the proper UV wavelengths, the compounds appear as dark spots against the fluorescent background. Alternatively, tocopherols and tocotrienols can be visualized by chromogenic spray reagents, such as the Emmerie-Engel reagent (2,2′-bipyridine-ferric chloride), or a more sensitive modified reagent, in which bipyridine is replaced with bathophenanthroline (17,20). Phosphomolybdic acid produces characteristic color reactions that can be used to distinguish β- and γ-tocopherol isomers (22). A solution of 20% antimony pentachloride in $CHCl_3$ produces characteristic color reactions for all four tocopherol analogs: reddish-yellow, yellowish-brown, green, and reddish-brown for α-, β-, γ, and δ-tocopherol, respectively (19). The color reaction given by o-dianisidine offers information regarding the presence of hydrogen or a methyl group at the position 5 of the chroman ring, a feature distinguishing γ- and δ-tocopherols from α-, and β-tocopherols (19,21). Charring, preceded by spraying with 10% copper(II) sulfate in 8% phosphoric acid (14), will visualize tocopherols and tocotrienols.

Table 3 Thin-Layer Chromatography

Sample preparation	Stationary support	Mobile Phase	Visualization	Quantitation	Comments	Reference (year)
Saponification	Commercial silica gel with fluorescence indicator	1-D. Benzene/ethanol, 99/1, dark 2-D. Hexane/EtOH, 9/1	110–120°C, 18–20 h	Densitometer: transmission, 270 nm	α-T in rat liver, serum	13 (1977)
Saponification	(a) Silica gel (b) Unactivated aluminum oxide	(a) Petroleum ether/diethyl ether/acetic acid, 90/10/1 (b) Benzene/diethyl ether, 50/50, in dark	0.004% 2,7-dichloro-fluorescein spray, UV at 254 nm	Elution with EtOH, colorimetric with bipyridine-$FeCl_3$ or bathophenan-throline-$FeCl_3$	α-, γ-, δ-T in feeds, oils, biological materials (β-T and γ-T comigrate)	15 (1967)
Extraction, saponification	Silica gel 60 HR, fluorescence indicator (0.003% sodium fluorescein)	1-D. Benzene/EtOH, 99/1, dark 2-D. Skellysolve B/EtOH, 9/1	UV light	Elution, colorimetric with bathophenanthroline-$FeCl_3$	α-, δ-T in retinas (β-T and γ-T comigrate)	16 (1975)
Saponification	Silica gel	1-D. Benzene/EtOH, 99/1 2-D. Hexane/EtOH, 9/1	Spray with ethanolic bathophenanthroline-$FeCl_3$	External standards applied to determine limit of detection	α-T in pig organs	20 (1975)
Extraction	Silica gel GF	Hexane/isopropyl ether, 85/15	100°C, 15 min, spray with 10% copper(II) sulfate phosphoric acid, char at 190°C, 10 min	Densitometer: 350 nm	α-, β-, δ-T and α-T3 in algal lipids (β- and γ-T comigrate)	14 (1984)
Two-step freezing in acetone, crystallization, extraction	Silica gel 60 with fluorescence indicator	Hexane/ethyl acetate, 92.5/7.5,3 times	Seven different visualization reagents, some used in combination	Elution, colorimetric with bipyridine-$FeCl_3$	α-, β-, γ-, δ-T and α-, β-, γ-, δ-T3 in oils and fats (γ-T and β-T3 comigrate), certain antioxidants comigrate with some homologs	17 (1976)
Extraction, crystallization	Silica gel G with fluorescence indicator (0.002% dichlorofluorescein)	1-D. Chloroform 2-D. Hexane/isopropyl ether, 80/20	UV light	Elution, colorimetric with bathophenanthroline-$FeCl_3$	α-, β-, γ-, δ-T and α-, β-, γ-, δ-T3 in cereals and plant oils (γ-T and β-T3 comigrate)	18 (1969)
Extraction, saponification	Silica gel G	1-D. Chloroform 2-D. Petroleum ether/isopropyl ether/acetone, 85/12/4	0.5% Bathophenanthro-line/0.2% $FeCl_3$ (EtOH) (1:1), 20% $SbCl_5$ in $CHCl_3$, 20% phosphomolybdic acid (EtOH), saturated o-dianisidine (acetic acid)	GC analysis	α-, β-, γ-, δ-T and γ-T3 in milk	19 (1975)

2.4 Quantitation

Off Plate

Vitamin E active compounds separated by TLC and visualized by non-destructive methods, such as fluorescence quenching, can be isolated from the TLC plate, usually by scraping off the silica gel containing the spots. The isolated compounds are then eluted from the gel and measured, either by the Emmerie-Engel reaction, in which tocopherols and tocotrienols reduce a bipyridine-ferric chloride solution to the colored ferrous complex, or in a more sensitive variation, in which batho-phenanthroline is substituted for bipyridine. Recovery of tocopherols from the isolated spots is often incomplete. To account for the losses and matrix effects, tocopherol-free triglycerides (16) or phospholipids (15,16) spiked with α-tocopherol were used as standards for the analysis of oils and grains (15) or rat tissue (15,16). Sometimes tocopherol standards were applied on the plate solely to identify tocopherols, while a second set of standards was prepared to calibrate the quantitative assay (16–18). To correct for background absorbance originating from the silica gel, unused portions of the same plate were scraped and eluted similar to tocopherol-containing spots (15–17).

Densitometry

For densitometry, tocopherols are converted to colored spots by chromo-genic spray reagents, such as the ones listed above. The optimal scanning wavelength depends on the color generated by the spray reagent. In the charring method employed by Hess and co-workers (13) tocopherols were oxidized to the respective quinones, by heating at 110–120°C, for 18–20 h, and scanned at 270 nm. Tocopherol acetates did not react under these conditions. Some authors report a good linear relationship between scanning peak areas and tocopherol concentration, though within a rather narrow concentration range of one order of magnitude or less (13,14). Hess et al. recommend that sets of standards bracket the concentration range of the samples to keep errors in accuracy below 10%. In the transmission mode, uneven thickness of the plate will affect fluorescence intensity. Commercial plates of uniform thickness minimize this problem (13).

2.5 Sample Preparation

Saponification

Saponification has been the preferred sample preparation method for TLC analysis. It involves heating of the sample in the presence of potassium hydroxide or sodium hydroxide, and accomplishes the hydrolysis of matrix lipids, most importantly triglycerides and phospholipids. Unlike the parent compounds, the hydrolysis products (fatty acids, glycerol) are hydrophilic and remain in the aqueous phase in a postsaponification, two-phase extraction. This decreases the load of material that extracts with tocopherol into the organic phase and is applied to the plate. Typically the sample is heated under reflux or in a pressure-tight vessel for 20–30 min at 70–100°C. Under these conditions, the labile tocopherols will degrade, unless protected from oxidation by nitrogen flushing (13,16), addition of antioxidants such as butylated hydroxytoluene (BHT) (20) or pyrogallol (13,16), limited exposure to light and rapid cooling of the reaction mixture after completion of the saponification (13,16). Subsequently, vitamin E is extracted from the reaction mixture with an unpolar organic solvent such as hexane (13,20) or ether (15). The fatty acid salts, formed during saponification, act as a detergent and may impede the extraction of vitamin E, causing poor recovery. This has been shown for the analysis of tocopherols from corn oil. δ-Tocopherol was most sensitive to the presence of fatty acids in the saponification mixture, followed by β- and γ-tocopherol and α-tocopherol, which showed the least effect at a given sample size (23). Tocopherol recovery from retinal lipids diminished at larger sample sizes, which caused a high fatty acid content in the reaction mixture (16). Recovery of α-tocopherol fell below 80% at fatty acid concentrations above 10 mg/ml in the aqueous saponification mixture. A calibration curve relating α-tocopherol recoveries to fatty acid concentration was constructed from saponified, α-tocopherol-spiked triglycerides and phospholipids and served to correct for effects of fatty acid content on α-tocopherol recovery. Large quantities of fatty acids were shown to impede chromatographic separation (13). In samples containing tocopheryl esters, either naturally or as a supplement, saponification will cause cleavage of the tocopheryl esters to the respective tocopherols (18). In animal feeds, tocopherol did not extract efficiently into ethyl ether until released from the matrix by saponification (24).

Direct Extraction

Tocopherols were extracted from cereals by Soxhlet extraction with acetone without saponification. Samples of various plant oils were first diluted with acetone and subsequently freed of triglycerides by cooling the solution in a dry ice/acetone bath and removal of solidified triglycerides by filtration (18). Recoveries for α-tocopherol and α-tocotrienol were 99%, compared to 91 and 83%, respectively, by saponification. A similar freezing technique was utilized on commercial vegetables and fats by freezing acetone solutions at -80°C (17). A single-phase extraction with acetone yielded good recovery of α-tocopherol from algae (14).

2.6 Applications

Tocopherols, tocotrienols, and tocopheryl esters in plant oils and cereal samples were isolated by an acetone extraction/freezing procedure and separated on a two-dimensional TLC system, capable of separating all tocopherol and tocotrienol homologs, as well as the tocopheryl esters. The content of vitamin E active species was determined from their reaction with bathophenanthroline-ferric chloride (18). Mueller-Mulot determined tocopherols and tocotrienols in 24 commercially available vegetable oils on one-dimensional TLC after sample cleanup by an acetone dilution/freezing technique. TLC, which required three successive developments of the plate, resolved all tocopherol and tocotrienol homologs except for β-tocotrienol and γ-tocopherol, which comigrated (17). Algal lipids from the *Euglena gracilis* strain Z were recovered by a single-phase extraction with acetone and separated on one-dimensional TLC with hexane/isopropyl ether (85/15). α-Tocopherol and α-tocotrienol, but not β- and γ-tocopherol, were separated and quantitated by densitometry at 350 nm after spraying the plate with 10% copper(II) sulfate in phosphoric acid and charring at 190°C. Calibration with tocopherol standards showed linear calibration curves for the densitometer peak response in concentration ranges between 0.1 and 2.4 μg for α-tocopherol, 0.2 and 1.2 μg for δ-tocopherol, 0.2 and 3.0 μg for γ-tocopherol, and 0.2 and 1.6 μg for α-tocotrienol (14). A densitometric method was created for the analysis of α-tocopherol in saponified rat liver and serum samples. Although α-tocopherol was the only homolog of interest, a two-dimensional separation system was necessary to separate coextracted quinols. To visualize tocopherols, they were converted to quinones by heating the plate in the presence of O_2 at 110–120°C for 18–20 h. This assay showed a linear relationship between amounts of α-tocopherol and densitometer peak areas in the 1–10 μg range at a scanning wavelength of 270 nm (13). Pig tissue samples were analyzed by TLC after saponification. α-Tocopherol was visualized by spraying the TLC plate with ethanolic bathophenanthroline-ferric chloride. A two-dimensional separation system was essential to separate α-tocopherol from other reducing substances from the unsaponifiable portion of pig liver tissue (20).

3. HIGH-PERFORMANCE LIQUID CHROMATOGRAPHY

3.1 General Considerations

The last decade saw a proliferation of HPLC techniques for the analysis of vitamin E. HPLC has surpassed GC by virtue of its greater flexibility and convenience in handling different sample matrices. It is easy to understand the need for such flexibility when one considers that vitamin E is analyzed in a variety of sample types that differ widely in both vitamin E content and complexity of the sample matrix. Matrices vary from pharmaceutical formulations, foods, and food additives to biological fluids and tissues, from the multivitamin tablet, to breakfast cereals, to retinal tissue. Sample preparation is a major part of any assay and its importance cannot be overstressed. Each matrix poses its own unique challenge, and sample preparation procedures must balance good recovery of the vitamin E active compounds and elimination of interferences with decomposition of the oxygen-sensitive tocopherols and tocotrienols during extensive sample cleanup. Chromatographic challenges in vitamin E analysis involve the separation of the tocopherol and tocotrienol homologs, tocopheryl esters, oxidation products, other fat-soluble vitamins such as retinol and carotenoids, and other matrix components, frequently triglycerides and cholesterol. Modern HPLC features like multiwavelength monitoring and gradient and flow programming offer convenience and speed, although at considerable cost. The choice of conditions for each assay is driven by the complexity of the matrix, the sample size, abundance of the various vitamin E active compounds, the efficiency of the extraction from the matrix and elimination of matrix components, and lastly the ability to afford feature-loaded HPLC equipment. Since tocopherol is a relatively nonpolar molecule without silanol sensitive functional groups, it chromatographs well on either reversed-phase or normal-phase silica-based columns without additives to control tailing. Reversed-phase systems enjoy more widespread use than normal-phase systems. Among the virtues of reversed-phase systems that make them a preferred choice over normal-phase systems are short equilibration times, ruggedness, and consistency of performance. The advantages of normal phase lie in its superior separation efficiency for structural isomers such as beta- and gamma-tocopherols. In addition, the unpolar normal-phase eluents are good solvents for lipid rich matrices, such as fats and oils. With proper choice of chromatographic conditions these samples can be analyzed on normal-phase systems with minimal sample preparation (25,26).

3.2 Separation Systems

Reversed Phase

Reversed phase is the separation system of choice in more than 70 percent of recently published procedures. This is understandable in light of the excellent reproductibility of retention times, fast equilibration, and superior ruggedness of reversed-phase columns over other stationary phases. On reversed phase, tocotrienols are eluted as a group ahead of the tocopherols. Within the two classes of vitamin E active compounds, the monomethyl-substituted homologs are eluted first, followed by dimethyl- and trimethyl- substituted homologs. This results in the following elution order: δ-tocotrienol, β- and γ-tocotrienol, α-tocotrienol, δ-tocopherol, β- and γ-tocopherol, and α-tocopherol, with the β- and γ-homologs coeluting (Fig. 2). This is in contrast to normal-phase systems

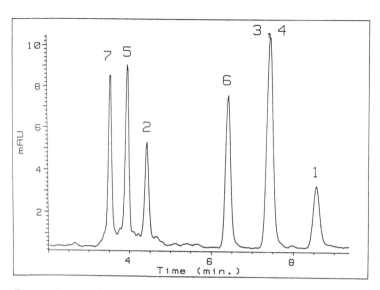

Figure 2 Separation of tocopherols and tocotrienols on a reversed-phase system. Chromatographic conditions: Zorbax ODS, 250 × 4.6 mm column dimensions, with an acetonitrile/methanol/dichloromethane (60/35/5) mobile phase, detection UV 295 nm, where 1 is α-T, 2 is α-T3, 3 is β-T, 4 is γ-T, 5 is γ-T3, 6 is δ-T, and 7 is δ-T3. (From Ref. 27 with permission.)

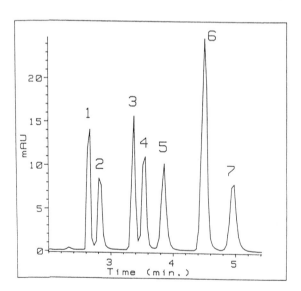

Figure 3 Separation of tocopherols and tocotrienols on a normal phase system. Chromatographic conditions: Zorbax SIL, 250 × 4.6 mm column dimensions, with a hexane/isopropanol (99/1) mobile phase, detection UV 295 nm, where 1 is α-T, 2 is α-T3, 3 is β-T, 4 is γ-T, 5 is γ-T3, 6 is δ-T, and 7 is δ-T3. (From Ref. 27 with permission).

where α homologs elute first, followed by β, γ, and δ homologs (Fig. 3) (27). Reversed-phase systems are uniquely compatible with electrochemical detection, which requires the presence of an electrolyte in the eluent solution, to support the redox reactions that are the basis for detection. Only reversed-phase eluents, typically mixtures of short-chain alcohols or acetonitrile with water, buffers, or salt solutions, are sufficiently polar to carry electrolytes. With few exceptions, reversed-phase systems for vitamin E employ octadecylsilane (ODS, C18) modified silica, in particle size ranges between 3 and 10 mm, and in column lengths from 6 to 30 cm, and internal diameters between 2 and 4.6 mm. Octylsilane silica (C8) is similar in performance but less retentive than C18 (28).

The highly lipophilic tocopherols are well retained on reversed-phase columns and require stong eluents. In about 70% of recently published procedures, mobile phases were either pure methanol or methanol/water mixtures containing up to 10% water. For the remainder, solvent choices included isopropanol/acetonitrile/water in a 50/30/20 volume ratio (29): acetonitrile/water/methanol, 49/3/48 (30); ethanol/water, 92/8 (31); acetonitrile/dichloromethane/methanol, 70/20/10 (32); acetonitrile/chloroform/isopropanol/water, 78/16/3.5/2.5 (33); methanol/ethanol, 1/9 or 3/7 (34); methanol/n-butanol/water, 87.4/10/2.6 (35); methanol/acetonitrile/chloroform, 25/60/15 (36), and 47/47/6 (37); and acetonitrile/methanol in various ratios (27).

Normal Phase

Normal-phase columns, though less convenient to employ, possess some unique advantages that might prescribe their use. In the case of tocopherol and related substances, normal-phase columns provide more selectivity and are generally superior for separations involving numerous isomers or related compounds (26,38–43). The isomeric beta- and gamma-tocopherols and -tocotrienols are effectively separated in following typical elution order: α-tocopherol, α-tocotrienol, β-tocopherol, β-tocotrienol, γ-tocopherol, γ-tocotrienol, δ-tocopherol, and δ-tocotrienol (Fig. 3) (25,27,44–46). Normal-phase systems are uniquely suitable for the direct analysis of cooking oils and fats, since the apolar normal-phase eluents are good solvents for these samples. Normal-phase eluents for the separation of vitamin E active compounds were composed of an alkane (hexane, heptane, isooctane) with a small amount of a polar modifier, either an alcohol (ethanol, methanol, isopropanol, butanol), an ether (tetrahydrofuran, methyl, t-butyl, isopropyl), or a chlorohydrocarbon (dichloromethane, chloroform). Among four modifiers—isopropanol, n-butanol, tetrahydrofuran, and dichloromethane—in a hexane mobile phase (27), Tan et al. found isopropanol to be most effective. Dichloromethane was too unpolar to elute the tocopherols, while tetrahydrofuran resulted in inconsistent separations. Between *n*-butanol and isopropanol, both of which eluted tocopherols effectively, isopropanol provided superior separations. The same authors also compared cyano, amino, and silica columns for their effectiveness in separating vitamin E active compounds. Cyano columns failed to separate β- and γ-homologs. Amino phase resolved the vitamin E species (23,46–48) but was less efficient than silica. Optimal resolution of all tocopherol and tocotrienol isomers was obtained with hexane/isopropanol, 98/2, on a Zorbax SIL silica column, 4.6 × 250 mm (27).

Gradient Elution

In general, isocratic elution is adequate to resolve vitamin E active compounds on reversed-phase or normal-phase systems. Gradient elution is employed in special cases, for example, to separate tocopherol oxidation products, such as tocopherolquinone and tocopherol dimer (49), or to speed up elution of strongly retained retinyl palmitate (50). Solvent gradients have been used for the separation of more complex mixtures. MacCrehan et al. resolved all-*trans*-retinol, 13-*cis*-retinol, α-tocopherol, γ-tocopherol, all-*trans*-β-carotene, *cis*-β-carotene, and α-carotene in a human plasma extract on a methanol/*n*-butanol/water solvent gradient on a reversed-phase system. Isocratic conditions had failed to resolve the retinols and elute the strongly retained carotenoids (35). Gradient elution has also been used in a "wash" mode to speed up elution of unidentified strongly retained compounds, either in the form of a flow gradient by a programmed increase in the flow rate (51) or as a step gradient (52) or linear solvent gradient (53) to a stronger eluent.

3.3   Detection

Absorbance Detection

Among the commercially available HPLC detectors, absorbance detection, fluorescence detection, and electrochemical detection have proven useful for vitamin E. The chroman ring system present in all vitamin E species gives rise to a UV absorbance maximum between 292 and 298 nm for the tocopherols and between 276 and 285 nm for the tocopheryl esters. Frequently 280 nm is chosen to accommodate inexpensive fixed-wavelength detectors. Mayne et al. detected α-tocopheryl acetate at 210 nm to minimize interference in chicken liver extracts containing a large amount of canthaxanthin (54). If other compounds such as vitamins A, D, or K were monitored in the same run, multiple-wavelength detection with multiple runs using fixed-wavelength detectors (55,56), or with single runs with multichannel detectors (37,44,57), programmable scanning detectors (33,35,39,58,59), or diode-array detectors (25,36,60) allowed to detect each compound with maximal sensitivity and selectivity at its absorbance maximum.

Fluorescence Detection

Compared to absorbance detection, fluorescence detection offers increased sensitivity and selectivity. The chroman ring system gives rise to fluorescence at 345 nm when excited at its absorbance maxima at 210 or 290 nm. The enhanced selectivity of fluorescence detection over absorbance detection can be exploited to simplify sample cleanup if the matrix components are not fluorescent at the chosen excitation and emission wavelengths (61). Tocopheryl esters, such as tocopheryl acetate, do not fluoresce (62), but can be cleaved to tocopherols by saponification (24,45,63). Fluorescence excitation wavelengths around 290 nm are widely used; a switch to excitation at the low UV maximum, however, may result in a major increase in sensitivity (64–67). The actual gain in sensitivity is somewhat dependent on the detector design. McMurray et al. shortened run times for the HPLC analysis of bovine and pig plasma on a C18 column with a methanol/water 97/3 (v/v) eluent by changing detection modes from absorbance to fluorescence, as late-eluting peaks, visible by absorbance detection, did not give a signal on the fluorescence detector. Tocopherol values by fluorescence detection were lower compared to absorbance, which is indicative of improved selectivity (68). By comparing detection limits of tocopherol homologs on a silica column, Taylor et al. demonstrated a 2.5- to 3.3-fold increase in sensitivity, for fluorescence with excitation at 290 nm (290 ex) and emission at 330 nm (330 em) versus absorbance at 292 nm (26).

Electrochemical Detection

Tocopherols and tocotrienols can be oxidized electrochemically at low potentials. This makes them suitable candidates for electrochemical detection (EC), which is the most sensitive and selective detection mode for tocopherols. Both amperometric and coulometric detectors have been used with good success in a potential range between +0.25 and +1.0 V. In amperometric detection, the electrochemical reaction, which occurs on a glassy carbon surface electrode, affects only a fraction of the eluting compound, while the porous graphite electrodes of coulometric detectors are capable of effecting a complete oxidation or reduction of an eluting species. Amperometric detectors have some practical advantages, like good accessibility of the electrode, low dead volumes, and easy maintenance, and enjoy more widespread use (35,52,71a–73,78,79,90). Coulometric detectors, on the other hand, offer some unique applications. At proper potential settings, coulometric cells can function as reactor cells (29,69,70). This was exploited by Edlund for the determination of coenzyme Q10 (Co Q10), coenzyme Q10H2 (Co Q10H2), and α-tocopherol in plasma and tissue samples. Using a series of three coulometric cells in an oxidation-reduction-oxidation configuration, the author poised Co Q10, Co Q10H2, and α-tocopherol all in a reduced state before they reached the last cell where they were oxidized and the resulting signal recorded (69). Murphy et al. measured tocopherol homologs and their corresponding quinones in extracts of tissue and plasma using a configuration of two cells in a reduction-oxidation mode. This two-cell system ensured that the compounds of interest were reduced when they reached the second cell, in which the compound was oxidized and the signal recorded. The setup allowed detection limits for tocopherols as low as 20 pg (70). Using both fluorescence (297 ex, 327 em) and amperometric detection (0.8 V vs. Ag/AgCl) to measure α-, γ, and δ-tocopherol in extracts of saponified feeds, Ueda determined the detection limit for tocopherols as 2.0 and 0.1 ng for fluorescence and amperometric detection, respectively, a 20-fold sensitivity gain by electrochemical (EC) detection (71a). In another application, amperometric detection could determine as little as 0.65 pg. α-tocopherol versus 2.4 ng for absorbance detection (295 nm), resulting in a sensitivity gain of three orders of magnitude (35). As mentioned previously, users of EC are mainly restricted to reversed-phase columns since electrochemical detection requires the presence of an electrolyte in the mobile phase. The electrolytes, either a perchlorate or acetate salt present in the concentration range of 5 to 50 mM, are soluble in most reversed-phase eluents, but insoluble in normal-phase eluents. Using normal-phase conditions Hiroshima et al. mixed an electrolyte solution of 0.1 M sodium perchlorate in ethanol:methanol (1:9, v/v) with the column effluent consisting of n:hexane/disopropyl ether (87.5/12.5 v/v) The detection limit was estimated at 1 ng (71).

3.4 Quantitation

For the quantitative determination of vitamin E active compounds both internal and external standardization are widely used. Internal standards are convenient to correct for losses and inaccuracies during sample preparation procedures. A good internal standard will closely match the analyte in its chemical and physical properties. This makes tocopherol isomers that are not present in the native sample the best candidates. Examples are δ-tocopherol (72,73), and γ-tocopherol (49). Structurally similar compounds such as α-tocopheryl acetate (26,28,31,33,36, 37,53,59,67,74,75) and tocol (30,35,46,64,71,76–81) are used most frequently. Retinyl acetate, which is structurally related to vitamin A rather than vitamin E, is a popular internal standard in analyses involving both vitamin E and A (55,58,60,82–84) but has also been used in the absence of vitamin A (57,85,86). The introduction of internal standards before or during sample preparation is a generally accepted means to correct for decomposition, resulting in incomplete recovery. This approach, however, will generate erroneous results if internal standard and analyte do not decompose at the same rate. Buttriss et al. determined that 85% of tocol, added as an internal standard, was lost during a 30-min saponification at 70°C, while loss of α-tocopherol and γ-tocopherol was only 5 and 15%, respectively. To correct for the differential loss between tocol and the tocopherols, the difference was entered as a correction factor in the internal standard calculation (64). Ueda et al. investigated uneven recoveries for tocol versus tocopherols in extracted, saponified tissue and blood samples. Among the many factors that affected the ratio of recoveries between tocol and tocopherols were the lipid content of the sample and the solvent composition of the extraction media. Uneven recoveries of internal standard and tocopherol were avoided either by adding tocol after saponification (71) or by replacing tocol with a synthetic internal standard, 2,2,5,7,8-pentamethyl-6-chromanol (23). In two-phase extractions, uneven distribution of the internal standard and tocopherol between aqueous and organic phase is a source of error that can be minimized by proper choice of internal standards. For the simultaneous measurement of retinol, tocopherols, carotenes, and carotenoids in extracted serum, Kaplan et al. employed three internal standards: retinyl acetate to calibrate for retinol, α-tocopheryl acetate to measure α- and γ-tocopherol and lycopene, and retinyl palmitate to calibrate for α- and β-carotene (33). In a comparison of merits of four internal standards by MacCrehan et al., tocol emerged as the best candidate, based on the following factors: a good signal on absorbance and EC detectors, good chromatographic resolution from other components, good peak shape, and stability (35).

3.5   Sample Preparation

Concepts

As a lipophilic substance, vitamin E is intimately associated with lipid components of the sample matrix. The various sample preparation procedures serve to liberate vitamin E from the sample matrix and extract it into a solvent that is compatible with the chromatographic system. The analyst strives to solubilize the portion of the sample containing the tocopherol and to reduce the load of detectable material that will travel through the column. In general, each mode of detection (UV, fluorescence, EC) can be paired with every type of sample preparation procedure. A more selective detector, however, can tolerate more matrix material in the sample, and thus simplify sample preparation. The sample preparation methods for vitamin E analysis fall into one or more of three categories: single-phase extraction with a miscible organic solvent, two-phase extraction with an alcohol and an immiscible organic solvent, and saponification, which reduces the load of organic extractables and cleaves tocopheryl esters.

Solvent Extraction

Solvent extraction procedures can be classified into single-phase extractions and two-phase extractions. In single-phase extractions, the sample is either dissolved or diluted in a water-miscible organic solvent such as alcohol or acetone. In biological samples single-phase extraction will eliminate proteins by precipitation. Other matrix materials, however, will remain in solution and may interfere in the chromatographic analysis of vitamin E. In two-phase extraction, the lipophilic vitamin E is extracted from an aqueous phase into a water immiscible organic solvent. In a first step, the aqueous sample is mixed with a water-miscible solvent, often ethanol, methanol, or isopropanol. After addition of the immiscible solvent, the phases will separate and vitamin E will partition into the organic phase together with other unpolar components such as triglycerides, phospholipids, or sterols. Among the wide variety of two-phase organic extraction procedures, the immiscible solvent is often hexane. Less commonly used are chloroform (43,47,48,65,62,76,80,85), ether (33,38,45,59,60), or higher alkanes (42,67,72,87). Alcohols are always an integral part of the two-phase extraction. They partition into aqueous and organic layers and serve to precipitate proteins as well as to facilitate the extraction of vitamin E. Alcohols frequently serve as carriers for the antioxidant or internal standard. Ethanol in excess of 30% in the aqueous layer, however, lowered the extraction efficiency for tocopherol in a two-phase organic extraction. In saponified tissue and blood samples, a level of 50% alcohol in the aqueous layer depressed recoveries by 70% for tocol (the internal standard), 15% for δ-tocopherol, and 1–2% for α-, β-, and γ-tocopherol. The addition of ethyl acetate to hexane improved the extraction efficiency for the internal standard (23). Mac-Crehan et al. have investigated the influence of the water-miscible solvent on extraction efficiency and found ethanol to be more effective than acetone, acetonitrile, methanol, and perchloric acid (35). For biological fluids and tissues, single-phase extractions may be more efficient than two-phase extractions. In a comparison of the two procedures for rodent tissues and plasma, a single-phase acetone extraction was superior over extractions using either ethanol/hexane or methanol/chloroform solvent systems (61).

Saponification

Saponification involves heating the sample in a strong alkali environment, to reduce the amount of organic extractables in a sample. This is accomplished by hydrolysis of triglycerides, phospholipids, and other lipid esters to more hydrophilic fatty acids and alcohols, which in a subsequent two-phase extraction will remain in the aqueous phase. This decreases the load of material that will extract with tocopherols into the organic phase and be injected into the analytical column. While this is generally desirable, it is not always necessary. Given a selective HPLC detector, the presence of large amounts of lipids that yield no signal is not necessarily detrimental, although column efficiency may be affected. Saponification procedures require prolonged heating of the sample or sample homogenate in aqueous potassium hydroxide at elevated temperatures, usually 70°C, or occasionally 80°C (66), 90°C (42), or 100°C (38,41,43,87,88). In a comparative study, reaction temperatures had little influence on tocopherol recovery (64). Heating times varied, but saponification efficiency was independent of time within a range of 5–40 min at 70°C (24). Saponification is always followed by an organic extraction to rid the sample of saponified material.

Alternatives to saponification that avoid the harsh conditions of high temperature and high pH were often used in samples of animal origin, such as plasma or tissue, and in foods fortified with vitamin E. Saponification is still universally employed in the analysis of endogenous tocopherols in plants.

Alternative Methods

A few equipment innovations that can supplant or augment extraction procedures are solid-phase extraction columns and coupled columns. Solid-phase extraction columns are short, disposable columns packed with resins chemically similar to those used in HPLC columns. Samples are applied to the columns, which are then washed to remove nonretained components. The analyte is eluted with a solvent, strong enough to displace it from the column, while leaving strongly retained components behind. The analyte is thereby isolated from both nonretained and strongly retained matrix components. With a wide variety of column resins and eluting solvent mixtures to choose from, the separation can be tailored to isolate the analyte from most matrix components. The procedure is fast, reproducible, and uses small volumes of solvent (28,87).

Coupled columns refer to a column setup where a valve is inserted between the precolumn and the analytical column. This allows the analyst to shunt nonretained as well as strongly retained components, eluting from the precolumn directly to waste, sparing the analytical column from undesired matrix components. The analyst can minimize sample cleanup this way, using the precolumn to make the initial cut of the sample (69).

Assessment of Recovery

The extent of extraction of vitamin E from the sample matrix is best determined by a recovery study. Typically a defined amount of standard is added to a sample to generate a "spiked" sample. The spiked sample is then prepared and analyzed in the same manner as a regular sample. The recovery is assessed from the difference between the expected (added) and the assayed vitamin E. During sample preparation, externally added vitamin E may be more accesible than vitamin E originating from the sample. This may lead to erroneous conclusions since the added analyte may be recovered from the sample while the native vitamin E is "locked up," as it were, in the matrix (24).

Utility of Antioxidants

Tocopherols are easily degraded during sample preparation procedures, especially in the presence of oxygen. The ease of oxidation of tocopherols is the basis of their biological activity. This feature is also exploited by electrochemical detection. During sample preparation, however, the oxidation of tocopherols will cause low recoveries and inaccurate results. By performing sample preparation promptly, in low light and at low temperatures, oxidation is minimized. Oxidation can be conveniently prevented by addition of antioxidants. In buccal mucosal extracts, tocopherol recovery varied from 10 to 80% in the absence of added antioxidant, while with addition of the antioxidant pyrogallol to the chloroform/methanol/water two-phase extraction, recoveries were near complete (94–103%) (76). Antioxidants were also necessary for complete recovery of α-tocopherol in the methanol/petroleum ether extraction of plasma or isolated red blood cells (59) and in the methanol/chloroform extraction of erythrocytes (80). Antioxidants ae universally employed to protect tocopherols in the harsh conditions of saponification. In addition to pyrogallol (23,24,43,45,59,62,64,71,76,77,80), ascorbic acid/ascorbate (24,30,34,39,41,51,61,63,65,66,87,88), butylated hydroxytoluene (34,35, 37,42,57,67,75,83,89), and ascorbyl palmitate (17) were used.

3.6 Applications

In multivitamin preparations vitamin E is present as the more stable α-tocopheryl acetate. Tocopheryl acetate is easily recovered from the tablet matrix by extraction with either reversed-phase eluents (44,85) or normal-phase eluents (44). For cooking oil, a simple dilution of the oil in mobile phase can be sufficient for direct analysis in a normal-phase system (25,26). The load of triglycerides in oils or fats can be lowered by saponification (41). This approach is limited, however, as high concentrations of fatty acid salts formed during saponification can interfere in the extraction of tocopherols (23,45,46) (Table 4).

Unlike foods and oils, in which vitamin E may exist in a variety of homologs, biological fluids and tissues contain predominantly α-tocopherol and only minor amounts of other homologs. For biological fluids

Table 4 High-Performance Liquid Chromatography: Vitamin Preparations, Standards, and Edible Oils

Sample preparation	Column mobile phase	Detection	Internal standard	Comments	Reference (year)
Add miscible organic solvent, clarify solution, inject	Partsil-10 silica, 4.6 × 250 mm (A), cyclohexane w/ 1.25% IPA μBondapack C-18, 3.9 × 300 mm (B), MeOH/H_2O, 90/10	UV/Vis, 325 nm	None	Vitamins E, A, and D	44 (1980)
	Ultrasphere silica, 4.6 × 250 mm, hexane/$CHCl_3$/IPA, 95/4.9/0.5	UV 292, 268, 292, 294, 298, 240 nm	None	Assay monitors α-T degradation	39 (1988)
	Whatman Partsil 5 silica, 4.6 × 250 mm, hexane/dibutylether/IPA, 90/10/0.05	UV 292 mn, FL 290 ex, 330 em	α-T acetate		26 (1981)
	Spherisorb C-18, 4.6 × 250 mm, gradient 85–100% MeOH in H_2O	UV 290 nm	γ-T	Separates α-T degradation components	49 (1984)
	Spheri-5 cartridge, 2.1 × 100 mm, RP-18, MeOH/H_2O 95/5 or silica, hexane/IPA 99.5/0.5	UV/vis 270, 300, 330 nm	None	Vitamins E, A, and D in vegetable oil	25 (1986)
	Spherisorb silica, 3 μm, 4.6 × 100 mm, hexane/IPA 99.8/0.2	UV 295 nm	None	Separates α-T, β-T, γ-T, δ-T	40 (1986)
	Zorbax, 4.6 × 250 mm, ODS, SIL, CN or NH_2 hexane/polar modifier, 99/1 or CH_3CN/ MeOH/CH_2Cl_2, 60/35/5	UV 295 nm	None	Separates α-T, α-T-3, β-T, -T, γ-T3, δ-T, δ-T3	27 (1989)
Add miscible organic solvent, saponify with KOH, 70–100°C for 5–30 min, extract with immiscible organic solution	Polygosil 60-5 silica, 4.6 × 250 mm, hexane/disopropyl ether, 90/10	FL 296 ex, 320 em	None	Saponification not necessary	41 (1985)

such as blood, plasma, serum, or milk, a two-phase extraction was adequate. Lang et al. used a detergent, sodium dodecyl sulfate, to disrupt the matrix and facilitate extraction of tocopherols and ubiquinones (34a, 34b). Saponification is rarely used for biological fluids (65), and satisfactory results can be achieved without it. For tissue and plasma samples, a single acetone extraction resulted in superior recovery, compared to a two-phase ethanol/hexane or methanol/chloroform extraction procedure. Acetone extraction involved addition of acetone and removal of insoluble material by centrifugation. Coextracted polar compounds did not interfere due to the selectivity of fluorescence detection (61). See Table 5 for a summary of separation systems for biological fluids.

For tissue samples, saponification is more common (23,33,45,46,64, 66,77). Alternatives to saponification are two-phase extractions in the presence of sodium dodecyl sulfate (34a, 34b, 70) and acetone extraction with subsequent cleanup by solid-phase extraction. The additional cleanup was found necessary as acetone extracts contain polar compounds, which would not partition into hexane or chloroform (28). Mostow et al. successfully analyzed tocopherols from crude acetone extracts without further cleanup by using HPLC conditions in which tocopherols were well resolved from polar matrix components. Strongly retained components were removed by gradient elution with methylene chloride (53). Nierenberg et al. analyzed tocopherol in feces after extraction of an aqueous slurry with acetonitrile/ethyl acetate/butanol (9/40/40) (57). For other tissues satisfactory results were obtained with a simple two-phase extraction of the aqueous homogenate (67,76,89). Analytical procedures for biological tissues are summarized in Table 6.

Solid food and animal feed products containing high amounts of fiber (grains, cereals, vegetables) present the most challenging matrix for efficient extraction of vitamin E (Table 7). For these samples homogenization with subsequent saponification is necessary to achieve a satisfactory recovery of vitamin E (24,38,42,43,45,54,62,63,71,87,88). Infant formula was analyzed in a multistep procedure, in which a first extraction with organic solvent was followed by saponification (43). McMurray et al. cautioned that on grassy animal feeds (hay, grass silage) extraction of vitamin E prior to saponification resulted in poor recovery (24). α-Tocopheryl acetate was successfully recovered from milk powder without saponification by a hexane/water extraction of the dry powder dispersed in dimethyl sulfoxide/dimethylformamide/chloroform (2/2/1) (51). α-Tocopheryl acetate and retinyl palmitate were quantitatively extracted from breakfast cereal by a straightforward chloroform/ethanol/water two-phase extraction (56). Extracts of α-tocopherol and α-tocopheryl acetate from fortified animal feeds were cleaned up by silica solid-phase extraction to remove pigments that interfered in an HPLC-UV analysis (87). Mayne et al. determined α-tocopherol in chicken liver by acetylation of extracted α-tocopherol. This derivatization was accomplished by treating dried extracts with acetic anhydride in pyridine with 4-(dimethylamino) pyridine added as catalyst. The reaction was stopped by addition of aqueous sodium bicarbonate and tocopheryl acetate was recovered by hexane extraction. This derivatization lengthened the retention time of tocopherol, moving it beyond the elution time of canthaxanthin. This approach is limited to UV detection since tocopheryl acetate does not yield a signal with fluorescence or electrochemical detection (54).

4. GAS CHROMATOGRAPHY OF VITAMIN E

4.1 General Considerations

For the gas chromatographic (GC) analysis of vitamin E, the transition from packed columns to capillary columns has brought more resolving power to separate isomeric tocopherols and tocotrienols, improved separation from interfering compounds, and lower detection limits. Capillary columns have evolved from coated columns to chemically bonded phases, which are more durable, and give more reproducible chromatography than coated capillary columns or packed columns. Tocopherols can be assayed by GC with or without prior derivatization. Tocopherols and their derivatives are conveniently monitored by flame ionization detectors. Mass spectrometric detection (GC-MS) provides additional identification of GC peaks through characteristic mass spectra and superior selectivity in the selected ion monitoring (SIM) mode.

4.2 Separation Systems

Stationary phases for packed-column gas chromatography of tocopherols ranged from nonpolar phases such as silicon gum rubber (91), silicon oil (92), Apiezon L (93), and SE-30 (94–98), to moderately polar OV-17 (19), SE-52 (99), and polar Silar-10C (100). Liquid phases were coated on acid/base-washed diatomaceous support materials, rendered inert by silanization. Popular support materials were GasChrom Q (93,95–97,100) and Chromosorb W (19,92,99). Historically, GC methods have separated tocopherols and tocotrienols except for β- and γ-isomers. Even by 1988, no packed-column GC method surveyed had adequately resolved β- and γ-tocopherol. Silicon oil phase separated tocopherols and tocotrienols from palm oil, but could not separate β and γ isomers of tocopherol or tocotrienol. In addition, δ-tocotrienol and α-tocopherol

Table 5 High-Performance Liquid Chromatography: Biological Fluids

Sample preparation	Column mobile phase	Detection	Internal standard	Comments	Reference (Year)
Add miscible organic solvent, clarify solution, inject	Ultrasphere ODS Minicolumn, 4.6 × 45 mm	EC T1 +0.18v, T2 +0.50 V, coulometric	None	EC discriminating enough to allow minimal sample cleanup and sensitive enough to require only a small amount of sample	29 (1983)
	LiChrosorb RP-18, 4.6 × 250 mm, MeOH/H$_2$O, 98/2	FL 295 ex, 340 em	None	Acetone extracts more α-T from tissue than CHCl$_3$ or hexane	61 (1983)
Add miscible organic solvent, extract with immiscible organic solvent, analyze organic phase	LiChrosorb R-18, 4.6 × 100 mm, 100% MeOH	UV 288 nm	Vitamin A acetate		85 (1988)
	μBondapack C-18, 3.9 × 300 mm, MeOH/H$_2$O, 95/5	UV 290 nm	α-T acetate		74 (1987)
	Superspher RP-18, 4 × 250 mm, CH$_3$CH/H$_2$O/MeOH, 49/3/48	UV 280 nm	tocol		
	Resolve C-18, 3.9 × 150 mm, EtOH/H$_2$O, 92/8, post-column derivatize with NaBH$_4$ in ethanol	α-T, UV 292 nm, vitamin K, FL 320 ex, 430 em	α-T acetate for α-T and cetyl naphthoate for vitamin K	α- and γ-T not separated, vitamin K measured	31 (1989)
	Silica Radial-PAK, 5 mm ID, n-hexane/isopropylether, 95/5	UV 280 nm	α-T acetate		75 (1986)
	Bio-Sil ODS-5S, 4.6 × 150 mm, MeOH/25 mM Na acetate, ph 5.0, 95/5	EC, 1.0 V	δ-T		72 (1985)
	μBondapack C18, 3.9 × 300 mm, MeOH/H$_2$O, 96/4	UV 290 nm	Retinyl acetate		82 (1982)
	Supleco C18, 4.6 × 150 mm, MeOH/50 mM Na perchlorate, 94/6	EC, 0.6 V	Tocol	Also measures retinol, small sample requirement	78 (1986)
	C18 MEOH/H$_2$O, 96/4	UV 290 nm	Retinyl acetate	α-T in serum, stable at -70°C for least 4 years	86 (1988)
	Nucleosil C18, 4.6 × 250 mm MeOH, 0.7% NaClO$_4$, 0.1% pyridine	EC, 0.9 V	Tocol		79 (1979)

Column	Detection	Internal standard	Notes	Ref. (year)
Biophase C18 CH$_3$CN/CH$_3$Cl/IPA/H$_2$O, 78/16/3.5/2.5	UV/vis 292, 490 nm	α-T acetate and retinyl palmitate	Multiple internal standards to correct for varying recovery	33 (1987)
Alltech NH$_2$ 4.6 × 250 mm, n-hexane/2-propanol, 98/2	UV 290 nm	None		47 (1986)
Zorbax ODS, 4.6 × 250 mm MeOH/H$_2$O, 99/1	FL 292 ex, 335 em	Tocol		80 (1983)
Vydac ODS, 4.6 × 250 mm either isocratic H$_2$O/MeOH/n-BuOH, 2.6/87.4/10, with step change in flow rate or gradient, same solvents with 15/75/10 going to 2/88/10, 20 mM ammonium acetate, pH 3.5, present in all solvent combinations	UV/vis 325, 295, 450 nm, EC +0.9 V	Tocol	α-T, retinol, and β-carotenes in serum, UV vs. EC, gradient vs. isocratic, one- vs. two phase extraction, saponification vs. no saponification	35 (1987)
Waters μBondpak C18, 3.9 × 300 mm, MeOH/H$_2$O, 97/3	UV 280 nm, FL 296 ex, 330 em	None	Spectrofluorescence, HPLC-UV, HPLC-fluorescence	68 (1979)
Waters Radial-Pak C18, 5 × 100 mm, step gradient, MeOH 8 min MeOH/CH$_3$CN/CH$_3$Cl, 47/42/11 for remainder	UV/vis 280 nm, 436 nm	Retinyl acetate	α-T, retinol, carotenes, lycopene in plasma	58 (1984)
Waters Radial-Pak C18, 5 × 100 mm MeOH/CH$_3$CN/CH$_3$Cl, 47/42/15	UV/vis 290, 325, 284, 470, 450 nm	α-T acetate	α-T, retinol, carotenes, lycopene	36 (1985)
H-P Hypersil ODS, 4.6 × 60 mm, 100% MeOH	UV/vis, 292, 305, 460 nm	Retinyl acetate	α-T, retinol, carotenes, lycopene	60 (1986)
Alltech NH$_2$, 4.6 × 250 mm, n-hexane/2-propanol, 92/2	UV 290 nm	None	α- and γ-T in milk	48 (1987)
Spherisorb ODS II, 4.6 × 150 mm, MeOH/H$_2$O, 96/4, with 50 mM Na perchlorate	EC, +0.4 to +1.0 V	None	α-T and α-T quinone, wash column with MeOH between injections	52 (1987)
CP Spher C18, 3 × 200 mm, 100% MeOH	UV 325 nm, FL 220 ex, 340 em	Retinyl acetate	α-T FL, retinol UV	83 (1986)
Nucleosil 5, C18, 3 × 120 mm, MeOH/H$_2$O, 95/5	UV 280, 340 nm	Retinyl palmitate	α-T and retinol	55 (1986)

Table 5 (Continued)

Sample preparation	Column mobile phase	Detection	Internal standard	Comments	Reference (Year)
	Regis ODS, 4.6 × 250 mm, MeOH/H$_2$O, 96/4	UV 215, 265, 292 nm	α-T acetate	α-T, β-T, γ-T, cholesterol, α-T quinone, antioxidant reduces conversion of α-T to α-T quinone during sample preparation	48 (1984)
	Spherisorb ODS-2, 4.6 × 100 mm, MeOH/CH$_3$CN/CHCl$_3$, 47/47/6	UV/vis 292, 325, 450 nm	α-T acetate	α-T, carotenes, retinol, lycopene and β-cryptoxanthin, multiple, wavelength detection enables differentiation of coeluting peaks	37 (1988)
	LiChrosorb RP-18 C18, 4.6 × 250 mm, MeOH/pyridine, 99.9/0.1 with 50 mM Na perchlorate	EC +0.7 V	δ-T	α-, β-, γ-T	73 (1984)
	RSIL, C18, 4.6 × 250 mm, 100% MeOH	UV 292 nm	Tocol	α-T and retinol	81 (1979)
	Zorbax ODS< 4.6 × 250 mm, 100% MeOH	UV 280 nm	Retinyl acetate	α-T and retinol	84 (1990)
	Spherisorb ODS-2, 4.6 × 100 mm, MeOH/1-propanol, 85/15, with 90 mM perchlorate	EC coulometric, UV 215 nm	Diethoxy analog of Q10	α-T, Q10, choesterol, coupled column	69 (1988)
Supelco LC-18, 4.6 × 150 mm, MeOH/H$_2$O, perchlorate	EC +0.6, UV/vis 94/6, 50 mM	tocol 313 nm	ECD for α-, β-, δ-, γ-T,	90 (1986) UV for retinol	
Add miscible organic solvent, saponify w/KOH, 70–100°C for 5–30 minutes, extract with immiscible organic solvent	Zorbax ODS, 4.6 × 250 mm, gradient MeOH/H$_2$O, 90/10, to EtOAc/IPA, 90/10	UV 300 nm	None	Vitamins A and E in plasma	50 (1989)
	μBondpak, C-18, 3.9 × 300 mm, MeOH/H$_2$O, 95/5	FL, 205 ex, 340 em	None	α-, β-, γ-, δ-T in plasma	65 (1979)

Table 6 High-Performance Liquid Chromatography: Biological Tissues

Sample preparation	Column mobile phase	Detection	Internal standard	Comments	Reference (Year)
Add miscible solvent, clarify solution, inject	Varian Micropak MCH-10 ODS, 4 × 300 mm, MeOH/H$_2$O, 95/5	UV 280 nm	α-T acetate	Step gradient to elute strongly retained compounds	53 (1985)
	Ultrasphere C8, 4.6 × 250 mm, 100% MeOH	UV 280 nm	α-T acetate	Solid-phase extraction for further cleanup	28 (1989)
Add miscible organic solvent, extract with immiscible organic solvent, analyze organic phase	Ultrasphere ODS, 4.6 × 250 mm, 100% MeOH	FL, 295 ex, 330 em	Tocol	α-T and retinol recovery greatly dependent on antioxidant	76 (1986)
	C18, 100% MeOH	UV 284 nm	None	α-T in rat retinas	89 (1984)
	Ultrasphere, ODS, MeOH/EtOH, 1/9, or 3/7 for more complex matrices, longer run time	UV 275 nm, EC +0.7 V	None	α-, γ-, and δ-T, ubiquinois, ubiquinones in blood, plasma, tissues, cell fractions, adjust MP to separate interferences according to the sample type	34, (1987)
	Waters μBondapak C18, 3.9 × 300 mm, MeOH/H$_2$O, 97/3	UV 275, 284 nm	Retinyl acetate	α-T and α-T acetate in feces	57 (1987)
	LiChrosorb SI-60-5 silica, 4.6 × 250 mm, heptane/IPA, 99.3/0.7	FL 215 ex, 320 em	α-T acetate	α-T < 4 min runtime	67 (1988)
	Altex Ultrasphere-ODS, 4.6 × 150 mm, IPA/CH$_3$CN/H$_2$O/TEA/HOAc, 60/20/19.4/0.5/0.1, pH 4.0	EC coulometric −0.70 V, +0.25 V	None	α-, δ-, γ-T, T-quinones	70 (1987)
Add miscible organic solvent, saponify with KOH, 70-100°C for 5–30 min, extract with immiscible organic solvent	Micropak SI-5, 4.5 × 150 mm, hexane/methyl t-butyl ether, 90/10	FL, 220 ex, 360 em	Tocol	α- and γ-T in rat liver. Correct for internal standard decomposition during saponification	64 (1984)
	Alltech C18, 100% MeOH	FL, 295 ex, 340 em	Tocol	α-T in adipose tissue	77 (1988)
	Whatman Partisil PXS ODS 10/25, hexane/2-propanol, 99/1	FL, 210 ex, 325 em	None	Acid wash of extract removes late-eluting interferences	66 (1983)
	Yanapack ODS-T C18, 4.0 × 250 mm or Nucleosil 5 NH2, 4.0 × 150 mm, reversed phase: MeOH with 50 mM perchlorate, normal phase: hexane/IPA, 99/1	Reversed phase: EC +0.8V, normal phase: FL	Tocol	Adipose tissues, low recovery at high fat content	46 (1987)
	Nucleosil 5 NH$_2$, 4.6 × 250 mm, hexane/IPA, 97/3	FL 297 ex, 327 em	2,2,5,7,8-Pentamethyl-6-chromanol	α-, β-, γ-, and δ-, optimize extraction by proper choice of solvents and volumes	23 (1987)

Table 7 High-Performance Liquid Chromatography: Food and Feed Grains

Sample preparation	Column mobile phase	Detection	Internal standard	Comments	Reference (year)
Add miscible organic solvent, extract with immiscible organic solvent, analyze organic phase	Zorbax ODS, 4.6 × 250 mm, 100% MeOH	FL 292 ex, 335 em	Tocol	Acetate esters not measured	62 (1986)
	Waters μPorasil 4 × 300 mm hexane/$CHCl_3$/EtOH, 85/15/0.15	UV 280, 313 nm, FL 360 ex, 415 em	None	α-T acetate and retinol palmitate in fortified cereal	56 (1979)
	Waters Rad-Pak silica, 8 mm ID hexane/IPA, 100/0.08	UV 280 nm, FL 295 ex, 335 em	None	α-T acetate in powdered milk, flow programming to hasten elution of late eluters	51 (1986)
Add miscible organic solvent, saponify with KOH, 70-100°C for 5-30 min, extract with immiscible organic solvent	Partisil-10 PAC 4 × 250 mm hexane/$CHCl_2$/IPA, 70/30/0.2	UV 292 nm	None	Solid-phase extraction as final cleanup	87 (1980)
	Chromegasphere SI 60, silica 4.6 × 150 mm, isooctane/THF, 97.5/2.5	FL 294 ex, 325 em	None	α-T, β-T, γ-, and δ-T α-, β-, γ-, and δ-T3	38 (1983)
	Rad-Pak silica or C18 MeOH, 100% or hexane/IPA, 99/1	FL 295 ex, 330 em	None		45 (1988)
	Waters μBondapak C18, 3.9 × 300 mm, MeOH/H_2O, 95/5	FL 296 ex, 330 em	None		63 (1979)
	Waters μBondapak C18, 3.9 × 300 mm, MeOH/H_2O, 95/5	FL 296 ex, 330 em	None		24 (1980)
	Spherisorb ODS C18, 3.2 × 250 mm MeOH/H_2O, 90/10	UV 280 nm	None	α-T, retinol in feeds	88 (1978)
	Yanapack ODS-T C18, 4.0 × 250 mm, MeOH with 50 mM perchlorate	ECD +0.8 V, FL 297 ex, 327 em	Tocol	α-, β-, γ-, and δ-T in feeds	71 (1985)
	Ultrasphere ODS, 4.6 × 250 mm MeOH/H_2O, 95/5	UV 210 nm	None	Acetylates α-T after saponification to separate from high canthaxanthin in sample	54 (1988)
	Ultrasphere-SI 4.6 × 250 mm hexane/IPA, 98.8/1.2	FL only info	None	α-T, γ-T, α-T3, γ-T3 and carotenoids in corn	42 (1987)
	LiChrospher SI 60 silica, 4.6 × 120 mm, hexane/IPA/EtOH, 100/1/0.5	FL 292 ex, 320 em	None	α-, β-, δ-T infant formula	43 (1989)

were not well separated. Nonsaponifiable material, such as β-sitosterol, interfered and was cleaned up by TLC (92). A 3% SE-30 packed column separated tocopheryl butyrate derivatives from steryl butyrates (97) but was unable to separate β- and γ-tocopheryl butyrates. Capillary columns have enabled the resolution of β- and γ-tocopherol homologs, and separation from interfering substances, such as cholesterol (101,102). In a direct comparison of packed and capillary columns, Marks demonstrated improved separation of deodorizer distillate on a capillary column, which eliminated the need for saponification, reduced analysis time from 2–3 h to 10 min, and increased precision. The capillary column improved the separation of β- and γ-tocopherol, and resolution of the internal standard from cholesterol (102). For capillary GC methods, the selection of liquid phases tended to be toward nonpolar phases DB-1 (103) and DB-5 (102,104,105), or the moderately polar phase Dexsil 400 (101). Lin et al. resolved all tocopherols as trimethysilyl (TMS) ethers on a 32-m PZ-176 capillary column (106). Separation of tocopherols and tocotrienols was achieved without derivatization on a 20-m OV-17 capillary (107). Separation of tocopherols from sterols, including sitosterol, stigmasterol, and cholesterol, in oil and fat samples was accomplished with a column coated with Dexsil 400 (101). See Table 8 for a summary of separation systems.

4.3 Detection

The flame ionization detector (FID) will detect tocopherols and tocotrienols with good sensitivity. FID can detect as little as 1 ng of α-tocopherol from a capillary column (103), or 20 ng of α-tocopherol from a packed column (91). No other type of detector is likely to replace the FID in routine use. Mass spectrometric (MS) detection allows unequivocal identification of tocopherols as demonstrated for the analysis of α-tocopherol in lung tissue (100) and ocular tissue (104), and was sensitive enough to detect 170 pg of α-tocopherol (100). α-Tocopherol was chromatographed after derivatization to its TMS ether and addition of deuterated α-tocopherol as internal standard. α-Tocopherol and internal standard were detected by selected ion monitoring (SIM) of their respective TMS ether ions at m/z 502, and at m/z 515 (100,104). In contrast to FID, SIM is a highly selective mode of detection. In rat lung, cholesterol TMS ether coeluted with α-tocopherol TMS ether from the GC column, but did not interfere with SIM of either α-tocopherol or deuterated internal standard. Nonderivatized tocopherol can be monitored at m/z 430, its molecular ion, as shown for rat liver samples (103).

Table 8 Gas Chromatography

Sample preparation	Derivatization	Stationary phase, column dimensions (type); temperature (°C)	Internal standard	Comments	Reference (year)
Extraction	Acetylation, silylation	1.5% SE-30 on Chromosorb W, 60–80 mesh, 0.45 m × 4 mm (packed); 250	Squalene	α-, γ-, δ-, and α-, γ-, δ-T acetate (β and γ-T not separate)	94 (1966)
Extraction	None	1978 AOAC conditions; 245–265	Hexadecyl hexadecanoate	α-T and α-T acetate in pharmaceuticals	108 (1979)
Extraction, saponification, column chromatography, 2-D TLC + extraction	None	2% OV-17 on Chromosorb WAW-DCMS, 80–100 mesh, 2 m × 3 mm (packed); 235	None	α-, β-, γ-, δ-T in milk (β- and γ-T co-elute)	19 (1975)
Saponification, purification by Kieselgel 60 chromatography	Silylation	5% Apiezon L on Gas-Chrom Q, 80–100 mesh, 1 m × 2.2 mm (packed); 260	Stigmasterol	α-T in chick liver	93 (1980)
Extraction, separation by column chromatography, TLC + extraction	None	3.8% silicone gum rubber on Diatoport S, 80–100 mesh, 1.22 m 3 × mm (packed); program 235–295	None	α-T, phytyl ubiquinone, phylloquinone, menaquinone in biological materials	91 (1969)
Extraction and/or purification by deactivated alumina	None	10% SE-30 on Aeropak 30, 100–120 mesh, 4 ft. × 3 mm (packed); 245	Dotriancontane	α-T and α-T acetate in multivitamin products	98 (1968)
Extraction and/or enzymatic digestion	None	5% SE-30 on Gas-Chrom Q, 80–100 mesh, 8 ft × 4 mm (packed); 265	Hexadecyl hexadecanoate	α-T and α-T acetate in feed concentrates	95 (1987)
Extraction and/or enzymatic digestion	None	5% SE-30 on Gas Chrom Q, 80–100 mesh, 6-8 ft × 4 mm (packed); 265	Hexadecyl hexadecanoate	α-T and α-T acetate in vitamin concentrates	96 (1988)

Sample preparation	Derivatization	Column conditions	Internal standard	Analytes (notes)	Ref. (year)
Saponification	Butyl esterification	3% SE-30 on Gas Chrom Q, 100–120 mesh, 6 ft × 5 mm (packed); 240	Cholesteryl isovalerate	α-, β-, γ-, and δ-T in vegetable oils (β- and γ-T co-elute)	97 (1977)
Saponification, TLC + extraction	None	2% Silicon oil on Chromosorb WAW-DMCS, 80–100 mesh, 1 m × 0.4 cm (packed); 235	Hexadecyl stearate	α-, δ-T, and α-T3 in palm oil (β- and γ-T and T3 coelute)	92 (1979)
Saponification	Silylation, acetates, propionates, butyrates	6% SE-52 on Chromosorb WAW-DMCS, 2.44 m × 4 mm (packed); 255	Hexadecyl hexadecanoate	α-, β-, γ-, δ-, sterols and steryl esters in vegetable oil distillates and residues (β- and γ-T coelute (best separation of isomers and interferers with propionates)	99 (1974)
Freeze-drying, microdissection	Silylation	3% Silar-10C on Gas-Chrom Q, 100–120 mesh, 2 m × 2 mm (packed); 230	Deuterated α-tocopherol	α-T in rat lung tissue, MS for ID	100 (1981)
Freeze-drying, microdissection	Silylation	D B – 5, 5 m (capillary); N/A	Deuterated α-tocopherol	α-T in ocular tissue, MS for ID	104 (1987)
Extraction, saponification, purification by column chromatography	None	0.25 μm DB-1, 15 m × 0.25 mm (capillary); program 220–270	Squalene	α-T and retinol and biological materials, MS for ID	103 (1988)
Saponification	Silylation	Dexsil 400, 50 m × 0.25 mm (capillary); 260	5,7-Dimethyl-tocol	α-, β-, γ-, and δ-T, campesterol, stigmasterol, sitosterol in fats and oils (tocotrienols resolved from the tocopherols, though β-, γ-T3 co elute)	101 (1983)
None	Silylation	0.25 μm DB-5, 30 m × 0.25 mm (capillary); programs 140–300, 300–320	Heptadecyl stearate	α-, β-, γ-, δ-, in deodorizer distillate	102 (1988)
Selective deacylation, separation by column chromatography	None	DB-5, 30 m (capillary); program 250–280	α-T acetate	α-, β, γ-, δ-T	105 (1984)

4.4   Quantitation

Quantitation is usually based on the excellent linear relationship of GC-FID peak areas to tocopherol concentration. A similar relationship exists between peaks from GC-MS detection and tocopherol concentration. Internal standardization is the preferred calibration method, as it allows to correct for losses during sample preparation procedures and variable injection volumes. Most accurate results are obtained when the internal standard is structurally closely related to α-tocopherol. For GC-MS deuterated α-tocopherol is a good choice. Thomas et al. found that the GC-MS peak area ratios of α-tocopherol to deuterated α-tocopherol were not equal to the weight ratio (100) and attributed this to the fact that α-tocopherol-d_{13} used as an internal standard was only one of the deuterated variants in the standard. The difference was corrected by calibration of peak ratios versus weight ratios. For accurate quantitation, the authors recommended to adjust the amount of internal standard to the expected endogenous α-tocopherol levels in the sample. A variety of internal standards were described for GC-FID methods. Only 5,7-dimethyltocol (101) is structurally related to tocopherols. Other internal standards were squalene (94,103), hexadecyl hexadecanoate (95–96,99,108), hexadecyl stearate (92), heptadecyl stearate (102), stigmasterol (93), and dotriacontane (98).

4.5   Sample Preparation

Freeze-Drying

Biological materials require sample preparation to liberate and extract vitamin E from the matrix prior to analysis. Saponification or derivatization are optional. For solid samples, such as plant and animal tissues, extraction or saponification is preceded by some form of homogenization, either mixing, grinding, or mincing. However, in some cases specific loci in a tissue were isolated for analysis. Thomas et al., for example, isolated specific portions of the rat lung (parenchyma, connective tissue, blood vessel walls, and the airway) after freeze-drying the whole organ and dissection under a microscope (100). Sections as small as 5 μg were obtained and extracted and derivatized to TMS ethers in one step. Stephens et al. used freeze-drying prior to microdissection on ocular tissues (104). α-Tocopherol in the prepared sections was then extracted and derivatized to TMS ethers in a single step.

Enzymatic Digestion

An AOAC method for the analysis of spray-formulated powders containing α-tocopheryl acetate requires an enzymatic digestion by protease (type XIV) to break down the sample matrix before extraction. Samples are incubated with protease at 60°C for 20–30 min prior to multiple single phase extraction with hexane (95,96).

Extraction

Single-phase or two-phase liquid extractions of the tocopherol from the sample matrix are straightforward and often sufficient. Examples of a single-phase extraction are benzene (98) or hexane (95,96,108) extractions of pharmaceutical products. Rat tissues were prepared with a modified Bligh-Dyer (109) single-phase extraction with dichloromethane, methanol, and sodium chloride (103). Butylated hydroxytoluene and EDTA were added to the extraction solvent to prevent α-tocopherol decomposition. Human milk was extracted with a two-phase system of ethanol, ethyl ether, and petroleum ether (19). For α-tocopherol acetate in feed concentrates, a Soxhlet extraction, with *n*-hexane/cyclohexane (1/1), preceded further dilution with *n*-hexane (95,96).

Saponification

As mentioned earlier (see section 2.5), saponification is useful in eliminating triglycerides and phospholipids from the sample matrix and to cleave tocopheryl esters. To protect vitamin E under high temperature and high pH, antioxidants such as ascorbic acid (92,93,97) and pyrogallol (19,101,103) are added. Temperatures ranged from 65 (103) to 100°C (by heating in a boiling water bath) (97). Exposure times ranged from 8 min (101) to 30 min (19,92,99). Slover et al. avoided the usual refluxing step to reduce α-tocopherol decomposition in oils and fats by placing the sample into a capped tube, and adding pyrogallol (antioxidant) and KOH under nitrogen. Saponification was complete after 8 min at 80°C. After saponification, samples are extracted into a water immissible solvent (19,92,93,97,99,101,103), derivatization is optional (93,97,99,101). It has been noted that the presence of fatty acids can affect the tocopherol recovery from postsaponification extraction, particularly δ-tocopherol. To improve recovery, a second extraction was performed, which increased δ-tocopherol recovery from 77 to 93% (101).

Chromatography

Some interferences can be effectively eliminated through column chromatography. Purification by column chromatography was performed following saponification (19,93,103) or direct extraction (91,98). Kormann purified saponified liver extracts in a 0.063–0.20 mm Kieselgel 60 column (150 × 10 mm) prior to derivatization (93). Sterols were removed from the unsaponifiable lipid portions of a digitonin-impregnated celite column (103). Unsaponifiable milk lipid was purified sequentially with alumina and passage through a Florisil column to remove free fatty acids (19). Aluminum oxide was effective in the removal of excipients in multivitamin products (98). TLC separation of the tocopherol homologs from interfering substances like sterols (92) is an alternative cleanup technique. Unlike column chromatography, TLC is capable of separating β- and γ-tocopherol homologs. This can be an advantage for packed-column GC, which cannot resolve β- and γ-tocopherol (92).

Derivatization

As tocopherols are thermally labile and decompose when exposed to high GC injector temperatures, underivatized tocopherols were applied to the GC column with cold on-column injection (103). Alternatively, derivatization of tocopherols can increase stability and volatility, shorten retention times, and improve peak shape. TMS ethers are the most common derivatives (93,94,99–102,104). They can be prepared in a straightforward manner by the addition of an equal volume of pyridine and a silylation reagent like bis(trimethylsilyl) trifluoroacetamide (BTSTFA), containing 1% trimethylchlorosilane (100). Unlike esterification procedures, which require heating at 100–130°C (94,97) and reaction times between 15 and 30 min (94,97), the TMS ether reaction is complete within 10–15 min at room temperature (100,104). Others tried acetates (94,99), propionates (99), or butyrates (97,99). Among these, propionate derivatives gave the better separation of tocopherols and sterols from interfering compounds (sterol hydrocarbons and ketones, glyceride esters) than acetates and butyrates in vegetable oil distillates and residues (99).

Selective Deacylation

Foster et al. describe a method to separate α-tocopheryl acetate in the presence of other tocopheryl acetates by deacetylation in pyrrolidine/dichloromethane at room temperature. Reaction rates for tocopheryl acetate isomers were highest for δ-tocopheryl acetate (15 min), followed by β- and γ-tocopheryl acetate (~2 h), while α-tocopheryl acetate was unreactive. α-Tocopheryl acetate was separated from β-, γ-, and δ-tocopherol through column chromatography. When tocopherols from soybean oil deodorizer distillate were acylated to hexanoates, deacylation was achieved in the same order, leaving α-tocopheryl hexanoate intact (105).

4.6   Applications

Specific portions of lung tissue (100) and ocular tissue (104) were analyzed with good sensitivity after freeze-drying and microdissection. The isolated sections were derivatized to TMS ethers by addition of silylation reagent without further sample treatment. α-Tocopherol was analyzed on Silar-10C (100) or DB-5 (104) capillary columns with retention times of 1.2 min (100) and 5 min (104), respectively, and monitored by mass spectrometric detection in the SIM mode. Unsaponifiable lipids from rat and tuna liver samples were cleaned up by column chromatography to remove sterols that interfered with the analysis of α-tocopherol and retinol on a 15-m DM-1 capillary column (103). Though FID responses were used for quantitation, GC-MS spectra were obtained to identify α-tocopherol. For the determination of α-tocopherol in chick liver, column chromatographic purification with Kieselgel 60 removed unspecified impurities preceding analysis of the TMS ethers on a column packed with 5% Apiezon L. Recovery of α-tocopherol added prior to saponification was 95% (93).

Vitamin E acetate oil concentrates were assayed on a 5% SE-30 packed column after dilution in hexane. Tocopherol and tocopheryl acetate isolated from feed concentrates were separated adequately on a packed 5% SE-30 column (95,96). Meijboom et al. used a TLC-GC method in an attempt to resolve all tocopherol and tocotrienols from palm oil, but were unable to separate the β and γ forms of tocopherols and tocotrienols (92). A packed-column separation of tocopheryl butyrates from steryl butyrates in saponified vegetable oil was described by Hartman. Though β- and γ-tocopheryl butyrates coeluted on a 3% SE-30 packed column, butyrates of cholesterol, campesterol, stigmasterol, and β-sitoserol were well separated from the tocopheryl derivatives (97). The analysis of deodorizer distillate from soybean oil was accomplished without saponification simply by derivatization of tocopherols to their TMS ethers and injection on a 30-m DB-5 capillary column. This procedure was able to separate sterols and other interferences from the tocopherols and was capable of resolving β- and γ-tocopherol (102). A packed-column method (99), in comparison, required saponification and showed an added increase in tocopherol content, which was attributed to the presence of the tocopheryl esters. Separation of tocopherols from major sterols in several edible oils and fats was accomplished with prior saponification on a 50-m Dexsil 400 capillary column (101).

Multivitamin preparations were analyzed for α-tocopheryl acetate without derivatization or saponification on a 10% SE-30 packed column. Tablets were extracted with benzene and purified through aluminum oxide to clean up formulation excipients. Dilution in tetrahydrofuran was sufficient for liquid multivitamin formulas. Creams were extracted with hexane from a heated aqueous emulsion and were purified on aluminum oxide. The purified hexane extract was evaporated to dryness and reconstituted with tetrahydrofuran for GC analysis (98).

5.   NEW DEVELOPMENTS AND FUTURE TRENDS

5.1   High-Performance Liquid Chromatography-Mass Spectrometry

Unlike gas chromatography-mass spectrometry combinations (GC-MS) which are well established, high-performance liquid chromatography-mass spectrometry (HPLC-MS) has proven technically more challenging. HPLC-MS interfaces that are capable of eliminating large amounts of solvents, such as thermospray and moving belt, have overcome many initial problems, but HPLC-MS remains limited to volatile mobile phase systems of low salt content, which makes many reversed-phase separations unfeasible. Also, samples matrices must be eliminated by either rigorous sample cleanup or column switching. Mass spectrometry detection, on the other hand, affords highly specific detection in the single ion monitoring (SIM) mode and unequivocal identification by means of a characteristic mass spectrum (110a). "Soft" ionization techniques like chemical ionization (CI), field desorption (FD), and fast atom bombardment (FAB) preserve the integrity of the tocopherols and make it possible to monitor the characteristic molecular ion. Van Der Greef et al. (110b) describe the determination of all tocopherol homologs and α-tocotrienol from maize germ oil by moving belt HPLC-MS on silica gel and EI and CI detection. The diluted oil sample was injected without prior cleanup. The bulk of triglycerides was diverted from the mass spectrometer through a switching valve.

5.2   Supercritical Fluid Chromatography

Supercritical fluid chromatography (SFC) commonly uses carbon dioxide above its critical temperature ($31°C$) and pressure (73 atm) to separate labile compounds on a variety of stationary phases. Supercritical carbon dioxide is a rather unpolar solvent, and organic modifiers such as methanol or ethanol are frequently added to increase solvent strength. Supercritical fluid extraction (SFE) is a mild and efficient extraction technique. The low temperature and oxygen-free environment of SFE are particularly suited for the extraction of labile lipids, such as vitamin E, from natural sources. Coupled SFE-SFC systems allow direct introduction of SFE extracts into an SFC system. Tocopherols were purified from wheat germ powder by SFE-SFC on a silica gel column with a carbon dioxide/ethanol mobile phase and separated into α-tocopherol and β-tocopherol fractions (111). Analytical SFC separations of tocopherols afford no advantage over HPLC techniques, which are more versatile and efficient. Coupled SFE-SFC, however, is an appealing preparative technique for the extraction of tocopherols in high purity from many natural sources under nondegrading conditions.

5.3 Separation of Stereoisomers

The presence of three chiral centers in the tocopherols gives rise to eight possible stereomers (Fig. 1 and Table 2). Natural tocopherols are synthesized in a highly stereospecific manner and occur only in the RRR configuration, while modern synthetic methods form a racemic mixture of some or all possible isomers (112). A partial separation of the stereomers of (all-*rac*)-α-tocopheol has been accomplished by GC of TMS ether (113) or methyl ether derivatives (114,115) on standard capillary columns and by HPLC of the acetate esters on noncommercial and commercial chiral phases (116,117). Vecchi et al. (116) attempted a complete separation of all stereomers on a chiral HPLC phase using a variety of tocopheryl esters and ethers. The successful system, however, was a combination of chiral HPLC and achiral capillary GC of the ethyl ethers. (All-*rac*)-α-tocopherol was first separated by HPLC into two groups of four isomers each, which differed in their stereochemistry at the achiral center C-2: the 2R and the 2S isomers. Subsequent capillary GC afforded a good separation of the isomers within each group. Pure synthetic preparations of the individual stereomers were used for peak identification and quantitative determination of all isomers.

5.4 Tandem Mass Spectrometry

In tandem mass spectrometry (MS/MS) the primary ionization and mass analysis of regular mass spectrometry is combined with a collision-induced fragmentation and a secondary mass analysis of a selected primary ion (parent ion). The specific mass and relative intensity of the secondary ions (daughter ions) identify the primary ion. This makes for a highly selective and sensitive analytical technique that is capable of analyzing compounds in complex mixtures with minimal sample cleanup. Tandem mass spectrometry still requires cleanup of bulk excipients. Walton et al. (118) have applied tandem mass spectrometry to a wide variety of vitamin E active compounds, including rare species such as 5- and 7-methyltocols. Tandem mass spectrometry with electrical ionization and a nitrogen gas collision chamber produced characteristic daughter ions for tocopherols and tocotrienols, while fragmentation patterns of isomeric methyltocols were very similar. Electrical ionization (EI) generated intense molecular ions, which were subsequently fragmented by collision with nitrogen gas. The fragmentation patterns of tocopherols and tocotrienols can be explained by a fissure of the oxygen-containing chroman ring and loss of the isoprenoid side chain (119). Tandem mass spectroscopy was used to demonstrate presence of δ-tocopherol and γ-tocotrienol in cyanobacteria strains (120).

5.5   New Possibilities for Vitamin E Analysis

Chromatographic techniques have been the mainstay of vitamin E
analytical methodology. Chromatography, like no other technique, is
able to separate and detect a multitude of closely related compounds
conveniently and reproducibly. The characterization and quantitative
determination of vitamin E active compounds will reach new horizons
with more sensitive and selective chromatographic methods. HPLC-MS
and HPLC-MS/MS (121) hold promise for sensitive and specific analyses
of vitamin E in complex biological matrices. Already, new vitamin E
active species, such as 5- and 7-methyltocols (122) and tocomonoenols
(123), have been described and there may be more to come. So far the
cost of mass spectrometric detection systems for HPLC has precluded
more widespread use. On the chromatographic front, smaller particle
size packing materials (3 μm silica) have increased the resolving power of
standard HPLC columns. A further increase in separation power can be
expected from capillary HPLC (124) and capillary SFC systems (125),
which by virtue of their low solvent flow rates will be more compatible
with mass spectrometric (MS) detectors. The advent of capillary HPLC
is currently limited by the lack of pumps capable of delivering flow rates
in the microliter per minute to nanoliter per minute range with the
necessary precision and detectors able to detect analytes in nanoliter elution volumes. The utility of normal- and reversed-phase capillary HPLC
was demonstrated on a prototype system (126). The β- and γ-tocopherol
isomers that do not separate on traditional reversed phase columns could
be resolved by reversed-phase capillary HPLC. Multidimensional HPLC,
as made possible by column switching, or HPLC-GC combinations will
widen the scope of vitamin E analysis by providing more resolving
power and the sensitivity of FID detection. The increased resolution
achievable by small-particle and capillary columns together with selective MS detectors will decrease the need for extensive sample cleanup
and yield more authentic analysis for labile vitamin E species.

   The recent advent of capillary electrophoresis (CE) has brought new
modes of separation to the analytical arena (127). In CE, known electrophoretic techniques such as free-zone electrophoresis, gel electrophoresis,
and isoelectric focusing were adapted to capillary systems, from which
the separated compounds can be eluted and detected with the convenience only known for HPLC. Traditional electrophoretic techniques
required aqueous media and charged compounds and thus were not
applicable to vitamin E. In an innovative application of CE, micellar
electrokinetic capillary chromatography (MECC) (127), micellar detergent solutions substitute for the aqueous buffer and electrokinetically
driven flow can elute compounds that do not carry a net charge. While

the applicability of MECC to vitamin E active compounds still remains to be demonstrated, MECC presents a novel concept for the analysis of vitamin E.

ACKNOWLEDGMENT

The authors wish to thank Maggie Neuner for her invaluable assistance with the preparation of this manuscript.

REFERENCES

1. H. M. Evans, G. O. Burr, and T. Althausen, *Memoirs of the University of California*, 8:1 (1927).
2. L. J. Machlin, in *Handbook of Vitamins* (L. J. Machlin, ed.), Marcel Dekker, New York, p. 99 (1984).
3. J. K. Lang and H. Esterbauer, in *Membrane Lipid Oxidation*, Vol. 3 (C. Vigo-Pelfrey, ed.), CRC Press, Boca Raton, FL, p. 265 (1990).
4. K. F. Gey, in *Elevated Dosages of Vitamins, Benefits and Hazards* (P. Waler, G. Brubacher, and H. Staehlin, eds.), Huber Publications, Toronto, p. 224 (1989).
5. G. W. Burton, K. H. Cheeseman, T. Doba, K. U. Ingold, and T. F. Slater, in *Biology of Vitamin E*, Ciba Foundation Symposium 101, Pitman, London, p. 4 (1983).
6. Nomenclature of Tocopherols and Related Compounds, *Pure Appl. Chem.*, 54:1507 (1982); *Eur. J. Biochem.*, 123:473 (1982).
7. K. E. Mason, P. E. Harris, *Biol. Symp.*, 12:459 (1947).
8. B. Parrish, *CRC Crit. Rev. Food Sci. Nutr.*, 13:161 (1980).
9. S. R. Ames, *Lipids*, 6:281 (1971).
10. J. Bauernfeind, in *Vitamin E, A Comprehensive Treatise* (L. J. Machlin, ed.), Marcel Dekker, New York, p. 99 (1990).
11. A. Emmerie and C. Engel, *Recl. Trav. Chim. Pays-Bas Belg.*, 58:283 (1939).
12. I. D. Desai, in *Vitamin E—A Comprehensive Treatise* (L. J. Machlin, ed.), Marcel Dekker, New York, pp. 67–98 (1980).
13. J. L. Hess, M. A. Pallansch, K. Harich, and G. E. Bunce, *Anal. Biochem.*, 83:401 (1977).
14. R. A. Ruggeri, T. R. Watkins, R. J. H. Gray, and R. I. Tomlins, *J. Chromatogr.*, 291:377 (1984).
15. D. C. Herting and E. E. Drury, *J. Chromatogr.*, 30:502 (1967).
16. J. Nishiyama, E. C. Ellison, G. R. Mizuno, and J. R. Chipault, *J. Nutr. Sci. Vitaminol.*, 21:355 (1975).
17. W. Mueller-Mulot, *J. AOCS*, 53:732 (1976).
18. C. K. Chow, H. H. Draper, and A. S. Csallany, *Anal. Biochem.*, 32:81 (1969).
19. H. Kobayashi, C. Kanno, K. Yamauchi, and T. Tsugo, *Biochim. Biophys. Acta*, 380:282 (1975).
20. M. Toulova, *Acta Vet. Brno*, 44:163 (1975).

21. K. J. Whittle and J. F. Pennock, *Analyst*, 92:423 (1967).
22. H. R. Bolliger and A. Konig, in *Thin-Layer Chromatography*, 2nd ed. (E. Stahl, ed.), Springer, New York, p. 286 (1967).
23. T. Ueda and O. Igarashi, *J. Micronutr. Anal.*, 3:185 (1987).
24. C. H. McMurray, W. J. Blanchflower, and D. A. Rice, *J. Assoc. Off. Anal. Chem.*, 63:1258 (1980).
25. M. Mulholland, *Analyst*, 111:601 (1986).
26. P. Taylor and P. Barnes, *Chem. Ind.*, 20:722 (1981).
27. B. Tan and L. Brzuskiewicz, *Anal. Biochem.*, 180:368 (1989).
28. H. R. Patel, S. P. Ashmore, L. Barrow, and M. S. Tanner, *J. Chromatogr.*, 495:269 (1989).
29. M. C. Castle and W. J. Cooke, *Ther. Drug Monit.*, 7:363 (1985).
30. A. Celardo, A. Bortolotti, E. Benfenati, and M. Bonati, *J. Chromatogr.*, 490:432 (1989).
31. B. E. Cham, H. P. Roeser, and T. W. Kamst, *Clin. Chem.*, 35:2285 (1989).
32. E. Grundel, M. Y. Jenkins, G. B. Mitchell, and S. R. Blakely, *FASEB J.*, 4:2230 (1990).
33. L. A. Kaplan, J. A. Miller, and E. A. Stein, *J. Clin. Lab. Anal.*, 1:147 (1987).
34a. J. K. Lang and L. Packer, *J. Chromatogr.*, 385:109 (1987).
34b. J. K. Lang, K. Gohil, and L. Packer, *Anal. Biochem.*, 157:106 (1986).
35. W. A. MacCrehan and E. Schoenberger, *Clin. Chem.*, 33:1585 (1987).
36. K. W. Miller and C-S. Yang, *Anal. Biochem.*, 145:21 (1985).
37. D. I. Thurnham, E. Smith, and P. S. Flora, *Clin. Chem.*, 34:377 (1988).
38. W. M. Cort, T. S. Vicente, E. H. Waysek, and B. D. Williams, *J. Agric. Food Chem.*, 31:1330 (1983).
39. Y. L. Ha and A. S. Csallany, *Lipids*, 23:359 (1988).
40. C-S. J. Shen and A. J. Sheppard, *J. Micronutr. Anal.*, 2:43 (1986).
41. A. J. Speek, J. Schrijver, and W. H. P. Schreurs, *J. Food Sci.*, 50:121 (1985).
42. E. J. Weber, *J. AOCS*, 64:1129 (1987).
43. T. Shenhsiu, T. F. Lee, C. C. Chou, and Q. K. Wei, *J. Micronutr. Anal.*, 6:35 (1989).
44. D. T. Burns and C. Mackay, *J. Chromatogr.*, 200:300 (1980).
45. H. E. Indyk, *Analyst*, 113:1217 (1988).
46. T. Ueda and O. Igarashi, *J. Micronutr. Anal.*, 1:15 (1987).
47. C. J. Lammi-Keede, *J. Pediatr. Gastroenterol. Nutr.*, 5:934 (1986).
48. P. A. Moffatt, C. J. Lammi-Keefe, A.M. Ferris, and R. G. Jensen, *J. Pediatr. Gastroenterol. Nutr.*, 6:225 (1987).
49. J-P. Koskas, J. Cillard, P. Cillard, *J. Chromatogr.*, 287:442 (1984).
50. J. L. Rudy, F. Ibarra, M. Zeigler, J. Howard, and C. Argyle, *LC-GC*, 7:969 (1989).
51. D. C. Woolard and A. D. Blott, *J. Micronutr. Anal.*, 2:97 (1986).
52. G. A. Pascoe, C. T. Duda, and D. J. Reed, *J. Chromatogr.*, 414:440 (1987).

53. N. D. Mostow, R. O'Neill, D. L. Noon, and B. R. Bacon, *J. Chromatogr.*, *344*:137 (1985).
54. S. T. Mayne and R. S. Parker, *J. Agric. Food Chem.*, *36*:483 (1988).
55. D. Cuesta Sanz and M. Castro Santa-Cruz, *J. Chromatogr.*, *380*:140 (1986).
56. W. A. Widicus and J. R. Kirk, *J. Assoc. Off. Anal. Chem.*, *62*:637 (1979).
57. D. W. Nierenberg, D. C. Lester, and T. A. Colacchio, *J. Chromatogr.*, *413*:79 (1987).
58. K. W. Miller, N. A. Lorr, and C-S. Yang, *Anal. Biochem.*, *138*:340 (1984).
59. D. D. Stump, E. F. Roth, Jr., and H. S. Gilbert, *J. Chromatogr.*, *306*:371 (1984).
60. D. B. Milne and J. Botnen, *Clin. Chem.*, *32*:874 (1986).
61. B. J. Zaspel and A. Saari Csallany, *Anal. Biochem.*, *130*:146 (1983).
62. J. Lehmann, H. L. Martin, E. L. Lashley, M. W. Marshall, and J. T. Judd, *J. Am. Diet. Assoc.*, *86*:1208 (1986).
63. C. H. McMurray and W. J. Blanchflower, *J. Chromatogr.*, *176*:488 (1979).
64. J. L. Buttriss and A. T. Diplock, *Methods Enzymol.*, *105*:131 (1984).
65. L. J. Hatam and H. J. Kayden, *J. Lipid Res.*, *20*:639 (1979).
66. C. G. Rammell, B. Cunliffe and A. J. Kieboom, *J. Liq. Chromatogr.*, *6*:1123 (1983).
67. H. Verhagen, B. Van Agen, G. J. Hageman, R. H. G. Beckers, and J. D. S. Kleinjans, *J. Liq. Chromatogr.*, *11*:2977 (1988).
68. C. H. McMurray and W. J. Blanchflower, *J. Chromatogr.*, *178*:525 (1979).
69. P. O. Edlund, *J. Chromatogr.*, *425*:87 (1988).
70. M. E. Murphy and J. P. Kehrer, *J. Chromatogr.*, *421*:71 (1987).
71a. T. Ueda and O. Igarashi, *J. Liq. Chromatogr.*, *1*:31 (1985).
71b. O. Hirashima, S. Ikenoya, M. Ohmae, and K. Kawabe, *Chem. Pharm. Bull.*, *29*:451 (1981).
72. P. P. Chou, P. K. Janes, and J. L. Bailey, *Clin. Chem.*, *31*:880 (1985).
73. M. Vandewoude, M. Claeys, and I. De Leeuw, *J. Chromatogr.*, *311*:176 (1984).
74. W. W. Borland and A. Shenkin, *Ann. Clin. Biochem.*, *24*:S1-111-S (1987).
75. J. E. Chappell, T. Francis, and M. T. Clandinin, *Nutr. Res.*, *6*:849 (1986).
76. N. R. Badcock, D. A. O'Reilly, and C. B. Pinnock, *J. Chromatogr.*, *382*:290 (1986).
77. G. J. Handelman, W. L. Epstein, L. J. Machlin, F. J. G. M. van Kuijk, and E. A. Dratz, *Lipids*, *23*:598 (1988).
78. M. Huang, G. J. Burckart, and R. Venkataramanan, *J. Chromatogr.*, *380*:331 (1986).
79. S. Ikenoya, K. Abe, T. Tsuda, Y. Yamano, O. Hirashima, M. Ohmae, and K. Kawabe, *Chem. Pharm. Bull.*, *27*:1237 (1979).

80. J. Lehmann and H. L. Martin, *Clin. Chem.*, 29:1840 (1983).
81. A. P. De Leenheer, V. O. R. C. De Bevere, M. G. M. DeRuyter, and A. E. Claeys, *J. Chromatogr.*, 162:408 (1979).
82. W. J. Driskell, J. W. Neese, C. C. Bryant, and M. M. Bashor, *J. Chromatogr.*, 20:439 (1982).
83. M. J. Russell, B. S. Thomas, and E. Wellock, *J. High Resolut. Chromatogr. Chromatogr. Commun.*, 9:281 (1986).
84. A. Sharma, *Ind. J. Exp. Biol.*, 28:780 (1990).
85. M. Amin, *J. Liquid Chromatogr.*, 11(6):1335 (1988).
86. E. W. Gunter, W. J. Driskell, P. R. Yeager, *Clin. Chim. Acta*, 175:329 (1988).
87. H. Cohen and M. R. Lapointe, *J. Assoc. Off. Anal. Chem.*, 63:1254 (1980).
88. P. Soederhjelm and B. Andersson, *J. Sci. Food Agric.*, 29:697 (1978).
89. D. F. Hunt, D. T. Organisciak, H. M. Wang, and R. L. C. Wu, *Curr. Eye Res.*, 3:1281 (1984).
90. M -L. Huang, G. J. Burckart, and R. Venkataramanan, *J. Chromatogr.*, 380:331 (1986).
91. G. H. Dialameh and R. E. Olson, *Anal. Biochem.*, 32:262 (1969).
92. P. W. Meijboom and G. A. Jongenotter, *J. AOCS*, 56:33 (1979).
93. A. Kormann, *J. Lipid Res.*, 21:780 (1980).
94. S. Ishikawa and G. Katsui, *J. Vitaminol.*, 12:106 (1966).
95. M. Labadie and C. E. Boufford, *J. Assoc. Off. Anal. Chem.*, 70:417 (1987).
96. M. Labadie and C. E. Boufford, *J. Assoc. Off. Anal. Chem.*, 71:1168 (1988).
97. K. T. Hartman, *J. AOCS*, 54:421 (1977).
98. F. P. Mahn, V. Viswanathan, C. Plinton, A. Menyharth, and B. Z. Senkowski, *J. Pharm. Sci.*, 57:2149 (1968).
99. D. K. Feeter, *J. AOCS*, 51:184 (1974).
100. D. W. Thomas, R. M. Parkhurst, D. S. Negi, K. D. Lunan, A. C. Wen, A. E. Brandt and R. J. Stephens, *J. Chromatogr*, 225:433 (1981).
101. H. T. Slover, R. H. Thompson, Jr., and G. V. Merola, *J. AOCS*, 60:1524 (1983).
102. C. Marks, *J. AOCS*, 65:1936 (1988).
103. C. R. Smidt, *J. Chromatogr.*, 434:21 (1988).
104. R. J. Stephens, D. S. Negi, S. M. Short, F. J. G. M. van Kuijk, E. A. Dratz, and D. W. Thomas, *Exp. Eye Res.*, 47:237 (1988).
105. C. H. Foster and E. B. Cross, *J. AOCS*, 61:1461 (1984).
106. S -N. Lin and E. C. Horning, *J. Chromatogr.*, 112:465 (1972).
107. F. Mordret and A. M. Laurent, *Rev. Fr. Corps Gras*, 25:245 (1978).
108. A. J. Sheppard and W. D. Hubbard, *J. Pharm. Sci.*, 68:98 (1979).
109. E. G. Bligh and W. J. Dyer, *Can. J. Biochem.*, 37:911 (1959).
110a. P. Newton, *LC-GC*, 8:706 (1990).
110b. J. Van der Greef, A. C. Tas, M.X. Ten Noever De Brauw, M. Hoen, G. Meijerhoff, and U. Rapp, *J. Chromatogr.*, 323:81 (1985).
111. M. Saito and Y. Yamauchi, *J. Chrom. Sci.*, 27:79 (1989).
112. O. Isler and G. Brubacher, *Vitamin E*, Georg Thieme Verlag, Stuttgart (1982).

113. H. T. Slover and R. H. Thompson, *Lipids*, *16*:268 (1981).
114. N. Cohen, C. G. Scott, C. Neukom, R. J. Lopresti, G. Weber, and G. Saucy, *Helv. Chim. Acta*, *64*:1158 (1981).
115. C. G. Scott, N. Cohen, P. P. Riggio, and G. Weber, *Lipids*, *17*:97 (1982).
116. M. Vecchi, W. Walther, G. Glinz, T. Netscher, R. Schmid, M. Lalonde, and W. Vetter, *Helv. Chim. Acta*, *73*:782 (1990).
117. H. Yamaguchi, Y. Itakura, and K. Kunihiro, *Iyakuhin Kekyu*, *15*:536 (1984).
118. T. J. Walton, C. J. Mullins, R. P. Newton, A. G. Brenton, and J. H. Beynon, *J. Chromatogr.* *425*:87 (1988).
119. S. E. Scheppele, R. K. Mitchum, C. J. Rudoph, K. F. Kinneberg and G. V. Odell, *Lipids*, *7*:297 (1972).
120. C. J. Mullins, T. J. Walton, R. P. Newton, J. H. Beynon, A. G. Brenton, and W. J. Griffiths, *Biochem. Soc. Trans.*, *14*:969 (1986).
121. J. Henion and T. Covey, in *Mass Spectrometry in Biomedical Research* (S. J. Gaskell, ed.), John Wiley & Sons, New York, p. 477 (1980).
122. J. F. Pennock, *Biochem. Soc. Trans.*, *11*:504 (1983).
123. A. Henry, R. Powls, and J. F. Pennock, *Biochem. J.*, *242*:367 (1987).
124. W. D. Pfeffer and E. S. Yeung, *J. Chromatogr.* *506*:401 (1990).
125. B. J. DeLuca, K. J. Voorhees, T. A. Langworthy, and G. Holzer, *J. High Resolut. Chromatogr. Chromatogr. Commun.*, *9*:182 (1986).
126. W. T. Wahyuni and K. Jinno, *J. Chromatogr.*, *448*:398 (1988).
127. J. D. Olechno, J. M. Y. Tso, J. Thayer, and A. Wainright, *Am. Lab.*, *22*:51 (1990).

4

VITAMIN K

Willy E. Lambert and André P. De Leenheer

Laboratory for Medical Biochemistry and Clinical Analysis,
State University of Ghent,
Ghent, Belgium

1. INTRODUCTION

Although some biochemical functions of vitamin $K_{1(20)}$ are already clear, several others remain to be elucidated. Chromatography played an important role in the isolation and characterization of this vitamin. Due to the complexity of the matrices and to the problems in the detection, the quantitation of endogenous vitamin $K_{1(20)}$ levels in humans, as well as the analysis of vitamin $K_{1(20)}$ in food samples, remains an analytical challenge. As a result, sample treatment and chromatography, followed by specific detection, are essential steps in vitamin $K_{1(20)}$ assays. The aim of this chapter is to rationalize this by reviewing the pertinent literature in this area, with special emphasis on applications to biosamples. We will focus mainly on the papers published after 1980.

1.1 Structures and Chemical Properties

All K-vitamers are derivatives of the same 2-methyl-1, 4-naphthoquinone structure. The number of isoprene units or the number of C atoms in the side chain can be used to characterize the molecules. Accordingly, MK-4 contains four isoprene units, or $K_{1(20)}$ has 20 carbon atoms in the side chain. Three molecules, each representative of a group of K-vitamers (Fig. 1), are described in more detail on the following page.

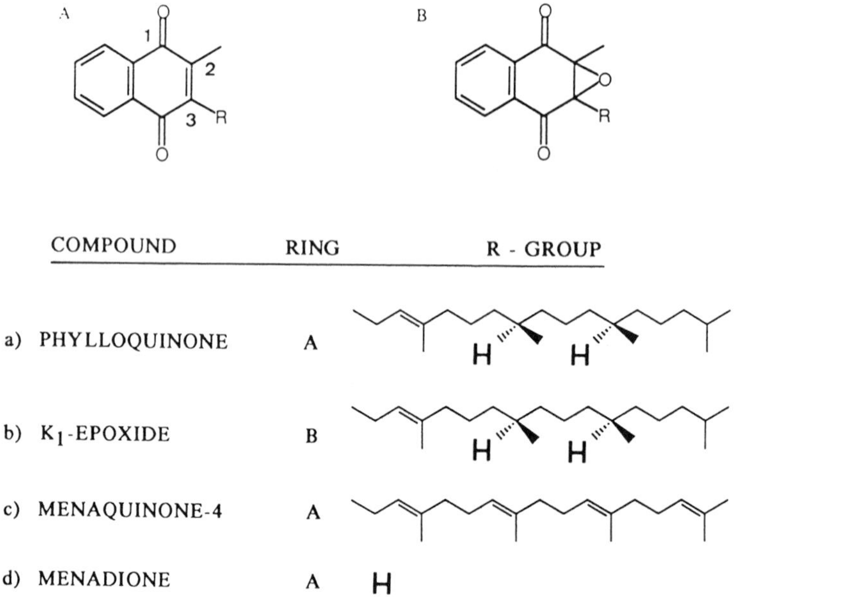

Figure 1 Structural formulas of some important K-vitamers: (a) phylloquinone, vitamin $K_{1(20)}$, 2-methyl-3-phytyl-1,4-naphthoquinone; (b) $K_{1(20)}$-epoxide; (c) menaquinone-4, 2-methyl-3-tetraprenyl-1,4-naphthoquinone; (d) menadione, 2-methyl-1,4-naphthoquinone.

1. Phylloquinone, 2-methyl-3-phytyl-1,4-naphthoquinone, or vitamin $K_{1(20)}$ is found in green plants. The side chain contains 20 carbon atoms (four isoprene units, three of them totally reduced). The stereochemistry of the chain of $K_{1(20)}$ is 2'-*trans*, 7'R and 11'R (Fig. 1a). Epoxidation of the double bond between carbons 2 and 3 of the naphtoquinone nucleus results in $K_{1(20)}$-epoxide (Fig. 1b). Vitamin $K_{1(20)}$ is insoluble in water, slightly soluble in alcohol, and readily soluble in ether, *n*-hexane, and chloroform. The molecule is destroyed in alkaline medium and is sensitive to daylight (isomer formation). On the other hand, the compound is stable in slightly acidic medium, under oxidizing conditions and in heat.

2. Menaquinone-*n*, 2-methyl-3-multiprenyl-1,4-naphthoquinone, or $K_2(n)$ is also called MK-*n*. Menaquinones are characterized by the polyprenyl side chain often containing a large number of isoprene units (up to 13), with *n* indicating the number of these units. Sometimes one or more isoprene units in the side chain are hydrogenated. This is the case in MK-9(II-H_2), in which the second isoprenoid group from the nucleus onward is hydrogenated. Menaquinones are

formed by bacteria (*Escherichia coli, Staphylococcus aureus*), and the all-*trans* configuration in the side chain is the most common (Fig. 1c). The physical and chemical properties of the menaquinones are comparable to those of phylloquinone.

3. Menadione, 2-methyl-1,4-naphthoquinone, or vitamin K_3, MK-o (Fig. 1d), does not occur in nature but has to be synthesized. In the body menadione is transformed to MK-4 by microorganisms or by alkylating enzymes (1). The water-soluble form, menadione sodium bisulfite (MSB), forms a complex with sodium bisulfite (MSBC) or with dimethylpyrimidinol (MPB). The latter compounds are often added to poultry feed (1).

For more detailed information about the chemical properties of these compounds we refer to the original articles by Suttie (1,2), Von Planta et al. (3), and Friedrich (4).

1.2 Biochemistry

Vitamin K was discovered by Hendrik Dam in an attempt to demonstrate the possible essential role of cholesterol in the diet of the chick. He reported hemorrhagic symptoms in chicks fed with an ether-extracted diet (5). The antihemorrhagic fat-soluble compound was called vitamin K_1 or phylloquinone. After the characterization and synthesis of vitamin $K_{1(20)}$, its mechanism of action was studied. It was shown that in mammals and birds, vitamin $K_{1(20)}$ is an essential cofactor in the post-translational carboxylation reaction of glutamic acid residues (GLU) to γ-carboxyglutamic acid residues (GLA) in a number of blood clotting factors (factors II, VII, IX, and X) (6) and also in some other proteins (e.g., protein C, protein S, and osteocalcin) (7–9). The adjacent carboxyl groups of these γ-carboxyglutamyl residues provide the vitamin K-dependent proteins with characteristic calcium- and phospholipid-binding properties that are essential for their activation and function (10). As already stated above, the molecular role of vitamin $K_{1(20)}$ in this carboxylation reaction has not yet been totally elucidated. Also in this area chromatographic techniques remain the method of choice for further study. Excellent reviews on the biochemistry and on the physiological function of vitamin $K_{1(20)}$ have been written by Suttie (2), Olson (11), and Vermeer (12).

2. THIN-LAYER CHROMATOGRAPHY

As a separation step, high-performance liquid chromatography (HPLC) has largely replaced the older thin-layer chromatographic systems

(TLC). However, in recent years TLC may have regained part of its lost importance. This is mostly attributable to the new developments such as high-performance thin-layer chromatography (HPTLC) and densitometry, eliminating some of the drawbacks inherent in classical TLC, such as low speed, poor sensitivity, and incompatibility with on-line quantitation. The pertinent literature up to 1983–1984 has been compiled in the first edition of this volume (13) and by recent reviews (14–16). Older review articles appeared in the late 1960s and the early 1970s (17–19).

2.1 Polar Inorganic Sorbents

Polar inorganic sorbents include silica, alumina, calcium and magnesium silicates, and diatomaceous earth, usually referred to as kieselguhr. The latter sorbents, however, are less frequently used than the polyvalent sorbents such as silica and alumina. Separation on silicic acid is based mainly on differences in polarity and is the method of choice for the isolation of naphthoquinones from other lipids and for the separation of geometric isomers. However, adsorption TLC does not distinguish between the different isoprenologs (menaquinones).

Silica gel H plates eluted with pure chloroform were successfully used by Baczyk et al. (20) in their study of the degradation of both vitamin D_2 and $K_{1(20)}$ exposed to ultraviolet (UV) light. Similarly, vitamin $K_{1(20)}$ was separated from α-tocopherol, β-carotene, and the vitamins A and D_2 in spinach. Here the silica plates were eluted with mixtures of petroleum ether:benzene (6:1, by volume) (21).

Silica gel layers can also be impregnated with 5-20% (w/w) silver nitrate. Compounds with double bounds in the side chain form complexes with the silver ions and show higher retention than their unsaturated counterparts. Consequently, argentation TLC easily separates saturated ($K_{1(20)}$), partly saturated [MK-n (H_n)], and fully unsaturated (MK-n) homologs from each other. However, the resolution between *cis* and *trans* isomers is almost completely lost (22). A typical eluent used for this separation is a mixture of light petroleum:chloroform:acetone (50:10:17, v/v).

Silver ions are not destructive for vitamin $K_{1(20)}$-related compounds and samples can easily be collected from the plates for further analysis. High-molecular-weight menaquinones, however, often show irreversible adsorption on TLC plates impregnated with $AgNO_3$ (23).

2.2 Modified Silica: Nonpolar Bonded Phases

Thin-layer plates with chemically bonded phases (e.g., C_2, C_8, C_{18}, phenyl) are also available and are very similar to the packing materials used for reversed phase HPLC. Consequently, mobile phases also consist of mixtures of water and an organic solvent (methanol, acetonitrile, or tetrahydrofurane). As an example, Collins et al. separated bacterial menaquinones on C_{18} reversed-phase plates eluted with a non-polar solvent mixture. In addition, they were able to separate demethyl menaquinones from their methylated analogs (24).

2.3   Detection and Quantification

A nondestructive way to visualize vitamin K-related compounds is based on fluorescence quenching. However, this procedure is not sensitive and serves only to localize the zones of interest. Spray reagents allow a more specific and a more sensitive detection of K vitamins. Their applications have been extensively reviewed by Lefevere et al. (13). Compositions such as 70% perchloric acid (25), 0.05% rhodamine B in ethanol, or 0.2% anilinonaphthalene sulfonic acid in methanol (22) are frequently used. However, they are destructive for the quinones.

Densitometric scanning (based on reflectance, transmission, simultaneous reflectance and transmission, fluorescence quenching, or fluorescence) has completely superseded both the visual scanning as well as the off-line quantitation after elution of the separated bands, especially in terms of sensitivity and speed of analysis (26). In addition, this technique allows the use of an internal standard resulting in improved precision. Without the introduction of this densitometric scanning, the enhanced resolution in HPTLC would be of no advantage. However, the explosive advance of HPLC in the past decades clearly explains the rapid decline in the number of applications of TLC not only in general, but also in the vitamin K area.

3.   HIGH-PERFORMANCE LIQUID CHROMATOGRAPHY

Since the introduction of microparticulate packing materials for high-performance liquid chromatography (HPLC), unprecedented improvements in column efficiency, resolution, sensitivity, and speed have been achieved. Modern liquid chromatography eliminates the risk of thermo-degradation and protects the compounds from light during the chromatographic run. The highly lipophilic and neutral character of the natural K vitamers renders them compatible with a multitude of HPLC systems (e.g., straight phase as well as reversed phase). Major problems that must be faced when analyzing vitamin K in biological materials include interferences by other lipids such as cholesterol, and the lack of assay sensitivity necessary to quantitate vitamin K down to the low picogram range. In the next section we will evaluate how the most recent papers (from 1980 onward) have dealt with these problems.

3.1 Isolation, Extraction, and Cleanup

Almost all research groups, independently from each other, arrived at similar experimental designs for the assay of vitamin $K_{1(20)}$ in biological samples. During all manipulations one should avoid contact with strong light and alkali (it is essential to remove all traces of detergents from glassware), and, as endogenous levels are in the picogram/per milliliter range, care should be taken to prevent contamination.

In human blood, vitamin $K_{1(20)}$ is transported by lipoproteins, more especially by the very-low-density lipoprotein fraction (VLDL) (27). In analyzing this matrix, denaturation of the lipoproteins is necessary before vitamin K-related compounds can be effectively extracted. In general, protein precipitation is very simple; however, there may be loss of the analyte by occlusion in the precipitate. Furthermore, when using strong acids, the analyte must be stable at the extreme pH values encountered. In our hands, addition of strong acids such as perchloric acid or tri-chloroacetic acid (1 ml, 5% v/v) to 1 ml of serum yielded very low and irreproducible recoveries. On the other hand, organic solvents that are miscible with water, such as ethanol, methanol, or isopropanol, are fre-quently used to denature the proteins. Denaturation is mostly performed by addition of double the amount of ethanol to the serum (Table 1). Other researchers used methanol (37) or isopropanol (38) for this pur-pose. Similar recoveries can be obtained using 80% (v/v) of methanol or 60% (v/v) of ethanol (39). By addition of double the amount of ethanol, a final percentage of 66 is reached. Further increase of the volume of ethanol lowers the recovery of vitamin $K_{1(20)}$ in the final extraction step with n-hexane. The highest recovery can be obtained with isopropanol; however, over 10% of isopropanol partitions into the n-hexane used for the extraction. In this way the evaporation time is increased and, more important, many polar compounds are coextracted and interfere in the chromatographic separation afterward.

Following this denaturation step, vitamin $K_{1(20)}$ can be extracted either in a monophasic procedure with a mixture of methanol and di-chloromethane (37,47,60) according to Bligh and Dyer (40), or by a biphasic extraction with n-hexane or n-pentane (Table 1). The Bligh and Dyer procedure results in a total extraction of all lipids but has several drawbacks, for example, formation of emulsion and difficulties in separating the lower layer from the extraction tube without contaminat-ing it with interfering material accumulating at the interface. From this point of view the n-hexane extraction procedure (2 min vortex mixing) is simpler and results in a clear upper layer that can be removed quite easily. Addition of 10–30% diethylether to the n-hexane increases the recovery but again can result in coextraction of interfering substances (41).

In the sample preparation of human milk, the denaturation step with ethanol is also frequently incorporated (Table 1) and the extraction is performed in a similar way as for serum samples, that is, with a nonpolar solvent such as n-hexane (42,43,45), pentane (46), or petroleum ether (42). Haroon and Shearer, however, preferred an extraction with chloroform and methanol (2:1, v/v) (47). To eliminate the large amount of triglycerides present in human milk samples, enzymatic hydrolysis with pancreas lipase can be incorporated (46,48,50,72). However, three of the above-cited research groups added a fairly high amount of 10 N NaOH to eliminate coextraction of the liberated acids into the organic layer. As mentioned earlier, phylloquinone is known to be unstable under these drastic alkaline conditions. It is well documented that in human milk the triglycerides (and also vitamin $K_{1(20)}$), are encapsulated by a membrane consisting of proteins and phospholipids (49). In addition, this membrane is inhibiting the hydrolytic action of pancreas lipase. Therefore, in our recently developed procedure for the analysis of vitamin $K_{1(20)}$ in human milk samples, we first treated the samples for two min in an ultrasonic bath to disrupt these fat globule membranes. Thereafter, enzymatic hydrolysis of the triglycerides can be performed more effectively (50). It is clear that for an enzymatic treatment of the samples several other parameters, such as the amount of lipase, Ca^{2+} ions and albumin, and pH, as well as reaction time and temperature, must be optimized.

The selectivity of the above described extractions with n-hexane or with methanol and chloroform or dichloromethane is rather low and many interfering lipophilic compounds are coextracted. This necessitates in almost all procedures for the analysis of vitamin $K_{1(20)}$ in serum and milk the use of two complementary HPLC systems displaying different retention mechanisms (e.g., adsorption and reversed-phase chromatography). In some cases, the first HPLC purification step is replaced by conventional column chromatography on silica gel (47) or on commercial silica (32) cartridges. Only a few research groups purify the serum extract on a reversed-phase system and use adsorption chromatography for the final analytical measurement (34,37,60). The chromatograms, however, clearly demonstrate that this is not the best choice. As an alternative, purification of the crude extract was also tried on hydroxyalkoxypropyl Sephadex (HAPS) (51).

Cham et al. (36) describe an additional washing of the n-hexane layer with methanol:water (9:1, v/v) to remove interfering (polar) com-

Table 1 Sample Preparation for Vitamin $K_{1(20)}$ Analysis

Sample volume (ml)	IS	Denaturation/ pretreatment (volume ratio)	Extraction (volume ratio)	Additional cleanup		Reference
				Column	Eluent (v/v)	
(a) Serum, Plasma						
6–13	$K_{1(20)}$-epoxide	Ethanol (2)	n-Hexane (4)	Partisil 5 25 × 0.5 cm	Hexane:diethyl ether (97:3)	29,56, 57
2	[³H]-$K_{1(20)}$	Ethanol (2)	n-Hexane (2.5)	Rsil 5 μm	Diisopropyl ether: n-hexane (3:97)	28,70
1.5	[³H]-$K_{1(20)}$	Ethanol (2)	n-Hexane (6)	μPorasil 30 × 0.39 cm 10 μm	Hexane:acetonitrile (99.8:0.2)	30,61, 68
0.1–0.6	Tocopheryl acetate	Methanol + 1% pyrogallol (1)	n-Hexane (7)	RadPak B 10 × 0.8 cm 10 μm	Isooctane:ethyl acetate (99:1)	53,58
1	MK-4 or chloro-$K_{1(20)}$	Methanol (1)	n-Hexane (5)	—	—	54
1	$K_{2(30)}$	Isotonic NaCl sol. (1) Isopropanol (3)	n-Hexane (10)	—	—	39
0.5	Eicosanyl naphthoate	Water (1) Isopropanol (3)	n-Hexane (12)	—	—	55
0.5	$K_{1(15)}$	1% Pyrogallol in ethanol (1)	n-Hexane (6)	Waters silica 5 μm	n-Heptane:ethyl acetate (99:1)	31,59
1	—	Methanol (3)	Methanol:dichloromethane (1:1, v/v) (2)	Sep-Pak C_{18}	Acetonitrile	37

1	—	Water (1) Ethanol (4)	n-Hexane (6)	Sep-Pak silica	n-Hexane:ether (97:3)	32,65
1	$K_{2(30)}$	Methanol (3)	Methanol:dichloromethane (1:1, v/v) (2)	Sep-Pak C_{18}	Acetonitrile	60
1	Dihydro $K_{1(20)}$	Ethanol (2)	n-Hexane (6)	Sep-Pak silica	n-Hexane:diethyl ether (97:3)	62
2	$K_{1(25)}$	Ethanol (2)	n-Hexane (3.7)	RoSil 5 μm 20 × 0.46 cm	n-Hexane:diisopropylether (98:5:1.5)	33,63, 64,69
0.25	$K_{1(25)}$	Ethanol (2)	n-Hexane (8)	NOVA-PAK C_{18} 10 × 0.8 cm	Acetonitrile: propan-2-ol: dichloromethane (68.5:22.2:9.3)	34
2	—	Water (0.5) Ethanol (1.5)	n-Hexane (2.5)	Sep-Pak silica	n-Hexane:diethyl ether (96:4)	66
1	$K_{2(30)}$	Ethanol (1)	n-Hexane-diethyl ether (1:1) (6)	Silica 20 × 0.5 cm	n-Hexane:benzene (1:2)	67
1	Dihydro $K_{1(20)}$	Ethanol (1) Water (1)	Petroleum ether (1) Diethyl ether (1)	μPorasil 33 × 0.78 cm 10 μm	Heptane:ethyl acetate (99:1)	41
0.05	$K_{1(25)}$	—	—	Bond-Elut C_8	Acetonitrile:iso-propanol:dichloro-methane (7:1:2)	52
1	Cetyl naphthoate	Ethanol (2)	Hexane (5)	—	Wash, with methanol: water (9:1)	36
0.5	$K_{1(25)}$	Ethanol (2)	n-Hexane (6)	Silica 25 × 0.4 cm 5 μm	n-Hexane:acetonitrile (99.85:0.15)	35

Table 1 (Continued)

Sample volume (ml)	IS	Denaturation/ pretreatment (volume ratio)	Extraction (volume ratio)	Additional cleanup Column	Additional cleanup Eluent (v/v)	Reference
(b) Milk and infant formula						
5–20	K_1-epoxide	—	Chloroform: methanol (2:1)	Kieselgel 60	Petroleum ether: diethyl ether (97:3)	47
				Partisil 5 25×0.46 cm	Hexane:dichloro- methane (8:2)	
50	—	0.2 M phosphate buffer, pH 7.7(4), + 2.5g lipase 1.5h, 37°C NaOH, 10N, (0.2) Ethanol (4)	n-Pentane (12)	—	—	72
20	—	(NH_4) OH (0.2) Methanol (3)	Dichloromethane (10), isooctane (5)	Apex silica 25×0.45 cm 5 μm	Isooctane:dichlo- romethane:isopro- panol (85:15:0.02)	73
10	α-Docosanyl naphthoate	Ethanol (2)	n-Hexane:ethyl ether (1:1) (10)	Kiesel gel 30×2 cm	n-Hexane:ethyl ether (97:3)	74
20	—	0.2 M phosphate buffer pH 7.7 (5) + 1 g lipase, 1.5h, 37°C NaOH, 10N, (0.05) Ethanol (5)	n-Pentane (15)	Nucleosil C_{18} (30 × 0.8 cm) 5 μm	Methanol:acetonitrile	46
1	—	Ethanol (1)	Sonication n-Hexane (10)	μPorasil 30×0.8 cm 10 μm	n-Heptane:ethyl acetate (99:1)	42

Sample	Vitamer	Treatment	Extraction	Column	Mobile phase	Ref.
1–2	$K_{2(30)}$	Ethanol (2)	n-Hexane (6)	Sep-Pak silica Spherisorb CN 25 × 0.5 cm 5 μm	n-Hexane:diethyl-ether (97:3) n-Hexane:dichloromethane (97:3)	44
1g		—	CO_2 supercritical fluid extraction	Silica	Dichloromethane:acetone (1:1)	76
0.5	$K_{1(25)}$	2 min ultrasonic, Tris buffer pH 7.7, lipase 1 mg/ml, 10 μl albumin, 20% 45 min, 37°C Ethanol (8) Water (4) 200 μl NH_3 Solution 5%	n-Hexane (15)	RoSil 5 μm 20 × 0.46 cm	n-Hexane:diisopropyl ether (98.5:1.5)	50
(c) Tissues, foods, and oils						
10 g Liver	K_1-epoxide	Ground with anhydrated Na_2SO_4	n-Hexane (5)	Sep-pak silica Partisil-5 silica 25 × 0.46 cm	n-Hexane:diethyl-ether (97:3) n-Hexane:dichloromethane (8:2)	77
4 g Placenta	—	Isopropanol (2.5)	n-Hexane (6)	Sep-pak silica	n-Hexane:diethyl-ether (97:3.5)	78
15 g Oil	—	Lipase (0.5) Phosphate buffer pH 5.5 (1.6) 15 h, 37°C Ethanolic KOH (3)	n-Pentane (10)	Alumina 14 × 1.5 cm	n-Hexane:diethyl-ether (93:7)	79
0.5 g Premix	—	DMSO (40) 30 min, 65°C	n-Hexane (50)	—	—	80

pounds coeluting with vitamin $K_{1(20)}$ in the reversed-phase chromatographic step.

All these additional cleanup steps remove as much extraneous triglycerides or polar compounds as possible, prior to the HPLC step, and provide cleaner separations and prolonged HPLC column life. Without this, adhering lipids alter retention times and produce spurious peaks.

It is clear that for the analysis of serum samples from patients supplemented with vitamin $K_{1(20)}$, a small volume of sample is sufficient, and less complicated cleanup procedures fullfil the requirements. In this way Kirk and Fell were able to extract vitamin $K_{1(20)}$ from 50 μl of serum by solid-phase extraction on a Bond Elut C8 column. Without further purification, the eluate was evaporated and injected on the analytical HPLC system (52).

3.2 Internal Standardization

Before describing the HPLC conditions, we would like to draw attention to the use of an internal standard (IS). For a complicated analysis with multiple chromatographic separations the choice of an appropriate IS is of the utmost importance. The IS compensates for losses during extraction, evaporation, redissolution, and injection of the sample and results in a control of each individual sample throughout the whole analytical procedure. General requirements such as structural analogy, absence in the matrix, stability, and extraction recovery similar to the compound of interest must be fulfilled. In addition, the IS should coelute with the vitamin $K_{1(20)}$ in all chromatographic purification steps, but must be separated from $K_{1(20)}$ in the final analytical chromatographic system. Also, during eventual postcolumn derivatization reactions, the IS should behave in exactly the same was as $K_{1(20)}$. Disregarding the use of an IS is certainly unacceptable for this type of analysis (32,37). Compounds such as tocopheryl acetate (53), eicosanyl naphthoate (55), cetyl naphthoate (36), and α-docosanyl naphthoate (74) do not fulfill the criterion of structural analogy. On the other hand, K_1 epoxide is a natural metabolite of $K_{1(20)}$, and this molecule can also be present in biosamples. An overview of all IS used in vitamin $K_{1(20)}$ analyses is also given in Table 1.

3.3 Adsorption Chromatography as a Cleanup Step

Although chromatography on open columns or on Sep-Pak silica cartridges removes lipids that are both less polar (e.g., hydrocarbons) and more polar (e.g., sterols, glycerides, fatty acids, and phospholipids) than vitamin $K_{1(20)}$ itself, many lipids, including cholesteryl esters, remain present. Most assay designs therefore include an extra purification step using adsorption chromatography before the final quantitation on an analytical HPLC column. Adsorption chromatography is the method of choice for the separation of different classes of lipids. Furthermore, the lipid-rich residue of the crude n-hexane extract can only be totally redissolved in the eluent of an adsorption HPLC system based on n-hexane, and certainly not in the eluent of a reversed-phase system consisting of methanol and water. As will be discussed in a later section, nonaqueous reversed-phase (NARP) chromatography is a valuable alternative.

The dimensions of the adsorption columns used for the cleanup of the samples are rather large (25–30 cm length, and 0.39–0.8 cm ID). Particle sizes of the silica are either 5 or 10 μm. Eluents for these adsorption systems are mainly based on n-hexane or n-pentane with a small percentage of a more polar organic modifier, such as diethyl ether, diisopropyl ether, acetonitrile, ethyl acetate, or dichloromethane (Table 1). Under these conditions, vitamin $K_{1(20)}$ and the internal standard elute quite close to each other (Fig. 2). In this way, a narrow fraction

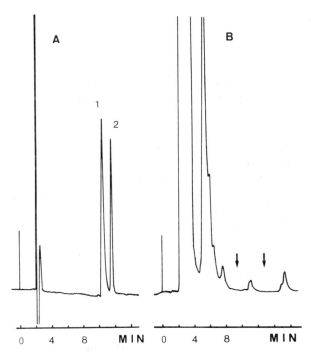

Figure 2 (A) Elution pattern of $K_{1(25)}$ (peak 1) and $K_{1(20)}$ (peak 2) standards on a RoSil 5 μm column eluted with an n-hexane: diisopropyl ether mixture (98.5:1.5, v/v); flow rate, 0.85 ml/min; detection, 252 nm. (B) Chromatographic run of a serum extract obtained under the same conditions. The arrows indicate the times of collection of the effluent.

can be collected and a lot of interfering compounds can be eliminated. The collected fraction is then concentrated to dryness and can be used for further analysis on the analytical reversed-phase system.

3.4 Analytical Reversed-Phase Chromatography

A large variety of packing materials can be used for the analytical reversed-phase chromatographic step (Table 2). In most cases, column dimensions are smaller than for the semipreparative adsorption chromatography and particle size is 5 μm in almost all systems. Eluents for these reversed-phase columns show a much larger variety than those for the adsorption chromatographic step. Ideally, when used with UV detection nonaqueous reversed-phase conditions are most suitable, because then all the lipids present in the collected fraction from the adsorption system can be easily redissolved. As these eluents have a high eluting power, highly retentive ODS packing materials are recommended (31,34, 47,52,54,59,77). When electrochemical detection (ECD) is used the addition of water is necessary to dissolve the supporting electrolyte ($NaClO_4$ or sodium acetate). With these semiaqueous mobile phases, the retention of the K vitamers drastically increases. To avoid these long retention times, the use of less retentive packings, such as octyl bonded phases, is advantageous. However, semiaqueous mobile phases are also used with C_{18} reversed-phase packing materials, as can be seen in Table 2 on the following pages.

As an alternative to the classical reversed-phase packing materials, a Japanese group investigated the chromatographic behavior of different fat-soluble vitamins, including vitamin $K_{1(20)}$, on polymer-based octadecyl bonded phases. By eluting a capillary fused silica column (50 × 0.053 cm) with a mixture of actonitrile:methanol (75:25), they were able to separate vitamins D_2, D_3, E, and $K_{1(20)}$ (81). These capillary systems, however, were not applied to the analysis of $K_{1(20)}$ in biosamples. On the other hand, a column of conventional dimensions (25 × 0.46 cm) packed with another polymer-based material (TSK gel ODS-120 T) was used for the determination of $K_{1(20)}$, K_1-epoxide, and MK-4 in human plasma (65) (Fig. 3).

3.5 Detection

As already mentioned, the procedures for the extraction and for the chromatography of the K vitamers from biosamples are very similar. Much larger variation, however, occurs in the detection procedures applied in the final measurement.

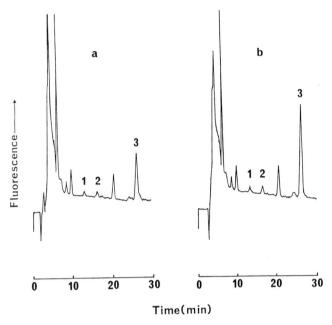

Figure 3 Elution of MK-4 (peak 1), K_1-epoxide (peak 2), and $K_{1(20)}$ (peak 3) from a TSK gel ODS-120T column eluted with a methanol:acetonitrile mixture (6:4, v/v) containing 0.25% sodium perchlorate. (a) Extract of 1 ml of plasma taken 12 h before a meal; (b) extract of 1 ml of human plasma taken 3 h after a meal (from Ref. 65).

UV detection

To detect vitamin $K_{1(20)}$ in column effluents, advantage can be taken of either its UV characteristics (λ_{max} 248 nm), its fluorescence after reduction to the corresponding hydroquinone, or its electrochemical properties.

Vitamin $K_{1(20)}$ displays a relatively poor UV absorbance ($\epsilon =$ 19,900 cm^2/mmol at 248 nm), which is hardly sufficient to detect and quantitate endogenous levels of vitamin $K_{1(20)}$ in plasma of approximately 500 pg/ml. In addition, 248 nm is a rather nonselective wavelength, and interferences are difficult to eliminate. Alternatively, several authors (Table 2) prefer detection at 254 nm, using a fixed-wavelength instrument. A better signal-to-noise ratio may partly compensate for the loss in absolute sensitivity, caused by working at this nonoptimal wavelength. Due to interfering compounds, results of earlier measurements of

Table 2 Final HPLC Step and Detection Modes for $K_{1(20)}$

Analytical HPLC			Detection		Reference
Column	Eluent (v/v)	Derivatization procedure	Mode	nm	
(a) Serum, plasma					
Octadecylsilane	?	—	UV	270	29
RP 18 LL 15 × 3.2 cm	Methanol	—	UV	248	28
		Methanol:acetate buffer (85:15) + ascorbic acid (1 mg/ml) Photochemical reaction	FL	320/420	70
		Reduction with NaBH₄ added postcolumn (37°C)	FL	320/420	70
μBondapak 30 × 0.39 cm 10 μm	Methanol:ethanol: water (37:57:8) + 0.04 M sodium perchlorate + 0.002% HClO₄	—	EC	−0.27 5 V	30
μBondapak C₁₈ 30 × 0.32 cm 10 μm	Methanol:water (95:5)	—	UV	254 and 280	53,58
Ultrasphere ODS 25 × 0.45 cm 5 μm	Acetonitrile: dichloromethane (70:30)	—	UV	254	54
Partisil-10 μm 25 × 0.45 cm	Hexane:acetonitrile (99.8:0.2)	—	UV	254	54
Hypersil-MOS 5 μm	0.03 M NaClO₄ in methanol:water (92.5:7.5)	EC reduction −0.4 V	Fl	320/420	39

Column	Mobile phase	Reduction/derivatization	Detection	Wavelength (nm)	Ref.
Nucleosil C$_{18}$ 15 × 0.46 cm 5 μm	0.6% (w/v) NaClO$_4$ in acetonitrile:isopropanol (9:1) + 0.07% HClO$_4$	EC reduction −1.4 V	Fl	330/430	55
Spherisorb octyl 25 × 0.5 cm, 5 μm	Methanol:0.05 M acetate buffer (99:1 or 95:5)	—	EC−1 V EC, redox, −1.3/0 V		56 44,57,75
Waters C$_{18}$ Resolve	Acetonitrile	—	UV	254 and 280	31,59
Lichrosorb Si 60 25 × 0.46 cm, 5 μm	Hexane:dioxane (99.75:0.25)	—	UV	248	37
Nucleosil C$_{18}$ 15 × 0.46 cm, 5 μm	0.25% NaClO$_4$ in ethanol:water (92.5:7.5)	EC reduction −0.55 V	Fl	320/430	32
Hypersil-MOS C$_8$ 12.5 × 0.46 cm 5 μm	0.03 M NaClO$_4$ in methanol:water (97:3)	EC reduction −0.9 V	Fl	330/435	60
Zorbax ODS 25 × 0.46 cm	30 mM Na acetate, pH 6 in ethanol:water (96.5:3.5)	EC reduction −0.65 V	Fl	340/430	61,68
Hypersil-ODS 25 × 0.46 cm 5 μm	2.0 M ZnCl$_2$, 1.0 M Na acetate, 1.0 M acetic acid in methanol:dichloromethane (80:20)	Reduction on Zn column 2 × 0.39 cm	Fl	248/418	62,71
RSIL C18 HL 15 × 0.32 cm 5 μm	Methanol:ethyl acetate (96:4)	Reduction with (CH$_3$)$_4$NB$_3$H$_8$ added postcolumn or incorporated in the eluent (75°C)	Fl	325/430	33,50,63 64,69

Table 2 (Continued)

Column	Analytical HPLC Eluent (v/v)	Derivatization procedure	Detection Mode	Detection nm	Reference
C_{18}, 4 μm	Acetonitrile:propan-2-ol:dichloromethane (68.5:22.2:9.3)	—	UV	270	34
TSK gel ODS-120T 20 × 0.46 cm 5 μm	0.25% NaClO$_4$ in methanol:acetonitrile (6:4)	EC reduction −0.8 V	Fl	320/430	65
Nucleosil 5 C_{18} 15 × 0.46 cm 5 μm	0.25% NaClO$_4$ in ethanol:methanol (1:4)	Reduction on RC-10 Pt column 10 × 0.4 cm	Fl	320/430	
Nucleosil 5 C_{18} 25 × 0.46 cm	Methanol:ethanol:water (1:2:0.06)	Postcolumn reduction on PtO$_2$ column 5 × 0.46 cm	Fl	254/430	
Hypersil MOS C_8 15 × 0.39 cm 5 μm	Methanol:0.03 M NaClO$_4$ in water (93:7)	EC reduction −1.0 V	Fl	240/418	41
Spherisorb RP-18 ODS 102 5 μm 10 × 0.21 cm	Acetonitrile:isopropanol:dichloromethane (7:1:2)	—	UV	248	52
Resolve C_{18} 15 × 0.39 cm 5 μ	Ethanol:water (92:8)	Reduction with NaBH$_4$	Fl	320/430	36
Waters XL octyl 7 × 0.46 cm 3 μm	5 mM NaClO$_4$ in acetonitrile:ethanol (95:5)	EC reduction −0.8 V	Fl	320/430	35
(b) Milk and infant formula					
Zorbax ODS	Methanol:dichloromethane (8:2)	—	UV	250	47,77

Column	Mobile phase	Treatment	Detection	Wavelength	Ref.
μBondapak C$_{18}$ 25 × 0.4 cm	Acetonitrile:methanol:THF:water (39:39:16:6)	—	UV	254	72
Spherisorb ODS 25 × 0.45 cm 5 μm	THF:methanol:water (27:67:6)	—	UV	254	73
YMC-Pack A-314 30 × 0.6 cm	Ethanol:water (99:1)	Reduction with NaBH$_4$ added postcolumn	Fl	320/430	74
Partisil ODS-2 25 × 0.46 cm 5 μm	0.05 M NaClO$_4$ in methanol:ethanol:60% HClO$_4$ (600:400:1.2)	—	EC −0.45 V/ +0.35 V		46
Waters Resolve C$_{18}$ 15 × 0.39 cm 5 μm	Acetonitrile	—	UV	254/270	42
μBondapak C$_{18}$ 15 × 0.39 cm 10μ	Acetonitrile:dichloromethane:0.025 M NaClO$_4$ in water (90:5:5)	—	EC-1.1 V		76
(c) Tissues, foods and oils					
TLC silica	Petroleum ether:ether (85:15)				
Nucleosil C$_{18}$ 15 × 0.46 cm 5 μm	Ethanol:water (92.5:7.5)	Reduction with NaBH$_4$ added postcolumn	Fl	320/430	78
C$_{18}$, 5 μm 15 × 0.46 cm	Methanol:acetonitrile:water (88:10:2)	—	UV	270	79
Rad-Pak 5 μm silica 10 × 0.8 cm	n-Hexane:2-propanol (99.9:0.1)	Photochemical decomposition	UV Fl	254 325/420	80
Rad-Pak 5 μm C$_{18}$ 10 × 0.8 cm	Methanol:water (96:4)				

the vitamin $K_{1(20)}$ in plasma often were much higher than the ones obtained with more selective detection procedures (28,37,53). Therefore, to obtain increased selectivity and sensitivity, other detection procedures were also investigated.

Electrochemical Detection

In 1979, Ikenoya et al. were the first to suggest amperometric detection of phylloquinone and structural analogs (82). Nevertheless, it took 4 years before Ueno and Suttie applied reductive electrochemical detection in the analysis of $K_{1(20)}$ in human serum (30). By applying a sufficiently negative potential to the electrode, the quinone moiety is reduced to the hydroquinone form, resulting in a current proportional to the amount of vitamin K reduced. However, extreme care must be taken to remove oxygen to eliminate high background currents and baseline drift. Another problem with reductive electrochemical detection is the passivation of the working electrode by species adsorbed to its surface, resulting in a decrease in sensitivity.

The introduction of a double-electrode system (redox mode) eliminates interference from oxygen (the reduction of this molecule being irreversible). By this technique vitamin $K_{1(20)}$ is reduced to the hydroquinone form on the first electrode, and the hydroquinone form is then reoxidized at the second electrode arranged in series. With thin-layer cells, however, only a small fraction (between 2 and 5%) of the analyte is reduced. This percentage is drastically increased (up to 100%) by the use of porous graphite electrodes with a flow-through design. However, this flow-through system is less easily passivated than thin-layer cells. Redox electrochemical detection not only results in an enhanced selectivity but also in a 10-fold increase in sensitivity (down to 50 pg/ml serum) as compared to the reductive electrochemical detection (56,57) (Fig. 4).

Both straight and reversed-phase systems, even combined with nonaqueous eluents, are compatible with electrochemical detection, provided that the mobile phase contains sufficient amounts of supporting electrolyte. The electrolytes are readily soluble in polar solvent systems. Therefore, most of the applications of electrochemical detection of vitamin $K_{1(20)}$ are based on reversed-phase chromatographic systems (Table 2). In one particular experiment, Langenberg tried also a straight-phase eluent by mixing the electrolyte solution with the column effluent postcolumn (38). However, he observed a serious loss in sensitivity as compared to the reversed-phase conditions.

Fluorescence Detection

A third option for detection of the K vitamers in HPLC is fluorescence detection. Since vitamin K does not exhibit native fluorescence, methods

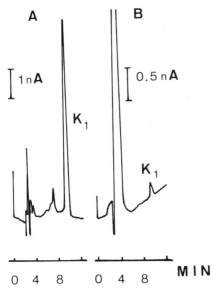

Figure 4 Chromatograms obtained for 1-ng injections of phylloquinone using LC-ECD in (A) redox mode and (B) reductive mode. Column: Spherisorb Octyl, 25 × 0.5 cm, 5 μm. Eluent:methanol:0.05 M acetate buffer, pH 3 (95:5, v/v) (from Ref. 57).

have been developed to prepare a fluorescent molecule. These include reduction of the molecule to the hydroquinone form either electrochemically or chemically, or photodecomposition of the different K vitamers. Each of these procedures will be described in the next paragraphs.

ELECTROCHEMICAL REDUCTION. In 1984, Langenberg (38) and Kusube et al. (55) used the coulometric detector as a postcolumn reactor to reduce phylloquinone to the fluorescent hydroquinone form. The cell volume of the electrochemical detector was only a few microliters, to minimize peak broadening. Vitamin $K_{1(20)}$ itself can be reduced at $-0.4\,V$; the reduction of K_1 epoxide, however, requires much lower potentials (lower than -1 V), resulting in high background currents. As a consequence, potentiostats were often overloaded and the potential was not well defined. By replacing the bipotentiostat with a simple potentiostat, Langenberg was able to quantitate K_1-epoxide in human serum (83) after treatment with coumarin anticoagulants. The method, however, was not sensitive enough to detect endogenous K_1-epoxide under normal physiological conditions. Later, also other research groups applied this electrofluorimetric technique for the quantitative determination of $K_{1(20)}$ alone (32,35,41,60,61) or together with K_1-epoxide (65). With this electrofluorimetric procedure combined with a column switching setup, Hirauchi et al. (65) were able to detect as little as 5 pg K_1-epoxide per injection for the standard, corresponding with a detection limit of 30 pg/ml (Fig. 3).

The combination of normal-phase chromatography with the electrofluorimetric method is more complicated (electrolyte has to be added postcolumn) and is inferior (lower quantum yield) to reversed-phase chromatography (38). Consequently, in all the above described procedures reversed-phase chromatographic conditions were used (Table 2).

CHEMICAL REDUCTION.   Chemical reduction of K vitamers can be performed either by a reagent that is added in solution or on a solid-phase reactor. In 1979, Abe et al. described a wet-chemical postcolumn reduction of $K_{1(20)}$ and of MK-4 with a solution of $NaBH_4$. The compounds were eluted from a C_{18} column with a mixture of ethanol:water (97:3) at a flow rate of 0.4 ml/min, and postcolumn an ethanolic solution of $NaBH_4$ was added (0.08%, w/v, 0.4 ml/min). The reduction was performed at room temperature in a stainless steel reaction coil (1 m × 0.8 mm ID). Later, also Sato et al. (74) and Cham et al. followed nearly the same procedure except for a slight increase in reaction temperature (up to 55°C) for the determination of $K_{1(20)}$ in milk and human serum, respectively (36). The drawbacks of the use of an aqueous mobile phase in the chromatography have already been described earlier in this chapter. In addition, it is well known that $NaBH_4$ decomposes quite rapidly in an aqueous solvent. For these reasons Lefevere et al. (70) applied a nonaqueous reversed phase system (100% methanol) while the reagent is added in ethanol. Under the described conditions (90 s reaction time at 37°C) maximal fluorescence is obtained. Another new aspect in this procedure concerns the air segmentation during the postcolumn reaction. Small air bubbles introduced by a peristaltic pump prevent peak broadening in the reactor. Before the reaction mixture can be directed to the detector cell the air bubbles have to be removed by a debubbler. The latter, however, often introduces such a high degree of band broadening that all resolution of the analytical column and of the postcolumn reaction system is lost.

In the wet-chemical postcolumn reduction we developed in 1986 (63) several of the above described drawbacks have been eliminated. First, a totally new reagent was used, that is, tetramethylammonium octahydridotriborate $[(CH_3)_4NB_3H_8]$. This reagent decomposes much more slowly than $NaBH_4$, but on the other hand, a higher temperature (up to 75°C) is necessary to initiate the reduction of K vitamers by this compound. Second, the reaction is performed in a "knitted coil" reactor (PTFE coil, 5 m × 0.5 mm ID) as developed by Engelhardt (84). The special geometric configuration of the reactor tubing minimizes band broadening and provides efficient mixing because the secondary flow pattern induces a rapid mass transfer. As a consequence, air segmentation is no longer necessary, and the instrumental setup can be substantially simplified by eliminating both the peristaltic pump (to introduce air bubbles) as well as the "debubbler" (to eliminate air bubbles before detection). It should be clear that also with this reagent several parameters, such as reagent concentration, reagent flow rate, reaction time, and temperature, must be optimized (83). Using this technique we were able to quantitate endogenous $K_{1(20)}$ in human serum (33) with a detection limit of 50 pg/ml. Our results were in good agreement with those reported by Shearer (29) and Langenberg (39) but substantially lower than the results obtained by using the less selective UV detection (28,37). While optimizing the reaction temperature we noted a drastic increase in reaction rate (or increased fluorescence) at higher temperatures, and only a slight formation of the fluorescent hydroquinone form at 20°C (Fig. 5.)

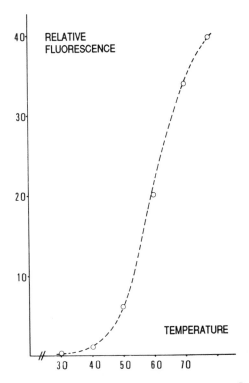

Figure 5 Reduction of vitamin $K_{1(20)}$: fluorescence yield in function of the reaction temperature. Reductant: $(CH_3)_4NB_3H_8$; concentration of the reagent: 6 mg/ml; eluent; methanol:ethyl acetate (96:4, v/v) (from Ref. 63).

This latter observation led to a new approach in which the reagent, $(CH_3)_4NB_3H_8$, was incorporated directly in the chromatographic eluent (6 mg/ml). Chromatography was performed at room temperature, thus preventing reduction of $K_{1(20)}$ during the separation step. After the analytical column, the effluent was passed through the knitted coil reactor kept at 75°C where the reaction takes place. Again the instrumental setup is simplified in that the reagent addition pump has been eliminated (Fig. 6). Furthermore, it was now possible to increase both the reaction time and the reagent concentration, resulting in a higher reaction yield and a lower limit of detection (30 pg/ml) (64). Under these conditions, however, K_1-epoxide is not reduced with a sufficient yield to allow quantitation of physiological levels of this molecule.

Reduction on a solid-phase reactor is a valuable alternative to the above described wet-chemical postcolumn thermoinduced reduction. As part of their efforts to eliminate oxygen from the eluent used in connection with electrofluorometric detection, Haroon et al. (62,71) remarked that a zinc oxygen-scrubber column was able to reduce quantitatively $K_{1(20)}$ in the presence of zinc ions. In this column, dry packed with zinc metal particles, they also observed the reduction of K_1-epoxide. Zinc chloride as well as the acetate buffer readily dissolve in the nonaqueous eluent system, which is another advantage. Later, two Japanese groups (66,67) also applied a solid phase reactor for the reduction of K vitamers. In both cases a platinum reduction column was used. In the latter report the eluent was a mixture of methanol:ethanol:water (1:2:0.06) saturated with H_2 gas. As no electrolytes were present, the problem of crystal formation in pump heads was avoided. However, the presence of water in the eluent represents a drawback of this procedure.

PHOTOCHEMICAL DECOMPOSITION. When irradiating vitamin K in solution, the molecule undergoes photodegradation to a number of compounds, for example, the hydroquinone form, which exhibit native fluorescence (70). Lefevere et al. used a custom-designed postcolumn photochemical reactor cell. A Teflon coil was placed around a water- or air-cooled 200-W Xe-Hg lamp. Enhanced fluorescence was found by addition of ascorbic acid (1 mg/ml) and an acetate buffer (pH 4) to the methanolic eluent. Ascorbic acid may thus act as a chemical reductant, protecting further oxidative decomposition of the formed hydroquinone. Under these conditions, Lefevere et al. were able to quantitate endogenous levels of vitamin $K_{1(20)}$. Later in 1988, Indyk applied the same photoinduced reduction followed by fluorescence detection (80). He also utilized a high-energetic 150-W Xe lamp, and the photochemical destruction took place instantaneously in the course of the normal passage of the eluent through the detector cell. In this approach, the

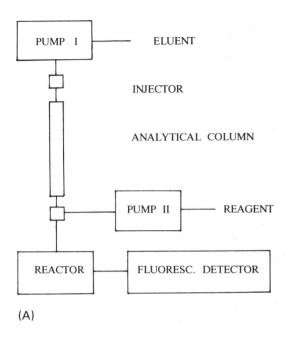

(A)

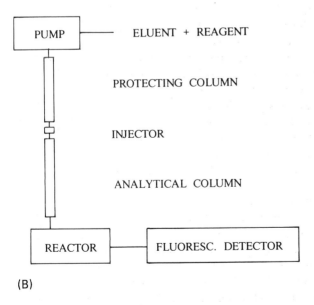

(B)

Figure 6 Instrumental setup for the analysis of K vitamers by wet-chemical reduction (A) with the reagent added by a second pump, or (B) with the reagent incorporated in the eluent.

obtained sensitivity was inadequate for the determination of physiological levels. The greatest advantage of the latter procedure certainly is its great simplicity as no reaction coil and no second pump are necessary.

3.6 Applications

As demonstrated in Tables 1 and 2, most of the above described procedures for chromatographic separation and detection were applied to the analysis of vitamin $K_{1(20)}$ in human plasma and serum, in milk and infant formulas, or in tissues, foods, and oils. In some papers the simultaneous determination of $K_{1(20)}$ together with the physiological metabolite K_1-epoxide has also been described. Although there still is a controversy about the exact fasting level of endogenous $K_{1(20)}$ in human serum, most of the selective detection procedures yield a reference interval between 200 and 1000 pg/ml (29,33,36,38,41,62,65). Less selective UV measurements clearly suffer from interferences and claim much higher values (28,53). The skewed distribution we found (28) was later confirmed by others (41,61). Likewise, several papers report the absence of any correlation between the vitamin $K_{1(20)}$ level in serum and age or sex (28,61,85). We also investigated the reference interval of vitamin $K_{1(20)}$ in children, and here also levels were below 1 ng/ml. They showed a skewed distribution, and again no correlation was seen between the observed values and the age or sex of the children (69). Almost simultaneously, a French group published very similar results (35).

Compared to the tremendous amount of papers on the chromatographic analysis of vitamin $K_{1(20)}$ itself, the number of papers on the determination of menaquinones by HPLC is rather limited. As there is a close structural analogy between vitamin $K_{1(20)}$ and the menaquinones, the same principles of chromatography and detection apply. The main problem in the analysis of menaquinones concerns the separation of different menaquinones (with isoprenyl chains largely differing in degree of saturation and chain length) in one single run and within a reasonable time. For this reason, several authors used two different eluents, the one with the highest eluting power being applied for the chromatography of MK-10 to MK-14 (Fig. 7) (88,89,91). Continuous-gradient elution was also used for the same purpose (90). As already mentioned detection can be performed in a similar way as for $K_{1(20)}$, that is, with UV detection (86,87,89) or with fluorescence detection after electrochemical (91) or chemical (88,90) reduction (Table 3). Using dual-electrode electrochemical detection (92), Shearer et al. confirmed earlier papers demonstrating that, in contrast to plasma, phylloquinone is not the major form of vitamin K in human liver. On the contrary, about 90% of the total liver reserve in adults comprises long-chain menaquinones (i.e., MK-7 to

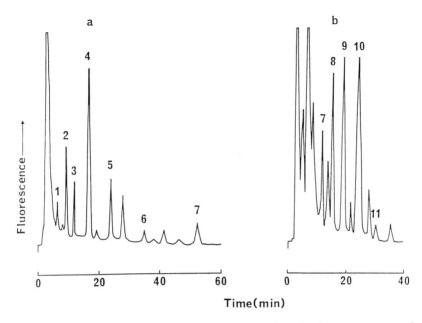

Figure 7 Reversed phase high-performance liquid chromatograms of an extract of bovine liver with different mobile phases: (a) 92.5% ethanol containing 0.25% sodium perchlorate; (b) 97.5% ethanol containing 0.25% sodium perchlorate. Peaks: 1, MK-4; 2, K_1; 3, MK-6; 4, MK-7; 5, MK-8; 6, MK-9; 7, MK-10; 8, MK-11; 9, MK-12; 10, MK-13; 11, MK-14. Electrochemical reduction followed by fluorescence detection (λ_{ex} 320 nm, λ_{em} 430 nm). Column: Nucleosil C_{18}, 5 μm, 15 × 0.46 cm ID (from Ref. 91).

MK-12). However, in the fetus and newborn the major liver form clearly is vitamin $K_{1(20)}$ itself. The much greater ratio of liver/plasma concentrations of menaquinones as compared to phylloquinone is indicative of the greater affinity of these more lipophilic menaquinones for liver membranes and also demonstrates their slower hepatic turnover.

The discovery and the characterization of the natural K vitamins (vitamin K_1 from plant origin and K_2 synthesized by bacteria) initiated a search for synthetic compounds with an equal physiological activity, but enhanced water solubility and/or stability. It was soon discovered that a methyl group in position 3 of the naphthoquinone nucleus and an unsubstituted benzene ring were essential for activity. The current belief is that this vitamin K_3 (menadione) is a provitamin that is metbolized in the liver to MK-4. For this reason, menadione is often added to animal feed. To improve its stability and absorption efficiency, the water-soluble derivative menadione sodium bisulfite is often used. HPLC conditions for

Table 3 Final HPLC Step and Detection Modes for Menaquinones

Column	Eluent (v/v)	Derivatization procedure	Detection mode (nm)	Reference
Lichrosorb RP 18 25 × 0.4 cm, 5 µm	Acetonitrile:THF (7:3)	—	UV (254)	86
Nucleosil 10 SA (Ag⁺) 25 × 0.46 cm	Methanol	—	UV (269)	86
Zorbax ODS 25 × 0.46 cm	Methanol:isopropyl ether (4:1)	—	UV (270)	87
Nucleosil C_{18} 15 × 0.46 cm, 5 µm	Ethanol:water (92.5:7.5) or (97.5:2.5)	Reduction with $NaBH_4$ added postcolumn	Fl (320/430)	88
Lichrosorb RP 18 25 × 0.46 cm	Methanol:1-chlorobutane (100:5) or (100:10)	—	UV (269)	89
Nucleosil C_{18} 25 × 0.46 cm, 5 µm	Methanol:ethanol (7:3) Gradient of methanol to 80% 2-propanol:ethanol (4:1) in 75 min	Reduction on Pt black column (RP-10, 1 × 0.4 cm)	Fl (320/430)	90
Nucleosil C_{18} 15 × 0.46 cm, 5 µm	Ethanol:water (92.5:7.5) or (97.5:2.5) with 0.25% $NaClO_4$	EC reduction −0.55 V	Fl (320/430)	91

the determination of vitamin K_3 are listed in Table 4. A water:ethanol or water:methanol mixture is often used to solubilize the menadione sodium bisulfite salt from the feed matrix. After treatment with aqueous Na_2CO_3 the bisulfite salt is destroyed, and the released menadione is extracted with a nonpolar solvent (e.g., n-hexane or n-pentane). Chromatography and detection are again performed in a way similar to the analysis of vitamin $K_{1(20)}$. Both electrochemical detection (95) and fluorescence detection after wet-chemical (93,94) or solid phase reactions (96) have been described (Fig. 8). Detection limits using these conditions are around 20 ng/g (93,96). By analogy to the analysis of vitamin $K_{1(20)}$ in milk and infant formula, one research group applied supercritical fluid extraction for the analysis of menadione in animal feed. Main advantages of this extraction method include its speed, the absence of light and air, and the simple removal of the extraction solvent. The major drawback of all of the procedures presented in Table 4 concerns the absence

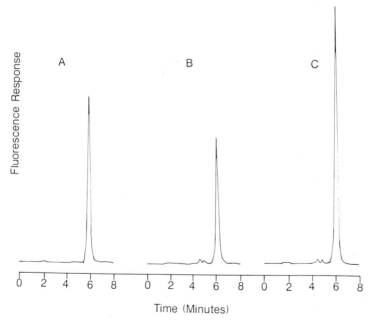

Figure 8   Typical HPLC-fluorescence chromatograms of (A) a 1-μg/ml MSB standard, (B) 1.00-g control synthetic animal feed, and (C) 1.00-g synthetic animal feed sample spiked with MSB at the 20-ppm level. Column: Supelcosil LC-18, 5 μm, 25 × 0.46 cm ID. Eluent: methanol:water (75:25, v/v). Postcolumn zinc reduction followed by fluorescence detection (λ_{ex} 325 nm, λ_{em} 425 nm) (from Ref. 96).

Table 4 Analysis of Synthetic K Analogues in Food

Sample preparation	Column	Eluent (v/v)	Derivatization	Detection	Reference
Water:ethanol (6:4) (96), 10% Tannin (4), n-Hexane (50), 10% Na_2CO_3 (20)	Hypersil ODS 25 × 0.46 cm 5 μm	Water:ethanol (4:6)	Reduction with $NaBH_4$ added postcolumn	Fl (325/425)	93
	Nucleosil C_{18} 15 × 0.46 cm 5 μm	Methanol:water (65:35)	Reduction with $NaBH_4$ added postcolumn	Fl (320/430)	94
Supercritical fluid CO_2 extraction, 8000 psi, 60°C, 20 min	μBondapak C_{18} 15 × 0.39 cm 10 μm	Acetonitrile:0.025 M aqueous $NaClO_4$ (90:10)	—	EC-0.75 V	95
Water:methanol (60:40) (10), 5% Na_2CO_3 (10), n-Pentane (30)	Supelcosil LC-18 25 × 0.46 cm 5 μm	Methanol:water (75:25)	Reduction on Zn column 2 × 0.2 cm	Fl (324/425)	96

of internal standardization. It should be clear, however, that in a complex analysis including extraction, purification, chromatography, and a postcolumn derivatization this is unacceptable.

4. GAS CHROMATOGRAPHY

Gas-liquid chromatography (GLC or GC) never became as popular for the analysis of K vitamers as it did for many other compounds of biomedical interest. Most papers deal with the separation and quantitation of standard mixtures of $K_{1(20)}$ and MK-n. Two excellent reviews on the early gas chromatographic work on vitamin K have been written by Sheppard et al. (97) and by Lefevere et al. (13). However, since that time, there has been little followup in this area. Two of the most obvious reasons for the relative unpopularity of GC are the high retention times and the possible on column degradation of the vitamin K-related compounds. Nevertheless, GC still displays some particularly interesting features for the vitamin K analysis. It can be applied in conjunction with specific and highly sensitive detection modes such as mass spectrometry (GC-MS), particularly selected ion monitoring (GC-SIM).

Bechtold and Jähnchen developed a GC method on a packed column for the quantitation of underivatized $K_{1(20)}$, K_1-epoxide, and menaquinone-4 in plasma (98). They used a 3% OV-17 column operated at 302°C with ECD. They applied this procedure to study the cyclic interconversion of vitamin $K_{1(20)}$ and K_1-epoxide in humans (99). Later, in 1984, the same group described the application of a fused-silica capillary column (25 × 0.32 mm ID) with a chemically bonded stationary phase (CP-Sil 5) operated at 285°C and again in conjunction with ECD. As compared to the packed column procedure the detection limit for the K vitamers was not improved. However, substantial chromatographic advantages were obtained, including better separation of the compounds of interest, longer column lifetime, and better reproducibility (100). In none of these studies, however, could endogenous vitamin $K_{1(20)}$ be quantitated in human plasma.

So far, there is only a very limited number of applications of mass spectrometry to the analysis of K vitamers. Guillaumont (101) reported a direct coupling between the HPLC and the MS apparatus by a moving-belt interface for the separation and the quantitation of cis- and trans-vitamin $K_{1(20)}$ using $K_{1(15)}$ as an internal standard. The separation was carried out on a Lichrosorb Si 60 5-μm column eluted with n-heptane:ethylacetate (99:1) at a flow rate of 50 μl/min. Electron impact mass spectra of $K_{1(20)}$ and of $K_{1(15)}$ are characterized by very intense molecular ion peaks at m/z 450 and 380, respectively. By monitoring these ions, a detection limit of 500 pg/ml was obtained for $K_{1(20)}$ in human plasma.

In a similar way, menaquinones are characterized by a molecular ion whose intensity decreases with increasing length of the side chain (102). Another fragment of major abundance, the base peak in some spectra, at m/z 225, is the stable oxonium ion, which increases in intensity with the size of the side chain. Both the molecular ion and the 225 ion were used to identify menaquinones extracted from human feces and purified on a high-performance liquid chromatographic system (88).

Owing to their higher volatility, GC analysis of synthetic K analogs (e.g., menadione) is less problematic than that of the natural K homologs ($K_{1(20)}$ as well as the group of menaquinones). Older GC analyses of these molecules have already been reviewed in an earlier edition of this work (13). Currently, LC methods have now clearly replaced GC analyses of these synthetic K vitamers.

5. FUTURE TRENDS

Improvements can be expected on each of the different steps of the analytical procedures for the determination of K vitamers in biosamples. New developments in sample preparation, separation, detection, and, in the case of K vitamers, postcolumn derivatizations will remain key issues in the 1990s.

As to the sample cleanup, one can expect that solid-phase extractions on minicolumns off-line, or on columns coupled on-line to the analytical system, will be investigated, with the aim of reducing sample size and analysis time. Automation of on-line purification on prepacked cartridges will also become one of the topics.

As to the chromatography, we believe that the applications of polymer-based stationary phases will steadily increase. Miniaturization of sample pretreatment will necessitate the use of narrow-bore columns and more sensitive detectors.

In an assay of K vitamers, enhanced detection sensitivity will depend on further developments in the postcolumn reaction systems. It is expected that the most significant developments in the vitamin K analysis will be in the area of "pumpless" reactions, which do not need a second pumping system to add the reagents, such as solid-phase reactors, electrochemical or thermoinduced reduction before fluorescence detection, and last but not least photochemical reactions. The pumpless nature of these procedures will enable the chromatographer to employ postcolumn reactions in a manner much simpler than in most cases today. With regard to postcolumn photochemical derivatization it is hoped that future studies will employ more wavelength-selective, narrow-bandpass light sources permitting more selective analyte photochemical derivatizations. Certainly, as a source laser light would greatly improve this selective photochemical derivatization. However, the high expenses involved in obtaining and focusing laser light sources presently limit their application.

As far as the other chromatographic techniques (e.g. TLC and GC) are concerned, we believe that in the future HPLC applications will largely supersede the GC applications.

Recently, TLC had a resurgence, possibly driven by the increasing need for the ability to screen large numbers of samples simultaneously, by the advent of more specialized layers (e.g., chiral phases, multiple-stationary phases, and sorbent-impregnated PTFE sheets), and by the availability of dedicated scanning densitometers. However, whether these new trends will also be applied to the analysis of K vitamers remains an open question.

REFERENCES

1. J. W. Suttie, in *Handbook of Lipid Research 2 "The Fat Soluble Vitamins"* (H. F. DeLuca, ed.), Plenum Press, New York, p. 211 (1978).
2. J. W. Suttie, in *Fat Soluble Vitamins. Their Biochemistry and Applications* (A. T. Diplock, ed.), Heineman, London, p. 225 (1985).
3. C. Von Planta, E. Billeter, and M. Kofler, *Helv. Chim. Acta*, 42:1278 (1959).
4. W. Friedrich, *Vitamins* (W. Friedrich, ed.), Walter de Gruyter, Berlin, New York, p. 287 (1988).
5. H. Dam, *Biochem. Z.*, 215:475 (1929).
6. J. Stenflo, P. Fernlund, W. Egan, and P. Roepstorff, *Proc. Natl. Acad. Sci. USA*, 71:2730 (1974).
7. W. Kisiel, *J. Clin. Invest.*, 64:761 (1979).
8. R. G. DiScipio and E. W. Davie, *Biochemistry*, 18:899 (1979).
9. P. V. Hauschka, J. B. Lian, and P. M. Gallop, *Proc. Natl. Acad. Sci. USA*, 72:3925 (1975).
10. C. T. Esmon, J. W. Suttie, and C. M. Jackson, *J. Biol. Chem.*, 250:4095 (1975).
11. R. E. Olson, *Annu. Rev. Nutr.*, 4:281 (1984).
12. C. Vermeer, *N. Comp. Biochem.*, 13:87 (1985).
13. M. F. Lefevere, A. E. Claeys, and A. P. De Leenheer, in *Modern Chromatographic Analysis of the Vitamins* (A. P. De Leenheer, W. E. Lambert, and M. G. M. De Ruyter, eds.) Marcel Dekker, New York, p. 201 (1985).
14. H. K. Lichtenthaler, in *Handbook of Chromatography: Lipids*, Vol. II (H. K. Mangold, ed.), CRC Press, Boca Raton, FL, p. 115 (1984).

15. B. Fried and J. Sherma, *Thin-Layer Chromatography, Techniques and Applications*, 2nd ed., Marcel Dekker, New York, p. 307 (1986).

16. A. P. De Leenheer, W. E. Lambert, and H. J. Nelis, *Handbook of Thin-Layer Chromatography* (J. Sherma and B. Fried, eds.), Marcel Dekker, New York, p. 993 (1990).

17. P. Sommer and M. Kofler, *Vitam. Horm.*, *24*:349 (1966).

18. H. R. Bolliger and A. König, in *Thin-Layer Chromatography, A Laboratory Handbook*, 2nd ed. (E. Stahl, ed.), Springer Verlag, Berlin, p. 259 (1969).

19. P. J. Dunphy and A. F. Brodie, *Methods Enzymol.*, *18C*:407 (1971).

20. S. Baczyk, L. Duczmal, I. Sobisz, and K. Swidzinska, *Mikrochim. Acta*, *2*:151 (1981).

21. L. Ersoy and R. Duden, *Lebensm.-Wiss. Technol.*, *13*:198 (1980).

22. H. K. Lichtenthaler, K. Börner, and C. Liljenberg, *J. Chromatogr.*, *242*:196 (1982).

23. Y. Haroon, M. J. Shearer, and P. Barkhan, *J. Chromatogr.*, *206*:333 (1981).

24. M. D. Collins, H. N. Shah, and D. E. Minnikin, *J. Appl. Bacteriol.*, *48*:227 (1980).

25. B. Rittich, M. Simek, and J. Coupek, *J. Chromatogr.*, *133*:345 (1977).

26. C. F. Poole and S. A. Schuette, in *Contemporary Practice of Chromatography*, (C. F. Poole and S. A. Schuette, eds.) Elsevier, Amsterdam, p. 619 (1984).

27. M. J. Shearer, P. Barkhan, and G. Webster, *Br. J. Haematol.*, *18*:297 (1970).

28. M. F. Lefevere, A. P. De Leenheer, A. E. Claeys, I.V. Claeys, and H. Steyaert, *J. Lipid Res.*, *23*:1068 (1982).

29. M. J. Shearer, S. Rahim, P. Barkhan, and L. Stimmler, *Lancet*, *ii*:460 (1982).

30. T. Ueno and J. W. Suttie, *Anal. Biochem.*, *133*:62 (1983).

31. L. Sann, M. Leclercq, J. Troncy, M. Guillaumont, M. Berland, and P. Coeur, *Am. J. Obstet, Gynecol.*, *153*:771 (1985).

32. K. Hirauchi, T. Sakano, and A. Morimoto, *Chem. Pharm. Bull.*, *34*:845 (1986).

33. W. E. Lambert, A. P. De Leenheer, and E. J. Baert, *Anal. Biochem.*, *158*:257 (1986).

34. M. Lucock, R. Hartley, and N. J. Wild, *J. Liq. Chromatogr.*, *10*:191 (1987).

35. F. Moussa, L. Dufour, J. R. Didry, and P. Aymard, *Clin. Chem.*, *35*:874 (1989).

36. B. E. Cham, H. P. Roeser, and T. W. Kamst, *Clin. Chem.*, *35*:2285 (1989).

37. A. Pietersma-de Bruyn and P. van Haard, *Clin. Chim. Acta*, *150*:95 (1985).

38. J. P. Langenberg and U. R. Tjaden, *J. Chromatogr.*, *305*:61 (1984).

39. J. P. Langenberg, Ph.D. Thesis, University of Leiden, Leiden, p. 44 (1985).

40. E. G. Bligh and W. J. Dyer, *Can. J. Biochem. Physiol.*, 37:911 (1957).

41. M. Guillaumont, M. Leclercq, H. Gosselet, K. Makala, and B. Vignal, *J. Micronutr. Anal.*, 4:285 (1988).

42. B. Fournier, L. Sann, M. Guillaumont, and M. Leclercq, *Am. J. Clin. Nutr.*, 45:551 (1987).

43. A. Yonekubo, I. Ichimaru, Y. Yamamoto, and F. Tsuchiya, *Igaku No Ayumi*, 126:1037 (1983).

44. R. von Kries, M. Shearer, P. T. McCarthy, M. Haug, G. Harzer, and U. Göbel, *Pediatr. Res.*, 22:513 (1987).

45. L. M. Canfield, G. S. Martin, and K. Sugimoto, in *Current Advances in Vitamin K Research* (J. W. Suttie, ed.), Elsevier, New York, p. 499 (1988).

46. H. Isshiki, Y. Suzuki, A. Yonekubo, H. Hasegawa, and Y. Yamamoto, *J. Dairy Sci.*, 71:627 (1988).

47. Y. Haroon, M. J. Shearer, S. Rahim, W. G. Gunn, G. McEnery, and P. Barkhan, *J. Nutr.*, 112:1105 (1982).

48. S. A. Barnett, L. W. Frick, and H. M. Balne, *Anal. Chem.*, 52:610 (1980).

49. S. Patton and T. W. Keenan, *Biochim. Biophys. Acta*, 415:273 (1975).

50. W. E. Lambert, O. Amédée-Manesme, M. Zheng, and A. P. De Leenheer, *Int. J. Vitamin Nutr. Res.*, 60:179 (1990).

51. J. N. Thompson, *Trace Organic Analysis: A New Frontier in Analytical Chemistry*, National Bureau of Standards, Gaithersburg, MD, publication 519, p. 279 (1979).

52. E. M. Kirk and A. F. Fell, *Clin. Chem.*, 35:1288 (1989).

53. M. Leclercq, M. Crozet, J. Durand, M. Bourgeay-Causse, and L. Sann, in *Chromatography in Biochemistry, Medicine* and *Environmental Research* (A. Frigerio, ed.), Elsevier, Amsterdam, p. 235 (1983).

54. A. C. Wilson and B. K. Park, *J. Chromatogr.*, 277:292 (1983).

55. K. Kusube, K. Abe, O. Hiroshima, Y. Ishiguro, S. Ishikawa, and H. Hoshida, *Chem. Pharm. Bull.*, 32:179 (1984).

56. J. P. Hart, M. J. Shearer, P. T. McCarthy, and S. Rahim, *Analyst*, 109:477 (1984).

57. J. P. Hart, M. J. Shearer, and P. T. McCarthy, *Analyst*, 110:1181 (1985).

58. L. Sann, M. Leclercq, A. Frederich, J. Bourgeois, M. Bethenod, and M. Bourgeay-Causse, *Dev. Pharmacol. Ther.*, 8:269 (1985).

59. L. Sann, M. Leclercq, M. Guillaumont, R. Trouyez, B. Bethenod, and M. Bourgeay-Causse, *J. Pediatr.*, 107:608 (1985).

60. P. M. M. van Haard, R. Engel, and A. L. J. M. Pietersma-de Bruyn, *Clin. Chim. Acta*, 157:221 (1986).

61. L. L. Mummah-Schendel and J. W. Suttie, *Am. J. Clin. Nutr.*, 44:686 (1986).

62. Y. Haroon, D. S. Bacon, and J. A. Sadowski, *Clin. Chem.*, 32:1925 (1986).

63. W. E. Lambert, A. P. De Leenheer, and M. F. Lefevere, *J. Chromatogr. Sci.*, *24*:76 (1986).
64. W. E. Lambert and A. P. De Leenheer, *Anal. Chim. Acta*, *196*:247 (1987).
65. K. Hirauchi, T. Sakano, T. Nagaoka, and A. Morimoto, *J. Chromatogr.*, *430*:21 (1988).
66. H. Hiraike, M. Kimura, and Y. Itokawa, *J. Chromatogr.*, *430*:143 (1988).
67. M. Shino, *Analyst*, *113*:393 (1988).
68. F. R. Greer, L. L. Mummah-Schendel, S. Marshall, and J. W. Suttie, *Pediatrics*, *81*:137 (1988).
69. W. E. Lambert, L. Vanneste, A. P. De Leenheer, and O. Amédée-Manesme, *Clin. Chem.*, *35*:671 (1989).
70. M. F. Lefevere, R. W. Frei, A. H. M. T. Scholten, and U. A. Brinkman, *Chromatographia*, *15*:459 (1982).
71. Y. Haroon, D. S. Bacon, and J. A. Sadowski, *J. Chromatogr.*, *384*:383 (1987).
72. M. P. Bueno and M. C. Villalobos, *J. Assoc. Off. Anal. Chem.*, *66*:1063 (1983).
73. S.-M. Hwang, *J. Assoc. Off. Anal. Chem.*, *68*:684 (1985).
74. T. Sato, M. Yahiro, K. Shimoda, Y. Asai, and M. Hamamoto, *J. Jpn. Soc. Nutr. Food. Sci.*, *38*:451 (1985).
75. J. P. Hart, M. J. Shearer, L. Klenerman, A. Catterall, J. Reeve, P. N. Sambrook, R. A. Dodds, L. Bitensky, and J. Chayen, *J. Clin. Endocrinol. Metab.*, *60*:1268 (1985).
76. M. A. Schneiderman, A. K. Sharma, K. R. Mahanama, and D. C. Locke, *J. Assoc. Off. Anal. Chem.*, *71*:815 (1988).
77. Y. Haroon and P. V. Hauschka, *J. Lipid Res.*, *24*:481 (1983).
78. H. Hiraike, M. Kimura, and Y. Itokawa, *Jpn. J. Hyg.*, *41*:764 (1986).
79. F. Zonta and B. Stancher, *J. Chromatogr.*, *329*:257 (1985).
80. H. Indyk, *J. Micronutr. Anal.*, *4*:61 (1988).
81. W. T. Wahyuni and K. Jinno, *Chromatographia*, *23*:320 (1987).
82. S. Ikenoya, K. Abe, T. Tsuda, Y. Yamano, O. Hiroshima, M. Ohmae, and K. Kawabe, *Chem. Pharm. Bull.*, *27*:1237 (1979).
83. J. P. Langenberg and U. R. Tjaden, *J. Chromatogr.*, *289*:377 (1984).
84. H. Engelhardt and U. D. Neue, *Chromatographia*, *15*:403 (1982).
85. M. J. Shearer, O. E. Crampton, P. T. McCarthy, and M. B. Mattock, *Haemostasis*, *16*:83 (1986).
86. B. M. Kroppenstedt, *J. Liq. Chromatogr.*, *5*:2359 (1982).
87. J. Tamaoka, *Methods Enzymol.*, *123*:251 (1986).
88. T. Sakano, T. Nagaoka, A. Morimoto, and K. Hirauchi, *Chem. Pharm. Bull.*, *34*:4322 (1986).
89. F. Fernandez and M. D. Collins, *FEMS Microbiol. Lett.*, *41*:175 (1987).
90. Y. Usui, N. Nishimura, N. Kobayashi, T. Okanoue, M. Kimoto, and K. Ozawa, *J. Chromatogr.*, *489*:291 (1989).
91. K. Hirauchi, T. Sakano, S. Notsumoto, T. Nagaoka, A. Morimoto, K. Fujimoto, S. Masuda, and Y. Suzuki, *J. Chromatogr.*, *497*:131 (1989).

92. M. J. Shearer, P. T. McCarthy, O. E. Crampton, and M. B. Mattock, in *Current Advances in Vitamin K Research* (J. W. Suttie, ed.), Elsevier, New York, p. 437 (1988).

93. A. J. Speek, J. Schryver, and W. H. P. Schreurs, *J. Chromatogr.*, *301*:441 (1984).

94. S. Notsumoto, T. Sakano, T. Nagaoka, A. Morimoto, K. Fujimoto, Y. Suzuki, K. Hirouichi, *Vitamins*, *62*:571 (1988).

95. M. A. Schneiderman, A. Sharma, and D. C. Locke, *J. Chromatogr. Sci.*, *26*:458 (1988).

96. S. M. Billedeau, *J. Chromatogr.*, *472*:371 (1989).

97. A. J. Sheppard, A. R. Prosser, and W. D. Hubbard, *J. Am. Oil Chem. Soc.*, *49*:619 (1972).

98. H. Bechtold and E. Jähnchen, *J. Chromatogr.*, *164*:85 (1979).

99. H. Bechtold, D. Trenk, T. Meinertz, M. Rowland, and E. Jähnchen, *Br. J. Clin. Pharmac.*, *16*:683 (1983).

100. H. Bechtold, F. Klein, D. Trenk, and E. Jähnchen, *J. Chromatogr.*, *306*:333 (1984).

101. M. Guillaumont, Ph.D. Thesis, Lyon, France, p. 123 (1987).

102. W. H. Elliot and G. R. Waller, in *Biochemical Applications of Mass Spectrometry*, (G. R. Waller, ed.), Wiley Interscience, New York, p. 513 (1972).

5

ASCORBIC ACID

Markku T. Parviainen and Kristiina Nyyssönen

University of Kuopio, Kuopio, Finland

1. INTRODUCTION

1.1 History

The first descriptions of the disease state called scurvy date back to ancient times. Scurvy was not only a devastating disease among the seafarers of the Middle Ages, but it ocurred also frequently on land, especially during war time with shortages of food. The association and the curative effect of fresh fruits and vegetables were recognized during the eighteenth century. Susceptibility of guinea pigs to scurvy was observed at the beginning of this century, leading to the development of a bioassay for the determination of antiscorbutic activity in foodstuffs. Later, the isolation was accomplished, and a structure of "hexuronic acid" and an empirical formula $C_6H_8O_6$ was suggested, leading eventually to the identification of vitamin C and its antiscorbutic activity. The vitamin was renamed ascorbic acid in 1933. Shortly thereafter Reichstein described the "classic Reichstein synthesis," which is still in use on an industrial scale.

Further historical background to the research leading to the discovery of vitamin C can be obtained from recent reviews (1,2).

Since the discovery of vitamin C, numerous assays for its determination in foods and biological tissues have been described in the literature.

The reader is advised to consult previous reviews, especially regarding nonchromatographic or early chromagraphic assay methods (3–5).

1.2 Chemistry

Ascorbic acid (2,3-endiol-L-gulonic acid-γ-lactone,AA) (Fig. 1), also called vitamin C or L-ascorbic acid, is a strongly reducing dibasic acid with a pK_1 of 4.1 and pK_2 of 11.8. It is easily oxidized (Fig. 1) by several agents (e.g., halogens, hydrogen peroxide, and others), especially in aqueous solutions, to form dehydroascorbic acid (DHA) via a semidehydroascorbic acid radical. This reaction is reversible, since dehydroascorbic acid can be reduced to ascorbic acid, for instance, by sulfur-containing agents like gluthathione. This reversible oxidation-reduction is the basis for many of the known biological functions of ascorbic acid.

The oxidation of AA to DHA is greatly favored by the presence of oxygen, heavy metal ions, especially Cu^{2+}, Ag^+, and Fe^{3+}, and by alkaline pH. The most important reactions of AA from the point of view of life involve the reduction of Fe^{3+}, and the superoxide anion $\dot{O}_2^+$, and the quenching of singlet oxygen $^1O_2$ (6).

DHA, in aqueous solution, is a hydrated bicyclic monomer (7). It is relatively hydrophobic, and less ionizable than AA, and therefore penetrates the cell membrane better. Dehydroascorbic acid in turn can be irreversibly oxidized to form diketogulonic acid (Fig. 1).

D-Isoascorbic acid, also called erythorbic acid (IAA), is a synthetic analog of AA, differing only in the configuration at carbon-5 (Fig. 2). IAA has been used in the food industry because it is not toxic, and it is effective as an antioxidant (8). Production of IAA is also cheaper than that of AA. The biological activity of IAA, on the other hand, is low

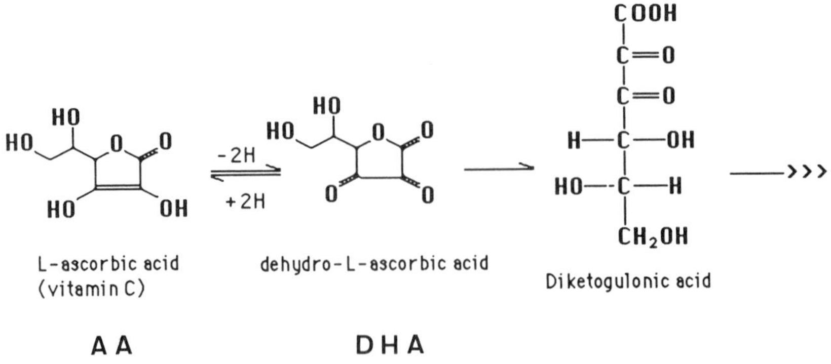

Figure 1   Oxidation and reduction of L-ascorbic acid (AA).

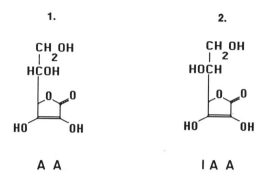

Figure 2 The structures of the isomers AA (L-ascorbic acid) (I) and IAA (D-isoascorbic acid or erythorbic acid) (II).

compared to that of AA. IAA has also been used as an internal standard in a number of chromagraphic analytical methods for AA (see section 3).

Some more complicated metabolites of AA (e.g., AA-2-phosphate, AA-2-sulfate, 2-O-methyl-AA, 6-deoxy-6-bromo-AA, 5-methyl-3,4-dihydroxytetrone) and their measurement are also of growing interest to nutritionists (5).

1.3 Physiology and Biochemistry

Biosynthesis

AA is widely biosynthesized in nature, particularly by chlorophyll-containing plants, and by animals, with the exception of a few mammalian and avian species (9). D-Glucose is used in animals as a source for the synthesis of AA. Figure 3 summarizes synthesis of AA in the liver. The last enzymatic reaction in the microsomal fraction of liver, the oxidation of L-gulono-γ-lactone to 2-oxo-L-gulono-γ-lactone by the enzyme L-gulonolactone oxidase (E.C. 1.1.3.8), is absent in primates and guinea pigs. Therefore, these species must obtain AA by dietary means, and the AA deficiency may lead to scurvy. Higher plants can use either D-glucose or D-galactose in their AA biosynthesis (9).

A wide variety of good AA sources has been summarized and listed by Friedrich (2). Potatoes and citrus fruits are quantitatively the most important sources of AA. The minimum AA requirement in humans to prevent scurvy is as low as 10 mg/day. The recommended dietary allowance of AA (10) in adolescents over 12 years old is 50 mg/day. However, an even higher recommendation of 100–200 mg/day has been suggested (11,12), since smoking, pregnancy, and stress, for example, are known to increase the requirement for AA.

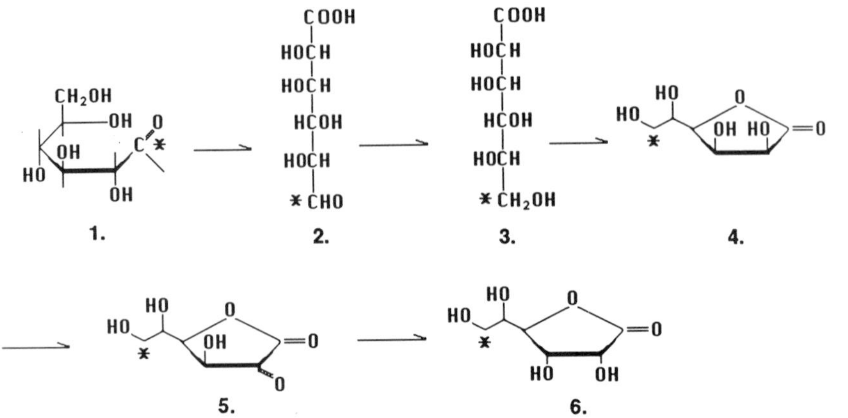

Figure 3 The mammalian biosynthesis of AA starting from ^{14}C-labeled D-glucose. Key: I, [1-^{14}C]-D-glucose; II, [1-^{14}C]-D-glucuronic acid; III, [6-^{14}C]-L-gulonic acid; IV, [6-^{14}C]-L-gulono-γ-lactone; V, [6-^{14}C]-L-2-oxo-gulono-γ-lactone; and VI, [6-^{14}C]-L-ascorbic acid.

Biological Functions and Mode of Action

AA is involed in a number of biochemical reactions, of which hydroxylations are best known. In these reactions, AA acts as an electron donor, and the product, monodehydroascorbic acid, is reduced back to AA by two hepatic microsomal enzymes: monodehydroascorbate reductase (E.C. 1.6.5.4) and ascorbate-cytochrome b_5 reductase (E.C. 1.10.2.1) (13). The electron transport reactions involving AA include the synthesis of collagen, the metabolism of cholesterol, the synthesis of catecholamines, and the hydroxylation of drugs.

Biosynthesis of collagen is clearly dependent on AA (14), which is one of the main pathways in which the vitamin participates. Many symptoms of scurvy, such as bleeding and delayed wound healing, can be attributed to the impairment of this function. The hydroxylation of procollagen on specific prolyl and lysyl residues by the enzymes prolyl hydroxylase (E.C. 1.14.11.2) an lysyl hydroxylase (E.C. 1.14.11.4) requires the presence of 2-oxoglutarate, Fe^{2+}, and AA as cofactors. The biosynthesis of carnitine belongs to a similar class of iron-AA-dependent hydroxylation pathways. Tyrosine degradation is also dependent on the presence of iron and AA.

Dopamine- β-monooxygenase (E.C. 1.14.17.1) is a copper-containing enzyme necessary for the hydroxylation of dopamine to form noradrenaline. This enzyme is located in the chromaffin cells of the adrenal medulla and adrenergic nerve endings. The chromaffin cells are also known to contain high concentrations of AA (15), which serves as an electron donor for the hydroxylations (16).

Other functions of ascorbic acid may include the reduction of plasma total cholesterol level and thus the reduction of the risk of atherosclerosis (17). It also appears to inhibit the formation of nitrosoamines (18), it may act as a modulator in mutagenesis and carcinogenesis (19), and it is probably involved in the functioning of the immune system (20). One of its most important functions is the reaction with active forms of oxygen (21), converting these to forms that are less toxic or nontoxic to the cell. One of the newest hypothesis concerns the modulatory effect of AA on blood pressure (22).

1.4 Analytically Important Properties

Crystalline AA and DHA are relatively stable in the presence of air, whereas in solution they are easily oxidized: they are most stable in acidic solutions and least stable in an alkaline environment. Degradation of vitamin C in solution is further dependent on the temperature, the presence or absence of oxygen, and the presence or absence of metal ions. In addition, the sample to be analyzed may contain several oxidation products of AA and DHA. Therefore, it is essential that the samples are suitably preserved immediately after they have been collected.

Stability of Ascorbic Acid in Standard Solutions and Biological Samples
AA standard solution of 5 mg/ml has a pH value of 3, so the stock standard can be made in distilled water. If dilute standard solutions are to be used, it is advisable to make the standard in acid, such as 5% *meta*-phosphoric acid (MPA) (23). A reducing agent such as homocysteine (24) or a chelating agent such as ethylenediamine tetraacetic acid (EDTA) (25) can be added to protect AA. Homocysteine and MPA, however, may interfere in the DHA assay in some chromatographic systems, if low ultraviolet (UV) detection wavelengths are used.

Acidification of the sample should be done promptly after sampling, and usually MPA or trichloroacetic acid (TCA) is used for this purpose. A plasma sample, for instance, is stable for at least 1 month when stored at $-80°C$ before analysis (23) if diluted promptly (i.e., in less than 30 min after sampling in 5% MPA, $1+9$, by volume). MPA has an additional advantage apart from the acidification of the sample and denaturation of the proteins: it chelates metals that act as catalysts in the oxidation of AA. Speek et al. (26) found that total vitamin C in whole blood was stable for eight days at $-20°C$, provided that ethyleneglycol-bis-(β-aminoethyl ether)-N,N,N',N'-tetraacetic acid (EGTA) and glutathione solution were immediately added to the blood sample. They used TCA for subsequent protein precipitation and acidification.

Kutnink and co-workers (27) and Ashoor et al. (25) added EDTA to the chromatographic mobile phase for further stabilization of AA (and IAA) against oxidation during chromatography. Margolis and Black (28) performed the analysis of AA in the presence of solvents that were purged with argon to reduce the oxygen content, and thus also to minimize the oxidation of AA during the chromatographic run. Margolis and Black also stabilized the deaerated solutions of AA with dithiothreitol (DTT). AA was stable in these solutions for at least 67 days when sealed under argon and stored at $-20°C$ (28).

Physical and Chemical Properties Useful in the Determination of Vitamin C

The detection of AA and DHA is somewhat difficult due to their unfavorable physiocochemical properties. For instance, the UV absorption maximum of DHA is at 210–227 nm (24,29), which limits the choice of the sample matrix, solvents, buffers, and other reagents used. Moreover, the low levels of DHA in most samples necessitate the use of other detection methods or indirect assays via AA for accurate quantitative work. The UV absorption of AA is strongly pH dependent: at pH 2 the absorption maximum is at 245 nm, and at pH 6.4 it is at 265 nm.

The reductive capabilities of AA can be especially exploited in the electrochemical detection methods (see section 3.3). DHA, however, is electrochemically inactive, and most DHA assays involve either the preliminary reduction of DHA to AA, and subsequent measurement of "total AA" (AA plus DHA), or the oxidation of AA to DHA, again followed by measurement of the "total AA." Differential measurement can be done by two measurements using high-performance liquid chromatography (HPLC) and UV detection: analyzing first the content of AA, and second that of "total AA." DHA can then be obtained by subtraction of AA from the "total AA" level (30). Another and more specific way of DHA measurement is based on complex formation. The ketone groups of DHA are reactive, and the addition of *ortho*-phenylenediamine (OPD) results in conversion to a quinoxaline fluorophor (31) (Fig. 4). The use of a dimethyl derivative of OPD increases the detection sensitivity even further (32).

2. PAPER AND THIN-LAYER CHROMATOGRAPHY

Paper (PC) and thin-layer chromatography (TLC) were applied in early analytical studies to increase selectivity in the analysis of AA and other similar chemical compounds. However, nowadays these methods have

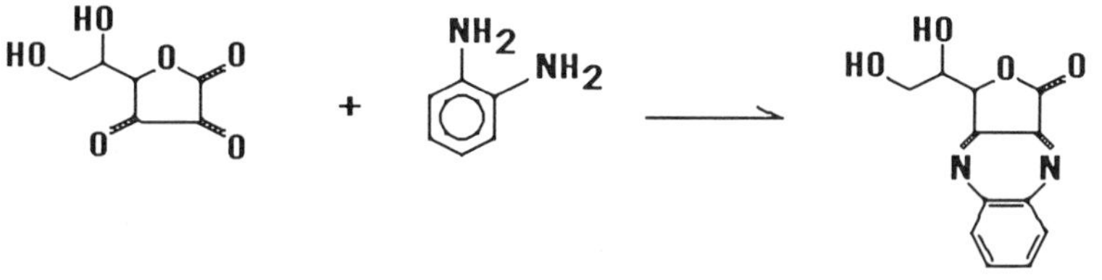

Figure 4 Reaction of DHA with o-phenylenediamine resulting in formation of a fluorophor quinoxaline.

little if any qualitative or quantitative use. The reader should therefore be referred to the review by De Ritter (33) for the PC applications.

Thin-layer chromatography, and especially high-performance thin-layer chromatography, should prove to have some advantages in the analysis of vitamin C compounds, especially in the food, pharmaceutical, and animal sciences. Quite recently Otsuka et al. (34) used TLC for the isolation and partial purification of the degradation products of 2,3-diketo-L-gulonic acid. For characterization, they used different spectrometric methods.

3. HIGH-PERFORMANCE LIQUID CHROMATOGRAPHY

3.1 Introduction

High-performance liquid chromatography (HPLC) has proven to be one of the most useful methods for the determination of ascorbic acid in foods (35–40), body fluids (23,27,35,41–46), tissues (44,47–51), and pharmaceuticals (32,52). However, spectrophotometric (53–56), fluorometric (57,58), or amperometric (59) determinations without any chromatographic steps are still widely used, especially in the assays of ascorbic acid in pharmaceuticals. Unlike the latter, biological samples more often contain unknown compounds that can interfere in spectrophotometric, fluorometric, or electrochemical detection if the method includes no chromatographic separation. Electrochemical or UV detection are the detection methods most often used for ascorbic acid HPLC determination.

3.2 HPLC Conditions

In neutral medium AA has a highly anionic character ($pK_1 4.17$) and can easily be chromatographed on HPLC using anion-exchange or reversed-phase columns. NH_2-bonded silica gel columns are the most popular among the weak anion-exchange methods. Bui-Nguyén (60) used a 10

μm NH$_2$-bonded column, and an isocratic mobile phase consisted of 75%
acetonitrile in potassium dihydrogen phosphate buffer, pH 4.4–4.7. This
method can detect IAA and AA from a fruit juice extract. Since the publication of this result, several reports have been published dealing with
the use of NH$_2$-bonded columns in the determination of AA, DHA, or
isoascorbic acid (23,24,29,42,61–63). Rather similar results to the
amino-bonded silica have been found with the use of a μBondapak/
carbohydrate column (64).

Liebes and co-workers (65) used strong anion-exchange column
material (Whatman Partisil 10 SAX) plus a guard column filled with
Whatman pellicular strong anion exchanger and gradient elution to separate AA from blood lymphocyte extracts. Later they published (66,67) a
description of a method for the determination of DHA, in addition to
that of AA, in lymphocytes. DHA was separated from AA by HPLC,
and this was followed by reduction with dithiothreitol, rechroma-
tography, and quantification as AA. In a recent study, Suzuki and
Fukuda (50) used a strong anion-exchange column (polymeric Mono Q,
Pharmacia, Sweden) with gradient elution. They separated AA and hex-
avalent chromium from rat lung tissue for toxicological purposes. Vanderslice and Higgs (68) used a Dionex strong anion-exchange resin in
their separation of AA and DHA.

Reversed-phase HPLC with octadecylsilane (ODS and C18) or octyl
(C8) columns is widely used for the quantitative estimation of AA, AA-
2-polyphosphate, DHA, and diketogulonic acid (26,27,30,36–40,44–
47,49,69–76). These reversed-phase columns have been used with and
without ion pairing. Quaternary ammonium compounds or tertiary
amines such as decyl- or octylamine are frequently used as ion-pairing
reagents in the mobile phase (27,29,38). Their action in the mobile phase
has been discussed in an earlier review (5). An ion-pairing technique is
useful when the analytes elute near the solvent front. Adding a reagent
that decreases the polarity of the analytes, or increases the polarity of the
stationary phase, improves the retention of the analytes. No ion pairing
is possible at low mobile-phase pH, due to ion suppression.

A macroporous copolymer of styrene and divinylbenzene is suitable
as a stationary phase for reversed-phase separations. Lloyd and her colleagues (40) describe the use of ion suppression chromatography with a
polymeric, macroreticular poly(styrene-divinylbenzene) HPLC packing
material (PLRP-S 100 Å, 5 μm, 25 cm × 4.6 mm ID) for the separation
of AA and IAA. UV detection was performed at 220 nm. NaH$_2$PO$_4$, 0.2
M (pH 2.14), was used as the mobile phase, which permitted the optimal
separation of AA and IAA. Small changes in pH and salt concentration
had a negligible effect on solute retentivity, and the eluent contained no
organic modifier. Obviously, a mobile-phase pH below the pK$_a$ of AA,

that is 4.17, is necessary for ion suppression reversed-phase separation. An excellent coefficient of variation of 0.5% for AA was found by Lloyd and co-workers (40) in their HPLC analysis of a relatively simple sample matrix such as orange juice.

Another recent development in column technology involves the use of a polymethacrylate material (RSpak DE-613, 6 μm, Showadenko, Japan; column size 15 cm $\times$ 6.5 mm ID) as described by Iriyama et al. (43). Using this column coupled with EC detection, these workers performed a simultaneous determination of AA and uric acid in several body fluids. The mobile phase consisted of 0.1 M K_2HPO_4-citric acid buffer, pH 4.6, containing 1 mM EDTA, and the column apparently operates on the basis of reversed-phase principles. Furthermore, Iriyama et al. (43) demonstrated an excellent sensitivity of 10 pg for AA in their HPLC.

3.3   Electrochemical Detection

Electrochemical (EC) detection of ascorbic acid is based on the oxidation of AA to DHA. An electrochemical detector usually consists of a thin-layer cell with a reference electrode, working electrode, and auxiliary electrode (77). In the oxidative reaction, a posivite constant voltage is applied between the working and reference electrodes. As the analyte flows through the cell, AA is oxidized to DHA, and electrons are released. The electric current produced can be measured. According to Faraday's law, the current is in direct proportion to the amount of analyte:

$$Q = nFN \tag{1}$$

where Q is the amount of electricity (coulombs), n is the number of electrons produced, and N is the amount of compound (moles).

The potential required to oxidize AA to DHA depends on the structure of the analytical cell, the type and condition of the working electrode, the composition of the mobile phase, and the temperature. The optimum potential for each type of electrochemical detector used in conjunction with certain HPLC conditions should be determined experimentally.

Wang and Hou (52) used an amperometric detector and found a potential of +0.60 V to be the most suitable for AA in their HPLC system. AA reached its limit current at +0.70 V, but that potential produces a high background current, which decreases the sensitivity of the detector. Iriyama et al. (43) used amperometry with a potential of +0.80 V for the determination of AA and uric acid in body fluids, whereas Kutnink et al. (27) used the same detector potential as Wang and Hou (52) for the measurement of AA, IAA, and uric acid in human plasma. Tsao et al. (78) determined ascorbic acid 2-sulfate, in addition to AA, in urine, and they used $+0.91$ V as the oxidizing potential. In an earlier study, Tsao and Salimi (47) separated IAA from AA by reversed-phase chromatography with amperometric detection. The chromatography system described by Tsao and colleagues (47,78) is capable of analyzing a number of more complicated metabolites of AA (e.g., AA-2-phosphate, AA-2-sulfate) in addition to AA and IAA. Honegger et al. (51) determined AA, cysteine, and glutathione in breast tissue using a potential as low as $+0.5$ V.

Hypothetically, DHA could be determined by electrochemical detection, since DHA is easily oxidized to diketogulonic acid in solution. In electrochemistry, however, DHA is rapidly hydrated to an electroinactive product. DHA can be assayed indirectly after reduction by homocysteine to AA prior to the electrochemical detection, as proposed by Behrens and Madére (44). These workers achieved separation using a 5-μm C18 reversed-phase column (25 cm $\times$ 4.6 mm ID), and a mobile-phase of 80 mM sodium acetate buffer, pH 4.8, containing 1 mM n-octylamine (ion-pair reagent), 15% methanol, and 0.015% MPA. The final pH of the mobile phase was 4.6, and $+0.7$ V was used as the oxidizing potential. They studied the applicability of this method to determine AA, DHA, and "total AA" in rat plasma and several tissues, and in selected foods (Fig. 5). An excellent correlation between HPLC EC and the 2,4-dinitrophenylhydrazine method for "total AA" was also shown (44). They only apparent drawback of this method is that two successive injections are needed. In the study by Baker et al. (69), AA was determined by HPLC with electrochemical detection, and OPD was used for producing a fluorescent derivative of DHA. In our opinion, this method seems to be rather laborious.

An exhaustively automated HPLC method combining EC and fluorometric detection of neurotransmitters, related compounds, AA, and uric acid in tissues was developed by Honegger and colleagues (49). A column-switching apparatus was included in their system, to allow the compounds to pass through one, two, or three reversed-phase columns as appropriate. The three columns were eluted simultaneously, and the total run time was 25 min. AA was detected electrochemically.

High sensitivity and selectivity have been claimed to be the major advantages of electrochemical detection. It has been suggested that the minimum detectable quantity is 10 pg (43), or 0.25 ng (27) for AA in body fluids. A detection limit around nanogram quantities has been suggested in food analysis (36). Behrens and Madére (44) showed that AA (and DHA) in rat plasma, tissues, and in several foods can be reproducibly detected and quantified at a detection limit of 50 pg.

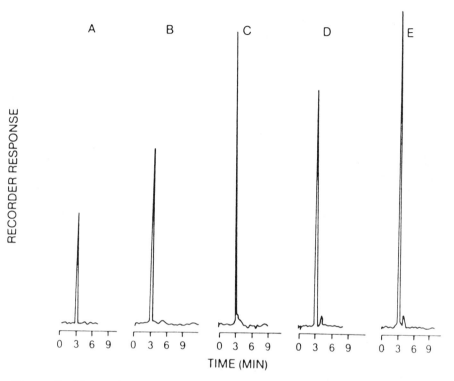

Figure 5 HPLC chromatogram for (A) 0.16 ng standard AA, (B) 0.25 ng AA in a tomato homogenate, (C) 0.25 ng AA in a tomato homogenate plus the 0.16 ng standard, (D) 0.36 ng AA in a tomato homogenate after incubation with homocysteine, and (E) same as (D) plus the 0.16 ng standard. The difference (D-B) represents the amount of DHA in tomato. HPLC conditions: column 5 μm C18 reversed phase (25 cm × 4.6 mm ID); mobile phase, 80 mM sodium acetate containing 1 mM n-octylamine, 15% methanol, and 0.015% MPA, pH 4.6; flow rate, 0.9 ml/min; electrochemical detection, +0.7 V oxidizing potential. From Ref. 44, with permission from Academic Press.

3.4   UV Detection

With regard to vitamin C analysis, ultraviolet (UV) detection has been frequently used both for foods, including fruits and vegetables (25,29,37–40), and for biological samples (23,24,29,42,45,46).

Doner and Hicks (29) described the weak anion-exchange HPLC separation of AA, IAA, and the corresponding dehydro forms plus diketogulonic acid and diketogluconic acid on aminopropyl bonded-phase silica. They achieved separation using an isocratic elution of a Zorbax NH₂ column (25 cm × 4.6 mm ID) with acetonitrile-0.05 M KH$_2$PO$_4$ (75:25, v/v). They used a sensitive refractive index detector to monitor the elution of the six compounds (Fig. 6). The detection limit was about 20 μg for AA,IAA, and DHA. For quantitative analysis of AA and IAA, Doner and Hicks used UV detection at 268 nm, with a lower limit of detection of less than 5 ng. Reduction of DHA and DHIAA in a duplicate sample with DTT allowed the indirect determination of these compounds as AA and IAA, respectively. To avoid reoxidation, DTT was also added to the mobile phase (1.0 mg/ml).

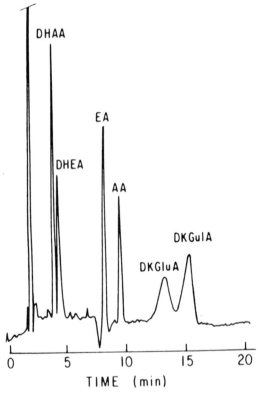

Figure 6 Chromatography of standard mixture (20 μl injected) of dehydroascorbic (DHAA, 160 μg), dehydroerythorbic (DHEA, 320 μg), erythorbic (EA, 160 μg), ascorbic (AA, 160 μg), diketoglukonic (DHGluA, 640 μg), and diketogulonic acid (DKGulA, 640 μg). HPLC conditions: column, Zorbax NH$_2$; mobile phase, 3:1 acetonitrile, 0.05 M KH$_2$PO$_4$; flow rate, 1.5 ml/min; refractive index detection, 16× attenuation; recorder chart speed, 0.25 cm/min. From Ref. 29, with permission from Academic Press.

Doner and Hicks (29) prepared their eluent mixture by gradually adding acetonitrile to prewarmed 0.05 M KH$_2$PO$_4$ in order to avoid salt precipitation. Apparently such precipitation was avoided in the study by Bui-Nguyén (60), who used the same eluent, by maintaining the column at 60°C. Heating the column also improved the separation of AA and IAA. Rose and Nahrwold (24) and Parviainen et al. (23) used a lower molar concentration of KH$_2$PO$_4$ (2.5 mM) at ambient temperature, which apparently lessens the probability of salt formation. With over 6 years of experience and after working with thousands of plasma samples, we have not seen any problems in our HPLC system due to salt formation. One reason might be the use of MPA in the samples and standards, which tends to acidify the eluent during sample injection and elution. Figure 7 exemplifies our method for AA analysis in plasma samples. Our

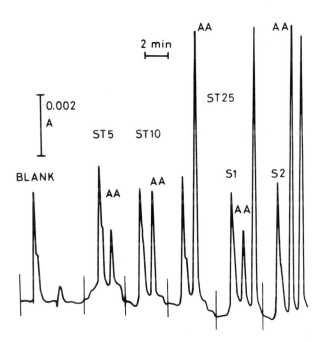

Figure 7 Separation of AA from plasma. Blank, 5% MPA injection; ST5, AA standard 5 mg/l; ST10, AA standard 10mg/l; ST25, AA standard 25 mg/l; S1, a normal plasma sample; same as S1 but AA (20 mg/liter) was added. Retention time of AA:2.4 min. HPLC conditions: column, Resolution-NH$_2$ 3 μm (Spherisorb S3NH$_2$ bulk packing; home-packed; dimensions: 150 mm × 4.6 mm ID); mobile phase, acetonitrile-0.0025 M KH$_2$PO$_4$ (75:25, v/v); flow rate 1.2 ml/min; UV detection 254 nm. Reprinted from Ref. 23, p. 2190.

detection limit for AA in human plasma is about 5 ng (23), which is similar to that in the study by Doner and Hicks (29), who had a less complex sample matrix. Furthermore, our method (23) has a good correlation and low bias compared to the conventional manual OPD fluorescence method as reference (linear regression equation: y(HPLC) = 1.035 × (OPD method) + 0.265; r = 0.93; n = 27).

Rose and Nahrwold (24) used UV detection at 240 nm and 254 nm for AA, and 210 nm for the detection of DHA. Parviainen et al. (23) used 254 nm, and Bui-Nguyén (67) used 268 nm for the detection of AA. The detection limits for AA and DHA were 0.5 and 10 μg, respectively, in the study by Rose and Nahrwold (24). Their conclusion is that adequate determination of total vitamin C is achieved by the conversion of DHA to AA with homocysteine and detection of the reduced form, because of the low UV detection sensitivity for DHA. However, Wimalasiri and Wills (68) successfully modified the method of Rose and Nahrwold (24) for the simultaneous analysis of AA and DHA in fresh fruit and vegetables. They used a μBondapak/carbohydrate column (30 cm × 4 mm ID), a mobile phase based on 70:30 (v/v) acetonitrile-water (containing 0.01 M ammonium dihydrogen phosphate, pH 4.3, adjusted with orthophosphoric acid), and dual UV wavelength detection at 254 nm (AA) and 214 nm (DHA). MPA was unsuitable as the extracting medium due to interference at lower wavelengths, whereas 3% citric acid proved to be a suitable medium for extraction. Coextractants from the sample matrix were an additional problem. They were removed by using C_{18} Sep Pak solid-phase extraction minicolumns. The chromatographic system of Wimalasiri and Wills (64) was capable of detecting 50 ng of AA at 254 nm, 200 ng at 214 nm, and 100 ng of DHA at 214 nm. These detection sensitivities are noticeably better than those described by Rose and Nahrwold (24), and proved to be low enough to allow the measurement of AA in all and DHA in most of the products.

A solid-phase extraction step with C_{18} Sep Pak was also included by Lavigne et al. (38) prior to HPLC in their AA analysis of goat's milk. Sanderson and Schorach (46) used two different preliminary purification and extraction methods prior to their HPLC method for AA and DHA in gastric juice. The gastric juice sample containing labeled AA, which was used to correct the analytical recovery, was passed through short Sephadex G-50 columns in order to remove mucus and large or medium molecular weight material. AA and DHA eluting in the first fraction were subjected to HPLC analysis. DTT was used for the reduction of DHA to AA, prior to the HPLC run. In the second purification method, perchloric acid precipitated samples were mixed with DTT and an internal standard (reductic acid) plus labeled AA to correct the analytical recovery. After the pH was brought to 6.5–7.0, the sample mixture was passed through a primed C_{18} Sep Pak. The eluate passing through contained "total AA," while other small UV absorbing molecules were retained. Sanderson and Schorach used Waters Nova-pak C_{18} compressed cartridges (10 cm × 8 mm ID) together with a guard column (Corasil C_{18} pellicular packing, 5 cm × 4.6 mm ID). The mobile phase consisted of 0.02 M $NH_4H_2PO_4$ buffer, pH 7.1-methanol (80:20, w/w), containing 0.62 g/liter tetrapentylammonium bromide. The UV detection wavelength was set to 270 nm.

The sensitivity (1 ng) of Sanderson and Schorach's method (46) approaches that of some HPLC EC methods. Their results were also in excellent agreement with the 2,4-dinitrophenylhydrazine method. Sanderson and Schorach used a new internal standard, reductic acid, which is an analog of AA. Furthermore, they used [^{14}C] AA to correct for any loss occurring during the extensive purification. Sanderson and Schorach are also concise in describing the problems that were encountered and the remedies to solve them. The first problem was due to complex mucous sample matrix that gradually deteriorated the chromatography. The second problem arose due to the building up of oxidizing sites on the column, or on the chromatographic system. The apparent drawbacks in our opinion are the complexity of the method and the fact that this method does not allow the simultaneous assay of AA and DHA.

Ziegler and colleagues (37) carried out a thorough investigation of the simultaneous assay of DHA and AA by reversed-phase HPLC, using a postcolumn reduction system. The successful separation of DHA and AA was achieved by a range of reversed-phase column materials, and DHA was reduced to AA with DTT in a postcolumn reaction system and detected as AA. Metaphosphoric acid (0.25%) was used as the mobile phase, and the postcolumn reagent consisted of trisodium phosphate dodecahydrate, sodium dihydrogen phosphate, and DTT, pH 7.6. The column and reaction coil were temperature controlled. Lower temperatures were favored because of stronger retardation and thus better separation. Both forms were detected at 267 nm with a sensitivity of 1.4 ng. The detection limit for DHA by direct UV detection at 225 nm was about 200 ng; thus it was enhanced by a factor of 140 by using the postcolumn system. A column switching valve was utilized for directing the column effluent either to the postcolumn reaction system or directly to the detector. Ziegler and colleagues (37) also demonstrate the applicability of a diode-array detector for on-line confirmation of the identity of the presumed AA peak in a standard and a sample (Fig. 8) of rose hip. The authors conclude that the method described provides for high sensitivity, selectivity, and accuracy and a short analysis time in the simultaneous assay of DHA and AA. The applicability of this promising method to the measurement of the DHA and AA content of foodstuffs

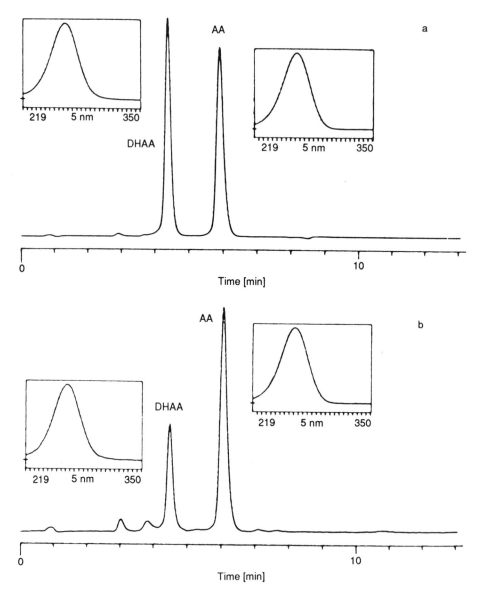

Figure 8 HPLC elution profiles of (a) a standard solution and (b) a rose hip sample containing 29% of DHA of the total vitamin C content (0.67% dry mass). Column: Lichrosorb RP-18 (5 μm; 25 cm × 4 mm ID); column temperature: 19°C; mobile phase (0, 25% MPA) flow rate 1.0 ml/min; postcolumn reagent (trisodium phosphate dodecahydrate, sodium hydrogen phosphate, and DTT, pH 7.6) flow rate 0.5 ml/min. The UV spectra of AA and reduced DHA were taken online during the chromatographic run. From Ref. 37, with permission from Elsevier Science Publishers.

and biological samples remains to be established. Lavigne et al. (38) also used diode-array detection in their multivitamin assay for vitamins B_1, B_2, and C in goat's milk.

We have developed an HPLC method for the quantification of DHA and AA in protein-free human milk, blood plasma, and leukocytes (buffy layer) (30). We used DL-homocysteine to convert the DHA to AA, which was measured by reversed-phase liquid chromatography with UV detection at 254 nm (Fig. 9). Table 1 summarizes the quantification results obtained for the different biological samples. The use of homocysteine for the reduction of DHA, and the subsequent measurement of AA, was initially described by Dennison et al. (79) for the determination of vita-

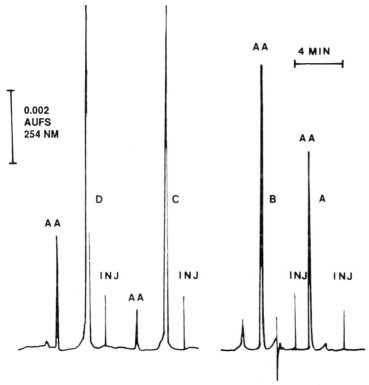

Figure 9 Representative chromatograms showing 20-μl injections of (A) AA standard (30 mg/l), (B) AA in filtered protein-free milk, (C) homocysteine-treated DHA standard (30 mg/l), and (D) a homocysteine-treated milk sample for "total AA" analysis. HPLC conditions: column, Nucleosil C_{18} 7 μm; mobile phase, 2 mmol/liter tetrabutylammonium hydroxide in water, pH 2.92; flow rate 1.5 ml/min; UV detection 254 nm. Reprinted from Ref. 30, p. 1723, by courtesy of Marcel Dekker, Inc.

Table 1 Normal Human AA and DHA Concentrations (Mean ± SEM) in Some
Biological Fluids and in Blood Leukocytes (30)

Sample	AA (mg/liter)	DHA (mg/liter)
Human milk (fresh) (n = 4)	54.3 ± 6.5	21.0 ± 9.1
Human milk (pasteurized) (n = 4)	8.6 ± 3.4	6.6 ± 2.4
Plasma (n = 23)	10.0 ± 0.8	0.16 ± 0.03
Blood leukocytes (n = 10)	0.21 ± 0.04 (mg/10^9 cells)	0.09 ± 0.03 (mg/10^9 cells)

min C in beverages. They used an amino column (μBondapak NH$_2$, 30
cm × 4 mm ID), a mobile phase composed of 50:50 (v/v) methanol-
0.25% KH$_2$PO$_4$ (pH 3.5), and UV detection at 244 nm. Behrens and
Madére (44) also applied a similar reduction procedure in their HPLC
EC method.

An assay at the nanogram level for AA in foods, using an Aminex
HPX-87 column (30 cm × 7.8 mm ID) connected to a MicroGuard ion
exclusion cartridge and using 0.009 N H$_2$SO$_4$ containing 0.05% EDTA as
eluent, was described by Ashoor and co-workers (25). UV detection was
conducted at 245 nm.

3.5 Fluorometric Detection

As previously pointed out, the simultaneous determination of AA and
DHA is difficult, because of the electrochemical inactivity of DHA or the
different UV absorption properties of AA and DHA.

The fluorescent assay by Speek et al. (26), which was modified from
that described by Keating and Haddad (70), consisted of the precolumn
derivatization of DHA with OPD to the quinoxaline derivative after the
oxidation of AA to DHA with ascorbic acid oxidase. The derivative was
then chromatographed on a reversed-phase column (ODS-Hypersil 3 μm,
8 cm × 4.6 mm ID) with a 20:80 (v/v) methanol-0.08 M KH$_2$PO$_4$ (pH
7.8) mobile phase, and was detected by fluorescence (excitation, 255 nm;
emission, 475 nm). This assay allows quantification of "total AA" (AA
plus endogenous DHA) in blood with a sensitivity of 0.2 μmol/liter. The
main limitation of this method is the relative instability of the quinoxaline derivative. VanderJagt and her collaborators (71) compared the

method described by Speek et al., (26) for "total AA" with an automated colorimetric method involving dichlorophenolindophenol (DCIP), and showed an excellent correlation but, not unexpectedly, somewhat lower results compared with the DCIP method. VanderJagt et al. (71) also measured the reduced AA using reversed-phase chromatography with an *n*-octylamine ion-pairing agent, and electrochemical detection. The AA and "total AA" levels showed close agreement, suggesting that only low levels of endogenous DHA are present in normal plasma. Speek and colleagues (72) utilized the same precolumn derivatization to analyze AA and IAA in foodstuffs, with a detection sensitivity of about 0.2 $\mu g/g$. Again, the quinoxaline derivatives of DHA and DHIAA were prepared, after the oxidation of AA and IAA with ascorbic acid oxidase. Omission of the enzymatic oxidation step permitted the exclusive determination of DHA and DHIAA present in the sample. Another precolumn derivatization reagent of DHA, 1,2-diamino-4,5-dimethoxybenzene, described by Iwata et al. (80) appears to yield even greater sensitivity than OPD.

Lopez-Anaya and Mayersohn (73) used a short reversed-phase C18 column (Ultrasphere ODS 3 μm, 7.5 cm × 4.6 mm ID, plus a 7.0 cm × 2.0 mm ID guard column packed with 10 μm polymeric PRP-1 with an ion-pair reagent (0.15 mM hexadecyltrimethyl ammonium bromide) in the mobile phase of 0.5 mM sodium acetate and 0.15 mM disodium EDTA dihydrate (pH 4.0) for the separation of AA and DHA in plasma and urine. The simultaneous quantification of both AA and DHA was done using fluorescence detection after a postcolumn reaction with 4,5-dimethyl-OPD. The postcolumn reagent also contained the oxidant, since AA must first be oxidized to DHA prior to the derivatization. The excitation wavelength was 365 nm, and the emission 440 nm. Isoascorbic acid was used as an internal standard, and the total run time was about 20 min (Fig. 10). The detection limit was 10 ng for AA and 4 ng for DHA. This method showed a good correlation with the methoxyaniline colometric method, and no apparent bias was observed.

Vanderslice and Higgs (68) have previously described a similar postcolumn detection system after the separation of AA and DHA with an anion-exchange resin (Dionex DA-X8-11) but using OPD as the derivatization reagent. The mobile phase consisted of 0.1 M citrate, 0.01 M NaCl, and 5 mM EDTA (pH 3.8), and two postcolumn reagent pumps were used. One pump was for the oxidizing reagent, and the other was for the fluorophor. The limit of detection was 20 ng for AA and 10 ng for DHA. A variety of foods including fruit juices, vegetables, and fruits were analysed by Vanderslice and Higgs (68), and their results agreed well with the manual fluorometric method in the "total AA" analysis.

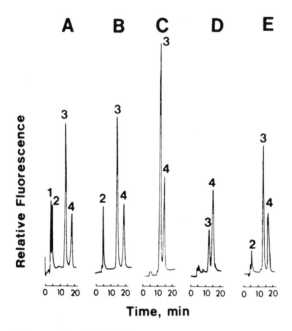

Figure 10   HPLC chromatograms of (A) standards in 10 g/liter MPA solution: DHIAA 5.0 mg/liter, DHA 5.0 mg/liter, AA 25.0 mg/liter, and IAA 10.0 mg/liter; (B) blank human urine diluted 1:3 with 10 g/liter MPA solution (DHA 4.4 mg/liter, AA 21.4 mg/liter and internal standard IAA 10.0 mg/liter; (C) human urine sample (diluted 1:50 with 10 g/liter MPA solution) obtained 3 h after a 1-g iv dose of AA (AA 21.9 mg/liter and internal standard IAA 10.0 mg/liter; (D) blank human plasma sample diluted 1:3 with 10 g/liter MPA solution (DHA 0.8 mg/liter, AA 4.7 mg/liter and internal standard IAA 10.0 mg/liter; and (E) human plasma sample (diluted 1:3 with 10 g/liter MPA solution) obtained 0.5 h after a 1-g iv dose of AA (DHA 1.9 mg/liter, AA 19.9 mg/liter, and internal standard IAA 10.0 mg/liter. Retention time (min): (1) DHIAA 4.60; (2) DHA 5.61; (3) AA 15.50; (4) IAA 19.90. From Ref. 79, with permission from the American Association of Clinical Chemistry.

A simultaneous determination of AA and DHA as described by Lunec and Blake (81) combines the UV and fluorometric detection methods. They measured AA and DHA in the serum and the synovial fluid of patients with rheumatoid arthritis after extracting the sample with MPA and stabilizing it with EDTA. OPD was added to the sample to react with DHA as described above, and the samples were injected on a Lichrosorb NH_2 column, eluted with 30:70 methanol-water. The elution of AA was monitored at 265 nm while the fluorescence of the DHA-quinoxaline derivative was also recorded. The detection limit for AA was

2.5 μmol/liter Lunec and Blake provide considerable data on the stability of AA and DHA during storage in MPA extracts. Both were stable for at least 1 month at $-25°C$. Furthermore, they argue that it is necessary to measure both active forms of vitamin C. The levels of DHA in normal plasma, however, were considerably higher than those obtained using other methods (30,71).

4. GAS-LIQUID CHROMATOGRAPHY

Gas-liquid chromatography (GLC) has provided increased sensitivity and selectivity for analytical work compared to PC and TLC. Sweeley et al. (82) were first to analyze AA as a timethylsilylether (TMS) derivative using a flame-ionization detector. Later, De Wilt (83) studied the TMS derivatives of sorbose, 2-keto-L-gulonic acid, and AA using gas chromatography-mass spectrometry (GC-MS) and found that AA is silylated to yield a tetra-TMS derivative. Pfeilsticker and co-workers (84) studied the structure of DHA in aqueous solution with different methods. They performed the GC analysis of DHA as a per-O-trimethylsilyl derivative. However, only relatively few applications on the quantitative analyses of AA in foods and pharmaceuticals exist, and these papers were published in the early 1970s.

Niemelä (85) used GLC to study the oxidative and nonoxidative alkali-catalyzed degradation of AA. He used an SE-54 silica-fused capillary column for the separation of the trimethylsilylated carboxylic acids obtained after the degradation of AA. The detection was done by flame ionization, and by mass spectrometry. His results demonstrate, a rapid and excellent separation of AA and a number of degradation products, of which many are also known as products of the AA in vivo metabolism. Over 50 compounds were detected, 32 of which could be identified as carboxylic acids (85). Threonic and oxalic acids were the main products after nonoxidative thermal and alkali-catalyzed degradation, with a considerable amount of isomerization to IAA. Threonic, oxalic, *threo*-2-pentulosonic, C-(*threo*-1,2,3-trihydroxypropyl)-tartronic, xylonic, glyceric, and lyxonic acids, in that decreasing order, were the main products in the oxidative alkali-catalyzed degradation of AA (Fig. 11). This method undoubedly holds promise as an excellent tool for the study in more detail of the degradation of AA and DHA.

5. FUTURE TRENDS

Recent developments in the assays of vitamin C compounds focus on multicomponent analyses, most often those of AA and DHA, and in some cases IAA is also measured. DHA and AA are regarded as the biologi-

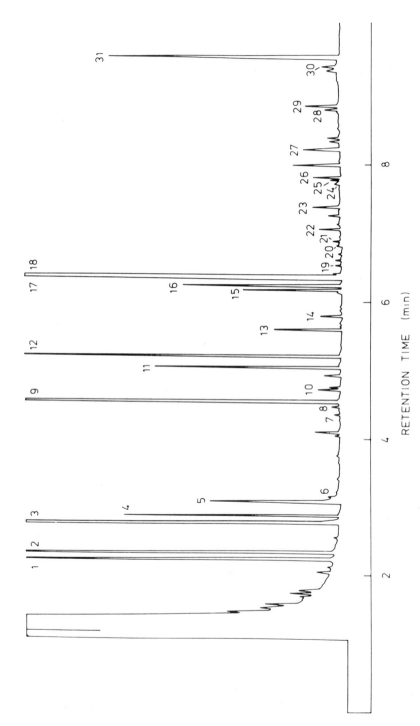

RETENTION TIME (min)

Figure 11

cally active vitamin C forms and thus demand, preferably, simultaneous assays.

The HPLC post-column oxidation/reduction systems in conjunction with UV,EC, or fluorometric measurement of AA in the photometrically or electrochemically active form, or as the fluorescent DHA-quinoxaline, combine specificity and selectivity in a much better way than the earlier HPLC and manual methods. The applicability of these methods, however, in animal, clinical, and nutrition sciences remains to be established.

If AA alone is the component of interest, one may choose a simple and rapid HPLC separation using weak anion-exchange chromatography or reversed-phase chromatography combined with UV or electrochemical detection, taking appropriate precautions in sample and standard handling. New chromatographic supports, especially polymeric stationary phases, show promise as interesting alternatives to the "classical" ones.

ACKNOWLEDGMENTS

We are grateful to Dr. Pekka Mäenpää, M.D., University of Kuopio, for his valuable advice, and we also thank Mr. Vivian Paganuzzi for revising our English.

REFERENCES

1. G. M. Jaffe, in *Handbook of Vitamins. Nutritional, Biochemical, and Clinical Aspects*, (L. J. Machlin, ed.), Marcel Dekker, New York, p. 201 (1984).
2. W. Friedrich, in *Vitamins*, W. De Gruyter, Berlin, pp. 931–932 (1988).

Figure 11   Separation on a SE-54 fused-silica capillary column (25 m × 0.32 mm ID) of the trimethylsilylated carboxylic acids obtained after oxygen-alkali treatment of AA at 110°C. 1, Lactic; 2, glycolic; 3, oxali; 4,3-hydroxypropanoic; 5, unidentified; 6, artifact; 7, succinic; 8,2-C-methylglyceric; 9, glyceric; 10, C-methytartronic; 11, tartronic; 12, 3-deoxytetronic; 13, dihydroxymalonic; 14, malic; 15, unidentified; 16, erythronic; 17, C-(hydroxymethyl) tartronic (minor component); 18, threonic; 19, erythraric; 20, threaric; 21, *threo*-2-pentulosonic; 22, C-(2-hydroxyethyl)tartronic; 23, 2-C-carboxy-3-deoxytetraric; 24, xylonic; 25, lyxonic; 26, C-(1,2-dihydroxyethyl) tartronic; 27, 2-C-carboxytetraric; 28, 2-C-carboxy-3-deoxypentraric; 29, ascorbic (AA); 30, C-(*erythro*-1,2,3-trihydroxypropyl)tartronic; and, 31, C-(*threo*-1,2,3-trihydroxypropyl)tartronic acid. The temperature program was 2 min at 110°C, 20°C/min to 230°C and 5 min at 230°C. The temperature of both the injection port and the detector was 260°C. From Ref. 85, with the permission from Elsevier Science Publishers.

3. L. A. Pachla, D. L. Reynolds, and P. T. Kissinger, *J. Assoc. Off. Anal. Chem.*, *68*:1 (1985).
4. M. H. Bui-Nguyén, in *Modern Chromatographic Analysis of the Vitamins* (A. P. De Leenheer, W. E. Lambert, and M. G. M. De Ruyter, eds.), Marcel Dekker, New York, pp. 267–301 (1985).
5. C. C. Tagney, *Prog. Clin. Biol. Res.*, *259*:331 (1988).
6. P. T. Chou and A. U. Khan, *Biochem. Biophys. Res. Commun.*, *115*:932 (1983).
7. H. Sapper, S. O. Kang, H. H. Paul, and W. Lohmann, *Z. Naturforsch.*, *37c*:942 (1982).
8. H. M. Goldman, B. S. Gold, and H. N. Munro, *Am. J. Clin. Nutr.*, *34*:24 (1981).
9. S. Lewin, in *Vitamin C: Its Molecular Biology and Medical Potential*, Academic Press, London, p. 105 (1976).
10. *RDA Recommended Dietary Allowances*, 9th ed., National Academy of Sciences, Washington, D.C. (1980).
11. D. Horning, *Trends Pharm. Sci.*, *3*:294 (1982).
12. L. Pauling, *Vitamin C and the Common Cold*, Freeman, San Francisco (1970).
13. W. Weis, *Ann. N.Y. Acad. Sci.*, *258*:190 (1975).
14. L. Tuderman, R. Myllylä, and K. Kivirikko, *Eur. J. Biochem.*, *80*:341 (1977).
15. D. Horning, *Ann. N. Y. Acad. Sci.*, *258*:103 (1975).
16. C. M. Visser, *Bioorg. Chem.*, *9*:261 (1980).
17. E. Ginter, P. Bobek, F. Kubec, J. Vozar, and D. Urbanova, *Int. J. Vitam. Nutr. Res.*, *Suppl.*, *23*:137 (1982).
18. W. H. Kalus and W. G. Filby, *Experientia*, *36*:147 (1980).
19. M. Shoyab, *Oncology*, *38*:187 (1981).
20. B. V. Siegel and B. Leibowitz, *Int. J. Vitam. Nutr. Res.*, *Suppl.* 23:9 (1982).
21. R. Sasaki, T. Kurokawa, and S. Tero-Kubata, *J. Gerontol.*, *38*:26 (1983).
22. J. T. Salonen, R. Salonen, M. Ihanainen, M. Parviainen, R. Seppänen, M. Kantola, K. Seppänen, and R. Rauramaa, *Am. J. Clin. Nutr.*, *48*:1226 (1988).
23. M. T. Parviainen, K. Nyyssönen, I. M. Penttilä, K. Seppänen, R. Rauramaa, J. T. S. Salonen, and C.-G. Gref, *J. Liq. Chromatogr.*, *9*:2185 (1986).
24. R. C. Rose and D. L. Nahrwold, *Anal. Biochem.*, *114*:140 (1981).
25. S. H. Ashoor, W. C. Monte, and J. Welty, *J. Assoc. Off. Anal. Chem.*, *67*:78 (1984).
26. A. J. Speek, J. Schrijver, and W. H. P. Schreurs, *J. Chromatogr.*, *305*:53 (1984).
27. M. A. Kutnink, J. H. Skala, H. E. Sauberlich, and S. T. Omaye, *J. Liq. Chromatogr.*, *8*:31 (1985).
28. S. A. Margolis and I. Black, *J. Assoc. Off. Anal. Chem.*, *70*:806 (1987).
29. L. W. Doner and K. B. Hicks, *Meth. Enzymol.*, *122*:3 (1986).
30. K. Nyyssönen, S. Pikkarainen, M. T. Parviainen, K. Heinonen, and I. Mononen, *J. Liq. Chromatogr.*, *11*:1717 (1988).

31. M. J. Deutsch and C. E. Weeks, *J. Assoc. Off. Anal. Chem.*, 48:1248 (1965).
32. G. Szepesi, *Z. Anal. Chem.*, 265:334 (1973).
33. E. De Ritter, *J. Assoc. Off. Anal. Chem.*, 48:985 (1965).
34. M. Otsuka, T. Kurata, and N. Arakawa, *Agric. Biol. Chem.*, 50:531 (1986).
35. L. A. Pachla and P. T. Kissinger, *Anal. Chem.*, 48:364 (1976).
36. N. Moll and J. P. Joly, *J. Chromatogr.*, 405:347 (1987).
37. S. J. Ziegler, B. Meier, and O. Sticher, *J. Chromatogr.*, 391:419 (1987).
38. C. Lavigne, J. A. Zee, R. E. Simard, and C. Gosselin, *J. Chromatogr.*, 410:201 (1987).
39. Y. Maeda, S. Ochi, T. Masui, and S. Matubara, *J. Assoc. Off. Anal. Chem.*, 71:502 (1988).
40. L. L. Loyd, F. P. Warner, J. F. Kennedy, and C. A. White, *J. Chromatogr.*, 437:447 (1988).
41. W. D. Mason, E. N. Amick, and W. Heft, *Anal. Lett.*, 13:817 (1980).
42. L. L. Hatch and A. Sevanian, *Anal. Biochem.*, 138:324 (1984).
43. K. Iriyama, M. Yoshiura, and T. Iwamoto, *J. Liq. Chromatogr.*, 8:333 (1985).
44. W. A. Behrens and R. Madére, *Anal. Biochem.*, 15:102 (1987).
45. R. R. Howard, T. Peterson, and P. R. Kastl, *J. Chromatogr.*, 414:434 (1987).
46. M. J. Sanderson and C. J. Schorach, *Biomed. Chromatogr.*, 2:197 (1987).
47. C. S. Tsao and S. L. Salimi, *J. Chromatogr.*, 245:355 (1982).
48. R. S. Carr, M. B. Bally, P. Thomas, and J. M. Neff, *Anal. Chem.*, 55:1229 (1983).
49. C. G. Honecker, W. Krenger, H. Langeman, and A. Kempf, *J. Chromatogr.*, 381:249 (1986).
50. Y. Suzuki and K. Fukuda, *J. Chromatogr.*, 489:283 (1989).
51. C. G. Honegger, J. Torhorst, H. Langemann, A. Kabiersch, and W. Krenger, *Int. J. Cancer*, 41:690 (1988).
52. E. Wang and W. Hou, *J. Chromatogr.*, 447:256 (1988).
53. M. E. Abdel-Hamid, M. H. Barary, E. M. Hassan, and M. A. Elsayed, *Analyst*, 110:831 (1985).
54. O. Lau, S. Luk, and K. Wong, *Analyst*, 112:1023 (1987).
55. F. Salinas and T. G. Diaz, *Analyst*, 113:1657 (1988).
56. U. Muralikrishna and J. A. Murty, *Analyst*, 114:407 (1989).
57. F. R. Visser, *J. Assoc. Off. Anal. Chem.*, 67:1020 (1984).
58. J. Peinado and F. Toribio, *Analyst*, 112:775 (1987).
59. A. G. Fogg, A. M. Summan, and M. A. Fernades-Arciniega, *Analyst*, 110:341 (1985).
60. M. H. Bui-Nguyén, *J. Chromatogr.*, 196:163 (1980).
61. L. W. Doner and K. B. Hicks, *Anal. Biochem.*, 115:225 (1981).
62. R. C. Rose and D. L. Nahrwold, *Anal. Biochem.*, 123:389 (1982).
63. R. C. Rose and M. J. Koch, *Anal. Biochem.*, 143:21 (1984).
64. P. Wimalasiri and R. B. H. Wills, *J. Chromatogr.*, 256:368 (1983).
65. L. F. Liebes, S. Kuo, R. Krigel, E. Pelle, and R. Silber, *Anal. Biochem.*, 118:53 (1981).

66. C. M. Farber, S. Kanengiser, R. Stahl, L. Liebes, and R. Silber, *Anal. Biochem.*, *134*:355 (1983).
67. R. L. Stahl, C. M. Farber, L. F. Liebes, and R. B. Silber, *Cancer Res.*, *45*:6507 (1985).
68. J. T. Vanderslice and D. J. Higgs, *J. Chromatogr. Sci.*, *22*:485 (1984).
69. J. K. Baker, J. Kapeghian and A. Verlangieri, *J. Liq. Chromatogr.*, *6*:1319 (1983).
70. R. W. Keating and P. R. Haddad, *J. Chromatogr.*, *245*:249 (1982).
71. D. J. VanderJagt, P. J. Garry and W. C. Hunt, *Clin. Chem.*, *32*:1004 (1986).
72. A. J. Speek, J. Schrijver and W. H. P. Schreurs, *J. Agric. Food Chem.*, *32*:352 (1984).
73. A. Lopez-Anaya and M. Mayersohn, *Clin. Chem.*, *33*:1874 (1987).
74. H. Langemann, J. Torhorst, A. Kabiersch, W. Krenger, and C. G. Honegger, *Int. J. Cancer*, *43*:1169 (1989).
75. L. L. Ibric, W. F. Benedict and A. R. Peterson, *In Vitro Cell Dev. Biol.*, *24*:669 (1988).
76. X. Y. Wang, M. L. Liao, T. H. Hung, and P. A. Seib, *J. Assoc. Off. Anal. Chem.*, *71*:1158 (1988).
77. K. Nyyssönen and M. T. Parviainen, *CRC Crit. Rev Clin. Lab. Sci.*, *27*:211 (1989).
78. C. S. Tsao, M. Young, and S. M. Rose, *J. Chromatogr.*, *308*:306 (1984).
79. D. B. Dennison, T. G. Brawley, and G. L. K. Hunter, *J. Agric. Food Chem.*, *29*:927 (1981).
80. T. Iwata, M. Yamagushi, S. Hara, and M. Nakamura, *J. Chromatogr.*, *344*:351 (1985).
81. J. Lunec and D. R. Blake, *Free Rad. Res. Commun*, *1*:31 (1985).
82. C. C. Sweeley, R. Bentley, M. Makita, and W. W. Wells, *J. Am. Chem. Soc.*, *85*:2497 (1963).
83. H. G. J. De Wilt, *J. Chromatogr.*, *63*:379 (1971).
84. K. Pfeilsticker, F. Marx, and M. Bockisch, *Carbohydr. Res.*, *45*:269 (1975).
85. K. Niemelä, *J. Chromatogr.*, *399*:235 (1987).

6

FOLIC ACID

Robert J. Mullin and David S. Duch

Wellcome Research Laboratories, Research Triangle Park,
North Carolina

1. INTRODUCTION

This section is a brief overview of folate biochemistry and cellular physiology oriented primarily toward mammalian species. A more complete review of these areas can be found in references 1–3. A series of nutritional studies with extracts from yeast, liver, and plants (4–7) led to the discovery of a group of closely related compounds and to the isolation of an essential nutrient that could serve as a growth factor for chicks and certain bacteria and that could be used for the treatment of macrocytic anemia. The factor isolated from spinach and other sources was first called folic acid by Mitchell et al. (7) and was subsequently characterized as N-[4-{[(2-amino-4-hydroxy-6-pteridinyl)methyl]amino}benzoyl] glutamic acid by Angier et al. (8).

1.1 Cellular Biochemistry of Folates

Studies in living organisms have shown that folate exists not as the fully oxidized species, folic acid, but predominantly as reduced forms with all essentially properties as the fully reduced tetrahydro derivatives (Fig. 1). Studies on the distribution of folate cofactors have shown that native folates are a family of compounds differing from each other in their state of reduction and the number of glutamate residues present. Tetrahydrofolate can be found substituted at the N^5 position to give the 5-methyl,

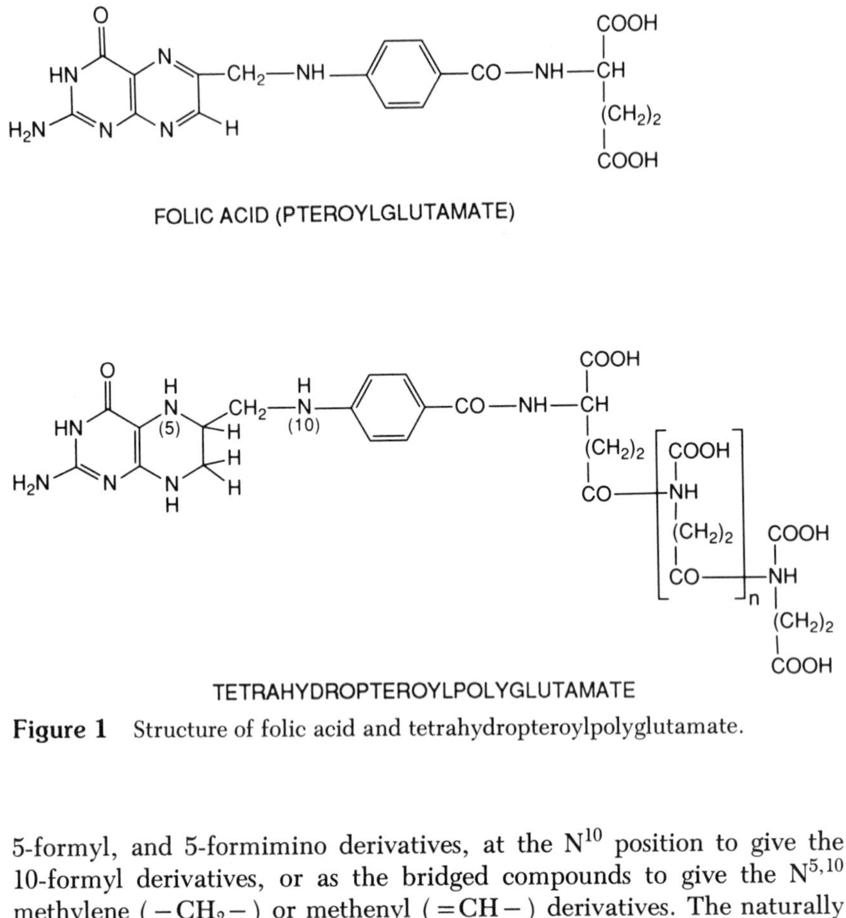

FOLIC ACID (PTEROYLGLUTAMATE)

TETRAHYDROPTEROYLPOLYGLUTAMATE

Figure 1 Structure of folic acid and tetrahydropteroylpolyglutamate.

5-formyl, and 5-formimino derivatives, at the N^{10} position to give the 10-formyl derivatives, or as the bridged compounds to give the $N^{5,10}$ methylene ($-CH_2-$) or methenyl ($=CH-$) derivatives. The naturally occurring folate cofactors also exist predominantly as polyglutamated compounds, containing from five to eight glutamate residues.

1.2 Transport of Folate Cofactors

Dietary folates must first be taken up by the intestine and, after passage through the circulatory system, by the cells where they are required. In both cases, uptake occurs by a carrier-dependent mechanism. Dietary folates exist predominantly in a polyglutamated conjugated form. Since the folate carrier transports the monoglutamate form of the cofactor, the folate polyglutamates must be hydrolyzed to the monoglutamate form by the enzyme folylpolyglutamate hydrolase, also known as conjugase (9,10). The distribution and characterization of hydrolases in the digestive system has been reviewed in depth (11).

Transport by the intestine has been characterized using a wide range of techniques, such as everted sacs and rings, isolated cells and membrane vesicles, and intestinal perfusion and loops. The transport system has been characterized as a pH-dependent, energy-dependent, carrier-mediated process at normal physiological concentrations of folates (12–14). In addition to folic acid, the intestinal transport system can transport reduced folates and folate analogs. The intestine is also capable of reduction of folic acid to tetrahydrofolate and conversion of tetrahydrofolate to 5-methyltetrahydrofolate (15–18). The circulating cofactor form has been shown to be 5-methyltetrahydrofolate, with the plasma containing the monoglutamate form and the cellular elements the polyglutamated derivative (19,20).

Cellular transport other than intestinal transport has been characterized to a large extent using tumor cells in culture. Entry of folates into cells has been shown to occur via a high-affinity carrier-mediated mechanism. The transport system allows transport of reduced folates and antifolates as well as folic acid, although the latter is transported at a much reduced rate (3,21,22). Efflux occurs by at least three routes, one of which is the influx carrier described above (23).

1.3   Interconversion and Utilization of Intracellular Folates

As discussed above, folates exist in nature primarily as polyglutamated derivatives rather than as monoglutamates. Since folates must be in the monoglutamate form to be transported into cells, polyglutamylation must occur after cell entry. This addition of glutamate residues is catalyzed by the enzyme folylpolyglutamate synthetase. Under normal physiological conditions folates exist predominantly as the penta- and hexaglutamates. Folylpolyglutamate synthetase has a broad specificity and can add glutamates to folates as well as antifolates, but studies suggest that tetrahydrofolate and/or 10-formyltetrahydrofolate may serve as the physiological substrate for the addition of the first glutamate. Higher-order polyglutamates appear to be generated from the tetrahydrofolate pool, since tetrahydrofolate polyglutamates are the only long-chain folate derivatives with detectable substrate activity (11,24).

Once inside the cell, folates can undergo interconversion to the various cofactor forms along with both reduction and oxidation (Fig. 2). Folate absorbed from the intestine is reduced to the tetrahydro level by dihydrofolate reductase. This enzyme also reduces dihydrofolate formed in the biosynthesis of thymidylate. With the exception of dihydrofolate reductase, folate-requiring enzymes function optimally with the polyglutamate forms of their folate cofactor. In general, studies on the distribution of the cofactor forms have shown that tetrahydrofolate, 10-

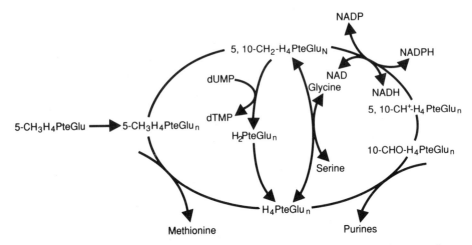

Figure 2 Metabolic interconversions of folate cofactors: CH_2-H_4PteGlu, N^5, N^{10}-methylenetetrahydrofolate; 5,10-CH^+-H_4PteGlu, 5,10-methenyltetrahydrofolate; 10-CHO-H_4PteGlu, 10-formyltetrahydrofolate; H_4PteGlu, tetrahydrofolate; H_2PteGlu, dihydrofolate; 5-CH_3-H_4PteGlu, 5-methyltetrahydrofolate. The subscript n refers to the number of glutamate residues in the molecule.

formyltetrahydrofolate, and 5-methyltetrahydrofolate are the cofactor forms present in the highest quantities in tissues and cells (2).

The *de novo* purine biosynthetic pathway has two reactions that are dependent on 10-formyltetrahydrofolate, GAR and AICAR transformylases. This cofactor is also used in the formylation of methionyl t-RNA. The cofactor 5,10-methylenetetrahydrofolate serves as both the reductant and the one-carbon donor in the biosynthesis of thymidylate from deoxyuridylate catalyzed by thymidylate synthase and is the cofactor for the conversion of glycine to serine by the enzyme serine hydroxymethyltransferase. The cofactor for the biosynthesis of methionine by methionine synthetase is 5-methyltetrahydrofolate. Reduced folates also participate in the catabolism of histidine as well as in specialized biochemical reactions in microorganisms (1,2).

2.   PAPER, THIN-LAYER, AND CONVENTIONAL CHROMATOGRAPHY

2.1   Paper and Thin-Layer Chromatography

Paper and thin-layer chromatography have not had wide acceptance as methods for the separation of folic acid and reduced folate cofactors. These separation methods were supplanted first by ion-exchange chromatography and subsequently by HPLC. The early uses of paper and thin-layer chromatography for the separation of folates have been reviewed (1,3).

2.2   Size Exclusion Chromatography

Chromatography on Sephadex G-10, G-15, and G-25 has been used to separate the various folate monoglutamate cofactors as well as the polyglutamated derivatives (25,26). Using Sephadex G-15 and G-25, Shin et al. (26) found that ionic strength had a marked effect on the elution of the cofactor forms. No separation of the monoglutamate derivatives occurred when water was used as the eluant. Interaction of the folates with the gel matrix increased as the ionic strength increased, resulting in a separation of at least some of the folate monoglutamates. A more complete separation of the cofactor forms required the use of more than one gel form. Increased separation of the folate polyglutamates was also obtained as the buffer strength was increased. These results indicate that the separation of the folate cofactors is not based solely on separation by size but is also dependent on ionic interaction with the matrix. These techniques have been used to characterize the folate pools in cobalamin-deficient L1210 cells and in normal diploid and SV40 transformed human fibroblasts (27,28). Other studies utilizing these techniques in combination with ion-exchange chromatography for the determination of folate levels in rat tissues have been described (29–31).

2.3   Ion-Exchange Chromatography

Ion-exchange chromatography on DEAE and TEAE celluloses, DEAE Sephadex, and QAE Sephadex has been used to separate the monoglutamate and polyglutamate forms of the folate cofactors and has yielded considerable information on the distribution and the metabolic role of folate cofactors in living organisms. These studies have been discussed in considerable detail in earlier reviews (1,2) and will not be discussed further here. These early studies served as the basis for the development of HPLC methods using ion-exchange resins for the separation of the monoglutamate and polyglutamate derivatives as well as for the determination of the polyglutamate chain lengths of folates (32–37). However, the use of ion-exchange resins in HPLC for the separation of folates was superseded by introduction of reversed-phase microparticulate resins.

3.   HIGH-PERFORMANCE LIQUID CHROMATOGRAPHY

Efforts directed toward the separation of folates by HPLC have generally been based upon one of two approaches, ion exchange or reversed-phase chromatography. A more recent development in the separation of folates by HPLC has been the use of a chiral stationary phase for the resolution of isomers at the carbon-6 position. For ease of discussion, analysis of folates by HPLC has been divided into three primary sections: sample preparation, separation methods, and methods of detection.

3.1 Sample Preparation

Methods of sample preparation that have been described in the literature vary considerably as a function of both the complexity of the sample, that is, pharmaceutical versus biological, and the expected folate content, that is, reduced versus nonreduced folates, folylpolyglutamates versus folylmonoglutamates. With this in mind, sample preparation methods have been segregated into three sections: methods for biological fluids, foods, and vitamins, methods for cultured cells, and methods for tissues.

Biological Fluids, Foods, and Vitamins

The detection method chosen for folate analysis dictates to some extent the level of sample preparation required. Sample preparation for methods using microbiological, fluorescence, or electrochemical detection is generally less stringent than for methods using UV absorbance. For plasma analysis most methods are designed to meet two criteria: reduction of protein content and preservation of the oxidation state of the folate sample. Various techniques for the reduction of protein content appear in the literature; the majority of these are based upon protein precipitation either by acidification (38–41), heating (40,42,43), or addition of an organic component (44–46). Several methods simply employ a reversed-phase cartridge to selectively extract folates directly from the plasma sample (39,47,48). Direct injection of plasma onto HPLC systems has also been described (49,50). Based upon the observation that plasma proteins are capable of considerable folate binding (42), it would seem prudent to disrupt this interaction prior to or during sample extraction. This may indicate that direct extraction on a reversed-phase cartridge or direct injection of plasma samples is inadvisable. The method chosen for protein precipitation should be a function of the expected folate content. The instability of 5-formyltetrahydrofolate to acidic conditions should rule out acidification as a precipitation option in those studies involving administration of 5-formyltetrahydrofolate. As an example, the appearance of additional HPLC peaks after acidification of 5-formyltetrahydrofolate has been described in the literature (39). In meeting the second criterion of sample preparation, the most common antioxidant employed has been ascorbic acid, generally at a concentration of 1 mg/ml (38,39,42–44,47,50). Reduced thiols such as mercaptoethanol (28,40,46) or dithiothreitol (41,43) have also been used as antioxidant, either alone (40,41,46) or in combination with ascorbic acid (38,43). Analysis of folates from whole blood is accomplished with similar methods (48). However, an additional problem, polyglutamation, must be addressed. Most HPLC methods have been designed for the analysis of folylmonoglutamates, whereas cellular folates appear as a mixture of polyglutamates. These must be converted to the monoglutamate level with folypolyglutamate hydrolase; the endogenous blood activity can be used for this step (48).

Preparation of milk samples for analysis of folate content requires the same process as described for plasma. Protein reduction has been accomplished by acidification in the presence of ascorbate and mercaptoethanol as antioxidants. Hog kidney folylpolyglutamate hydrolase (51) has been used to convert polyglutamates to the monoglutamate species (52). Following filtration, the sample may be injected directly for HPLC analysis. Urine samples following administration of 5-formyltetrahydrofolate have also been analyzed by HPLC (39,50,53). Following collection with ascorbic acid at a concentration of 1 mg/ml, samples have been analyzed directly or with simple dilution when necessary.

Various folate-fortified materials such as milk and soy-based infant formula (54–56), corn and oat flakes (54,56), vitamin mixtures (57,58), and animal diets (59,49) have been analyzed for folate content. The methods generally involve mechanical disruption followed by dissolution of the sample in buffer. These methods use direct injection of clarified supernatant (49,57,58) or concentration and purification of the sample on an ion-exchange cartridge prior to analysis (55,56,59).

3.2 Cultured Cells

Sample preparation for folate analysis of cultured cells is similar to that used for plasma except that folylpolyglutamates must be hydrolyzed to monoglutamates. An additional obstacle to the analysis of cellular folates is one of quantitation. With cellular folates being below the sensitivity level of most detection methods, the introduction of a radiolabeled folate source is required to allow detection and quantitation. Typically either folic acid or 5-formyltetrahydrofolate has been the source of folate for introduction of radiolabel. Most methods described in the literature represent variations of two established methods (60,61). The first of these methods, described by Matherly et al. (60), is based upon the extraction of cellular folates with heat precipitation at 90°C in pH 7.2 maleate buffer containing 1% mercaptoethanol while maintaining the sample under N_2. The sample is then digested with chicken pancreas folylpolyglutamate hydrolase overnight at 37°C. The folylpolyglutamate hydrolase is inactivated and protein is removed with a second heating step. Recovery of standard folates can be seen in Table 1. Methylenetetrahydrofolate does not survive this method intact, 25% of the 10-formyltetrahydrofolate is converted to 5-formyltetrahydrofolate, and an additional 10% is converted to 5,10-methenyltetrahydrofolate. A second method, described by Allegra et al. (61), extracts the folate fraction and precipitates proteins in 2% ascorbate, 2% mercaptoethanol, pH 6.0 at 90°C. Following digestion with hog kidney folylpolyglutamate hydrolase (62) and a second protein precipitation by heating, the folates are concentrated and partially purified by extraction on a C18 cartridge. Recovery of standard folates again can be seen in Table 1. Upon examination of several methods, Kashani and Cooper (63) recommended heat precipitation of protein at 100°C in pH 6.5 phosphate buffer containing 0.2 M mercaptoethanol, and digestion with rat serum folylpolyglutamate hydrolase, followed by protein precipitation with methanol and freeze drying. However, recovery values for this method were not reported.

3.3 Tissues

Methods used for the preparation of tissue samples for folate analysis are similar to those described above for cultured cells. All of the methods discussed here for tissue preparation employ heating steps to precipitate the bulk of the tissue protein. The methods differ considerably as to when the heating step takes place. In three methods (62,64,65), samples are heated immediately after gross tissue disruption and are then homogenized. The intent of the early heating step is twofold: rapid inactivation of

Table 1 Percent Recovery of Folate Standards

Folate[a]	Percent Recovery						
10-CHO-H$_4$PteGlu		85	55	65	69	59	
H$_4$PteGlu	95	91	80	68	80	58	94
5-CHO-H$_4$PteGlu	105	26	123		79	60	68
H$_2$PteGlu		45			56	62	
PteGlu		84			73	66	88
5-CH$_3$-H$_4$PteGlu	93	100	89	>90	94	69	89
Reference	(66)	(64)	(67)	(60)	(65)	(61)	(51)

[a] 10-CHO-H$_4$PteGlu, 10-formyltetrahydrofolate; H$_4$PteGlu, tetrahydrofolate; 5-CHO-H$_4$PteGlu, 5-formyltetrahydrofolate; H$_2$PteGlu, dihydrofolate; PteGlu, folic acid; 5-CH$_3$-H$_4$PteGlu, 5-methyltetrahydrofolate.

any enzymatic activity which could lead to interconversion of the folate pools, and protein precipitation. Three alternative methods (51,66,67) start with tissue homogenization and follow with heat precipitation at a later time. The extreme of this approach (66,67) calls for an overnight incubation of the homogenate at 37°C at pH 4.0 to allow for conversion of folates to monoglutamates by endogenous folylpolyglutamate hydrolase activity. This approach would seem to risk extensive interconversion of folate pools, but the reported recovery of standards added to liver extract (Table 1) indicates that this is not the case. All of the above methods include ascorbate as an antioxidant at a typical concentration of 1% (w/v). The majority of the methods (62,64,65,67) also include mercaptoethanol at concentrations ranging from 50 mM to 1.5 M. Folate extraction is carried out at slightly acidic conditions. The apparent reasons for this choice include stability of ascorbic acid, optimal pH of the conjugase activity employed, and avoidance of alkaline pH, which upon heating can result in the conversion of 10-formyltetrahydrofolate to tetrahydrofolate (1). Various sources for hydrolase activity have been used for tissue folate digestion. They include rat plasma (65), rat liver (64), hog kidney (62), and endogenous enzyme (66,67). All appear to be adequate, although there may be an advantage with rat plasma due to its activity at neutral pH and ease of preparation. In each of the methods discussed here, the hydrolase activity is heat precipitated prior to preparation of the sample for HPLC analysis. The complexity of this latter step is a function of the detection method used and can be as simple as centrifugation and filtration for those methods based upon microbiological detection. For methods based upon spectral detection using either UV or fluorescence, interfering materials must be removed. The general approach in the literature involves chromatography of the sample on an ion-exchange resin that retains the folate sample. Various matrices have been used, including quaternary amine cartridges (51,66,67) and Dowex 50 (64). An extension of this latter method (68) includes a C18 cartridge to concentrate and further purify the folate sample. The recovery of added standard folates with these methods can be seen in Table 1. Tissue folate levels determined using the above methods are presented in Table 2.

3.4 Separation Methods

The number of folate cofactor forms, variable polyglutamate chain lengths, and instability of many of the reduced derivatives have made separation of these complex mixtures extremely difficult. Although many techniques such as electrophoresis, gel exclusion, and paper and thin-layer chromatography have been investigated to affect separation, only

Table 2   Liver Folate Content

Rat

Folate	Percent folate						
Strain[a]	W	S-D	S-D	S-D	S-D	S-D	?
10-CHO-H$_4$PteGlu[b]		2.8	0.9	1.03	3.0		7.21
H$_4$PteGlu	3.61	11.46	1.3	5.7	4.64	9.64	8.01
5-CHO-H$_4$PteGlu	1.27	2.79		1.34	1.04	7.1	2.2
5-CH$_3$-H$_4$PteGlu	7.69	10.2	3.54	7.34	5.13	5.51	5.38
SUM	12.57	27.3	5.77	15.41	13.82	22.3	22.8
Reference	(66)	(62)	(64)	(67)	(65)	(51)	(81)

Mouse

Folate				
Strain	CD-1	C57/B1	C57/B1	S-W
10-CHO-H$_4$PteGlu	0.855	1.14	16.1	6.4
H$_4$PteGlu	3.38	11.26	6.4	42.9
5-CHO-H$_4$PteGlu			3.4	
5-CH$_3$-H$_4$PteGlu	4.89	4.13	4.7	11.6
SUM	9.07	16.53	30.6	60.9
Reference	(64)	(64)	(57)	(100)

Primate

Folate		
Species	Human	Cynomolgus monkey
10-CHO-H$_4$PteGlu	3.3	10.5
H$_4$PteGlu	6.5	7.4
5-CHO-H$_4$PteGlu		
5-CH$_3$-H$_4$PteGlu	6.0	7.6
SUM	15.8	25.5
Reference	(100)	(100)

[a] S-D, Sprague-Dawley; S-W, Swiss-Webster; W, Wistar; ?, not reported.

[b] 10-CHO-H$_4$PteGlu, 10-formyltetrahydrofolate; H$_4$PteGlu, tetrahydrofolate; 5-CHO-H$_4$PteGlu, 5-formyltetrahydrofolate; H$_2$PteGlu, dihydrofolate; PteGlu, folic acid; 5-CH$_3$-H$_4$PteGlu, 5-methyltetrahydrofolate.

two methods have been widely used in studies on the distribution and characterization of folate pools. Substantial information has been gathered using conventional ion-exchange chromatography. With the advent of HPLC, use of ion-exchange mediums was adapted to this system, but was eventually supplanted by the use of reversed-phase microparticulate resins as the separation medium.

Ion-Exchange HPLC

Ion-exchange-based HPLC methods for the resolution of the various folate derivatives represent for the most part an extension of low-pressure conventional chromatographic techniques on DEAE resins. These methods are based on both weak (32) and strong (33,34,53) ion exchangers. In general ion-exchange-based HPLC methods for folate analysis have not received continued interest and would not be considered routine.

Reversed-Phase HPLC

A review of the reversed-phase HPLC methods for chromatographic analysis of folic acid and its monoglutamated derivatives represents a significant challenge since the methods employed are nearly as numerous as the research groups in the field (see Table 3). The majority of work in this area has been carried out with a C18 stationary phase (38, 39,42,44,45,47–50,52,57–60,62–67), although C8 (61,79) and phenyl (40,41,46,51,80) phases have also been used. Methods have also been described for the use of C18 and phenyl phases in series (54). The diversity of methods stems primarily from optimization for the anticipated sample composition and secondarily from the requirements of the detection systems employed. The chemical structure of folates presents a minor problem for reversed-phase HPLC due to the presence of the carboxyl functions of glutamic acid. These ionic species must be masked in some fashion to allow for interaction with a nonpolar stationary phase. In general this has been accomplished by one of two methods. Either an acidic mobile phase is employed to protonate the carboxyl function, or an ion-pairing reagent is employed to mask the carboxyl function. These two approaches generate species that differ in hydrophobicity; the ion pair interacts more strongly than the protonated folate with a nonpolar phase. As a result of this difference those methods employing ion-pairing reagents, such as tetrabutylammonium salts, hexanesulfonate, or octanesulfonate, generally require higher methanol content in the mobile phase than those methods with an acidic mobile phase (Table 3).

MULTIVITAMIN ANALYSIS. Several methods have been described for the analysis of folic acid from multivitamin preparations (55, 70,71,73,75,79), and the majority use an ion-pairing reagent, either hexanesulfonate (79), octanesulfonate (70,75), or tetrabutylammonium hydroxide (71). On the basis of speed, the method of Dong et al. (79) appears superior: six water-soluble vitamins, including ascorbic acid, niacin, niacinamide, pyridoxine, folic acid, and riboflavin, can be resolved in just over 6 min. An alternative method (70), with an analysis time of 60 min, is capable of resolving thiamine, riboflavin sodium phos-

Table 3 Reversed-Phase HPLC Systems for the Separation of Folylmonoglutamates

Mobile phase[a]	Elution	Reference
C18 column		
3% ACN,4% MeOH,0.5M NH$_4$H$_2$PO$_4$,pH 3.5	Isocratic	47
5% ACN, ph 5, NaH$_2$PO$_4$	Isocratic	69
6% ACN, 100 mM Na acetate, pH 5.7	Isocratic	59
8% ACN, 10 mM KH$_2$PO$_4$, 1% OSA, 0.5% TEA, pH 2.8	Isocratic	70
10.5% ACN, 30 mM NaH$_2$PO$_4$, pH 2.0	Isocratic	66
16% ACN, 0.13% TBAOH, 0.005% EDTA, KH$_2$PO$_4$, pH 7.6	Isocratic	57
5% MeOH, 25 mM NaH$_2$PO$_4$, pH 7	Isocratic	49
6% MeOH, 4% ACN, 10 mM Na acetate, pH 4.5	Isocratic	71
18% MeOH, 5 mM TBAP	Isocratic	62
20% MeOH, 5mM TBAP, 0.1M NaH$_2$PO$_4$, pH 4.5	Isocratic	72
20% MeOH, 5mM TBAP, 10 mM NH$_4$H$_2$PO$_4$, pH 6.8	Isocratic	64
20% MeOH, 50 mM TBAP, KH$_2$PO$_4$, pH 6.8	Isocratic	52
20% MeOH, 100mM NaH$_2$PO$_4$, pH 6.0	Isocratic	73
24% MeOH, 0.3% TBAOH, 15 mM NaH$_2$PO$_4$, pH 7.0	Isocratic	58
25% MeOH, 5 mM TBAP, H$_3$PO$_4$, pH 6.5	Isocratic	74
30% MeOH, 5 mM TBAP, pH 7	Isocratic	44
55% MeOH, 0.85% NaH$_2$PO$_4$, 0.065% OSA	Isocratic	75
ACN:0.1% KH$_2$PO$_4$, pH 4.2–5.2	Gradient	50
ACN:16 mM NaH$_2$PO$_4$, mM TBAP, pH 6	Gradient	67
ACN:NH$_4$H$_2$PO$_4$, pH 2.5–2.9 with TFA	Gradient	42
ACN:0.1 M Na acetate, pH 5.5	Gradient	48
ACN:0.1 M Na acetate, pH 5.5	Gradient	38
ACN:0.1 M Na acetate, pH 5.5	Gradient	60
ACN:10 mM NH$_4$ formate, pH 3.5	Gradient	39
MeOH:4 mM TBAOH, pH5.5	Gradient	45
MeOH:5 mM TBAP	Gradient	76
EtOH:1 mM TBAP	Gradient	63
EtOH:5 mM TBAP, 5 mM mercaptoethanol	Gradient	77
EtOH:7 mM TBAP, 1 mM ascorbate	Gradient	65
EtOH:10 mM TBAP, pH 7.55	Gradient	78
C8 column		
15% MeOH, 5 mM TBAP, pH 5.5 or 7.4	Isocratic	61
15% MeOH, 5 mM hexanesulfonate, 1% HOAc, 0.1% TEA	Isocratic	79
Phenyl column		
1.2% MeOH, 100 mM KH$_2$PO$_4$, 5 mM TBAP, pH 7.0 and 0.5% MeOH, 36 mM NaClO4, 1.3 mM KH$_2$PO$_4$, pH 7.0	Isocratic	80
15% MeOH, 50 mM KH$_2$PO$_4$, 100 μM EDTA, pH 3.5	Isocratic	46
15% MeOH, 50 mM·KH$_2$PO$_4$, pH 3.5	Isocratic	41
ACN: 33mM NaH$_2$PO$_4$, pH 2.3	Gradient	51

[a] TBAOH, tetrabutylammonium hydroxide; TBAP, tetrabutyl ammonium phosphate; ACN, acetonitrile; MeOH, methanol; BME, mercaptoethanol; TEA, triethylamine; TFA, trifluroacetate; OSA, octanesulfonic acid.

phate, caffeine, sodium benzoate, and cyanocobalamin in addition to the six components mentioned above (Fig. 3). Multivitamin analysis represents an optimal situation for folate analysis since only the relatively stable folic acid species is present, and its concentration is considerably higher than that seen in biological samples. The usefulness of these methods for biological samples is unknown.

FOOD ANALYSIS. A number of foods, including cornflakes (54), infant formula (54–56), milk (52,81), animal diets (59), cabbage, and oat flakes (56) have been analyzed for folate content. There does not appear to be any trend toward a common method. Tetrabutylammonium phosphate was employed as an ion-pairing reagent in two of these studies (52,81), and two of the methods where vitamin-fortified materials were being analyzed (55,59) were optimized for detection of folic acid.

PLASMA ANALYSIS. Folate analysis of normal human plasma represents a considerable challenge, since normal levels are between 5 and 10 ng/ml (11–22 pmol/ml). Direct analysis of normal plasma folates has been accomplished via electrochemical (41,46,47) fluorescent (72), and UV (48) detection. A number of methods with UV detection (38–40,42–45,49,50,68,82) have been designed for analysis of plasma following administration of exogenous folates and appear to lack the sensitivity required for analysis of normal plasma folates. Alternative detection methods may allow for extension of these methods to the levels required for plasma analysis.

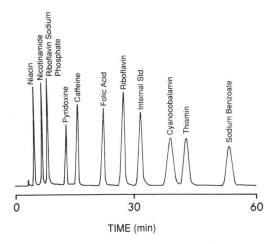

Figure 3 Resolution of a vitamin mixture by HPLC. Reversed-phase separation of a vitamin mixture on a C18 column. The mobile phase was comprised of acetonitrile, 0.01 M potassium dihydrogen phosphate, triethylamine (8:91.5:0.5 v/v) with 5 mM sodium octanesulfonate, pH 2.8. Taken from Maeda et al. (70).

Generally two stationary phases, either C18 or phenyl, have been employed for plasma folate analysis, with the C18 phase being the more widely employed. Three methods have also described the use of a C8 stationary phase (40,41,46). The majority of the methods described do not employ ion-pairing reagents; only five of the above methods use tetrabutylammonium salts (43–45,68,82). The most common methods achieve resolution through the use of an acidic mobile phase (pH 2.5 to 5.5) with low organic solvent content on a C18 column. Isocratic (47) or gradient (38,39,42,48,50) chromatography has been used. Two methods use a neutral mobile phase, one employing 1% methanol isocratically to allow for retention on a C8 column (49). In the second method, the sample is loaded onto a C18 column in the absence of methanol and a mobile phase containing 5% methanol is used for elution (49).

ANALYSIS OF INTRACELLULAR FOLATE POOLS. Analysis of intracellular folates represents a complex analytical problem since eight potential parent species are present (folic acid, dihydrofolate, tetrahydrofolate, 10-formyltetrahydrofolate, 5-formyltetrahydrofolate, 5,10-methylenetetrahydrofolate, 5,10-methenyltetrahydrofolate, 5-methyltetrahydrofolate) in variable states of polyglutamation. No one method has proven capable of resolving the numerous potential species. With the exception of one recent method (81), the polyglutamate issue has been sidestepped through employment of folylpolyglutamate hydrolase treatment of samples prior to chromatographic analysis. While surrendering potentially valuable information, this digestion reduces all species to monoglutamates, which can then be analyzed using methods similar to those discussed above. In general, only cells from tissue culture or animal tissues have been studied for their intracellular folate content. Since both represent the same challenge in terms of chromatography, they will be considered as one topic in this section.

As was the case for analysis of plasma, methods for the analysis of complex mixtures of intracellular folates can be split into two categories, those that employ the ion-pairing reagent tetrabutyl ammonium phosphate (61–65,67) and those that do not (51,60,66). Ion-pairing methods generally are carried out on a C18 column using mobile phases with near-neutral pH and organic content in the range of 12-20% (Table 3). Similar methods based upon a C8 column have also been described (61). Figure 4 represents a typical chromatogram produced according to the method of Duch et al. (64). One major difference seen in methods using paired ion separation appears in the latter stages of chromatography with the elution of dihydrofolate, folic acid, and 5-methyltetrahydrofolate. Subtle differences in chromatography result in these peaks eluting with differing degrees of resolution and, in some cases, a different order. The basis for these differences is unclear since these methods vary

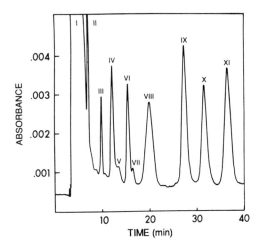

Figure 4   HPLC separation of folate cofactors. Folates were chromatographed on a C18 column with a mobile phase of 10 mM ammonium dihydrogen phosphate, 5 mM tetrabutylammonium phosphate, containing 22% methanol. A mixture of folates in 0.1% sodium ascorbate containing 10 mM mercaptoethanol was injected onto the column. Peak I, ascorbate, 5,10-methenyltetrahydrofolate; peak II, mercaptoethanol; peak III, p-aminobenzoylglutamic acid; peak IV, 28 ng N^{10}-formyltetrahydrofolate; peak V, N^{10}-formyldihydrofolate; peak VI, 18.8 ng tetrahydrofolate; peak VII, N^{10}-formylfolic acid; peak VIII, 12.5 ng N^{5}-formyltetrahydrofolate; peak IX, 12.5 ng dihydrofolate; peak X, folic acid; peak XI, 25 ng N^{5}-methyltetrahydrofolate. Taken from Duch et al. (65).

in column manufacturer, concentration of ion-pairing reagent, pH of the mobile phase, and organic content. Of those methods that do not use ion pairing, two (60,66) use fluorescence detection and employ acidic mobile phases (pH < 2.3) to enhance sensitivity. These methods are used to detect only tetrahydrofolate, 5-methyltetrahydrofolate, and 5-formyltetrahydrofolate. It is not clear how the remaining folate species would behave in these systems. Another non-ion-pairing method (60) employs a mobile phase of pH 5.5 and elutes standard folates with relatively low organic concentration. On the basis of resolution, total run time (including equilibration for gradient methods), and expense of necessary hardware, the method of Duch et al. (64) appears superior. Employing a conventional steel column, this method is capable of baseline resolution of 10-formyltetrahydrofolate, tetrahydrofolate, 5-formyltetrahydrofolate dihydrofolate, folic acid, and 5-methyltetrahydrofolate in that respective order in less than 40 min under isocratic conditions. This method eliminates column equilibration and simplifies and lowers the cost of necessary hardware. With this method, 5,10-methenyltetrahydrofolate-elutes with ascorbic acid but the former typically is not present due to its instability at neutral pH. 5,10-Methylenetetrahydrofolate, which generally does not survive sample processing (60,64) and is converted to tetrahydrofolate, will coelute with folic acid by this method if injected directly.

Separation of Stereoisomers

Recent advances in the development of chiral stationary phases (83) have led to the development of methods capable of resolving the C-6 isomers of the N^5-substituted tetrahydrofolate derivatives (84,85). These methods are based upon the interaction of these species with a bovine serum albumin-based matrix. This methodology has been adapted to the analysis of biological samples (43). This methodology is presently restricted to the analysis of N^5-substituted tetrahydrofolate derivatives, since other fully reduced folate species lack the stability to remain intact under the conditions used (R. Mullin, unpublished observation).

3.5 Methods of Detection

Four methods, based on UV absorbance, fluorescence, electrochemical, and microbiological measurements, have been described for the detection of folates following chromatography. Since each method has its strengths and weaknesses, they will be discussed separately here.

UV Absorbance

The most common method for detection of folates following HPLC has been UV absorbance (38–42,44,45,48,49,57–60,62,64,67,69–71,74–80). With molar extinction coefficients in the range of $30,000M^{-1}\,cm^{-1}$ (1), folates are readily detectable. The typical wavelength chosen for detection has been 280 nm (40,48,49,55,62,74,77,78). However, additional methods are based upon detection at 284 nm (64), 300 nm (45), and 304 nm (45). Diode array detectors have also recently been used for detection (67,81). The detection levels for UV absorbance have been reported to be as low as 0.8 and 0.5 pmol for 5-formyltetrahydrofolate, respectively, with a gradient elution method for plasma analysis (39). However, gradient elution methods designed for the resolution of one folate species generally report limits of detection in the range of 2 to 5 pmol (40,48,49,79). Those methods designed for the resolution of multiple folate species have somewhat reduced sensitivities, most likely due to larger peak widths; reported limits of sensitivity are in the range of 10–40 pmol for a mixture of standard folates (45,55,62,77). The most sensitive methods based on UV detection are adquate for direct analysis of plasma samples. Most of the UV detection methods described above may be used for tissue folate analysis. However, because of the lack of selectivity of this detection method, samples must be purified prior to analysis. Unless considerable precautions are taken and numerous controls are routinely used there is the likelihood that artifactual data may be generated.

Fluorescence

Several methods that use fluorescence detection of folates have been described (51,52,54,66,72). Fluorescence detection is considerably more selective and somewhat more sensitive than UV detection. The most sensitive of these methods (51) uses native fluorescence at pH 2.3 with excitation at 290 nm and emission at 365 nm and reports detection limits of 0.16, 0.03, and 0.31 pmol for tetrahydrofolate, 5-methyltetrahydrofolate, and 5-formyltetrahydrofolate, respectively. However, using similar methods, others report detection limits 5- to 10-fold higher (66,72). Folic acid is also detectable by fluorescence, but only following conversion to a pterin fragment with HTH dry chlorine by a postcolumn reaction (51,54). These methods are apparently capable of routine detection in the range of 1 pmol. The principal drawback of analysis using fluorescence is that native fluorescence appears to be limited to tetrahydrofolate, 5-formyltetrahydrofolate, and 5-methyltetrahydrofolate. Two frequently studied intracellular materials, dihydrofolate and 10-formyltetrahydrofolate, cannot be studied with this method. For detection by fluorescence methods 10-formyltetrahydrofolate is routinely converted to 5-formyltetrahydrofolate. However, this would eliminate fluorescence detection of 10-formyltetrahydrofolate as an option in experiments involving 5-formyltetrahydrofolate as a source of exogenous folates. At this time, fluorescence detection of tissue folates requires considerable precolumn sample preparation (51,54,66).

Electrochemical Detection

Electrochemical detection of folates with amperometric electrodes perhaps represents the forefront of detection sensitivity, with tetrahydrofolate, 5-methyltetrahydrofolate, 10-formyltetrahydrofolate, 5-formyltetrahydrofolate and folic acid having respective minimum detectable levels of 6.8, 2.2, 265,317, and 181 fmol (46). However this method has only been successfully employed for the detection of 5-methyltetrahydrofolate in plasma (41,46,47) and PteGlu in vitamin preparations (73). Electrochemical detection has been unsuitable for analysis of tissue samples due to considerable background interference (52). Development of a method to remove interfering materials, which to a large extent appears to be ascorbic acid (52), could make this the detection method of choice for folate analysis. However, in its present state, electrochemical detection does not represent an attractive method due to considerable background signal in biological samples.

Microbiological Assay

Though it was one of the first assay methods used, the microbiological assay for folates is still widely used as a method of detection, due in large part to the sensitivity of the method. This assay is based on the early observations that folates stimulated the growth of *Lactobacillus casei* and *Streptococcus faecalis*. The history of the development of this assay has been reviewed (1,2) and detailed aspects of the assay itself have been presented (87). The differential assay for mixtures of folates uses *Lactobacillus casei*, *Streptococcus faecalis*, and *Pediococcus cerevisiae*. The relative activities of the various folate cofactors for these organisms are illustrated in Table 4. In general, *L. casei* responds to all of the com-

Table 4   Relative Activity of Various Forms of Folic Acid for Assay Organisms[a]

Compound	Streptococcus faecalis	Lactobacillus casei	Pediococcus cerevisiae[c]
Folic acid (PteGlu[d])	+[b]	+	−
Pteroyldiglutamic acid	+	+	−
Pteroyltriglutamic acid	−	+	−
Pteroylheptaglutamic acid	−	−	−
H_4PteGlu	+	+	+
5-HCO-H_4PteGlu	+	+	+
10-HCO-H_4PteGlu	+	+	+
5,10-CH=H_4PteGlu	+	+	+
5-CH_3-H_4PteGlu	−	+	−
Pteroic acid	+	−	−
10-HCO-PteGlu	+	+	−
10-HCO-H_2PteGlu	+	+	−

[a] From Stokstad and Thenen (88).

[b] Plus indicates activity of 70–100% of folic acid on a molar basis for *S. faecalis* and *L. casei* and 70–100% of the activity of 5-HCO-H_4PteGlu for *P. cerevisiae*. Minus indicates activiey of less than 5%.

[c] Only leucovorin (5-HCO-H_4PteGlu) is oxygen stable, but all four tetrahydrofolic acid derivatives are active in the aseptic ascorbate assay method.

[d] PteGlu, folic acid; H_4PteGlu, tetrahydrofolate; 5-CHO-H_4PteGlu, 5-formyltetrahydrofolate; 10-CO-H_4PteGlu, 10-formyltetrahydrofolate; 5,10-CH-H_4PteGlu, 5,10-methenyltetrahydrofolate; 5-CH_3H_4PteGlu, 5-methyltetrahydrofolate, 10-CHO-PteGlu, 10-formylfolic acid, 10-CHO-H_2PteGlu, 10-formyldihydrofolate.

monly occurring forms of the folate cofactors including di- and trigluta-mates. *Streptococcus faecalis* does not respond to 5-methyltetrahydro-folate or to folates having more than one glutamate residue. *Pediococcus cerevisiae* responds to folates other than 5-methyltetrahydrofolate. Since all of the test organisms do not respond to the higher polyglutamates, the glutamate residues must first be removed by treatment of the extracts with conjugase. Differences in growth are determined by measurement of turbidity on a colorimeter.

Further refinements of the original assay have increased the speed, utility, and sensitivity of this assay. Automated methods were developed for use of the assay in clinical laboratories to increase the number of samples that could be handled (89–91). In contrast to the long times required in the standard microbiological assay, the continuous-flow automated method described by Tennant (89) required a total incuba-tion period of only 4 h. The growth response to folates was determined by measuring the rate of reduction of 2,3,5-triphenyl tetrazolium chloride. A comparison of the automated methods with the standard assay indicated that the results obtained were similar using both methods (92). Antibiotic-resistant test organisms have also been used to eliminate the need for aseptic conditions (89,90,93), and in other studies (94–96) antifolate test organisms have been used to measure folate levels in the presence of these inhibitors. The importance of the proper control of pH in this assay has also been discussed (93,97). More recently, modifications of the standard assay have been described (98,99) that use 96-well micro-titer plates and a microtiter plate reader for the measurement of folate levels. These methods are less labor intensive, allow the assay of large numbers of samples, have a sensitivity of 10 fmol, which is 10-fold greater than the sensitivity of the standard assay, and all folates exhibit similar growth stimulation of the test organism.

4. FUTURE TRENDS

In light of the number of methods available for the resolution of folyl-monoglutamates (Table 3) there does not seem to be considerable need for continued improvement in this area. Improvements in the area of detection, either fluorescent or electrochemical in nature, offer the larg-est potential. With increased selectivity the need for sample processing beyond extraction and conversion to monoglutamates could be elim-inated, greatly simplifying analysis. This level of sample processing has been achieved for microbiological analysis, but the time- and labor-intensive nature of the microbiological assay is a limiting factor in the widespread acceptance of this method.

The bulk of the methodology discussed here is applicable only to folylmonoglutamates. Considerable important biological data is sacrificed with the hydrolysis of polyglutamates to the monoglutamate forms, since these species are typically the true biological cofactors. Currently one method that has had limited use but carries considerable potential is that of direct HPLC analysis of complex folylpolyglutamate samples (81). With a sample preparation method based upon extraction of folates on immobilized milk folate binding protein and an HPLC method capable of partially resolving folates based upon both substitution and degree of polyglutamation, Selhub and co-workers generated data on the folate pools of rat liver comparable to that achieved by conventional methods (Table 2). Analysis of the HPLC eluant does require a diode array detector and mathematical digestion of the spectral data to resolve poorly separated folate species of similar degrees of polyglutamation. Presently, versions of this method have not been demonstrated in additional laboratories.

A relatively recent method (86) for folate analysis based upon a competitive enzyme-linked ligand sorbent assay may represent a novel direction in the area of folate detection. With a sensitivity of 20 fmol for 5-methyltetrahydrofolate, this method should be capable of detection equal to the methods described above. However, the detection limits for standard folates are not clear, but the authors do indicate weak interaction with 5-formyltetrahydrofolate. No data for the detection of 10-formyltetrahydrofolate are given.

REFERENCES

1. R. L. Blakley, *The Biochemistry of Folic Acid and Related Pteridines*, North Holland, Amsterdam (1969).
2. R. L. Blakley and S. J. Benkovic, *Folates and Pterins, Volume 1 Chemistry and Biochemistry of Folates*, John Wiley and Sons, New York (1984).
3. R. L. Blakley and S. J. Benkovic, *Folates and Pterins, Volume 3, Nutritional, Pharmacological and Physiological Aspects*, John Wiley and Sons, New York (1984).
4. L. Wills, *Br. Med. J.*, *1*:1059 (1931).
5. E. L. R. Stokstad and P. D. V. Manning, *J. Biol. Chem.*, *125*:687 (1938).
6. E. E. Snell and W. H. Peterson, *J. Bacteriol.*, *39*:273 (1940).
7. H. K. Mitchell, E. E. Snell, and R. J. Williams, *J. Am. Chem. Soc.*, *63*:2284 (1941).
8. R. B. Angier, J. H. Boothe, B. L. Hutchings, J. H. Mowat, J. Semb, E. L. R. Stokstad, Y. SubbaRow, C. Waller, D. B. Cosulich, M. J. Fahrenbach, M. E. Hultquist, E. Kuh, E. H. Northey, D. R. Seeger, J. P. Sickels, and J. M. Smith, Jr., *Science*, *103*:667 (1946).
9. C. E. Butterworth, Jr., C. M. Baugh, and C. Krumdieck, *J. Clin. Invest.*, *48*:1131 (1969).

10. C. M. Baugh, C. L. Krumdieck, H. J. Baker, and C. E. Butterworth, Jr., *J. Clin. Invest.*, *50*:2009 (1971).

11. J. J. McGuire and J. K. Coward, in *Folates and Pterins, Volume 1, Chemistry and Biochemistry of Folates* (R. L. Blakley and S. V. Benkovic, eds.), John Wiley and Sons, New York, p. 135 (1984).

12. J. Selhub, G. J. Dhar, and I. H. Rosenberg, *Pharm. Ther.*, *20*:397 (1983).

13. I. H. Rosenberg, J. Zimmerman, and J. Selhub, *Chemioterapia*, *4*:354 (1985).

14. H. M. Said and R. Redha, *Biochem. J.*, *247*:141 (1987).

15. P. F. Nixon and J. R. Bertino, *N. Engl. J. Med.*, *286*:175 (1972).

16. W. B. Strum, *Biochim. Biophys. Acta*, *554*:249 (1979).

17. J. Selhub, G. M. Powell, and I. H. Rosenberg, *Am J. Physiol. 246*:G515 (1984).

18. J. Selhub, H. Brin, and N. Grossowicz, *Eur. J. Biochem.*, *33*:433 (1973).

19. V. Herbert, A. R. Larrabee, and J. M. Buchanan, *J. Clin. Invest.*, *41*:1134 (1962).

20. J. M. Noronha and V. S. Aboobaker, *Arch. Biochem. Biophys.*, *101*:445 (1963).

21. I. D. Goldman, *Ann. NY. Acad. Sci.*, *186*:400 (1971).

22. M. Dembo and F. M. Sirotnak, in *Folate Antagonists as Therapeutic Agents, Volume 1, Biochemistry, Molecular Actions and Synthetic Design* (F. M. Sirotnak, J. J. Burchall, W. B. Ensminger, and J. A. Montgomery, eds.), Academic Press, New York, p. 173 (1984).

23. G. B. Henderson and E. M. Zevely, *J. Biol. Chem.*, *259*:1526 (1984).

24. D. J. Cichowicz and B. Shane, *Biochemistry*, *26*:513 (1987).

25. J. Kas and J. Cerná, *J. Chromatogr.*, *124*:53 (1976).

26. Y. S. Shin, K. U. Buehring, and E. L. R. Stokstad, *J. Biol. Chem.*, *247*:7266 (1972).

27. K. Fujii, T. Nagasaki, and F. M. Huennekens, *J. Biol. Chem.*, *257*:214 (1982).

28. R. M. Hoffman, D. W. Coalson, S. J. Jacobsen, and R. W. Erbe, *J. Cell Physiol.*, *109*:497 (1981).

29. Y. S. Shin, M. A. Williams, and E. L. R. Stokstad, *Biochem. Biophys. Res. Commun. 47*:35 (1972).

30. Y. S. Shin, K. U. Buehring, and E. L. R. Stokstad, *Arch. Biochem. Biophys.*, *163*:211 (1974).

31. M. J. Conner and J. A. Blair, *Biochem. J.*, *186*:235 (1980).

32. L. S. Reed and M. C. Archer, *J. Chromatogr.*, *121*:100 (1976).

33. R. W. Stout, A. R. Cashmere, J. K. Coward, C. G. Hawath, and J. R. Bertino, *Anal. Biochem.*, *71*:119 (1976).

34. S. K. Chapman, B. C. Greene, and R. R. Streiff, *J. Chromatogr.*, *145*:302 (1978).

35. B. Shane, *Am. J. Clin. Nutr.*, *35*:599 (1982).

36. A. R. Cashmore, R. N. Dreyer, C. Hawath, J. O. Knipe, J. K. Coward, and J. R. Bertino, *Methods Enzymol.*, *66*:459 (1980).

37. M. A. Archer and L. A. Reed, *Methods Enzymol.*, *66*:452 (1980).

38. B. Payet, G. Fabre, N. Tubiana, and J. P. Cano, *Caner Chemotherap. Pharmacol.*, *19*:313 (1987).

39. O. Van Tellingen, H. R. Van Der Woulde, J. H. Beijnen, C. J. T. Van Beers, and W. J. Nooyer, *J. Chromatogr.*, *488*:379 (1989).

40. M. Tani and K. Iwai, *J. Chromatogr.*, *267*:175 (1983).

41. M. D. Lucock, R. Hartley, and R. W. Smithells, *Biomed. Chromatogr.* *3*:58 (1989).

42. E. M. Newman, J. A. Straw, and J. H. Doroshow, *Cancer Res.*, *49*:5755 (1989).

43. L. R. Laughman, W. D. Brenkmann, K. A. Stydnicki, E. D. Morgan, M. Collier, V. B. Knick, D. S. Duch, R. Mullin, and R. Ferone, *Cancer*, *63*:1031 (1989).

44. F. Trave, Y. M. Rustum, N. J. Petrelli, L. Herrera, A. Mittelman, C. Frank, and P. J. Creaven, *J. Clin. Oncol.*, *6*:1184 (1988).

45. J. A. Straw, D. Szapary, and W. T. Wynn, *Cancer Res.*, *44*:3114 (1984).

46. M. Kohashi, K. Inoue, H. Sotobayashi, and K. Iwai, *J. Chromatogr.*, *382*:303 (1986).

47. B. K. Birmingham and D. S. Greene, *J. Pharm. Sci.*, *72*:1306 (1983).

48. K. Hoppner and B. Lampi, *Nutr. Rep. Int.*, *27*:911 (1983).

49. C. Wegner, M. Trotz, and H. Nau, *J. Chromatogr.*, *378*:55 (1986).

50. J. A. Straw, J. M. Covery, and D. Szapary, *Cancer Res.*, *41*:3936 (1981).

51. J. F. Gregory, D. B. Sartain, and B. P. F. Day, *J. Nutr.*, *114*:341 (1984).

52. D. L. Holt, R. L. Wehling, and M. G. Zeece, *J. Chromatogr.*, *449*:271 (1988).

53. J. Lankelma, E. Van Der Kleijn, and M. J. Jansen, *J. Chromatogr.*, *182*:35 (1980).

54. B. P. Day and J. F. Gregory, *J. Agric. Food Chem.*, *29*:374 (1981).

55. K. Hoppner and B. Lampi, *J. Liq. Chromatogr.*, *5*:953 (1982).

56. J. F. Gregory, B. P. F. Day, and K. A. Ristow, *J. Food Sci.*, *47*:1568 (1982).

57. I. J. Holcomb and S. A. Fusari, *Anal. Chem.*, *53*:607 (1981).

58. W. H. Tafolla, A. C. Sarapu, and G. R. Dukes, *J. Pharm. Sci.*, *70*:1273 (1981).

59. G. W. Schieffer, G. P. Wheeler, and Carolyn O. Cimino, *J. Liquid Chromatogr.*, *7*:2659 (1984).

60. L. H. Matherly, C. K. Barlowe, V. M. Phillips, and I. D. Goldman, *J. Biol. Chem.*,. *262*:710 (1987).

61. C. J. Allegra, R. L. Fine, J. C. Drake, and B. A. Chabner, *J. Biol. Chem.*, *261*:6478 (1986).

62. K. E. McMartin, V. Virayotha, and T. R. Tephly, *Arch. Biochem. Biophys.*, *209*:127 (1981).

63. S. A. Kashani and B. A. Cooper, *Anal. Biochem.*, *146*:40 (1985).

64. D. S. Duch, S. W. Bowers, and C. A. Nichol, *Anal. Biochem.*, *130*:385 (1983).

65. S. D. Wilson and D. W. Horne, *Anal. Biochem.*, *142*:529 (1984).

66. J. C. Gounelle, H. Ladjimi, and P. Prognon, *Anal. Biochem.*, *176*:406 (1989).

67. T. Rebello, *Anal. Biochem.*, *166*:55 (1987).

68. R. J. Mullin, B. R. Keith and D. S. Duch, in *The Expanding Role of Folates and Fluoropyrimidines in Cancer Chemotherapy* (Y. Rustum and

J. J. McGuire, eds.), Plenum Press, New York, p. 25 (1988).
69. J. A. Montgomery, T. P. Johnston, H. J. Thomas, J. R. Piper, and C. Temple, *Adv. Chromatogr.*, *15*:169 (1977).
70. Y. Maeda, M. Yamamoto, K. Owada, S. Sato, T. Masui, and H. Nakayawa, *J. Assoc. Off. Anal. Chem.*, *72*:244 (1989).
71. C. Paveenbampen, D. Lamontanaro, J. Moody, J. Zarembo, and C. Rehim, *J. Pharm Sci.*, *75*:1192 (1986).
72. P. Giulidori, M. Galli-Kienle, and G. Stramentinoli, *Clin. Chem.*, *27*:2041 (1981).
73. E. Wang and W. Hou, *J. Chromatogr.*, *447*:256 (1988).
74. M. Fawaz, M. Novovitch, and J. Alary, *Ann. Pharm. Fr.*, *46*:121 (1988).
75. M. Amin and J. Reusch, *Analyst*, *112*:989 (1987).
76. B. A. Allen and R. A. Newman, *J. Chromatogr.*, *190*:241 (1980).
77. S. D. Wilson, and D. W. Horne, *Proc. Natl. Acad. Sci. USA*, *80*:6500 (1983).
78. D. W. Horne, W. T. Briggs, and C. Wagner, *Anal. Biochem.*, *116*:393 (1981).
79. M. W. Dong, J. Lepore, and T. Tarumoto, *J. Chromatogr.*, *442*:81 (1988).
80. R. N. Reingold and M. F. Picciano, *J. Chromatogr.*, *234*:171 (1982).
81. Sellub J., *Anal. Biochem.*, *182*:84 (1989).
82. S. Arbuck, H. O. Douglass, F. Trave, S. Milliron, M. Baroni, H. Nava, L. J. Emrich, and Y. M. Rustum, *J. Chem. Oncol.*, *5*:1150 (1987).
83. S. Allenmark, *J. Liq. Chromatogr.*, *9*:425 (1986).
84. K. E. Choi and R. L. Schilsky, *Anal. Biochem.*, *168*:398 (1988).
85. I. W. Wainer and R. M. Stiffin, *J. Chromatogr.*, *424*:158 (1988).
86. I. S. Hansen and J. Holm, *Anal. Biochem.*, *172*:160 (1988).
87. O. D. Bird, and V. M. McGlohon, in *Analytical Microbiology* (F. Kavanazh, ed.), Vol. 2, Academic Press, New York, p. 409 (1972).
88. E. L. R. Stokstad and S. W. Thenen, in pp. 387.
89. G. B. Tennant, *J. Clin. Pathol.*, *30*:1168 (1977).
90. R. E. Davis, D. J. Nichol, and A. Kelley, *J. Clin. Pathol.*, *23*:47 (1970).
91. G. Calvin, G. L. Gibson, and D. W. Neill, *J. Clin Pathol.*, *24*:18 (1971).
92. J. E. O'Donnell, G. B. Tennant, and B. M. Jones, *J. Clin. Pathol.*, *30*:1175 (1977).
93. I. Chanarin, R. Kyle, and J. Stacey, *J. Clin. Pathol.*, *25*:1050 (1972).
94. B. M. Mehta and D. J. Hutchinson, *Cancer Chemother. Rep.*, *59*:935 (1975).
95. B. M. Mehta and D. J. Hutchinson, *Cancer Treat. Rep.*, *61*:1657 (1977).
96. B. M. Mehta, A. L. Gisolic, D. J. Hutchinson, A. Vrenberg, M. G. Kellick, and G. Kosen, *Cancer Treat. Rep.*, *62*:345 (1978).
97. D. R. Phillips and A. J. A. Wright, *Br. J. Nutr.*, *47*:183 (1982).
98. E. M. Newman and J. F. Tsai, *Anal. Biochem.*, *154*:509 (1986).
99. D. W. Horne and D. Patterson, *Clin. Chem.*, *34*:2357 (1988).
100. F. C. Johlin, C. S. Fortman, D. D. Ngheim, and T. R. Tephley, *Mol. Pharmacol.*, *31*:557 (1987).

7

NICOTINIC ACID
AND NICOTINAMIDE

Katsumi Shibata and Tatsuhisa Shimono

Teikoku Women's University, Osaka, Japan

1. INTRODUCTION

1.1 History

Pellagra (which is now recognized as the set of symptoms related to niacin deficiency) was first reported as "Mal de la Rose" by Casal in 1735. The term "pellagra," consisting of a synthesis of the Italian word from "pelle" (skin) and "agra" (rough), was introduced by Frapolli in 1771. This disorder persisted in southern Europe and the southern United States until the early 1900s. The occurrence of pellagra was associated with corn consumption, although pellagra was initially believed to be an infectious disease. Goldberger's team (1) showed in 1915 that pellagra could not be transmitted to healthy people and it was postulated that the disease was attributable to a deficiency of a nutrient, the so-called pellagra-preventing factor. In 1937, Elvehjem et al. (2) showed that nicotinic acid cured the black tongue of dogs (similar symptom of human pellagra) and isolated nicotinamide as a pellagra-preventing factor from liver. In 1938, Spies et al. (3) showed that administration of nicotinic acid would cure pellagra, and it was gradually accepted that pellagra was caused by a nicotinic acid or nicotinamide deficiency. The pellagragenic effect of corn is now considered to be due to nicotinic acid in a form not released by digestion. It is bound with glucose, imbedded in a glycopeptide (4). Alkali, or even ammonia vapor, will release the vitamin in a form useful to humans and animals (4). The fact that Central America diets do not cause pellagra, in spite of a very high corn content, has been attributed to cooking the corn in lime as part of tortilla preparation.

Pyridine-3-carboxylic acid (nicotinic acid) was first discovered as an oxidation product of nicotine by Huber in 1867 (5). In 1873, Weidel (6) described the elemental analysis and crystalline structure of salts and other derivatives of nicotinic acid in some detail. Nicotinic acid was first isolated from rice bran by Suzuki (7) in 1912 and from yeast by Funk (8) in 1913. But, these investigators did not know the antipellagra activity of nicotinic acid. Pyridine-3-carboxamide (nicotinamide) was first isolated from liver as an antipellagra factor in 1937 by Elvehjem et al. (2) as described above. NAD^+ and $NADP^+$ were discovered as cozymase of alcohol fermentation and as a hydrogen-transporting coenzyme by Harden and Young (9) in 1904 and by Warburg and Christian (10) in 1934, respectively. Subsequently, nicotinamide was found to be an integral part of NAD^+ (11) and $NADP^+$ (12). Over 350 enzymes require NAD^+ and $NADP^+$ as coenzyme.

1.2 Chemical Properties

Nicotinic Acid

Nicotinic acid has been designated as pyridine-3-carboxylic acid, pyridine-β-carboxylic acid, PP (pellagra-preventing) factor, vitamin PP, or antipellagra vitamin. The structure of nicotinic acid is given in Fig. 1. Nicotinic acid ($C_6H_5O_2N$, molecular weight = 123.11) forms colorless, nonhygroscopic needles and is stable in air. It sublimes without decomposition at 234–237°C. It is amphoteric; the pK_a values are 4.9 and 2.07. The pH of a saturated aqueous solution is 2.7. One gram dissolves in 60 ml water and in 80 ml ethanol. It is freely soluble in boiling water, boiling alcohol, alkali hydroxides, and carbonates, and soluble in propylene glycol. It is insoluble in diethyl ether. Aqueous nicotinic acid can be autoclaved for 10 min at 120°C without decomposition. Furthermore, nicotinic acid is stable even when autoclaved in 1–2 N mineral acid or alkali. The molar absorptivity is 2800 M^{-1} cm^{-1} at 260 nm in 50 mM potassium phosphate buffer, pH 7.0.

Nicotinamide

Nicotinamide is known as pyridine-3-carboxamide, nicotinic acid amide, pellagramine, pyridine-β-carboxylic acid amide, and vitamin PP. The structure of nicotinamide is given in Fig. 1. Nicotinamide ($C_6H_6ON_2$, molecular weight = 122.12) has a melting point of 129–131°C. It is a colorless, crystalline compound that crystallizes as needles from benzene. One gram dissolves in 1 ml water, in 1.5 ml ethanol, and in 10 ml glycerol. Nicotinamide dissolves in acetone, chloroform, and butanol, but is only slightly soluble in diethyl ether and benzene. In neutral solution it is very stable. However, nicotinamide is converted into nicotinic acid in 1 N mineral acid and alkali when heated at 100°C. A 10 % (w/v) solution

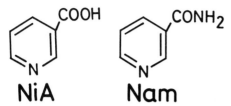

Figure 1   Structures of nicotinic acid (NiA) and nicotinamide (Nam).

in water has a neutral pH and can be autoclaved for 10 min at 120°C without decomposition. The molar absorptivity is 3300 at 260 nm in water.

Nicotinamide Adenine Dinucleotide (NAD^+)

NAD^+ has been designated as diphosphopyridine nucleotide (DPN), co-enzyme I, factor V, codehydrogenase I, Harden's coferment, cozymase I, and codihydrase. NAD^+ ($C_{21}H_{27}O_{14}P_2$, molecular weight = 663.4) (inner salt) is a very hygroscopic white powder and is freely soluble in water. A 1% solution has a pH of about 2.

Nicotinamide Adenine Dinucleotide Phosphate ($NADP^+$)

NADP is known as triphosphopyridine nucleotide (TPN), coenzyme II, Warburg's coferment, codehydrogenase II, cozymase II, and phosphoco-zymase. $NADP^+$ ($C_{21}H_{28}N_7O_{17}P_3$, molecular weight = 743.44) (inner salt) is a grayish-white powder. It is soluble in water, or in methanol, but much less soluble in ethanol, and practically insoluble in diethyl ether and ethyl actate.

Stability of NADH (Reduced NAD^+) and NADPH (Reduced $NADP^+$)

NADH and NADPH are rapidly destroyed in acid (99% loss in 0.6 min) in 0.02 N HCl (13). However, NADH and NADPH are very stable in alkali (13). Although directly stable to alkali, NADH and NADPH tend to oxidize after long periods of time (13). NADH could be stored for nearly 3 months without decomposition at pH 9.1 either at 4°C or −20°C.

Stability of NAD^+ and $NADP^+$

Alkali accelerates the rate of destruction of NAD^+ and $NADP^+$ (13). However, NAD^+ and $NADP^+$ are stable in acidic conditions. Aqueous solutions are stable for about 1 week. When these solutions are neutral-ized, they are stable for about 2 weeks of 0°C.

1.3   Biochemistry

Biosynthesis

NAD^+ is biosynthesized via four pathways as shown in Fig. 2: (I) nicotinic acid → nicotinic acid mononucleotide → nicotinic acid adenine

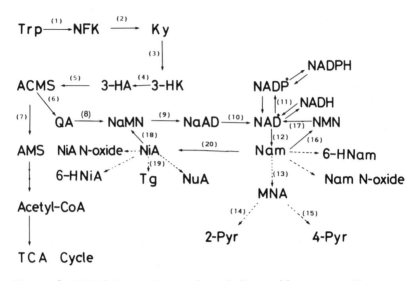

Figure 2 NAD$^+$ biosynthesis and catabolism. Abbreviations: Trp = trypto-phan, NFK = N-formylkynurenine, Ky = kynurenine, 3-HK = 3-hydroxykynurenine, 3-HA = 3-hydroxyanthranilic acid, ACMS = α-amino-β-carboxymuconate-ϵ-semialdehyde, AMS = α-aminomuconate-ϵ-semialdehyde, QA = quinolic acid, NaMN = nicotinic acid mononucleotide, NaAD = nicotinic acid adenine dinucleotide, NAD$^+$ = nicotinamide adenine dinucleotide, NADP$^+$ = nicotinamide adenine dinucleotide phosphate, NADH = reduced nicotinamide adenine dinucleotide, NADPH = reduced nicotinamide adenine dinucleotide phosphate, MNA = N^1-methylnicotinamide, 2-Pyr = N^1-methyl-2-pyridone-5-carboxamide, 4-Pyr = N^1-methyl-4-pyridone-3-carboxamide, Nam N-oxide = nicotinamide N-oxide, 6-HNam = 6-hydroxynicotinamide, NuA = nicotinuric acid, Tg = N^1-methylnicotinic acid (trigonelline), NiA N-oxide = nicotinic acid N-oxide, 6-HNiA = 6-hydroxynicotinic acid. Enzymes: (1) trypto-phan oxygenase (EC 1.13.11.11), (2) formydase (EC 3.5.1.9), (3) kynurenine 3-hydroxylase (EC 1.14.13.9), (4) kynureninase (EC 3.7.1.3), (5) 3-hydroxyanthranilic acid oxygenase (EC 1.13.11.6), (6) nonenzymatic, (7) aminocarboxymuconate-semialdehyde decarboxylase (EC 4.1.1.45), (8) quino-linate phosphoribosyltransferase (EC 2.4.2.19), (9) NaMN adenylyltransferase (EC 2.7.2.18), (10) NAD$^+$ synthetase (EC 6.3.5.1), (11) NAD$^+$ kinase (EC 2.7.1.23), (12) NAD$^+$ glycohydrolase (EC 3.2.2.5), (13) nicotinamide methyl-transferase (EC 2.2.1.1), (14) 2-Pyr-forming MNA oxidase (EC 1.2.3.1), (15) 4-Pyr-forming MNA oxidase (EC number is not given), (16) nicotinamide phos-phoribosyltransferase (EC 2.4.2.12), (17) NMN adenylyltransferase (EC 2.7.7.1), (18) nicotinate phosphoribosyltransferase (EC 2.4.2.11), (19) nicotinic acid methyltransferase (EC 2.7.1.7), and (20) nicotinamidase (EC 3.5.1.19). Solid line, biosynthesis; dotted line, catabolism.

dinucleotide $\rightarrow NAD^+$, (II) nicotinamide $\rightarrow$ nicotinamide mononucleotide $\rightarrow NAD^+$, (III) nicotinamide $\rightarrow$ nicotinic acid $\rightarrow$ nicotinic acid mononucleotide $\rightarrow$ nicotinic acid adenine dinucleotide $\rightarrow NAD^+$, and (IV) quinolinic acid $\rightarrow$ nicotinic acid mononucleotide $\rightarrow$ nicotinic acid adenine dinucleotide $\rightarrow NAD^+$. In the four NAD^+ biosynthetic pathways, pathways II and IV are physiologically important. Quinolinic acid is synthesized from an essential amino acid tryptophan.

Table 1 shows the $[NAD^+ + NADPH]$ (14) and total nicotinamide (15) levels in various tissues of rats.

Catabolism

NAD^+ is catabolized mainly through five pathways as shown in Fig. 2: (I) $NAD^+ \rightarrow$ nicotinamide $\rightarrow$ MNA $\rightarrow$ 2-Pyr, (II) $NAD^+ \rightarrow$ nicotinamide $\rightarrow$ MNA $\rightarrow$ 4-Pyr, (III) $NAD^+ \rightarrow$ nicotinamide $\rightarrow$ nicotinamide N-oxide, (IV) $NAD^+ \rightarrow$ nicotinamide $\rightarrow$ nicotinic acid $\rightarrow$ nicotinuric acid, and (V) $NAD^+ \rightarrow$ nicotinamide $\rightarrow$ nicotinic acid $\rightarrow$ N^1-methylnicotinic acid (trigonelline). In rats, pathway II mainly functions, and in humans pathway I. Pathway V functions in mushrooms, shellfish, and plants, but not in mammals.

1.4   Physiological Function

Pellagra-Preventing Factor

Pellagra is a typical hypovitaminosis disorder. A sufficient supply of niacin to humans or animals totally prevents the symptoms of pellagra. This disorder is characterized by three main symptoms: dermatitis, diarrhea,

Table 1   NAD (NAD^+ + NADH) and Total Nicotinamide (Free Nicotinamide + NAD^+ + NADH + $NADP^+$ + NADPH) Levels in Various Tissues of Rats

	NAD^+ + NADH[a]	Total nicotinamide[a]
Liver	753 ± 12	1559 ± 42
Kidney	616 ± 30	1061 ± 35
Small intestine	219 ± 24	453 ± 15
Spleen	144 ± 13	504 ± 13
Heart	599 ± 26	1047 ± 16
Brain	271 ± 26	457 ± 13
Testis	154 ± 9	241 ± 6
Muscle	574 ± 20	677 ± 14
Lung	106 ± 9	391 ± 22
Pancreas	233 ± 17	352 ± 7
Blood	95 ± 3	136 ± 4

[a] Values are means $\pm$ SEM for five rats, as nmol/g fresh weight.

and dementia. A number of nonspecific symptoms precede the actual clinical manifestation, such as anorexia, weakness, and maldigestion. The minimum requirement of niacin is about 4.5 mg/100 kcal.

Biochemical Function

The biochemical function of nicotinic acid and nicotinamide actually comes down to that of NAD^+ and $NADP^+$ as coenzymes of dehydrogenases. The latter function in oxidation-reduction systems is well known.

Further, NAD^+ is a substrate in non-oxidation/reduction reactions, such as ADP-ribosylation. The enzyme poly (ADP-ribose) synthetase presents in the nuclei of eukaryotes, and catalyzes the transfer of ADP-ribose of NAD to form a polymer of ADP-ribose attached to a protein acceptor.

1.5   Pharmacological Function

Reduction of Serum Cholesterol and Triglycerides by Nicotinic Acid

The first report that large doses of nicotinic acid reduce serum cholesterol levels in humans appeared in 1955 by Altschul (16). Several subsequent studies indicated that nicotinic acid lowers plasma triglycerides as well. However, its use has been limited by the well-known flushing of the face that results from large doses. The conclusions reached by a collaborative research group (17) indicated that it is a safe drug, and that it causes a 22% lowering of plasma cholesterol and a 52% lowering of plasma triglycerides. The mechanism by which nicotinic acid lowers plasma cholesterol and triglycerides is not known. Some authors suggest that the synthesis of lipoprotein is reduced in the liver as a result of reduced lipolysis in the adipose tissue (18,19). Nicotinamide does not possess this pharmacological function.

Vasodilatation by Nicotinic Acid

Nicotinic acid is used as a vasodilator. The flush reaction to nicotinic acid, which occurs very rapidly, is highly characteristic. The biochemical mechanism of the vascular response to nicotinic acid is not well understood. However, some reports suggest that nicotinic acid somehow enhances the biosynthesis or release of prostaglandin E_1, which stimulates adenylate cyclase and raises the level of cAMP (20,21). Wilson and Douglass (22) reported that the amount of nicotinic acid per injection should be below 200 mg because the injection of 250 mg nicotinic acid to humans causes very severe flushing.

Nicotinamide in the Prevention of Diabetes

The intraperitoneal injection of streptozotocin to mouse, rat, monkey, and dog induces diabetes. However, when a large amount of nicotinamide is administered before the administration of streptozotocin, the streptozotocin-induced diabetes is inhibited. This is also effective when nicotinamide is administered within 2 h after the streptozotocin administration (23,24). The NAD$^+$ content in β cells of Langerhans islands in the pancreas is reduced by the administration of streptozotocin. However, this decrease does not occur after prior administration of a large amount of nicotinamide (25,26). The decrease in NAD$^+$ content by streptozotocin is attributable to the stimulation of poly (ADP-ribose) synthetase in the β cells (27). Nicotinic acid does not possess this preventive effect.

2. PAPER AND THIN-LAYER CHROMATOGRAPHY AND ION-EXCHANGE CHROMATOGRAPHY

2.1 Introduction

Paper and thin-layer chromatography have not been used for separation of unlabeled nicotinic acid and nicotinamide because of low sensitivity and low resolution. These compounds are rather determined by high-performance liquid chromatography (HPLC) and gas chromatography (GC). However, these chromatographic techniques are still useful for the separation of labeled compounds.

Ion-exchange chromatography is still used for preparative purification of nicotinic acid and nicotinamide and their related compounds. Ion-exchange systems can separate a large number of substances, but require long analysis times.

2.2 Paper and Thin-Layer Chromatography

Table 2 shows R$_f$ values of nicotinic acid and nicotinamide and their derivatives in different eluents. (Abbreviations used in the balance of this chapter are identified in Table 2). The detection is performed by illumination under short-wavelength UV light (257.3 nm).

2.3 Ion-Exchange Chromatography

Separation of the Intermediates of Niacin-NAD$^+$ Biosynthetic Pathway on a Dowex 1-Formate Column

Figure 3 shows the elution profile of NMN, nicotinic acid, NAD$^+$, NaMN, NaAD, quinolinic acid, NADP, and ADP-ribose on a Dowex 1-formate, X2 column (29 cm × 0.8 cm ID) (28,29). The elution was carried out by application of a formic acid concave-concentration gradient $0.01\ N \rightarrow 0.25\ N \rightarrow 2\ N \rightarrow 6\ N$. The mixing chamber initially contained 250 ml of water. The detection was at 260 nm.

Table 2 Values of Nicotinic Acid and Nicotinamide and Their Metabolites in Paper and Thin-Layer Chromatography[a]

	Paper chromatography							Thin-Layer chromatography			
	(I)*1	(II)*1	(III)*1	(IV)*1	(V)*1	(VI)*1	(VII)*2	(I)*3	(II)*3	(VIII)*3	(IX)*4
NADP+	0.02	0.24	—	0	—	—	0	0.03	0.50	0.70	—
NAD+	0.15	0.40	0.62	0	—	—	0	0.13	0.61	0.58	—
NaAD	0.16	0.26	0.64	0	—	—	0	0.15	0.52	0.57	—
NMN	0.18	0.42	0.28	0	—	—	0	0.11	0.63	0.73	—
NaMN	0.20	0.23	0.48	0	—	—	0	0.13	0.47	0.75	—
Nam	0.81	0.84	0.81	0.61	0.70	—	0.25	0.87	0.88	0.45	—
NiA	0.64	0.71	0.74	0.27	0.11	—	0.49	0.77	0.82	0.55	0.32
QA	0.33	0.53	0.65	0.36	—	—	0.20	—	—	—	—
MNA	0.67	0.81	—	0.10	0.04	0.08	0.39	—	—	—	—
Tg	0.63	0.66	—	0.06	—	—	—	—	—	—	0.53
Nam N-oxide	0.70	0.76	—	0.29	0.30	—	—	—	—	—	0.56
NiA N-oxide	0.62	0.52	—	0.10	—	—	—	—	—	—	0.67
2-Pyr	0.80	0.85	—	0.52	0.52	—	—	—	—	—	0.81
4-Pyr	0.70	0.85	—	0.46	0.44	—	—	—	—	—	0.44
NuA	0.62	0.66	—	0.12	0.04	0.55	—	—	—	—	—
Reference	74	75	74	74	76	76	77	*5	*5	*5	78

[a] Solvent system: (I) 1 M ammonium acetate: 95% ethanol (3:7, pH 5.0); (II) isobutyric acid:ammonia:water (66:1.7:33); (III) pyridine:water (2:1); (IV) upper layer of n-butanol:acetone:water (45:5:50); (V) upper layer of n-butanol saturated with 3% ammonia; (VI) upper layer of n-butanol saturated with water:pyridine (60:1); (VII) upper layer of ethyl acetate:formic acid:water (60:5:35); (VIII) the solvent consists of 600 g ammonium sulfate in 0.1 M sodium phosphate: 2% n-propanol (pH 6.8); (IX) isopropanol:conc. HCl:water (70:15:15). Substrates: *1, Whatman no. 1 paper, ascending chromatography; *2, Toyo no. 50 paper, ascending chromatography; *3, MN 300G cellulose plate, ascending chromatography; *4, silica gel 60/Kieselguhr F254, ascending chromatography; *5, K. Shibata, unpublished data. Abbreviations: NaAD = nicotinic acid adenine dinucleotide; NMN = nicotinamide mononucleotide; NaMN = nicotinic acid mononucleotide; Nam = nicotinamide; NiA = nicotinic acid; Tg = trigonelline = N^1-methylnicotinic acid; Nam N-oxide = nicotinamide N-oxide; NiA N-oxide = nicotinic acid N-oxide; MNA = N^1-methylnicotinamide; QA = quinolinic acid; 2-Pyr = N^1-methyl-2-pyridone-5-carboxamide; 4-Pyr = N^1-methyl-4-pyridone-3-carboxamide; NuA = nicotinuric acid.

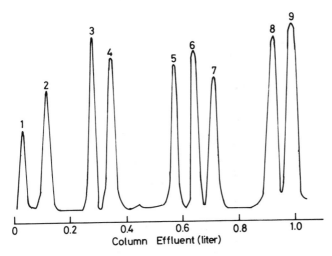

Figure 3 Ion-exchange chromatographic separation of the substances involved in biosynthesis of NAD^+ on a conventional column of Dowex 1-X2 formate. Elution was conducted under gravity. Peaks: 1, void peak, Nam; 2, NMN; 3, NiA; 4, NAD^+; 5, NaMN; 6, NaAD; 7, QA; 8, $NADP^+$; 9, adenosine diphosphate-ribose. For abbreviations, see Figs. 1 and 2. The elution was carried out by application of a formic acid concave concentration gradient 0.01 N (150 ml) → 0.25 N (250 ml) → 2 N (400 ml) → 6 N (400 ml). The mixing chamber initially contained 250 ml of water. The detection was at 260 nm.

Separation of Niacin Metabolites on a Dowex 1-Formate Column

Figure 4 shows the elution profile of MNA, N^1-methylnicotinic acid, nicotinamide N-oxide, 4-Pyr, 2-Pyr, nicotinamide, 6-hydroxynicotinamide, nicotinic acid, nicotinuric acid, and 6-hydroxynicotinic acid on a Dowex 1-formate X4 column (73.6 cm × 0.9 cm ID) (30). Gradient elution was done with ammonium formate-formic acid or various pH values and ion strengths. Detection was performed by UV absorption at 254 nm.

3. HIGH-PERFORMANCE LIQUID CHROMATOGRAPHY

3.1 Introduction

Total niacin (nicotinic acid + nicotinamide) in food is still measured by the microbiological method using *Lactobacillus planturum* or by the colorimetric method. However, these methods suffer from several disadvantages; nicotinic acid and nicotinamide are not distinguished because of hydrolysis before the determination, the microbiological method is time-consuming, and the reproducibility is rather low, whereas the

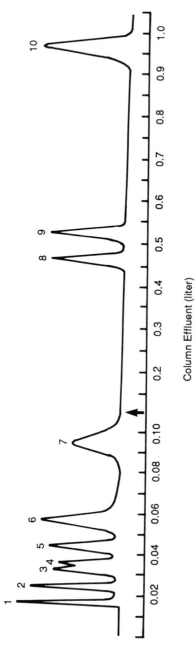

Figure 4 Ion-exchange chromatographic separation of the substances involved in catabolism of NAD^+ on a conventional column of Dowex 1-X4 formate. Elution was conducted at 0.2 ml/min with water for the first 110 ml (arrow) and at 1 ml/min with ammonium formate-formic acid of various pH and ion strength thereafter. Peaks: 1, MNA; 2, Tg; 3, Nam N-oxide; 4, 4-Pyr; 5, 2-Pyr; 6, Nam; 7, 6-HNam; 8, NiA; 9, NuA; 10, 6-HNiA. For abbreviations, see Figs. 1 and 2.

colorimetric method has low sensitivity and the reagents required are harmful and unstable. Reversed-phase chromatographic systems are now the most popular, simple, and precise method.

3.2   Nicotinic Acid and Nicotinuric Acid

Nicotinic acid is used as a drug; however, nicotinuric acid is not. Nicotinuric acid is a detoxified metabolite of nicotinic acid and is only detected in urine when a large amount of nicotinic acid is administered.

Biosamples

In 1978, Hengen et al. (31) measured nicotinic acid and nicotinuric acid in plasma and urine with reversed-phase high-performance liquid chromatography. The preparation of plasma and urine extracta is time-consuming (two extractions with organic solvents and evaporation to dryness are included) and losses during these procedures are likely. This method requires fairly large amounts of plasma (0.5 ml), and the analytical methods for urine and blood are different. In 1982, McKee et al. (32) measured nicotinamide, MNA, 2-Pyr, nicotinic acid, and nicotinuric acid in urine with HPLC using a linear ion-pair mobile-phase gradient. This method was very fascinating at first glance, but was impractical for the measurement of nicotinic acid and nicotinuric acid in biological samples owing to interfering peaks. In 1984, Tsuruta et al. (33) reported a sensitive method for the determination of nicotinic acid in serum, in which nicotinic acid is reacted with N, N'-dicyclohexyl-O-(7-methoxycoumarin-4-yl)methylisourea (DCCI) in acetone to give the corresponding fluorescent 4-hydroxymethyl-7-methoxycoumarin esters. The compound is separated by reverse-phase HPLC on LiChrosorb RP-18 with isocratic elution using aqueous acetonitrile containing a small amount of sodium 1-hexanesulfonate as a mobile phase. This method requires 100 μl of serum. This method might be superior, but DCCI is not commercially available and phosgene is needed for the synthesis of DCCI. In 1988, Shibata (34) reported a simultaneous measurement of nicotinic acid and nicotinuric acid in blood and urine by a reversed-phase HPLC. This method is the most reliable and practical. A chromatogram of a reference mixture of nicotinic acid and nicotinuric acid is described in Fig. 5. The detection limits of nicotinic acid and nicotinuric acid were 10 pmol (1.23 ng) and 10 pmol (1.80 ng), respectively, at a signal-to-noise ratio of 5:1.

The chromatograms of extracts of blood samples before and after nicotinic acid administration to rats (25 mg injected intraperitoneally) are shown in Figs. 6A and B, respectively. Nicotinic acid and nicotinuric acid were not detected in blood (obtained from tail vein) before the

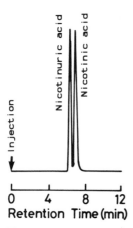

Figure 5   Chromatogram of a reference mixture of nicotinic acid and nicotinuric acid. Conditions: column, Chemcosorb 5-ODS-H (150 mm × 4.6 mm ID, particle size 5 μm; obtained from Chemco Scientific Co., Osaka, Japan); mobile phase, 10 m*M* potassium phosphate buffer (pH 7.0) containing 5 m*M* tetra-*n*-butylammonium bromide-acetonitrile (100:9, v/v); flow-rate, 1 ml/min; detection wavelength, 260 nm; column temperature, 25°C.

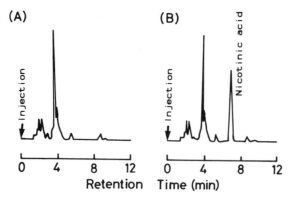

Figure 6   (A) Chromatogram of the extract of rat blood before the nicotinic acid administration. (B) Chromatogram of the extract of rat blood, 0.5 h after the nicotinic acid administration (25 mg of nicotinic acid per rat dissolved in 1 ml of sterile saline was injected intraperitoneally). For conditions, see Fig. 5.

nicotinic acid injection. After the nicotinic acid injection, only nicotinic acid was detected in blood. The chromatograms of extracts of urine samples before and after nicotinic acid injection are shown in Figs. 7A and B, respectively. Nicotinic acid and nicotinuric acid were not detected in urine before the nicotinic acid injection.

Food

Nicotinic acid is contained mainly in plant food such as coffee, cereals, and seeds, but not in animal foods such as fish, pork, beef, and chicken (animal food contains nicotinamide). There are no reports about the determination of nicotinic acid in plant food.

Coffee contains appreciable amounts of nicotinic acid. Nicotinic acid contents in roasted coffees and instant coffees are in the range of 9.5–26.3 mg per 100 g (35) and about 24 mg per 100 g (36), respectively. In 1985, Trugo et al. (37) reported the measurement of nicotinic acid in instant coffees. Chromatograms of reference nicotinic acid and the extract of instant coffee are shown in Fig. 8. The detection limit of nicotinic acid was 0.8 nmol (8.1 µg).

Tyler et al. (38) reported a determination of nicotinic acid in cereal samples by reversed-phase HPLC with a UV method using a reversed-phase column.

3.3   Nicotinamide, N'-Methyl-2-pyridone-5-carboxamide (2-Pyr), and N^1-Methyl-4-pyridone-3-carboxamide (4-Pyr)

Nicotinamide is present in pork, beef, chicken, and fish. 2-Pyr and 4-Pyr are the major metabolites in nicotinic acid and nicotinamide excreted in

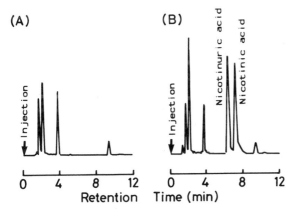

Figure 7   (A) Chromatogram of the extract of rat urine before the nicotinic acid administration. (B) Chromatogram of the extract of rat urine excreted 0.5 h after the nicotinic acid injection (25 mg/rat). For conditions, see Fig. 5.

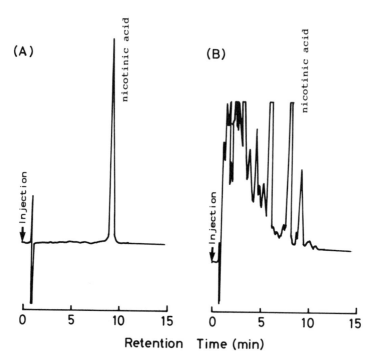

Figure 8 (A) Chromatogram of a reference nicotinic acid. (B) Chromatogram of the extract of instant coffee. Conditions: column, Spherisorb ODS-2 (150 mm × 5 mm ID, obtained from Phase Separation Ltd., UK); mobile phase, 5 mM tetra-n-butylammonium hydroxide (pH adjusted to 7.0 with 4 M sulfuric acid)-methanol (92:8, v/v); flow rate, 1.5 ml/min; detection wavelength, 254 nm; column temperature, ambient.

urine. The contents of 2-Pyr and 4-Pyr in blood are below the limit of detection (39). The HPLC methods for analysis of nicotinamide and the related compounds are summarized in Table 3. Shibata et al. (40) reported the simultaneous measurement of nicotinamide, 2-Pyr, and 4-Pyr. This method is commonly applicable not only to urine and pharmaceutical preparations but also to biological materials and foods. Chromatograms of a reference mixture of isonicotinamide (used as an internal standard), nicotinamide, 2-Pyr, and 4-Pyr and of extracts of rat urine, human urine, rat liver, and of the extract of multivitamin preparations are shown in Fig. 9. The detection limits for nicotinamide, 2-Pyr, and 4-Pyr were 10 pmol (1.22 ng), 2 pmol (304 pg), and 2 pmol (304 pg), respectively, at a signal-to-noise ratio of 5:1.

Daily urinary excretion of nicotinamide, 2-Pyr, and 4-Pyr in rats, mice, guinea pigs, hamsters, and humans is given in Table 4.

3.4 NAD$^+$, NADH, NADP$^+$, and NADPH

Chromatographic analysis of NAD$^+$, NADH, NADP$^+$, and NADPH is
not practical because these compounds are not stable. In biological
materials they are usually measured by enzymatic methods (41,42).
However, HPLC analysis of pyridine nucleotide coenzymes in rat liver
has been reported. Chromatograms of an extract of rat liver are shown
in Figs. 10 and 11 (43). In our laboratory, standard NAD$^+$, NADPH,
NADP$^+$, and NADPH have been reported using HPLC as shown in Fig.
12 (unpublished data).

3.5 N^1-Methylnicotinamide (MNA)

Kutnink et al. (44) reported an isocratic reversed-phase HPLC-UV
method for the determination of MNA in human urine. A method for
urinary MNA and 2-Pyr using isocratic reversed-phase HPLC UV detection method after a simple anion-exchange cleanup procedure has been
described by Carter (45). However, UV detection suffers from sensitivity.
In 1987, Shibata (46) developed a highly sensitive HPLC method with
fluorescence detection. MNA was reacted with acetophenone in a
strongly alkaline medium at 0°C in the presence of a large amount of
isonicotainamide. After 10 min formic acid was added and the mixture
was kept at 0°C for another 15 min. The mixture was heated in a boiling
water bath for 5 min. The reaction product, 1-methyl-7-phenyl-1,5-
dihydro-5-oxo-1,6-naphthyridine, was analyzed by HPLC. When acetophenone is omitted from the mixture, the reaction product is not formed.
A large amount of isonicotinamide was added to protect MNA from
the deamidation reaction, yielding N^1-methylnicotinic acid. N^1-
Methylnicotinic acid did not react with acetophenone. This approach
can be applied to liver and blood extracts as well as to urine (47). The
detection limit was 0.01 pmol (1.37 pg as MNA) at a signal-to-noise ratio
of 5:1. Chromatograms of reference MNA and MNA in urinary extracts
are shown in Fig. 13. Daily urinary excretion of MNA in rats, mice,
guinea pigs, hamsters, and humans is given in Table 4.

3.6 Nicotinamide N-Oxide

Nicotinamide N-oxide is synthesized from nicotinamide, probably in the
liver, and excreted into the urine. Nicotinamide N-oxide is detected only
in rodents such as rats, mice, guinea pigs, and hamsters (48,49). The
nicotinamide N-oxide content of rat and mouse liver was below the limit
of detection (unpublished data). A method for the determination of
nicotinamide N-oxide has been reported by Shibata (50). Chromatograms of reference nicotinamide N-oxide and an extract of rat urine are

Table 3 HPLC Determination of Nicotinamide in Biosamples

Reference	Source	Pretreatment	Column	Mobile phase	Detection	Detection limit	Other compounds detected simultaneously
De Vries (1980) (78)	Plasma Urine	Sep Pak C18 cartridge	μBondpak C_{18} (250 × 4 mm) LiChrosorb RP-18 (300 × 4 mm)	4.446 g Dioctylsulfo-succinate/1450 ml of water + 1050 ml of methanol	254 nm	0.1 mg/liter (plasma) 1.0 mg/liter (urine)	Isonicotinic acid (IS) Nicotinic acid Nicotinuric acid Isonicotinamide (IS)
McKee (1982) (32)	Urine	Filtration through 0.2-μm membrane filter	Ultrasphere-ODS (150 × 4.6 mm)	Linear gradient: A,10 mM KH_2PO_4 containing 10 mM PSA*1 and 10 mM TMA*2 (pH 3.3) B,100 ml of 10 mM PSA and 10 mM TMA + 900 ml of acetonitrile	254 nm	0.1 μg/injection	Nicotinic acid MNA Nicotinuric acid 2-Pyr
Kitada (1982) (79)	Meat	MeOH extraction	LiChrosorb RP-8 (250 × 4 mm)	0.03 M Potassium phosphate buffer (pH 7.0): MeOH (9:1) + 5 mM TBA*3	260 nm	0.5 mg/100 g meat	Nicotinic acid
Fujimoto (1987) (80)	Meat	MeOH extraction, alumina column	UnisilQ C-18-5 (250 × 4.6 mm)	100 mM Sodium acetate + 1 mM TBA:MeOH (76:24)	254 nm	Not described	Nicotinic acid

Reference	Sample	Extraction	Column	Mobile phase	Detection	Detection limit	Compounds
Takatsuki (1987) (81)	Meat	Water extraction, deproteinization with zinc sulfate	μBondpak C$_{18}$ (300 × 3.9 mm)	10 mM PIC-B7*4	263 nm	1 mg/100 g meat	Nicotinic acid
Oishi (1988) (82)	Meat	MeOH extraction, Sep-Pak alumina N cartridge	LiChrosorb RP-18 (300 × 4 mm) (particle size, 5 μm)	0.1 M Sodium acetate containing 10 mM TBA (pH 5): MeOH (10:2)	261 nm	0.5 mg/100 g meat	Nicotinic acid
Shibata (1988) (40)	Urine Blood Tissues Meat Drug	Diethyl ether extraction	Chemcosorb 7-ODS-L (250 × 4.6 mm) (particle size 7 μm)	10 mM KH$_2$PO$_4$ (pH 3.0): acetonitrile (96:4)	260 nm	1.22 ng/injection	Isonicotinamide (IS) 2-Pyr 4-Pyr
Hamano (1989) (83)	Meat	Boiled water extraction	Partisil SCX (250 × 4.6 mm)	50 mM Phosphate buffer (pH 3.0)	260 nm	4 ng/injection	Ascorbic acid Sorbic acid Nicotinic acid

[a] Key = *1 PSA = 1-pentanesulfonic acid sodium salt. *2 TMA = tetramethylammonium chloride. *3 TBA = tetra-n-butylammonium bromide.
*4 PIC-B7 = heptane sulfonic acid, adjusted to pH 3.5 with phosphoric acid.

Table 4 Daily Urinary Excretion (μmol/day) of Nicotinic Acid and Nicotinamide and Their Catabolic Metabolites[a]

	Human[*1]	Rat[*2]	Mouse[*3]	Hamster[*3]	Guinea pig[*3]
Nicotinamide	ND	0.51 ± 0.03	0.18 ± 0.03	0.58 ± 0.04	0.10 ± 0.03
MNA	31 ± 12	0.85 ± 0.09	0.16 ± 0.04	0.13 ± 0.02	0.35 ± 0.01
2-Pyr	60 ± 27	0.78 ± 0.09	0.20 ± 0.06	0.27 ± 0.06	2.60 ± 0.09
4-Pyr	7 ± 3	9.78 ± 9.27	0.10 ± 0.04	0.13 ± 0.03	0.10 ± 0.01
Nicotinamide N-oxide	ND	0.13 ± 0.01	0.35 ± 0.04	0.20 ± 0.04	0.10 ± 0.03
Nicotinic acid	ND	ND	ND	ND	ND
Nicotinuric acid	ND	ND	ND	ND	ND

[a] Key: [*1], Values are means ±SD (n = 84), cited from Ref. 84. [*2], Values are means ±SEM (n = 5), cited from Ref. 85. [*3], Values are means ±SEM (n = 4–5), cited from Ref. 49.

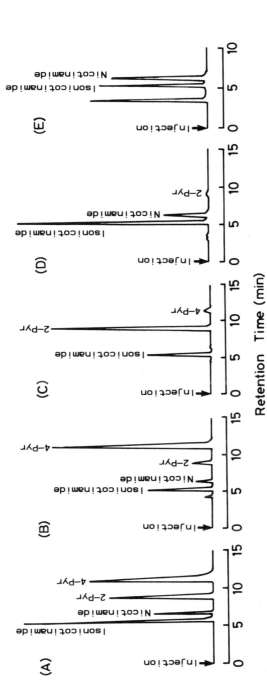

Figure 9 (A) Chromatogram of a reference mixture of isonicotinamide, nicotinamide, 2-Pyr, and 4-Pyr. (B) Chromatogram of the extract of rat urine. (C) Chromatogram of an extract of human urine. (D) Chromatogram of an extract of rat liver. (E) Chromatogram of the extract of multivitamin complex. Conditions: column, Chemcosorb 7-ODS-L (250 mm × 4.6 mm ID, particle size 7 μm; obtained from Chemco Scientific Co.); mobile phase, 10 mM potassium dihydrogenium phosphate, monobasic (pH adjusted to 3.0 by addition of conc. phosphoric acid), plus acetonitrile (96:4, v/v); flow rate, 1 ml/min; detection wavelength, 260 nm; column temperature, 25°C.

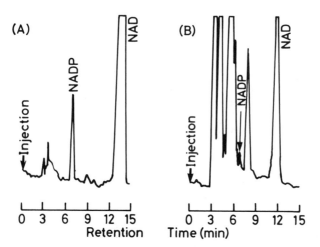

Figure 10 (A) Chromatogram of a reference mixture of NAD and NADP. (B) Chromatogram of an extract of rat liver. Conditions: column, μBondpak C$_{18}$ (obtained from Waters Associates, Milford, MA); mobile phase, 0.2 M ammonium phosphate buffer (pH 5.25)-methanol (97:3, v/v); flow rate, 1.1 ml/min; detection wavelength, 254 nm; column temperature, ambient.

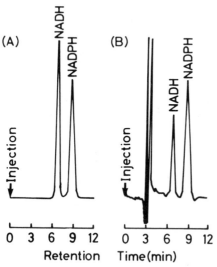

Figure 11 (A) Chromatogram of a reference mixture of NADH and NADPH. (B) Chromatogram of an extract of rat liver. Conditions: column, μBondpak C$_{18}$; mobile phase, 0.2 M ammonium phosphate buffer (pH 6.0)-methanol-trimethylamine (82:17.87:0.13); flow rate, 1.1 ml/min; detection wavelength, 340 nm; column temperature, ambient.

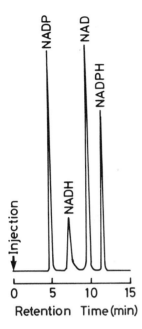

Figure 12 Chromatogram of a reference mixture of NAD^+, $NADP^+$, NADH, and NADPH. Conditions: column, Chemcosorb 5-ODS-H (150 mm × 4.6 mm ID, particle size 5 μm); mobile phase, acetonitrile in 25 mM potassium dihydrogenium phosphate (pH 4.5) increasing linearly from 1 to 7% at 0.4%/min; flow rate, 1 ml/min; detection wavelength, 260 nm, column temperature, 25°C.

shown in Fig. 14. Chloroform was used to extract nicotinamide N-oxide from urine saturated with potassium carbonate. The detection limit for nicotinamide N-oxide was 2 pmol (276 pg) at a signal-to-noise ratio of 5:1. 2-Pyr and 4-Pyr could also be extracted completely, the two compounds eluting at around 8 min under the present HPLC conditions (Fig. 14B). When this sample was subjected to the HPLC system for simultaneous analysis of nicotinamide, 2-Pyr, and 4-Pyr (Fig. 9), the peak of nicotinamide N-oxide overlapped partly with an unknown peak. However, under the present analytical condition, nicotinamide N-oxide was eluted without interfering peaks. Nicotinamide was also partly extracted in this process and eluted at about 10 min (Fig. 14B). Nicotinamide N-oxide eluted at the same time even when sodium 1-octanesulfonate was omitted from the mobile phase, although, identification of the peak of nicotinamide N-oxide was easier in the presence of sodium 1-octanesulfonate than in its absence, because no interfering peaks were eluted at the elution time of nicotinamide N-

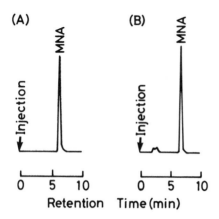

Figure 13 (A) Chromatogram of 1-methyl-7-phenyl-1,5-dihydro-5-oxo-1,6-naphthyridine from a reference MNA. (B) Chromatogram of 1-methyl-7-phenyl-1,5-dihydro-5-oxo-1,6-naphthyridine from MNA in rat urine. Conditions: column, Chemcosorb 300–7SCX (150 mm × 4.6 mm ID, particle size 7 μm); mobile phase, 31.25 mM potassium dihydrogenium phosphate (pH 4.5)-acetonitrile (80:20, v/v); flow rate, 1 ml/min; excitation and emission wavelength of 382 nm and 440 nm; column temperature, 25°C.

oxide. Daily urinary excretion of nicotinamide N-oxide in rats, mice, giunea pigs, and hamsters is given in Table 4.

3.7 N^1-Methylnicotinic Acid (Trigonelline)

Trigonelline (N^1-methylnicotinic acid) was named after the leguminous plant *Trigonella foenum graecum* L. (fenugreek), from which the compound was first isolated and characterized (51). In plant cells, N^1-methylnicotinic acid functions as a "G2 factor," which promotes cell arrest in the G2 stage of the cell cycle (52). However, N^1-methylnicotinic acid is inactive in mammalian cells; for example, when a large amount of N^1-methylnicotinic acid was fed to weanling rats, the body weight gain was not affected compared with the control (53). All of the administered N^1-methylnicotinic acid was recovered unchanged from urine (53).

The HPLC determination of N^1-methylnicotinic acid has been reported by Trugo et al. (54). Chromatograms of a reference mixture of N^1-methylnicotinic acid, theobromine, theophylline, and caffeine and an extract of instant coffee are shown in Fig. 15.

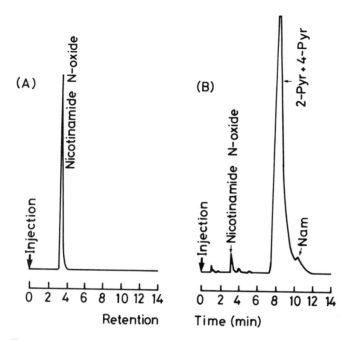

Figure 14 (A) Chromatogram of reference nicotinamide N-oxide. (B) Chromatogram of an extract of rat urine. Conditions: column, Chemcosorb 5-ODS-H (150 mm × 4.6 mm ID, particle size 5 μm); mobile phase, 10 mM potassium dihydrogenium phosphate (pH adjusted to 3.0 by the addition of conc. phosphoric acid) containing 0.1 g/liter 1-octanesulfonate-methanol (100:4, v/v); flow rate, 1 ml/min; detection wavelength, 260 nm; column temperature, 25°C.

3.8 Others

Quinolinic Acid and Nicotinic Acid N-Oxide

Standard quinolinic acid and nicotinic acid N-oxide can be determined by the HPLC system described under in section 3.2 (34). Nicotinic acid N-oxide and quinolinic acid were eluted at around 3.5 and 10.0 min, respectively, as shown in Fig. 16. Nicotinic acid N-oxide is not detected in biological materials. Quinolinic acid is synthesized not only from tryptophan in mammals (55) but also from aspartic acid and dihydroxyacetone phosphate in microorganisms (56). Therefore, quinolinic acid is the key intermediate in the de novo NAD^+ biosynthetic pathway. Furthermore, quinolinic acid has been shown to excite nerve cells in rodents and primates on iontophoretic application (57), and intracere-

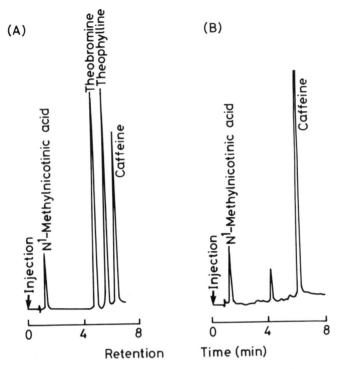

Figure 15 (A) Chromatogram of a reference mixture of N^1 = methylnicotinic acid, theobromine, theophylline, and caffeine. (B) Chromatogram of an extract of instant coffee. Conditions: column, Spherisorb ODS (250 mm × 5 mm ID, particle size 5 μm); mobile phase, methanol in 15 mM tripotassium citrate buffer (pH 6.0) increasing linearly from 0 to 60% at 10%/min; flow rate, 2 ml/min; detection wavelength, 272 nm; column temperature, probably ambient.

bral injection of quinolinic acid in rats results in selective "axon-sparing" neuronal lesions (58). The quinolinic acid content in biological materials is very low, so its content cannot be measured by this HPLC method. The GC-MS method would be suitable for the determination of quinolinic acid as described in section 4.2.

6-Hydroxynicotinic Acid and 6-Hydroxynicotinamide

6-Hydroxynicotinic acid and 6-hydroxynicotinamide were found as urinary excretion metabolites in rats following intraperitoneal injection of nicotinic acid-7-^{14}C and nicotinamide-7-^{14}C (59). The acid was eluted after about 6 min in the HPLC system as in Fig. 9 (unpublished data). 6-Hydroxynicotinic acid is available from commercial sources but 6-

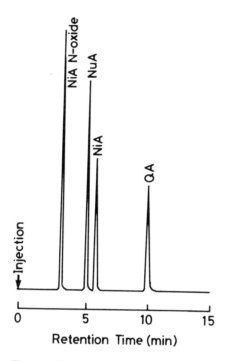

Figure 16   Chromatogram of a reference mixture of nicotinic acid N-oxide, nicotinuric acid, nicotinic acid, and quinolinic acid. For conditions, see Fig. 5.

hydroxynicotinamide is not. Therefore, the determination of 6-hydroxynicotinamide using HPLC has not been reported.

NaMN, NMN, and NaAD

NaMN, NMN, and NaAD are intermediates in the biosynthesis of NAD^+. The contents of these substances in biological materials are very low. Determinations of these substances have not been reported. However, in our laboratory, the purity of standard NaMN, NMN, and NaAD is routinely checked by HPLC as demonstrated in Fig. 17 (unpublished data).

4.   GAS CHROMATOGRAPHY

4.1   Introduction

Nicotinamide and nicotinic acid are insufficiently volatile to be analyzed directly by GC. However, after suitable derivatization their GC analysis becomes feasible.

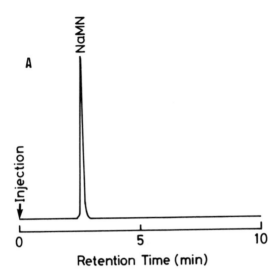

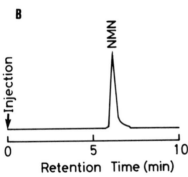

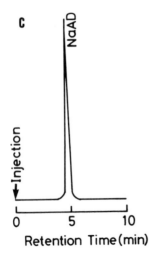

4.2   Nicotinamide

Tanaka et al. (60) reported that the determination of nicotinamide as 3-cyanopyridine after dehydration by heptafluorobutyric anhydride was performed by GC with flame ionization detection and using a column of 5% OV-17 on Chromosorb W AW DMCS at 130°C. The minimum detectable amount of 3-cyanopyridine was ~2.0 μg. Nicotinamide in foods was extracted with acetonitrile without the need for a cleanup stage.

4.3   Quinolinic Acid

Quinolinic acid was identified as a metabolite of tryptophan in the rat by Henderson and Hirsch in 1949 (61). Quinolinic acid has been known to be a key intermediate of the tryptophan-NAD$^+$ and aspartate + dihydroxyacetone phosphate-NAD$^+$ pathways since the clear demonstration in vitro by Nishizuka and Hayaishi in 1963 (55). It has been proved that quinolinic acid is transformed into nicotinic acid mononucleotide in the presence of 5-phosphoribosyl-1-pyrophosphate by quinolinate phosphoribosyltransferase (55). In 1978, Lapin (57) first reported that quinolinic acid induced seizures when injected directly into the brains of mice. Later, quinolinic acid was shown to increase neuronal activity when ionophoretically applied to neurons in rats cerebral cortex, striatum, and hippocampus (58,62,63). Now quinolinic acid is known as a potent neurotoxin and as a precursor of NAD$^+$ in the liver.

GC analysis of nonvolatile compounds such as quinolinic acid requires a derivatization step. Heyes and Markey (64) have reported quantification of quinolinic acid in rat brain, whole blood, and plasma after quinolinic acid derivatization to its hexafluoroisopropyl (HFIP)

Figure 17   (facing page)   (A) Chromatogram of reference nicotinic acid mononucleotide (NaMN). Conditions: column, Tosoh TSKgel ODS-80TM (150 mm × 4.6 mm ID, particle size 5 μm, obtained from Tosoh Corporation, Tokyo, Japan); mobile phase, 10 mM potassium phosphate (pH adjusted to 3.0 by the addition of conc. phosphoric acid)-acetonitrile (98:2, v/v); flow rate, 1 ml/min; detection wavelength, 260 nm; column temperature, 25°C. (B) Chromatogram of reference nicotinamide mononucleotide (NMN). Conditions: column, Shimadzu PNH$_2$-10/S2504 (250 mm × 4.0 mm ID, obtained from Shimadzu, Kyoto, Japan); mobile phase, 10 mM potassium dihydrogenium phosphate (pH 4.5); flow rate, 1 ml/min; detection wavelength, 260 nm; column temperature, 35°C. (C) Chromatogram of reference nicotinic acid adenine dinucleotide (NaAD). Conditions: column, Shimadzu PHN$_2$-10/S2504 (250 mm × 4.0 mm ID); mobile phase, 250 mM potassium dihydrogenium phosphate (pH 4.5); flow rate, 1 ml/min; detection wavelength, 260 nm; column temperature, 45°C.

ester and GC electron-capture negative ionization (CI) MS with [^{18}O] quinolinic acid as an internal standard. Negative CI efficiently forms a characteristic molecular anion, and consequently negative CI GS/MS has higher sensitivity than electron impact (EI) ionization GC/MS. The chromatograms of selected ion recording of QA-HFIP and [^{18}O]QA-HFIP at m/z 467 and 471 with packed and capillary columns are shown in Figs. 18 and 19, respectively. The minimum detectable limit of quinolinic acid for standards at signal-to-noise ratio of 10:1 was 30 fmol on packed columns and 3 fmol on capillary columns.

    Quinolinic acid concentrations in whole blood and plasma were about 170 and 362 pmol/ml. Two hours after tryptophan (0.370 mmol/kg) administration, quinolinic acid increased in whole blood 135-fold, in plasma 74-fold, and in frontal cortex 23-fold.

5. FUTURE TRENDS

The quantification of the acids such as quinolinic and nicotinic acids proceeds into two stages. The first stage consists of extraction and concentration of the compounds from biomaterials. This procedure is so complicated that the reproducibility of the recovery of the target compound is poor in some cases (e.g., recovery of quinolinic acid). The progress of computer technology will make it possible to use automated sample pretreatment systems (e.g., autoinjector with pretreatment function for HPLC and/or advanced automated sample processor) or by a laboratory robot (e.g., a robot system for HPLC or an automatic preparation system for HPLC) with high reproducibility.

    The second stage is the instrumental analysis of target compounds. Quantitation of low amounts of quinolinic acid and nicotinic acid con-

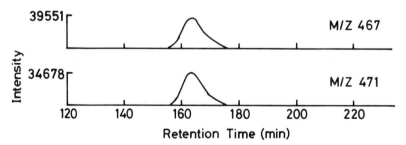

Figure 18   Selected ion recording of QA-HFIP and [^{18}O]QA-HFIP at m/z 467 and 471. Sample: rat cerebral cortex including the [^{18}O]QA internal standard. QA = quinolinic acid. HFIP = hexafluoroisopropanol. Conditions: column, SP-2401 (1.5 m × 1.5 mm ID, obtained from Supelco Inc., Bellefonte, PA); column temperature, 115°C; carrier gas, methane; flow rate, not described.

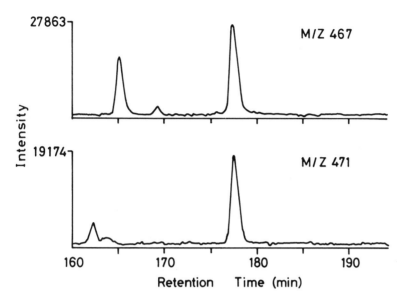

Figure 19   Selected ion recording of QA-HFIP and [^{18}O]QA-HFIP at m/z 467 and 471. Sample, rat frontal cortex including the [^{18}O]QA internal standard. Conditions, column, DB-5 (30 m × 0.25 mm ID, obtained from J and W Scientific, Folsom, CA); column temperature, 95°C for 1 min → 170°C, 30°C/ min; carrier gas, helium; flow rate, not described; sample injection, splitless injection mode.

tinues to be a challenge. In HPLC derivatization is required to increase the detector sensitivity. Evidently, for GC purposes the derivative should be volatile and thermostable. Many derivatizing agents that react with carboxyl groups have been produced for both HPLC and GC (e.g., 65–67); the application of these agents will be further and thoroughly investigated. These developments will enable trace analysis of quinolinic acid and nicotinic acid by the use of HPLC with fluorescence detector, electrochemical detector, and MS and by GC with electron capture, thermionic, and negative CI MS detection devices.

For quantification of the radioactive compounds, HPLC with radiochemical detection has already been developed. Undoubtedly, the latter technique also has potential to become popular (e.g., 68).

As for separation columns, capillary columns will more frequently be used in HPLC, as is already the case in GC. In addition, multidimensional column chromatographic systems combined with different columns for pretreatment and separation of target compounds appear to be useful (69).

For the analysis of ion compounds, capillary electrophoresis seems powerful as a complementary method in HPLC. For the analysis of non-ionic compounds, micellar electrokinetic chromatography might be useful as well. Terabe et al. (70) and Fujiwara et al. (71) analyzed water-soluble vitamins including nicotinamide and nicotinic acid by this method. Finally, supercritical fluid chromatography (SFC) might become the third powerful method for analysis of bioorganic compounds in addition to HPLC and GC (72,73).

REFERENCES

1. J. Goldberger, C. H. Waring, and D. G. Willits, *Public Health Rep.*, *30*:3117 (1915).
2. C. A. Elvehjem, R. J. Madden, F. M. Strong, and D. W. Wooley, *J. Am. Chem. Soc.*, *59*:1767 (1937).
3. T. D. Spies, C. Cooper, and M. A. Blankenhorn, *J. Am. Med. Assoc.*, *110*:622 (1938).
4. E. Kodicek and P. W. Wilson, *Biochem. J.*, *76*:27p (1960).
5. C. Huber, *Ann. Chem. Pharm.*, *141*:271 (1867).
6. H. Weidel, *Ann. Chem. Pharm.*, *165*:328 (1873).
7. U. Suzuki, T. Schimamura, and S. Odaka, *Biochem. Z.*, *43*:89 (1912).
8. C. Funk, *J. Physiol.*, *46*:173 (1913).
9. A. Harden and W. J. Young, *J. Physiol.*, *32*:Proc., Nov. 1 (1904).
10. O. Warburg and W. Christian, *Biochem. Z.*, *274*:112 (1934).
11. H. von Euler, H. Ahlers, and F. Schlenk, *Z. Physiol. Chem.*, *124*:113 (1936).
12. O. Warburg and W. Christian, *Biochem. Z.*, *275*:464 (1935).
13. O. H. Lowry, J. V. Passonneau, and M. K. Rock, *J. Biol. Chem.*, *236*:2756 (1961).
14. K. Shibata, *Vitamins (Jpn.)*, *61*:39 (1987).
15. K. Shibata, H. Matsuo, and K. Iwai, *Agric. Biol. Chem.*, *51*:3429 (1987).
16. R. Altschul, H. Hoffer, and J. D. Stephen, *Arch. Biochem.*, *54*:558 (1955).
17. Coronary Drug Project Research Group, *J. Am. Med. Assoc.*, *231*:360 (1975).
18. B. Vessley, H. Lithell, I. -B. Gustafsson, and J. Berg, *Atherosclerosis*, *33*:457 (1979).
19. S. M. Grundy and G. L. Vega, *Am. J. Med.*, *83*: (suppl. 5B): 9 (1987).
20. R. G. G. Anderson, G. Aberg, R. Brattsand, E. Ericsson, and L. Lundholm, *Acta Pharmacol. Toxicol.*, *41*:1 (1977).
21. W. S. Phillips and S. L. Lightman, *Lancet*, *1*:754 (1981).
22. D. W. S. Wilson and A. B. Douglass, *Biol. Psychiatr.*, *21*:974 (1986).
23. W. E. Dulin and B. M. Wyse, *Proc. Soc. Exp. Biol. Med.*, *130*:992 (1969).

24. W. Stauffacher, I. Burr, A. Gutzeit, D. Veleminsky, and A. E. Renold, *Proc. Soc. Exp. Biol. Med.*, *133*:194 (1970).

25. P. S. Schein, D. A. Cooley, M. G. Anderson, and T. Anderson, *Biochem. Pharmacol.*, *22*:2625 (1973).

26. T. Anderson, P. S. Schein, M. G. McMenamin, and D. A. Cooney, *J. Clin. Invest.*, *54*:672 (1974).

27. H. Yamamoto and H. Okamoto, *Biochem. Biophys. Res. Commun.*, *95*:474 (1980).

28. H. Ijichi, A. Ichiyama, and O. Hayaishi, *J. Biol. Chem.*, *241*:3701 (1966).

29. T. Negishi and A. Ichiyama, *Vitamins (Jpn.)*, *40*:38 (1969).

30. C. Bernofsky, *Anal. Biochem.*, *96*:189 (1979).

31. N. Hengen, V. Seiberth, and M. Hengen, *Clin. Chem.*, *24*:1740 (1978).

32. R. W. McKee, Y. A. Kang-Lee, M. Panaque, and M. E. Swedseid, *J. Chromatogr.*, *236*:309 (1982).

33. Y. Tsuruta, K. Kohashi, S. Ishida, and Y. Ohkura, *J. Chromatogr.*, *309*:309 (1984).

34. K. Shibata, *Agric. Biol. Chem.*, *52*:2973 (1988).

35. E. B. Hughes and R. F. Smith, *J. Soc. Chem. Ind.*, *65*:284 (1946).

36. P. Okungbowa, M. C. F. Ma, and A. S. Truswell, *Proc. Nutr. Soc.*, *36*:1A (1977).

37. L. C. Trugo, R. Macrae, and N. M. F. Trugo, *J. Micronutr. Anal.*, *1*:55 (1985).

38. T. A. Tyler and R. R. Shrago, *J. Liq. Chromatogr.*, *3*:269 (1980).

39. K. Shibata and H. Matsuo, *Vitamins (Jpn)*, *63*:569 (1989).

40. K. Shibata, T. Kawada, and K. Iwai, *J. Chromatogr.*, *424*:23 (1988).

41. K. Shibata and K. Murata, *Nutr. Int.*, *2*:177 (1986).

42. K. Shibata and K. Tanaka, *Agric. Biol. Chem.*, *50*:2941 (1986).

43. T. F. Kalhorn, K. E. Thummel, S. D. Nelson, and J. T. Slattery, *Anal. Biochem.*, *151*:343 (1985).

44. M. A. Kutnink, H. Vannucchi, and H. E. Sauberlich, *J. Liq. Chromatogr.*, *7*:969 (1984).

45. E. G. Carter, *Am. J. Clin. Nutr.*, *36*:926 (1982).

46. K. Shibata, *Vitamins (Jpn.)*, *61*:599 (1987).

47. K. Shibata, *Vitamins (Jpn.)*, *62*:225 (1988).

48. K. Shibata, H. Taguchi, and Y. Sakakibara, *Vitamins (Jpn.)*, *63*:369 (1989).

49. K. Shibata, H. Kakehi, and H. Matsuo, *J. Nutr. Sci. Vitaminol.*, *36*:87 (1990).

50. K. Shibata, *Agric. Biol. Chem.*, *53*:1329 (1989).

51. E. Jahns, *Ber. Dtsch. Chem. Ges.*, *18*:2518 (1985).

52. D. G. Lynn, K. Nakanishi, S. L. Patt, J. L. Occolowitz, S. Almedia, and L. S. Evans, *J. Am. Chem. Soc.*, *100*:7759 (1978).

53. K. Shibata and H. Taguchi, *Vitamins (Jpn.)*, *61*:493 (1987).

54. L. C. Trugo, R. Macrae, and J. Dick, *J. Sci. Food Agric.*, *34*:300 (1983).

55. Y. Nishizuka and O. Hayaishi, *J. Biol. Chem.*, *238*:PC483 (1963).

56. S. Nasu, F. Diwicks, S. Sakakibara, and R. K. Gholson, *J. Biol. Chem.*, 257:626 (1982).
57. I. P. Lapin, *J. Neutral Trans.*, 32:37 (1978).
58. R. Schwarcz, W. O. Whetsell, and R. M. Mangano, *Science*, 219:316 (1983).
59. Y. C. Lee, R. K. Gholson, and N. Raica, *J. Biol. Chem.*, 244:3277 (1969).
60. A. Tanaka, M. Iijima, Y. Kikuchi, Y. Hoshino and N. Nose, *J. Chromatogr.*, 466:307 (1989).
61. L. M. Henderson and H. M. Hirsch, *J. Biol. Chem.*, 181:667 (1949).
62. T. W. Stone and M. N. Perkins, *Eur. J. Pharmacol.*, 72:411 (1981).
63. M. N. Perkins and T. W. Stone, *J. Pharmacol. Exp. Ther.*, 226:551 (1983).
64. M. P. Heyes and S. P. Markey, *Anal. Biochem.*, 174:349 (1988).
65. N. J. Bertrand, A. W. Ahmed, B. Sarrasin, and V. N. Mallet, *Anal. Chem.*, 59:1302 (1987).
66. J. Goto, H. Miura, M. Inada, T. Nambara, T. Nakagawa, and H. Suzuki, *J. Chromatogr.*, 452:119 (1988).
67. N. Nimura, T. Kinoshita, T. Yoshida, A. Uetake, and C. Nakai, *Anal. Chem.*, 60:2067 (1988).
68. K. Shibata, H. Taguchi, H. Nishitani, K. Okumura, Y. Shimabayashi, N. Matsushita, and H. Yamazaki, *Agric. Biol. Chem.*, 53:2283 (1989).
69. R. W. Frei and K. Zech (eds.), *Selective Sample Handling and Detection in High-Performance Liquid Chromatography*, part A, Elsevier Science, Amsterdam (1988).
70. H. Nishi, N. Tsumagari, T. Kakimoto, and S. Terabe, *J. Chromatogr.*, 465:331 (1989).
71. S. Fujiwara, S. Honda, and S. Honda, *J. Chromatogr.*, 447:113 (1988).
72. R. M. Smith (ed.), *Supercritical Fluid Chromatography*, Royal Society of Chemistry, London (1988).
73. B. A. Charpentier and M. R. Sevenants (ed.), *Supercritical Fluid Extraction and Chromatography*, American Chemical Society, Washington, DC (1988).
74. Y. Nishizuka and O. Hayaishi, *J. Biol. Chem.*, 238:3369 (1968).
75. Y. Hagino, S. J. Lan, C. Y. Ng, and L. M. Henderson, *J. Biol. Chem.*, 243:4980 (1968).
76. S. Chaykin, M. Dagani, L. Johnson, and M. Samli, *J. Biol. Chem.*, 240:932 (1965).
77. H. Taguchi, H. Takamizawa, M. Muto, Y. Shimabayashi, and K. Iwai, *Vitamins (Jpn.)*, 52:363 (1978).
78. J. X. DeVries, W. Gunthert, and R. Ding, *J. Chromatogr.*, 221:161 (1980).
79. Y. Kitada, M. Inoue, K. Tamase, M. Imou, A. Hasuike, M. Sasaki, and K. Tanigawa, *Eiyo to Shokuryo*, 35:121 (in Japanese) (1982).
80. T. Fujimoto and M. Moribe, *Fukuoka-shi Eisei Shikenshoho*, 12:60 (in Japanese) (1987).

81. K. Takatsuki, S. Suzuki, M. Sato, K. Sakai, and I. Ushizawa, *J. Assoc. Off. Anal. Chem.*, 70:698 (1987).
82. M. Oishi, E. Amakawa, T. Ogiwara, N. Taguchi, K. Onishi, and M. Nishijima, *Shokuhin Eiseigaku Zasshi*, 29:32 (in Japanese) (1988).
83. T. Hamano, Y. Mitsuhashi, N. Aoki, and S. Yamamoto, *J. Chromatogr.*, 457:403 (1989).
84. K. Shibata and H. Matsuo, *Am. J. Clin. Nutr.*, 50:114 (1989).
85. K. Shibata and H. Matsuo, *Agric. Biol. Chem.*, 53:2031 (1989).

8

VITAMIN B$_1$: THIAMINE

Takashi Kawasaki

Hiroshima University School of Medicine,
Hiroshima, Japan

1. INTRODUCTION

1.1 History

The history of the discovery of thiamine in 1897 and the subsequent developments in its research field up to 1940 have been briefly reviewed by Gubler (1).

Before the discovery of thiamine (1897) by Eijkman as an antipolyneuritis factor in rice bran, Takaki (1885) had already succeeded to eliminate beriberi (thiamine hypovitaminosis) from Japanese navy ships by feeding the crew with a diet containing a high ratio of proteins to carbohydrates (2).

In 1911, Funk first isolated the antiberiberi principle in a crude form from rice bran extracts and named it "vitamine" because it supposedly contained an amine function. As is well known, this name was later adopted in general to designate the whole class of trace nutritional factors. In 1926, Jansen and Donath succeeded in isolating and crystallizing the active substance from rice bran extracts. Ten years later Williams and his group (3) presented the chemical formula for vitamin B$_1$, achieved the first chemical synthesis of the biologically active material, and proposed the name of thiamine.

As to the physiological functions of thiamine, Peter et al. (4) first demonstrated the very low consumption rate of oxygen by thiamine-deficient pigeon brain homogenates when incubated with glucose. Later, the same group clearly showed a recovery of oxygen consumption when thiamine was added to the homogenates (5). Lohmann and Schuster (6) in 1937 discovered thiamine pyrophosphate (TPP) as the active coenzyme form of the vitamin in yeast pyruvate decarboxylase. This work lay at the basis of the elucidation of the biochemical function of thiamine.

1.2 Chemical Properties

The chemical structure of thiamine is shown in Fig. 1. A pyrimidine moiety (2-methyl-4-amino-5-hydroxymethylpyrimidine) and a thiazole moiety (4-methyl-5-hydroxyethylthiazole) are connected by a methylene group. The double-salt form of thiamine with hydrochloric acid ($C_{12}H_{17}N_4OSCl \cdot HCl$; molecular weight 337.28) is readily soluble in water, less soluble in methanol and glycerol, nearly insoluble in ethanol, and insoluble in ether and benzene (7).

Thiamine in water is most stable between pH 2 and 4 and unstable at alkaline pH; it is heat labile with its decomposition dependent on pH and exposure time to heat (8).

The structures of phosphate esters of thiamine are also shown in Fig. 1. Thiamine monophosphate (TMP), thiamine pyrophosphate (TPP), and thiamine triphosphate (TTP) are commonly found in organisms. About 80–90% of the total thiamine content in cells is TPP, the coenzyme form of thiamine. In some animal tissues, especially pig skeletal muscle (9) and chicken white skeletal muscle (10), TTP is present in an extremely high amount (70–80% of total thiamine, i.e., thiamine plus thiamine phosphate esters). However, TTP has no coenzyme activity. Thiamine pyrophosphate in dried state is stable for several months when stored at a low temperature in the dark. In solution, TPP is unstable and partially decomposes to TMP and/or thiamine when stored for several months at pH 5 and 38°C. However, TPP in solution at pH 2–6 and at 0°C is stable for 6 months (11). In an aqueous solution TTP is stable for at least 6 months when stored at −80°C. Aqueous TPP solutions stored at −20°C have even a better stability.

For the chemical determination of thiamine, thiochrome (Thc) is the most important compound. Its structure is shown in Fig. 1. Thiochrome is quantitatively formed from thiamine by alkaline oxidation with cyanogen bromide (12) or potassium ferricyanide (13–16). It is a highly fluorescent compound. Thiamine phosphate esters are also quantitatively converted to thiochrome phosphate esters without affecting the phosphate bond: thiochrome mono-, pyro-, and triphosphate are referred to as ThcMP, ThcPP, and ThcTP, respectively.

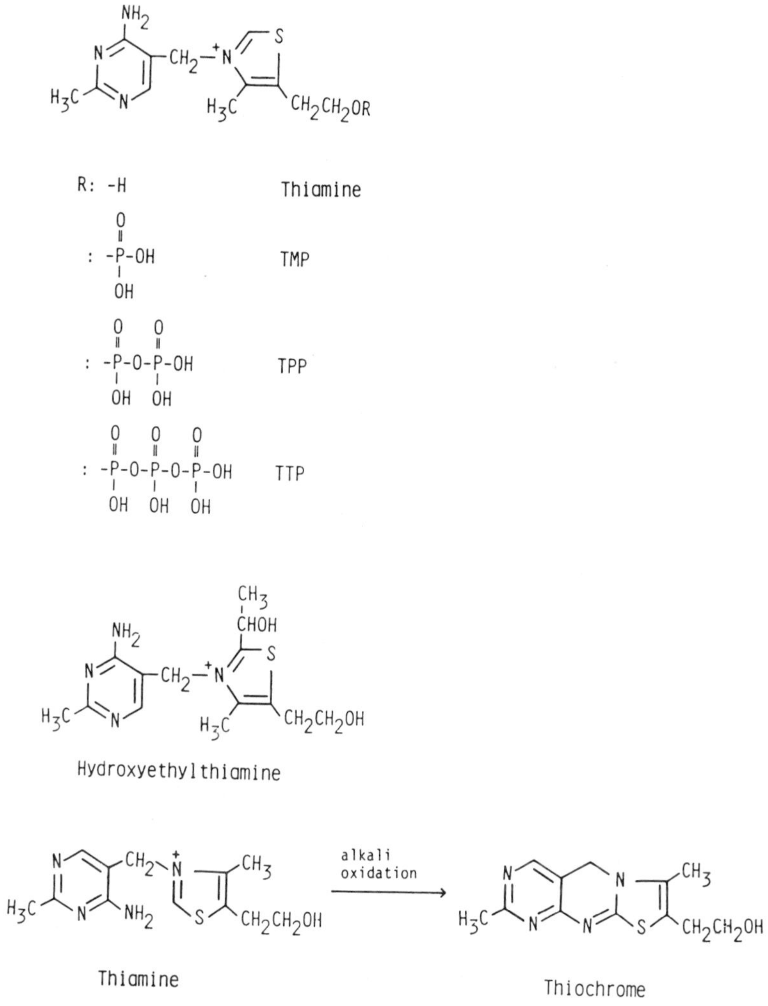

R: -H   Thiamine

   : $-\overset{\overset{O}{\|}}{\underset{\underset{OH}{|}}{P}}-OH$ TMP

   : $-\overset{\overset{O}{\|}}{\underset{\underset{OH}{|}}{P}}-O-\overset{\overset{O}{\|}}{\underset{\underset{OH}{|}}{P}}-OH$ TPP

   : $-\overset{\overset{O}{\|}}{\underset{\underset{OH}{|}}{P}}-O-\overset{\overset{O}{\|}}{\underset{\underset{OH}{|}}{P}}-O-\overset{\overset{O}{\|}}{\underset{\underset{OH}{|}}{P}}-OH$ TTP

Hydroxyethylthiamine

Thiamine   Thiochrome

Figure 1 Structures of thiamine and its related compounds.

Thiochrome and its phosphates are fluorescent at a pH above 8, and all of these have identical excitation maxima at 375 nm and nearly identical fluorescence maxima at 432–435 nm (17,18) as shown in Fig. 2.

Alkaline solutions (pH > 9) of thiochrome and its phosphates are stable at least for 3 days at room temperature. ThcPP and ThcTP in 0.1 N HCl solution are converted quantitatively to ThcMP upon heating above 95°C for 10 min (H. Sanemori and T. Kawasaki, unpublished observation).

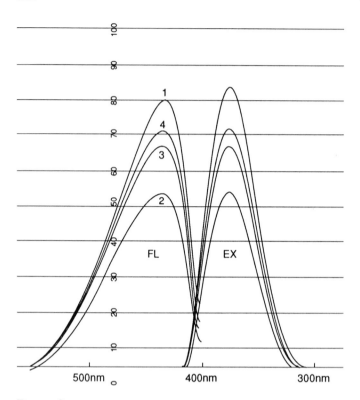

Figure 2 Excitation and fluorescence spectra of thiochrome compounds. Thiochrome (Thc) derivatives were prepared from the corresponding thiamine derivatives by alkaline BrCN oxidation: (1) Thc; (2) ThcMP; (3) ThcPP; and (4) ThcTP. (From Ref. 18.)

Hydroxyethylthiamine, a derivative of thiamine, is found in cells in the form of hydroxyethyl-TPP (19). It is converted to the corresponding thiochrome derivative by alkaline potassium ferricyanide oxidation, but not by alkaline BrCN oxidation (20). This difference in oxidation property is useful for its determination. Factors affecting a cyanogen bromide-based assay of thiamine include drugs and phosphatases used for treating biological samples (21).

1.3   Biochemistry

Absorption

Intestinal thiamine transport has been studied mainly by the everted sac method or tissue accumulation method (22,23). The results obtained suggest that thiamine is absorbed actively against a concentration gradient at low concentrations (less than 2 μM), and that thiamine at concentrations above 2 μM is absorbed by diffusion (24–26). The relationship of thiamine transport across the brush-border membrane and its phosphorylation to TPP has not been clarified (23). Although several studies support the idea that there is a close relationship between transport and phosphorylation (27–30), other studies question the role of phosphorylation in transport (25,31). Resolving this relationship using everted intestinal sacs or rings is technically difficult since coupling of thiamine metabolism to the transport process should always be taken into consideration.

To study the mechanism of thiamine entry through the membrane, brush-border membrane vesicles were prepared from guinea pig jejunum. The vesicles contained no thiamine pyrophosphokinase (EC 2.7.6.2) but had Na$^+$ gradient-dependent amino acid transport systems (32,33). With these preparations, Hayashi et al. (34) obtained evidence that thiamine is transported by simple diffusion and that a specific carrier system is not involved in thiamine transport in the small-intestinal brush-border membrane of the guinea pig. More recently, Rindi et al. (35) showed an involvement of a specific carrier for thiamine, catalyzing facilitated transport of thiamine in brush-border membrane vesicles of rat small intestine. After passing through the brush-border membrane by simple or facilitated diffusion, thiamine is accumulated as TPP by thiamine pyrophosphokinase in the cytoplasm (25,27,36).

Metabolism

Thiamine is metabolized to TPP by thiamine pyrophosphokinase in animal cells. This enzyme has been purified from liver (37), brain (38–40), and heart (41,42). It is also present in parsley leaves (43), yeast (44), and *Paracoccus denitrificans* (45,46). In *Escherichia coli*, thiamine is metabolized to TPP by a two-step reaction catalyzed by thiamine kinase (EC 2.7.1.89) (47,48) and TMP kinase (EC 2.7.4.10) (48–50). Thiamine pyrophosphate is further metabolized to TTP in yeast (51) and rat brain (52,53), but its enzymatic conversion by brain preparations is disputed by Schrijver et al. (54). The observation that extremely high amounts of TTP are present in pig (9) and chicken (10) skeletal muscles led us to study the biosynthesis of TTP from TPP in these tissues. The results obtained indicate that cytosolic adenylate kinase (EC 2.7.4.3) catalyzes TTP formation from TPP in vitro (55,56) as well as in vivo (10). However, this does not exclude the possibility of the existence of another enzyme involved in TTP biosynthesis.

The ratio of the cellular concentration of TTP to TPP is a good indicator of differences in thiamine metabolism between chicken white (fast-twitch) and red (slow-twitch) muscle. The ratio in the former is 5.0

and in the latter 0.4, the concentration of total thiamine being equal in both types (10). Differences in thiamine metabolism between the white and red mammalian muscles, as well as differences in cellular localization of thiamine phosphate esters, have been reported by Matsuda et al. (57,58).

Physiological Functions

Thiamine has to be converted to TPP before exerting its physiological function as a coenzyme in cells. Thiamine pyrophosphate functions as a coenzyme for several important enzymes in carbohydrate and amino acid metabolism (59), including pyruvate dehydrogenase (EC 1.2.4.1), oxoglutarate dehydrogenase (EC 1.2.4.2), transketolase (EC 2.2.1.1), branched-chain α-keto acid dehydrogenase (EC 1.2.4.4), pyruvate decarboxylase (EC 4.1.1.1), and carboxylate carboligase (EC 4.1.1.47).

In oxidative decarboxylation of pyruvate and oxoglutarate, as shown in Fig. 3, TPP functions as a carrier of "active aldehyde" to form the intermediates, hydroxyethyl-TPP and α-hydroxy-β-carboxypropyl-TPP, which are finally transferred to coenzyme A (CoA) to form acetyl-CoA and succinyl-CoA, respectively.

Thiamine is known to affect nerve functions as an antipolyneuritis factor. There are many reports on the effects of thiamine on nerve conductance or neurotransmission (52,60–63). However, the exact mechanism of neurological function is not known. Neither has the role of TTP

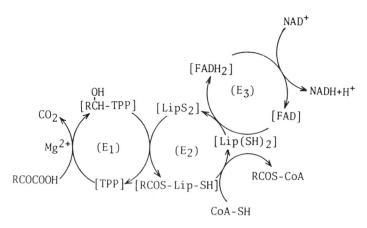

Figure 3 The mechanism of oxidative decarboxylation of α-keto acids. E_1, α-keto acid dehydrogenase; E_2, lipoate acyltransferase; E_3, lipoamide dehydrogenase. R: CH_3-, $HOOC-CH_2CH_2$-; R-CH(OH)-TPP, "active aldehyde"; $LipS_2$, lipoate; Lip (SH)2, dihydrolipoate; RCOS-Lip SH, 6-acyldihydrolipoate; [ ], coenzymes bound to the enzyme proteins.

been elucidated as yet. Schoffeniels et al. (64–66) suggested that TTP may be involved in some kind of anion transport mechanism.

2. THIN-LAYER CHROMATOGRAPHY

2.1 Paper Chromatography

The presence of TTP in rat liver has been first reported by Rossi-Fanelli et al. (67) using paper partition chromatography (PPC). This is a pioneering study of PPC in separating thiamine phosphates in a biological material, but the TTP fraction was heavily contaminated by TPP. Siliprandi and Siliprandi (68) developed several methods to separate thiamine phosphates, including PPC, starch column chromatography, ion-exchange chromatography, paper electrophoresis, starch column electrophoresis, and cellulose column electrophoresis.

A good PPC separation of thiamine phosphates was obtained at the 50-μg level in three different solvent systems (68): I, n-propanol-H_2O-1 M acetate buffer, pH 5 (70:20:10); II, n-propanol-0.5 M acetate buffer, pH 4.5 (60:40); and III, n-propanol-H_2O-1 M acetate buffer, pH 5 (65:25:15). PPC was run by an ascending method for 15–30 h and each spot on the paper was detected under UV light after spraying with an alkaline ethanolic $K_3Fe(CN)_6$ solution. To quantitate the thiamine compounds separated by PPC, each portion of the paper strip corresponding to the spots of thiamine compounds was cut out and eluted with water. The eluates were subjected to photometry at 270 nm. This approach allowed quantitation of 10 μg of each thiamine compound (68).

A microassay for thiamine, TMP, and TPP after separation by PPC was reported to yield a detection limit of approximately 0.02 μg (60 pmol) of thiamine (69). This detection limit is still at least three orders of magnitude higher than the one obtained by high-performance liquid chromatography with fluorescence detection (section 3.2).

Kiessling (70) measured the amounts of TTP in rat liver and brain by use of PPC combined with a microbiological method: in the liver the levels of TPP and TTP were 5.88 and 0.09 μg/g wet weight, respectively, whereas in the brain levels of 2.70 and 0.044 μg/g wet weight were found.

2.2 Thin-Layer Chromatography

Two-dimensional thin-layer chromatography (TLC) was applied to separate thiamine and its metabolites and precursor compounds, including hydroxyethylthiamine, pyrimidine and thiazole fragments of thiamine, carboxylic acid and sulfonic acid derivatives of the pyrimidine moiety, and N'-methylnicotinamide (71). The amounts of the compounds applied were 0.1–8 μg. Most of the TLC procedures have been used to analyze thiamine in pharmaceutical preparations (72–75).

In these assays thiamine was separated from riboflavin, pyridoxine, nicotinamide, and p-aminobenzoic acid (73) and, in addition, from Ca-pantothenate, choline, inositol, and cyanocobalamin (75) at the levels of 20–250 μg (73) and of 4–10 mg (75). Solvent systems used were (a) glacial acetic acid-acetone-methanol-benzene (volume ratio not specified) (73) and (b) chloroform-ethanol-water (50:25:1) (75). UV detection was carried out at 246 nm.

2.3   Other Techniques

A systematic study to separate thiamine phosphate esters by ion-exchange chromatography was carried out by Siliprandi and Siliprandi (68). They described conditions for the quantitation of chemically synthesized TMP, TPP, and TTP in detail, and proposed the use of paper chromatography for qualitative separation and ion-exchange chromatography for quantitation of these phosphate esters. However, both fractions of TPP and TTP separated by the ion-exchange chromatography were shown to be highly active toward yeast apodecarboxylase (68), which indicated TPP contamination of the TTP fraction. Furthermore, in this method, high concentrations (millimolar levels) were used. This procedure is therefore not directly applicable to the separation of thiamine phosphate esters in animal and plant tissues that normally have micromolar amounts of the phosphate esters.

Quantitative assay conditions for thiamine and its phosphates in animal tissues were first described by Rindi and de Giuseppe (76). Thiamine and TMP coeluted from the column and were then separately determined after incubation in the presence or absence of phosphatase. The method consisted of two procedures: removal of impurities in the extracted materials by chromatography on a charcoal column treated with cholesteryl stearate, and subsequent separation of thiamine compounds by anion-exchange column chromatography on Dowex 1 × 8. The recovery of thiamine obtained after treatment on the charcoal column averaged 95%. The contents of thiamine and its phosphate esters in rat tissues are given in Table 1.

The analytical method of Rindi and de Giuseppe (76) was modified by Koike et al. (77). They found the conditions described by Rindi and de Giuseppe inconsistent for separating TTP from TPP, but successfully used Dowex 1 × 4, as shown in Fig. 4. Thiamine and TMP eluted together in peak 1 (Fig. 4.). They were then separately determined by the thiochrome method (12) after incubation of the eluate with or without Taka-diastase. The contents of thiamine, TMP, TPP, and TTP

Table 1 Contents of Thiamine and Its Phosphate Esters in Rat Tissues[a]

Compound	Brain (5)		Heart (5)		Kidney (7)		Liver (6)	
	µg/g	%	µg/g	%	µg/g	%	µg/g	%
Thiamine	0.11±0.08	4.4±0.10	0.16±0.01	2.3±0.35	0.22±0.02	6.2±0.45	0.24±0.01	3.5±0.15
TMP	0.30±0.09	11.5±0.25	0.41±0.05	5.9±0.91	0.35±0.06	9.8±1.42	0.66±0.01	9.4±0.43
TDP	2.61±0.15	78.9±1.18	7.44±0.44	86.0±0.06	3.47±0.13	78.6±1.62	6.81±0.44	77.9±1.28
TTP	0.19±0.02	5.0±0.19	0.57±0.04	5.6±0.48	0.27±0.0	5.2±0.24	0.92±0.13	9.0±1.48

[a] Values are expressed as micrograms of each compound per gram weight of tissue. The values given are means ±SE. The numbers in parentheses are the number of determinations. The percentages show the thiamine content of each fraction as a percentage of the total thiamine of the tissue. From Ref. 76.

327

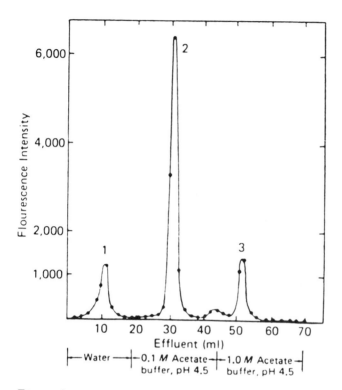

Figure 4 Chromatogram of thiamine and its phosphate esters in the rat liver: (1) Thiamine and TMP; (2) TPP; and (3) TTP. (From Ref. 77.)

in rat liver were 0.75, 0.77, 7.37, and 1.09 μg/g wet weight, respectively. These results are in good agreement with those of Rindi and de Giuseppe (76). The recovery of thiamine and of its phosphates added separately to tissue extracts was 91.0 and 81.0–83.3%, respectively (77).

The analytical method described by Koike et al. (77), however, is not adequate for the analysis of many biological samples. The charcoal column pretreatment and ion-exchange column chromatography are technically difficult and require a fairly long completion time. The charcoal treatment requires special techniques that can cause problems of reproducibility of results.

A similar separation method, especially for TPP and TTP in liver, was reported by Parkhomenko et al. (78). They used a Sephadex cation-exchange column without charcoal pretreatment. Thiamine monophosphate and thiamine eluted into the same fraction, but the authors stated that the separation of TMP and thiamine by this method was not their aim. This method, using a Sephadex cation exchanger, also requires 24 h for completion of the elution of TMP with a recovery of 90–100% of TPP and TTP applied to the column. The minimum amount of thiamine phosphate esters detected by this method was calculated to be about 1 μg (approximately 2 nmol for each ester).

The formation of a TPP artifact during ion-exchange column chromatography on a Dowex 1 × 8 in the formate form was demonstrated (79). This artifact formation was prevented by the substitution of formate by acetate. The resulting single-column procedure developed was able to separate thiamine and its phosphates in micromolar amounts.

3. HIGH-PERFORMANCE LIQUID CHROMATOGRAPHY

3.1 Introduction

High-performance liquid chromatography (HPLC) has been developed in recent years for the analysis of drugs, biological materials, and metabolites. The analysis of thiamine by HPLC has been reported for pharmaceutical preparations (84–86), foods (89–95), urine (92,96,97), and blood (96–101). These methods, however, involved analysis of free thiamine and not thiamine phosphate esters. Since thiamine exists mostly as TPP in biological materials, samples were first treated with Taka-diastase or acid phosphatase to hydrolyze TPP to thiamine (89,91,93–95,97–101).

The determination of thiamine and its phosphates by LC was reported by Gubler and Hemming (102), Kawasaki and his associates (18,103–105), Kimura et al. (106,107), Schoffeniels's group (108,109), Iwata et al. (110), and Brunnekreeft et al. (111).

3.2 Analytical Systems

Stationary Phase

There are many kinds of stationary phases used for analysis by LC. Porous silica particles chemically bound to a monomolecular octadecyl layer, such as μBondapak C$_{18}$, are most frequently used in reversed-phase LC. As an improved reversed-phase sorbent, a poly(styrene-divinylbenzene) resin can be used within an extended pH range of 1–13 because of its chemical stability (109). LiChrosorb NH$_2$ found applications for thiamine (101) as well as thiamine phosphate esters (9,18,103–105). A strong cation exchange resin was also used in the early 1970s for high-speed chromatographic separation of thiamine in pharmaceutical preparations (112,113).

Mobile Phase

The mobile phase used in HPLC is dependent on the hydrophobicity of the compounds. In reversed-phase liquid chromatography (LC), appropriate mixtures of methanol and water (or buffer solution), with or without ion-pair chromatography (IPC) reagents, are used.

Detection

The detection of thiamine compounds in the eluate is carried out either spectrophotometrically, usually at 254 nm, or fluorometrically.

In fluorometric detection, two different procedures are used. First, samples containing thiamine compounds are converted precolumn to thiochrome compounds and then chromatographed (9,18,96,97, 101,103–105,109–111). In the second procedure, samples are first directly chromatographed and then thiamines in the eluate are converted postcolumn to thiochrome compounds using reagents for alkaline oxidation (93–95,98–100,102,106,107). Although different postcolumn fluorogenic oxidation systems were described by different authors, the principle is always the same. For example, the effluent from the column is mixed with 0.01% potassium ferricyanide in 15% NaOH, which is sent to a mixing coil by a proportioning pump at the rate of 0.3 ml/min. Thiochrome fluorescence in the mixture is then measured (98,106).

The excitation wavelength for the fluorometric detection is usually 365–375 nm, while the emission wavelength is usually 425–435 nm.

The detection limit depends on the method used. Fluorometric detection is much more sensitive than its spectrophotometric counterpart. The latter method is suitable for analysis of large quantities of thiamine in pharmaceutical preparations and foods: the detection limit is approximately 2 ng or 6 pmol as thiamine hydrochloride (92). On the other hand, the detection limit by the fluorometric method is 0.05 pmol or 17 pg as thiamine hydrocholoride (103–105). In more recent studies the minimum detectable amount of thiamine was reported to be 5 fmol (101,109). Fluorescence detection is more suitable for the analysis of thiamine in biological materials such as cells, blood, and urine. For example, total plasma thiamine of 0.5 nmol/l is the lowest limit of detection by fluorescence (101). Kimura et al. (98) could analyze the total thiamine content of blood using only a 100-μl sample.

The time required for completion of chromatography is usually less than 10 min, and in some cases less than 25 min (84–87,89–91,96–98,102,103,107,110).

Precision

In all analytical systems listed above, the recovery of thiamine added to the sample is 100 ±10%, and the coefficient of variation is 1–5%.

Internal Standard

As internal standard, either salicylamide (100) or anthracene (97) has been used. These compounds, which are not related to thiamine in structure but have fluorescence characteristics comparable to those of thiochrome, have been used only to compensate for variability in the volume injected into the column. In other studies, thiochrome compounds derived from authentic thiamine and its phosphates are used as calibration standards for the analysis of thiamine phosphates (18,103–105), since the fluorescence intensity of thiochrome phosphates varies considerably (see Fig. 2) (18).

3.3 Thiamine

Pharmaceutical Preparations

Reversed-phase HPLC systems were recently applied for the simultaneous assay of thiamine and other water-soluble vitamins in multivitamin preparations. No special treatment of the sample was required before chromatography.

Kirchmeier and Upton (84) and Walker (85) have used similar HPLC systems to separate thiamine from nicotinamide, riboflavin, and pyridoxine in multivitamin preparations: a μBondapak C18 column was used with a mobile phase of methanol-hexane sulfonate-acetic acid, followed by UV detection at 270 and 254 nm, respectively. The detection limit of standard thiamine was relatively high: 90 ng (84) and 400 ng (85), respectively.

In more recent procedures (87,88), the mobile phases in the reversed-phase systems were optimized. With 0.2 M ammonium phosphate buffer (pH 5.1), Kothari and Taylor (87) could separate folate, pyridoxine, nicotinamide, and thiamine in this order in 20 min, followed by vitamin B$_{12}$ and riboflavin. The latter two compounds eluted after a step gradient to 30% aqueous methanol. This procedure has the advantage of separating completely at least nine coenzyme forms of water-soluble vitamins, including TPP. A similar mobile phase composed of methanol-water (50:50) was used by Amin and Reusch (88) in connection with a LiChrosorb RP-18 column to separate thiamine, pyridoxine, vitamin B$_{12}$, and riboflavin in 3 min, as shown in Fig. 5. The detection limit at 254 nm is 5 ng (15 pmol) for thiamine and 10–20 ng for the other three vitamins, with a coefficient of variation of less than 4%.

Foods

Thiamine was analyzed by HPLC in rice (91,93), cereals (90,92,94,95), meat (89,95), and other by-products. In these systems, thiamine could be determined simultaneously with riboflavin and niacin.

Samples, in either 0.1 N HCl or 0.1 N H$_2$SO$_4$, were autoclaved for 30 min and then subjected to enzymatic hydrolysis with Taka-diastase and papain (89,91). The filtrate was then chromatographed. The system used for rice and rice products (91) was as follows: column, μBondapak

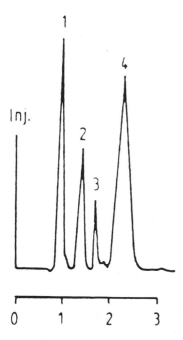

Figure 5 Typical separation of four vitamins from capsules. Peaks 1–4 are thiamine, pyridoxine, vitamin B$_{12}$, and riboflavin, respectively. (From Ref. 88.)

C18; detection, ultraviolet (UV) 254 nm; mobile phase, methanol-glacial acetic acid-H$_2$O-PIC 5-PIC 7 (390:10:600:25:25, v/v). Recovery data for samples of rice measured by both the HPLC and the American Association of Cereal Chemists (AACC) method (114) showed no significant variation at levels of both 1 and 5% probability. The detection limit for thiamine was 30 ng.

The HPLC system for cereals (90) is quite similar to that for rice (91), with minor exceptions. The mobile phase was a mixture of 12.5% acetonitrile and 87.5% 10 mM phosphate buffer (pH 7.0) containing 5 mM heptane sulfonate.

The HPLC system was modified to determine thiamine in meat and meat products (89). The sample filtrate was oxidized to thiochrome by the alkaline ferricyanide method and the thiochrome was extracted with isobutyl alcohol. Aliquots of the extract were chromatographed using a Spherisorb silica column and chloroform-methanol (90:10, v/v) as the mobile phase. Detection was performed fluorimetrically. The recovery values ranged between 84.4 and 94.2%, and the detection limit for thiamine was 0.05 ng (0.15 pmol).

A simultaneous determination of thiamine and riboflavin in food by LC with postcolumn derivatization was recently described (94,95). Extraction of thiamine and riboflavin from foods and enzymatic digestion of the extract were carried out according to the AOAC methods (1980). After filtration, an aliquot (50–100 μl) was injected on a μBondapak C18 column and eluted with methanol-water (40:60, v/v) containing 5 mM PIC B6. Riboflavin fluorescence in the eluate was detected directly at 360 nm (excitation) and 500 nm (emission). Thiamine in the eluate was then passed in a reaction coil and reacted with an alkaline ferricyanide solution, to convert thiamine to thiochrome, and determined at 360 nm (excitation) and 425 nm (emission). This procedure could be successfully used for determining the two vitamins in a wide range of foods including raw meats, processed meats, cereal products, fruits, and vegetables (95).

Clinical Specimens

HPLC is useful for the analysis of thiamine in clinical specimens such as urine and blood, because it is quick, accurate, and highly sensitive. A urinary thiamine assay by HPLC was first reported by Roser et al. (96). In this assay, urinary thiamine was passed through a Decalso cation-exchange column to remove interfering compounds, eluted with 3.4 M KCl, and then converted to thiochrome by alkaline potassium ferricyanide. The reaction mixture was extracted with i-butanol. The extract was then chromatographed in the following system: column, silica (LiChrosorb Si); mobile phase, methanol-diethyl ether (22:88, v/v); detection, fluorescence.

Without submitting urine to a cation-exchange column, Yasuda et al. (97) directly oxidized urinary thiamine with alkaline BrCN solution to thiochrome, extracted the latter with n-butyl alcohol and then analyzed it by HPLC using a reversed-phase C18 column with methanol-water (95:5, v/v) as the mobile phase, followed by fluorescence detection (excitation at 375 nm; emission at 435 nm). The recovery was 102–109 % with an intra-assay and interassay coefficient of variation (C.V.) of 1.2 and 5.4 %, respectively. The average amount of thiamine excreted into 24-h urine was 181 μg (97).

The determination of thiamine in blood by HPLC with either precolumn or postcolumn derivatization is valuable to assess the thiamine status in humans, because of its sensitivity, specificity, reproducibility, speed, and simplicity. Most procedures determine total thiamine in blood after hydrolysis of the phosphates with an appropriate phosphatase (96–101). Other HPLC methods (109,111,115) were used to quantitate thiamine and its phosphates in blood separately, total thiamine being the sum of the individual levels (111,116).

Yasuda et al. (97) deproteinized human whole blood (1 ml) with trichloroacetic acid, adjusted the pH of the supernatant to 4.5, and treated the extract with Taka-diastase. The free thiamine thus formed was converted to thiochrome by alkaline BrCN oxidation. The thiochrome extracted into n-butyl alcohol was analyzed by reversed-phase (Nucleosil C18) HPLC with methanol-water (95:5, v/v) and fluorescence detection (excitation, 375 nm; emission, 435 nm). The method gave a good recovery of 98.6–104.8%, a C.V. of 5.6%, and a detection limit of 3 ng (10 pmol) thiamine per milliliter of blood.

Schrijver et al. (99) described a reliable postcolumn derivatization HPLC method for total thiamine in whole blood. Two milliliters of whole blood was deproteinized with trichloroacetic acid, neutralized with sodium acetate buffer to a final pH of 4.5, and then treated with Taka-diastase for 2 h at 45°C. After centrifugation, the clear supernatant was used for direct HPLC analysis. A LiChrosorb Si-100 column (250 × 4.6 mm; 10 μm) was used and 240 μl of the extract was injected onto the column, eluted with a mobile phase composed of 40 mM Na_2HPO_4-30 mM KH_2PO_4 and ethanol (87:13, v/v), at pH 6.8.

The effluent was mixed with the thiochrome reagent [1.2 mM $K_3Fe(CN)_6$-1.8 M NaOH] in a reaction coil, followed by fluorescence detection (excitation, 367 nm; emission, 430 nm). The concentration of thiamine in the original sample was calculated from the peak area versus a thiamine standard.

The within-assay and between-assay coefficients of variation for the determination of total thiamine in whole blood were 4.2 and 4.4%, respectively. The between-assay analytical recovery of TPP added to blood samples was 99.9 ±11.7% (mean ±SD). The analysis of samples from 98 normal volunteers, not matched for age and sex, revealed an overall range for total thiamine of 70–185 nmol/l blood, with a mean value of 115 nmol/l blood. The frequency distribution of total thiamine in these blood samples is shown in Fig. 6. Using a distribution-free method (117) with the limits of percentiles of 2.5 and 97.5% and a reliability of 95%, a "normal" range of 95–155 nmol of total thiamine/l blood was obtained (99). J. Schrijver extended the number of analyses of total thiamine in whole blood to 598 normal volunteers and obtained a value of 129.2 ±21.9 nmol/l blood (personal communication). This HPLC method could also be applied to the analysis of thiamine in plasma and erythrocytes.

Kimura et al. (98) described an HPLC method with postcolumn derivatization for blood thiamine. Samples were hydrolyzed with Taka-diastase, chromatographed through an adsorption column (Shodex-OH) with a mobile phase of 0.2 M NaH_2PO_4, and then detected fluorometrically after an automated oxidation reaction on the eluate with alkaline

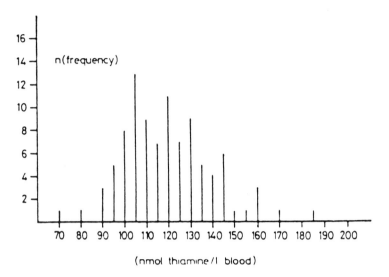

Figure 6 Frequency distribution of total thiamine in whole blood samples of normal healthy Dutch volunteers (n=98). (From Ref. 99.)

potassium ferricyanide. This method requires only 0.1 ml blood, and showed 90–100% recovery of added thiamine and a good correlation (r = 0.94) of the data with those obtained by the ordinary BrCN assay method (12). Thiamine concentration in human blood was 46.2 ±2.3 µg/l by this method (n = 20).

A similar HPLC method with a postcolumn derivatization system was used for the analysis of total thiamine in human whole blood as well as in serum, cerebrospinal fluid, and milk (100). The HPLC system consisted of a µBondapak column and the mobile phase was a mixture of methanol-50 mM sodium citrate buffer pH 4.0 (45:55, v/v) plus 10 mM sodium 1-octanesulfonate. Two milliliters blood was needed. The minimum detectable amount was 60 fmol of thiamine. The intra-assay and interassay coefficients of variation were 2.3% and 3.9%, respectively. The recovery of TPP added to blood samples was 98.7%.

The total thiamine content in whole blood of 56 healthy volunteers determined by this method ranged from 71 to 185 nmol/liter with a mean value of 117 nmol/liter. The reference range calculated by means of the distribution-free method (117) was found to be 88–157 nmol of total thiamine/liter blood (100).

Weber and Kewitz (101) reported a sensitive HPLC method for thiamine in human plasma, based on precolumn oxidation of thiamine to thiochrome followed by HPLC separation and fluorescence detection. The method includes a disadvantageous step to extract the thiochrome into isobutanol, but, on the other hand, has a detection limit as low as 5 fmol. Plasma isolated from blood samples was deproteinized and the supernatant obtained after centrifugation was neutralized before hydrolysis with acid phosphatase. The free thiamine formed was oxidized to thiochrome with $HgCl_2$ and then alkalinized. The thiochrome was extracted with isobutanol and then analyzed on the HPLC system: column, LiChrosorb NH_2 (120 × 4.6 mm; 5 μm); mobile phase, methanol-diethyl ether (25:75, v/v); detection, fluorescence (excitation, 365 nm; emission, 440 nm). The minimum sample volume required for the assay was 0.3 ml of plasma and the minimum plasma concentration detectable was 0.5 nmol of thiamine/liter (0.17 μg/liter). Plasma levels of thiamine in 91 volunteers ranged from 6.6 to 43 nmol/liter, showing a mean of 11.6 nmol/liter. This HPLC method was used to study the pharmacokinetics of thiamine excretion into urine after intravenous or oral dosing (101).

3.4   Thiamine Phosphate Esters

Straight-Phase Liquid Chromatography

The first complete separation of thiamine and thiamine phosphate esters in straight-phase liquid chromatography (LC) was reported by Kawasaki's group (18,103). The analytical system consisted of LiChrosorb NH_2 (250 × 4.6 mm ID; 10 μm) as the stationary phase and acetonitrile-90 mM potassium phosphate buffer, pH 8.4 (60:40, v/v), as the mobile phase. Detection was carried out fluorometrically (excitation, 375 nm; emission, 430 nm) at room temperature.

Applied samples were thiochrome, ThcMP, ThcPP, and ThcTP, which were formed from thiamine and the corresponding phosphate esters by alkaline BrCN oxidation. This oxidation was carried out by mixing a 1.6-ml sample with 0.2 ml of 0.3 M BrCN and 0.2 ml of 1 M NaOH. It is also important to prepare a blank by reversing the order of BrCN and NaOH addition according to the method of Fujiwara and Matsui (12). Since the intensity of thiochrome fluorescence depends on the pH and reaches a steady level at a pH above 8 (17,18), the mobile phase should contain an alkaline buffer. The detection limit of this system was 1 pmol for each of the thiamine phosphates (18). However, this sensitivity was insufficient to determine quantities of TTP in rat brain unless 40 μl of the sample was injected (103).

Improved instrumentation to reduce the detection limit is now used in our laboratory (105). The main change has been the replacement of the fluorescence detector, which improved the detection limit to 0.05 pmol for thiamine and its phosphates. The stationary and mobile phases are identical to those described above, and a spectrofluorimeter equipped with a mercury lamp as a light source is used at 365 nm for excitation and 430 nm for emission.

The volume of the original sample to be oxidized is now routinely 160 µl, which is mixed with 20 µl of 0.3 M BrCN and then 20 µl of 1 M NaOH. The injection volume of the oxidized sample is 10 µl, which is sufficient to detect TTP in most animal tissues. The concentrations of thiamine and its phosphates in the samples were calculated from the peak area (mV · s) by use of a computer connected on-line. Thiamine, TMP, TPP, and TTP in the original sample are detected in this order as the thiochromes within 7 min.

The capacity factor (k′) is determined at different concentrations of potassium phosphate buffer (pH 8.4) containing a constant percentage of acetonitrile (40%). As shown in Fig. 7, the k′ values obtained in the range of 75–100 mM buffer are satisfactory for the separation of thiamine phosphates, with 90 mM being optimal. When the ratio of acetonitrile to 75 mM potassium phosphate buffer (pH 8.4) was varied from 10:90 to 60:40, the k′ values for each thiamine and its phosphates remained less than 5.0, but the fluorescence intensity of thiochrome compounds increased 2.5-fold. Based on these results, the mobile phase for

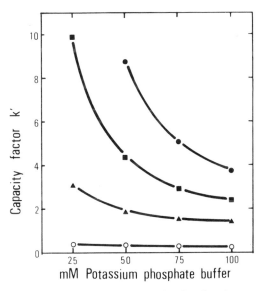

Figure 7 Capacity factor (k′) for thiochrome and its phosphates separated by the improved straight-phase LC system. Concentrations of potassium phosphate buffer (pH 8.4) are varied at a fixed ratio of acetonitrile to the buffer (60:40, v/v); ○, thiochrome (Thc); ▲, ThcMP; ■, ThcPP; ●, ThcTP.

the straight-phase LC system is composed of acetonitrile-90 mM potassium phosphate buffer, pH 8.4 (60:40, v/v).

A chromatogram for Thc, ThcMP, ThcPP, and ThcTP (1 pmol each) obtained with the improved straight-phase LC system is illustrated in Fig. 8. The resolution factors (R_s) calculated from the widths and retention times are 2.4 for Thc-ThcMP, 1.6 for ThcMP-ThcPP, and 2.1 for ThcPP-ThcTP, respectively. These values of R_s indicate a complete separation of each peak, as seen in Fig. 8. The detection limit of thia-

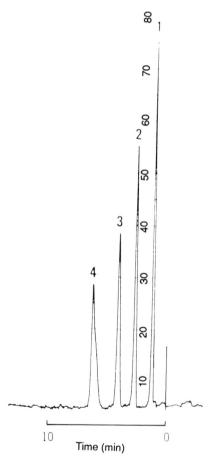

Figure 8 Chromatogram of thiochrome and its phosphate esters analyzed by the improved straight-phase LC system. Thiochrome (Thc) and its phosphates were prepared from thiamine and its phosphates by alkaline BrCN oxidation; (1) Thc; (2) ThcMP; (3) ThcPP; and (4) ThcTP (1 pmol each).

mine and its phosphates is 0.05 pmol, which is consistent with that in the reverse-phase HPLC system (104) equipped with the same fluorometer.

This straight-phase LC system has been successfully employed isocratically to determine thiamine phosphates, especially TTP, in biological materials (9,10; see also Fig. 11) as well as TPP or TTP after enzymatic hydrolysis (10,55,56).

Reversed-Phase Liquid Chromatography

A reversed-phase LC system with precolumn derivatization to thiochromes for thiamine and its phosphates was first described by Kawasaki et al. (104). In this system TTP elutes first, followed by TPP, TMP, and finally thiamine. Since then, many reversed-phase LC systems (107–111,115) have been described with either pre- (108–111) or postcolumn derivatization (107,115).

In our LC system, thiamine compounds are converted to thiochromes by alkaline BrCN oxidation prior to separation. An ODS column is used as the stationary phase and 2.5% N,N-dimethylformamide (DMF)-25 mM potassium phosphate buffer (pH 8.4) as the mobile phase. The detector is identical to that used in the improved straight-phase LC system. After completion of ThcMP elution, the mobile phase is changed to 25% DMF-25 mM potassium phosphate buffer (pH 8.4) for elution of Thc.

The capacity factors (k') were calculated for ThcMP, ThcPP, and ThcTP by varying the ratio of DMF to potassium phosphate buffer (25 mM, pH 8.4) or by varying the buffer concentration with a fixed concentration of DMF (2.5%). The k' values ranged from 1.8 to 6.0 in 2.5% DMF-25 mM potassium phosphate buffer (pH 8.4) (104), suggesting the suitability of the mobile phase for separation of thiamine phosphates. The resolution factors (R_s) for ThcTP-ThcPP and ThcPP-ThcMP in this system were 1.6 and 2.2, respectively, when calculated from the chromatogram shown in Fig. 9. The detection limit of thiamine and its phosphates was 0.05 pmol (104).

A reversed-phase LC of thiamine phosphates followed by postcolumn fluorogenic oxidation was described by Kimura et al. (107), although the application data for biological materials were not included. A μBondapak C_{18} column was used with a mobile phase of a 0.2 M sodium phosphate-phosphoric acid buffer (pH 4.3). The effluent was oxidized by the system and detected fluorometrically (98,106).

Schoffeniels et al. applied a reversed-phase LC system for thiamine and its phosphates with precolumn derivatization by alkaline $K_3Fe(CN)_6$ (108) to tissues. They used an ODS column as the stationary phase and gradient elution with 25 mM phosphate buffer (pH 8.4)/methanol. The gradient program was as follows: after being kept for 1 min at 10%, the

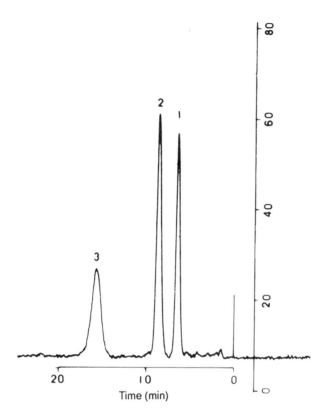

Figure 9 Chromatogram of thiochrome and its phosphate esters separated by reversed-phase LC. Thiochrome (Thc) phosphates were prepared from thiamine phosphates by alkaline BrCN oxidation: (1) ThcTP; (2) ThcPP; and (3) ThcMP. (From Ref. 104.)

methanol concentration was raised to 100% in 3 min, and then 6 min after the injection of the sample the initial 10% was restored. Detection was carried out fluorometrically (excitation 390 nm, emission 475 nm). ThcTP, ThcPP, ThcMP, and Thc eluted in this order within 14 min with a detection limit of 0.05 pmol each. The method was suitable for the determination of thiamine compounds in neural tissues (108).

The same group (109) subsequently modified and improved this HPLC method by using a styrene-divinylbenzene reversed-phase column (PRP-1) eluted isocratically. The main advantage of the PRP-1 reversed phase compared to silica-based reversed phase is its stability over the pH range 1–13. The determination of thiamine phosphates by precolumn derivatization must be carried out above a pH of 8.0 of the mobile phase

(18). Only under these conditions are thiochrome phosphates fluorescent. At alkaline pH, however, silica-based sorbents rapidly deteriorate. The isocratic elution is carried out in two different modes: the mobile phase contains 10% methanol for the determination of thiochrome phosphates and 10% tetrahydrofuran (THF) for thiochrome. The elution was completed in 14 min. As compared to previous methods, the detection limit was lowered (108), to 10 fmol for thiochrome phosphates and 5 fmol for thiochrome. This modified HPLC method has been applied to the analysis of thiamine and TMP in human serum (109).

Another reversed-phase LC system with precolumn derivatization has been reported by Iwata and his group (110). Thiamine and its phosphates were converted to fluorophores by alkaline cyanogen bromide. The thiochromes were injected in a neutralized solution on an ODS silica column. The mobile phase, containing 100 mM Na$_2$HPO$_4$ · H$_3$PO$_4$ buffer (pH 2.5) and methanol (92:8), was mixed postcolumn for alkalinization with 0.2 M NaOH-70% methanol, followed by fluorescence detection. The elution of these four thiochromes was completed in 30 min, and the detection limit was 0.1 pmol for thiamine phosphate esters and 0.05 pmol for thiamine. This method has been used for the determination of thiamine and its phosphates in animal tissues, especially in skeletal muscles (57,58).

An HPLC method optimized for the simultaneous determination of thiamine and its phosphates in whole blood has been reported by Brunnekreeft et al. (111). The method includes precolumn derivatization with alkaline K$_3$Fe(CN)$_6$ and gradient elution with mixtures of 140 mM phosphate buffer (pH 7.0), methanol, $tert$-butylammonium hydroxide, and dimethylformamide. This gradient method is a modification of the method of Bontemps et al. (108). An ODS column was used and detection was performed fluorometrically (excitation 367 nm, emission 435 nm). The total run time was 15 min, and the minimum detectable amount was 0.5 nmol/l for thiamine as well as its phosphates.

3.5 Applications

Tissue Contents of Thiamine and Its Phosphates

To determine thiamine and its phosphates at low concentrations in cells and tissues, pretreatment with charcoal is necessary to concentrate the compounds and to remove impurities interfering in the analysis (77,78). The method to detect thiamine in food involves enzymatic hydrolysis of thiamine phosphates to thiamine before LC separation. The straight-phase and reversed-phase LC systems are preferred over charcoal or enzymatic treatments because they can analyze tissue thiamine compounds simply by conversion of thiamine to thiochrome before chromatography. An example of a procedure to determine the tissue content of thiamine and its phosphates is described.

Male Wistar rats weighing 250–300 g were sacrified by decapitation, and the liver and brain were immediately removed. Approximately 200 mg of the tissue was weighed and homogenized in 5 volumes of 10% trichloroacetic acid (TCA) by use of a Polytron 20 ST at 4°C. After centrifugation for 15 min at 16,000 × g, the supernatant was extracted at least three times with the same volume of ether to remove TCA. The water layer obtained, 0.4 ml, was mixed with 50 μl 0.3 M BrCN and then with 50 μl 1 M NaOH. In blank experiments, 50 μl 1 M NaOH was first added to 0.4 ml of the water layer and mixed, followed by the addition of 50 μl 0.3 M BrCN. An aliquot of both the oxidized sample and the blank was injected onto the column and chromatographed in the improved straight-phase LC system.

Chromatograms of thiamine and its phosphates analyzed by the improved straight-phase LC system are shown in Figs. 10 (liver) and 11 (brain). Good separation of peaks 1, 2, 3, and 4, representing thiamine, TMP, TPP, and TTP, respectively, is evident. Although unidentified peaks can be seen in the sample, no peaks appear in the region of TTP. Blank sample peaks are subtracted from test sample peaks, as described by Fujiwara and Matsui (12). Cellular concentrations of thiamine and its phosphates can then be calculated (Table 2).

When the contents of thiamine phosphates in guinea pig and pig tissues were determined with the same LC system, an extremely high concentration of TTP, averaging 70% of total thiamine (26.1 nmol/g wet weight), was detected in adult pig skeletal muscle (9). In one extreme case 88.7% of the total thiamine (19.6 nmol/g wet weight) was present as TTP. The chromatogram is shown in Fig. 12. Chicken white skeletal muscle was also found to contain a high TTP to total thiamine ratio (70% at a total level of 1.9 nmol/g wet weight), while in chicken red muscle this ratio averaged 30% for the same amount of total thiamine (10).

The reversed-phase LC was also successfully applied to the analysis of animal tissues (104). A chromatogram of thiamine phosphates in rat liver is shown in Fig. 13. Although not indicated, thiamine was eluted by changing the mobile phase to 25% DMF-25 mM potassium phosphate buffer (pH 8.4). When 0.2 pmol of ThcTP was cochromatographed with the oxidized sample, the recovery was 103% (Fig. 13). Cellular concentrations of TTP, TPP and TMP in different tissues determined by reversed-phase LC (104) agree with those determined by straight-phase LC (Table 2). This reversed-phase LC system allows detection of a sharp peak of tissue TTP without any interfering peak in the blank (Fig. 13).

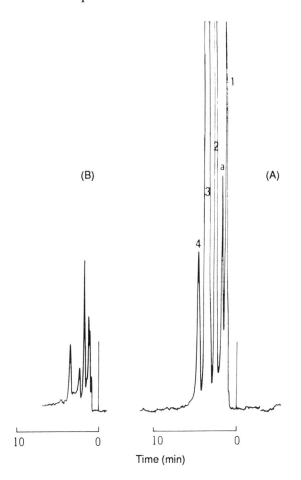

Figure 10   Elution pattern of thiamine and its phosphates in rat liver analyzed by the improved straight-phase LC system: (A) sample; (B) blank; (1) thiamine; (2) TMP; (3) TPP; (4) TTP; and (a) unidentified peak.

With the reversed-phase LC method described above (110), Matsuda et al. determined the contents of thiamine and its phosphates in various tissues of different animals (57,58). Total thiamine and TPP levels in the brain and kidney were significantly higher in the particulate fraction than in the soluble one, while those in the liver, soleus muscle (red muscle), and EDL (extensor digitorum longus: white muscle) muscle were markedly lower in the former fraction than in the latter.

TTP was localized in the particulate fraction in the brain, heart and kidney, while in the liver, soleus, and EDL muscles it occurred mainly

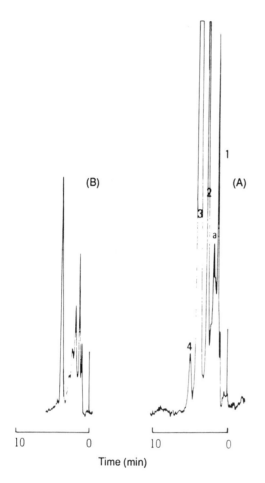

Figure 11 Elution profile of thiamine and its phosphates in the rat brain analyzed by the improved straight-phase LC system: (A) sample and (B) blank. Symbols are the same as in Fig. 10.

in the soluble fraction. In the pig skeletal muscle, especially in the white muscle, the soluble fraction contained TTP to the extent of 77% of total thiamine (Table 3), correlating well with the results reported elsewhere (9). Thiamine phosphates in these muscles were localized solely in the soluble fraction, and the TPP concentration was higher in the soleus than in the EDL (58).

Determination of Thiamine and Its Phosphates in Blood

As described above (section 3.3), the determination of total thiamine in blood specimens is important to assess thiamine status in humans as an

Table 2 Contents of Thiamine and Its Phosphate Esters in Rat Tissues[a]

Compound	Liver (nmol/g wet weight)	Brain (nmol/g wet weight)
Thiamine	1.45 ± 0.72 (4.8)	0.34 ± 0.13 (5.3)
TMP	3.98 ± 1.87 (13.2)	1.27 ± 0.60 (19.6)
TPP	24.02 ± 4.49 (79.7)	4.83 ± 0.49 (74.5)
TTP	0.68 ± 0.10 (2.3)	0.04 ± 0.02 (0.6)
Total thiamine	30.13	6.48

[a] Values represent the mean ± SD for five rats. The numbers in parentheses refer to percentages of total thiamine.

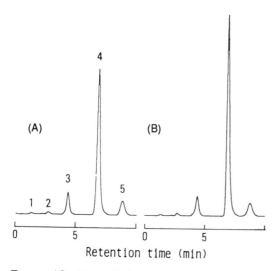

Figure 12 Typical chromatogram of thiamine phosphates in an extract of pig skeletal muscle: A, skeletal muscle extract; B, A plus 1 pmol of authentic TTP converted to ThcTP; 1, thiamine; 2, TMP; 3, TPP; 4, TTP; 5, unknown. (From Ref. 9.)

indicator for thiamine deficiency. Most of the LC methods include a hydrolysis step of the blood sample with an appropriate phosphatase before the LC step (96–101). Some of the other methods determine thiamine and its phosphates in blood specimens directly without enzymatic hydrolysis (109,111,115,116,118). Total thiamine is obtained by summing the levels of these thiamine forms (109,111,115,116).

Warnock (118) determined TPP in erythrocyte hemolysates by LC with precolumn derivatization using alkaline BrCN and fluorescence

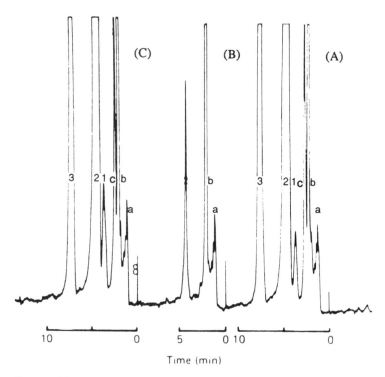

Figure 13 Chromatogram of thiamine phosphate esters in the rat liver: (A) sample; (B) blank; (C) sample plus 0.2 pmol ThcTP; (1) TTP; (2) TPP; (3) TMP; (a and b) peaks in the blank; (c) unidentified peak. (From Ref. 104.)

Table 3 Thiamine and Its Phosphate Esters in Soluble and Particulate Fractions of Pig Red and White Muscles[a]

	Content (pmol/mg protein)				
	Total	TTP	TDP	TMP	Thiamine
Red					
Soluble	330.2	164.7	132.6	23.7	9.2
Particulate	15.24	4.63	8.84	1.61	0.16
White					
Soluble	116.9	89.7	24.2	1.7	1.3
Particulate	12.27	1.80	9.72	0.75	ND

[a] Values are means of two determinations. From Ref. 58.

detection. The stationary phase was Bondapak-NH$_2$ and the mobile phase consisted of methanol-100 mM potassium phosphate buffer (pH 7.5) (50:50, v/v). A mean TPP value of 123 ±27 ng/ml packed normal human erythrocytes was obtained, which is consistent with results obtained previously using an enzymatic method (119).

A reversed-phase LC method with postcolumn derivatization (107) was used by Kimura and Itokawa (115) to determine thiamine and its phosphates in blood of humans as well as of various animals. Human whole blood was shown to contain TPP in the highest concentration, followed by TTP, and TMP and thiamine in undetectable amounts. TPP was calculated to be 70% of the total thiamine content while TTP accounted for 30%. This ratio of TTP to total thiamine in human whole blood is quite high compared to 1.5% (111) and 3.5% (116) obtained in other studies.

More recently, Brunnekreeft et al. (111) also reported the determination of thiamine and its phosphates in human whole blood. Sixty-five samples were obtained from healthy volunteers. The mean level (±SD) of TPP was 120 ±17.5 nmol/liter versus 4.1 ±1.6 nmol/liter, for TMP, and 4.3 ±1.9 nmol/liter for thiamine. For TTP, levels were all below 4.0 nmol/liter. Total thiamine calculated was 132 nmol/liter (mean), which is in good agreement with the results reported by Schrijver et al. (99; also personal communication).

We also analyzed the content of thiamine and its phosphates in human blood by straight-phase LC with precolumn derivatization (105). Blood samples were obtained from 12 healthy volunteers after a 12-h fasting period. The mean (±SD) values in nmol/liter were 2.23 ±1.24 for TTP, 51.6 ±8.01 for TPP, 4.77 ±1.24 for TMP, 5.39 ±2.58 for thiamine, and 64.0 ±7.90 for total thiamine (116). The mean total thiamine is lower than what has been described by others (99,111), which is probably due to the fasting conditions before blood sampling.

Thiamine Metabolism in Animal Tissues

To study the cell metabolism of thiamine and its phosphates, a disulfide derivative of thiamine, thiamine tetrahydrofurfuryldisulfide (TTFD) hydrochloride, was injected intraperitoneally into rats at 25 mg/kg body weight. The animals were sacrificed at various times after injection, and their livers were assayed for changes in thiamine and thiamine phosphate levels. Concentrations were determined by straight-phase LC. Patterns of changes in the contents of thiamine compounds are shown in Fig. 14.

The concentration of thiamine rapidly rose to a peak level 1 h after injection and then decreased fairly rapidly. This was followed by a rise in TPP levels, which were one-third lower than the maximal thiamine level. Thiamine pyrophosphate remained at the plateau for 2 h before

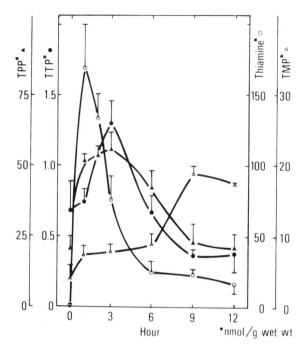

Figure 14   Profile of changes in content of thiamine and its phosphates in the liver of rats injected intraperitoneally with thiamine tetrahydrofurfuryldisulfide: ○, thiamine; △, TMP; ▲, TPP; ●, TTP. (From Ref. 120.)

gradually decreasing. The concentration of TTP, after an initial lag time, rose to a maximum peak concentration 3 h after injection. These results indicate a net increase of TTP in vivo, followed by a rapid reduction in concentration (120). It is clear that the HPLC technique used in this experiment was quite adequate to study thiamine metabolism.

4.   GAS CHROMATOGRAPHY

4.1   Introduction

Gas chromatography (GC) is a fast, selective, and sensitive analytical method that is useful for relatively volatile compounds. The polar nature and low volatility of thiamine prohibit its direct analysis at temperatures at which it is stable. Derivatization of thiamine prior to GC analysis is therefore required. Hilker and Mee (80) reported a GC analysis of trifluoroacetyl derivatives of thiamine and TPP on a polar stationary phase, ethylene glycol adipate. They obtained a separation of TPP (t_r 3.6 min) from coeluting thiamine and thiochrome (t_r 7.4 min). The detection limit was less than 0.5 μg (1.5 nmol) for thiamine. Analyzing 20 μl of rat plasma, thiamine and TPP were detectable. This procedure remains, however, qualitative (80).

Dwivedi and Arnold (81) were the first to report the GC determination of thiamine after cleavage with NaHSO$_3$ to 4-methyl-5-(2-hydroxyethyl)thiazole, a relatively volatile compound. However, the procedure suffered from the need to maintain the column at low temperatures to prevent decomposition of the thiazole.

Echols et al. (82) modified the procedure of Dwivedi and Arnold by using a flame-ionization detector (FID) and a nitrogen phophorus detector (NPD) as part of internal and external standard methods, respectively. They determined the thiamine content in pharmaceutical vitamin formulations. With the same GC system, Echols et al. (83) could determine thiamine amounts in meat, vegetables, and cereals.

4.2 Procedures for Determination

A procedure used for the determination of thiamine in meat (83) is briefly described.

Meat was homogenized in 0.1 M HCl and heated at 100°C for 1 h, cooled, and adjusted to a pH of 4.5–5. The mixture was then subjected to enzymatic hydrolysis with mylase 100 and papain for 4 h at 45–50°C. To cleave thiamine to 4-methyl-5-(2-hydroxyethyl)thiazole, NaHSO$_3$ or Na$_2$SO$_3$ was added, the pH was readjusted to 4–5, and the mixture was again heated at 100°C for 2 h. After the addition of trichloroacetic acid (TCA), the mixture was chilled and filtered. The filtrate was adjusted to a pH of 11–12 and then extracted with chloroform, which was evaporated to dryness. The residue was taken up in 1 ml of the internal standard solution and the latter was concentrated to 0.5 ml. The resulting sample was stored for analysis.

The internal standard used was 2-(hydroxyethyl)pyridine (I), dissolved in methanol (2 mg/ml) and diluted appropriately. The calibration standard was 4-methyl-5-(2-hydroxyethyl)thiazole (II), which was obtained commercially or by cleavage of thiamine with NaHSO$_3$, as described above. The calibration was done by use of aliquots of the standard solution of compound II, which were mixed with an aliquot of compound I and then chromatographed by GC at an appropriate temperature. The difference in the retention times of compounds I and II is quite clear and can vary from less than 1 to 5 min, depending on the temperatures. The concentration of a given standard obtained by the cleavage of thiamine agreed within 5% with a calibration standard of the same concentration prepared from compound II.

Values obtained for the meat analyses by the GC method are given in Table 4 and compared with those obtained by the Official AOAC

Table 4   Thiamine Contents in Meats[a]

		GC method		AOAC method
Type	μg/5g	μg/5 g plus 20 μg thiamine	μg/g	μg/g
Calf liver	25.3 ± 4.0	46.1 ± 5.9	5.1 ± 0.8	4.5 ± 0.9
Pork liver	20.2 ± 2.0	42.3 ± 3.8	4.0 ± 0.4	3.4 ± 0.5
Pork chops	54.6 ± 1.6	74.2 ± 2.1	10.9 ± 0.3	8.8 ± 0.8
Chicken	7.2 ± 1.5	28.2 ± 0.2	1.4 ± 0.3	1.8 ± 0.2
Ground beef	10.5 ± 0.9	30.5 ± 2.4	2.1 ± 0.2	1.5 ± 0.3

[a] From Ref. 83.

method (AOAC, 1980). Deviation from the experimental mean of ten trials was usually within ±10%. The detection limit of this GC method for thiamine is 0.8 μg/ml (82), corresponding to 2.4 pmol injected.

Advantages of the GC method are its simplicity, ease of standardization, and lack of cleanup steps in the sample preparation. Disadvantages are the relatively large amount of sample required and the inability to separate thiamine phosphate esters.

5. FUTURE TRENDS

High-performance liquid chromatography is a useful technique for the quantitative determination of thiamine and its phosphate esters not only in pharmaceutical preparations but also in biological materials, especially clinical specimens.

HPLC systems have rapidly proliferated since the first edition of this book. The detection limit for thiamine as well as thiamine phosphates as obtained with fluorescence detection is now in the fmol range. This allows the accurate determination of these compounds in human blood samples.

TTP was found to be the predominant thiamine form (approximately 70% of total thiamine) in pig skeletal muscle (9,58) and in chicken white muscle (10). TTP can be analyzed both by straight-phase LC (9,10) and reversed-phase LC (58). The biological role of TTP remains to be elucidated.

The analysis of total thiamine in human whole blood is important to assess thiamine deficiency. This can be carried out successfully by LC either with or without enzymatic hydrolysis. Reversed-phase LC (111) and straight-phase LC (116) are both useful for this purpose.

Finally, LC systems should be developed for a simultaneous determination of thiamine and other water-soluble vitamins in clinical specimens to assess multivitamin deficiencies.

REFERENCES

1. C. J. Gubler, in *Handbook of Vitamins: Nutritional, Biochemical and Clinical Aspects* (L. J. Machlin, ed.), Marcel Dekker, New York, p. 245 (1984).
2. K. Takaki, *Lancet*, *1*, 1369, 1451 (1906).
3. R. R. Williams and J. K. Cline, *J. Am. Chem. Soc.*, *58*, 1504 (1936).
4. N. Gavrilescu and R. A. Peters, *Biochem. J.*, *25*, 1397 (1931).
5. N. Gavrilescu, A. P. Meiklejohn, R. Passmore, and R. A. Peters, *Proc. R. Soc.*, *Ser. B*, *110*, 431 (1932).
6. K. Lohmann, and P. Schuster, *Biochem. Z.*, *294*, 188 (1937).
7. *Merck Index*, 11th ed. (S. Budavari, ed.), Merck & Co., Rahway, NJ, p. 1464 (1989).
8. B. C. P. Jansen, in *The Vitamins*, 2nd ed., Vol. 5 (W. H. Sebrell, Jr. and R. S. Harris, eds.), Academic Press, New York, p. 99. (1972).
9. Y. Egi, S. Koyama, H. Shikata, K. Yamada, and T. Kawasaki, *Biochem. Int.*, *12*, 385 (1986).
10. K. Miyoshi, Y. Egi, T. Shioda, and T. Kawasaki, *J. Biochem.*, *108*, 267 (1990).
11. S. Yurugi, in *Experimental Procedures in Biochemistry*, Vol. 13, *Vitamins & Coenzymes*, Japan Biochemical Society, Kagakudojin, Tokyo, p. 60 (1975).
12. M. Fujiwara and K. Matsui, *Anal. Chem.*, *25*, 810 (1953).
13. F. Bergel and A. R. Todd, *Chem. Ber.*, *68*, 2257 (1935).
14. F. Bergel and A. R. Todd, *J. Chem. Soc.*, 1601 (1936).
15. F. Bergel and A. R. Todd, *J. Chem. Soc.*, 365 (1937).
16. D. J. Hennesy and L. R. Cerecedo, *J. Am. Chem. Soc.*, *61*, 179 (1939).
17. W. Hamanaka, *Vitamins*, *32*, 576 (1965).
18. K. Ishii, K. Sarai, H. Sanemori, and T. Kawasaki, *Anal. Biochem.*, *97*, 191 (1979).
19. M. Morita, Y. Nishibe, and T. Mineshita, *J. Vitaminol. (Kyoto)*, *14*, 67 (1968).
20. Y. Shibata, *J. Biochem.*, *59*, 76 (1966).
21. D. T. Wyatt, M. Lee, and R. E. Hillman, *Clin. Chem.*, *35*, 2173 (1989).
22. G. Rindi and U. Ventura, *Physiol. Rev.*, *52*, 821 (1972).
23. R. C. Rose, *Annu. Rev. Physiol.*, *42*, 157 (1980).
24. A. M. Hoyumpa, H. M. Hiddleton, F. A. Wilson, and S. Schenker, *Gastroenterology*, *68*, 1218 (1975).
25. T. Komai, K. Kawai, and H. Shindo, *J. Nutr. Sci. Vitaminol.*, *20*, 163 (1974).
26. U. Ventura and G. Rindi, *Experientia*, *21*, 645 (1965).
27. V. Basilico, G. Ferrari, G. Rindi, and G. D'Andrea, *Arch. Int. Physiol. Biochim.*, *87*, 981 (1979).

28. G. Rindi and G. Ferrari, *Experientia, 33*, 211 (1977).
29. G. Rindi and U. Ventura, *Experientia, 23*, 175 (1967).
30. U. Ventura, G. Ferrari, R. Tagliabue, and G. Rindi, *Life Sci., 8*, 699 (1969).
31. T. Komai and H. Shindio, *J. Vitaminol. (Kyoto), 18*, 55 (1972).
32. K. Hayashi, S. Yamamoto, K. Ohe, A. Miyoshi, and T. Kawasaki, *Biochim. Biophys. Acta, 601*, 654 (1980).
33. O. Satoh, Y. Kudo, H. Shikata, K. Yamada, and T. Kawasaki, *Biochim. Biophys. Acta, 985*, 120 (1989).
34. K. Hayashi, S. Yoshida, and T. Kawasaki, *Biochim. Biophys. Acta, 641*, 106 (1981).
35. D. Casirola, G. Ferrari, G. Gastaldi, C. Patrini, and G. Rindi, *J. Physiol., 398*, 329 (1988).
36. G. Cusaro, G. Rindi, and G. Sciorelli, *Int. J. Vitaminol. Nutr. Res., 47*, 99 (1977).
37. Y. Mano, *J. Biochem., 47*, 283 (1960).
38. L. R. Johnson and C. J. Gubler, *Biochim. Biophys. Acta, 156*, 85 (1968).
39. J. W. Peterson, C. J. Gubler, and S. A. Kuby, *Biochim. Biophys. Acta, 397*, 377 (1975).
40. T. Wakabayashi, *Vitamins, 52*, 223 (1978).
41. M. Hamada, *J. Jpn. Biochem. Soc., 41*, 837 (1969).
42. Z. Suzuoki, K. Furuno, K. Murakami, T. Fujita, T. Matsuoka, and K. Takeda, *J. Nutr., 94*, 427 (1968).
43. H. Mitsuda, Y. Takii, K. Iwami, and K. Yasumoto, *J. Nutr. Sci. Vitaminol., 21*, 189 (1975).
44. Y. Kaziro, *J. Biochem., 46*, 1523 (1959).
45. H. Sanemori, Y. Egi, and T. Kawasaki, *J. Bacteriol., 126*, 1030 (1976).
46. H. Sanemori and T. Kawasaki, *J. Biochem., 88*, 223 (1980).
47. A. Iwashima, H. Nishino, and Y. Nose, *Biochim. Biophys. Acta, 258*, 333 (1972).
48. H. Nakayama and R. Hayashi, *J. Bacteriol., 112*, 1118 (1972).
49. H. Nishino, *J. Biochem., 72*, 1093 (1972).
50. H. Nishino, A. Iwashima, and Y. Nose, *Biochem. Biophys. Res. Commun., 45*, 363 (1971).
51. T. Yusa, *Plant Cell. Physiol., 2*, 471 (1961).
52. Y. Itokawa and J. R. Cooper, *Biochim. Biophys. Acta, 196*, 274 (1970).
53. J. H. Pincus, Y. Itokawa, and J. R. Cooper, *Neurology, 19*, 841 (1969).
54. J. Schrijver, T. Dias, and F. A. Hommes, *Neurochem. Res., 3*, 699 (1977).
55. H. Shikata, S. Koyama, Y. Egi, K. Yamada, and T. Kawasaki, *Biochem. Int., 19*, 933 (1989).
56. H. Shikata, Y. Egi, S. Koyama, K. Yamada, and T. Kawasaki, *Biochem. Int., 18*, 943 (1989).
57. T. Matsuda, H. Tonomura, A. Baba, and H. Iwata, *Comp. Biochem. Physiol., 94B*, 399 (1988).
58. T. Matsuda, H. Tonomura, A. Baba, and H. Iwata, *Comp. Biochem. Physiol., 94B*, 405 (1988).

59. L. O. Krampitz, *Annu. Rev. Biochem.*, *38*, 213 (1968).
60. R. L. Barchi, in *Thiamine* (C. J. Gubler, M. Fujiwara, and P. M. Dreyfus, eds.), John Wiley and Sons, New York, p. 283 (1976).
61. L. Eder and Y. Dunant, *J. Neurochem.*, *35*, 1278 (1980).
62. H. P. Gurtner, *Helv. Physiol. Pharmacol. Acta (Suppl.)*, *11*, 1 (1961).
63. A. Von Muralt, *Vitam. Horm.*, *5*, 93 (1947).
64. L. Bettendorf, P. Wins, and E. Schoffeniels, *Biochem. Biophys. Res. Commun.*, *154*, 942 (1988).
65. L. Bettendorf, C. Grandfils, P. Wins, and E. Schoffeniels, *J. Neurochem.*, *53*, 738 (1989).
66. L. Bettendorf, P. Wins, and E. Schoffeniels, *Biochem. Biophys. Res. Commun.*, *171*, 1137 (1990).
67. A. Rossi-Fanelli, N. Siliprandi, and P. Fasella, *Science*, *116*, 711 (1952).
68. D. Siliprandi and N. Siliprandi, *Biochim. Biophys. Acta*, *14*, 52 (1954).
69. L. M. Lewin, and R. Wei, *Anal. Biochem.*, *16*, 29 (1966).
70. K. H. Kiessling, *Biochim, Biophys. Acta*, *46*, 603 (1961).
71. Z. Z. Ziporin and P. P. Waring, *Methods Enzymol.*, *18A*, 86 (1970).
72. C. Levorato and L. Cima, *J. Chromatogr.*, *32*, 771 (1968).
73. T. Bican-Fister and V. Drazin, *J. Chromatogr.*, *77*, 389 (1973).
74. W. Schlemmer and E. Kammerl, *J. Chromatogr.*, *82*, 143 (1973).
75. S. A. Ismaiel and D. A. Yassa, *Analyst*, *98*, 816 (1973).
76. G. Rindi and L. de Giuseppe, *Biochem. J.*, *78*, 602 (1962).
77. H. Koike, T. Wada, and H. Minakami, *J. Biochem.*, *62*, 492 (1967).
78. J. M. Parkhomenko, A. A. Rybina, and A. G. Khalmuradov, *Methods Enzymol.*, *62*, 59 (1979).
79. A. D. Gounaris and M. Schulman, *Anal. Biochem.*, *102*, 145 (1980).
80. D. M. Hilker and J. M. L. Mee, *J. Chromatogr.*, *76*, 239 (1973).
81. B. K. Dwivedi and R. G. Arnold, *J. Food Sci.*, *37*, 889 (1972).
82. R. E. Echols, J. Harris, and R. T. Miller, Jr., *J. Chromatogr.*, *193*, 470 (1980).
83. R. E. Echols, R. H. Miller, W. Winzer, D. J. Carmen, and Y. R. Ireland, *J. Chromatogr.*, *262*, 257 (1983).
84. R. L. Kirchmeier and R. P. Upton, *J. Pharm. Sci.*, *67*, 1444 (1978).
85. M. C. Walker, B. E. Carpenter, and E. L. Cooper, *J. Pharm. Sci.*, *70*, 99 (1981).
86. R. B. H. Wills, C. G. Shaw, and W. R. Day, *J. Chromatogr. Sci.*, *15*, 262 (1977).
87. R. M. Kothari and M. W. Taylor, *J. Chromatogr.*, *247*, 187 (1982).
88. N. Amin and J. Reusch, *J. Chromatogr.*, *390*, 448 (1987).
89. C. Y. W. Ang and F. A. Moseley, *J. Agric. Food Chem.*, *28*, 483 (1980).
90. J. F. Kamman, T. P. Labuza, and J. J. Wartesen, *J. Food Sci.*, *45*, 1497 (1980).
91. R. B. Toma and M. M. Tabekhia, *J. Food Sci.*, *44*, 263 (1979).
92. D. M. Hilker and A. J. Clifford, *J. Chromatogr.*, *231*, 433 (1982).
93. H. Ohta, T. Baba, Y. Suzuki, and E. Okada, *J. Chromatogr.*, *284*, 281 (1984).
94. D. J. Mauro and D. L. Wetzel, *J. Chromatogr.*, *299*, 281 (1984).

95. P. Wimalasiri and R. B. H. Wills, *J. Chromatogr.*, *318*, 412 (1985).
96. R. L. Roser, A. H. Andrist, Y. H. Harrington, H. K. Naito, and D. Lonsdale, *J. Chromatogr.*, *146*, 43 (1978).
97. K. Yasuda, R. Ikeda, and A. Kawada, *Clin. Pathol.* (Japanese), *29*, 564 (1981).
98. E. Kimura, T. Fujita, and Y. Itokawa, *Clin. Chem.*, *28*, 29 (1982).
99. J. Schrijver, A. J. Speek, J. A. Klosse, H. J. M. VanRijn, and W. H. P. Schreurs, *Ann. Clin. Biochem.*, *19*, 52 (1982).
100. J. P. M. Wielders and C. J. K. Mink, *J. Chromatogr.*, *277*, 145 (1983).
101. W. Weber and H. Kewitz, *Eur. J. Clin. Pharmacol.*, *28*, 213 (1985).
102. C. J. Gubler and B. C. Hemming, *Methods Enzymol.*, *62*, 63 (1979).
103. K. Ishii, K. Sarai, H. Sanemori, and T. Kawasaki, *J. Nutr. Sci. Vitaminol.*, *25*, 517 (1979).
104. H. Sanemori, H. Ueki, and T. Kawasaki, *Anal. Biochem.*, *107*, 541 (1980).
105. T. Kawasaki, *Methods Enzymol.*, *122*, 15 (1986).
106. E. Kimura, T. Fujita, S. Nishida, and Y. Itokawa, *J. Chromatogr.*, *188*, 417 (1980).
107. E. Kimura, B. Panijpan, and Y. Itokawa, *J. Chromatogr.*, *245*, 141 (1982).
108. J. Bontemps, P. Phillippe, L. Bettendorff, J. Lombet, G. Dandrifosse, and E. Schoffeniels, *J. Chromatogr.*, *307*, 283 (1984).
109. L. Bettendorff, C. Grandfils, C. DeRycker, and E. Schoffeniels, *J. Chromatogr.*, *382*, 297 (1986).
110. H. Iwata, T. Matsuda, and H. Tonomura, *J. Chromatogr.*, *450*, 317 (1988).
111. J. W. I. Brunnekreeft, H. Eidhof, and J. Gerrits, *J. Chromatogr.*, *491*, 89 (1989).
112. K. Callmer and L. Davies, *Chromatographia*, *7*, 644 (1974).
113. R. C. Williams, D. R. Baker, and J. A. Schmit, *J. Chromatogr. Sci.*, *11*, 618 (1973).
114. AACC, *Approved Methods of the AACC*, 7th ed., American Association of Cereal Chemists, St. Paul, MN (1962).
115. M. Kimura and Y. Itokawa, *J. Chromatogr.*, *332*, 181 (1985).
116. Y. Egi, and T. Kawasaki, manuscript in preparation.
117. C. L. Rumke, and P. D. Bezemer, *Ned. Tijdschr. Geneeskd.*, *116*, 1559 (1972).
118. L. G. Warnock, *Anal. Biochem.*, *126*, 394 (1982).
119. L. G. Warnock, C. R. Prudhomme, and C. Wagner, *J. Nutr.*, *108*, 421 (1978).
120. H. Sanemori and T. Kawasaki, *Experientia*, *38*, 1044 (1982).

9

FLAVINS

Peter Nielsen

Universitätskrankenhaus Eppendorf,
Hamburg, Germany

1. INTRODUCTION

1.1 History

More than 100 years ago, a fluorescent compound was isolated first from whey, and later from different biological materials, giving rise to several names such as lactochrome, ovoflavin, or lactoflavin. When it became clear that the yellow pigments, isolated from different sources, had a common structure, the new compound was named riboflavin (vitamin B_2) [for historical review see Wagner-Jauregg (1) and Hemmerich (2)].

In the years between 1933 and 1935 the structure and the main chemical reactions of riboflavin were studied and the chemical synthesis was performed. About the same time the coenzyme forms, flavin mononucleotide (FMN) and flavin adenine dinucleotide (FAD), were isolated in pure form and the structures were determined. After the Second World War, the epoch of flavin biochemistry began. Many flavoproteins were isolated and their fascinating physicochemical properties were studied.

Succinate dehydrogenase was the first enzyme found with the prosthetic group (FAD) covalently bound to the protein. It is clear now that a significant part of the total amount of flavin in the organism is covalently bound (mainly via carbon atom 8α). Another milestone in flavin research was the characterization of the flavosemiquinones, the first example of a stable flavin radical. In addition to riboflavin, FMN, and FAD, a number of flavin analogs with biological activities have been found in microorganisms and plants. Among these, the coenzyme factor F_{420} isolated from methanogenic bacteria should be mentioned, which has 5-deazaflavin as its chromophore.

1.2 Chemical Properties

Riboflavin, 7,8-dimethyl-10-(1'-D-ribityl)isoalloxazine (Fig. 1), is a yellow-green, light-sensitive compound, and is widely distributed in animal and plant cells.

In biological systems, the two coenzyme forms FMN and FAD (chemical structure: see Fig. 1) are predominant. The terms "flavin mononucleotide" and "flavin adenine dinucleotide" are actually incorrect, because FMN is no nucleotide and FAD is no dinucleotide. However, these names are still accepted. Some authors use the name riboflavin also to designate the coenzyme form of the vitamin and take vitamin B2 as a general term. In this text, the names riboflavin (RF), FMN, and FAD will be used as specific terms. Some basic physicochemical properties of these flavins are outlined in Table 1.

FAD can be hydrolyzed to form FMN and finally riboflavin, whereas the none-glycosidic bonding between the isoalloxazine ring and the ribityl side chain withstands hydrolysis.

Based on their unique tricyclic isoalloxazine structure (benzene, pyrimidine, and pyrazine ring), the reactivity of flavin compounds in chemical and biochemical reactions is very complex (for a recent general review see Ref. 3), and only some reactions that are important for the analysis of flavin compounds can be mentioned in this text.

Riboflavin and FMN are very sensitive to UV light (4). The effective photolysis of riboflavin is a complex, pH-dependent reaction, which results in the formation of 60–70 % lumiflavin in basic solutions or lumichrome in neutral or slightly acid solutions as the main component (Fig. 2). In contrast to riboflavin, lumiflavin can be extracted from biological samples with chloroform and measured photometrically (at 450 nm). The lumiflavin method has been widely used (see section 3.2) for analytical riboflavin determination in various sources.

When protected from light, riboflavin is rather stable in neutral and slightly acidic solutions. In basic solution, the pyrazine ring is opened to form 1,2-dihydro-6,7-dimethyl-2-oxo-D-ribityl-3-chinoxalincarbone acid and urea (5).

In acidic solution, a migration of the phosphate group in the 5'-position of FMN has to be considered that, starting from pure riboflavin 5'-phosphate, yields the formation of significant amounts of riboflavin

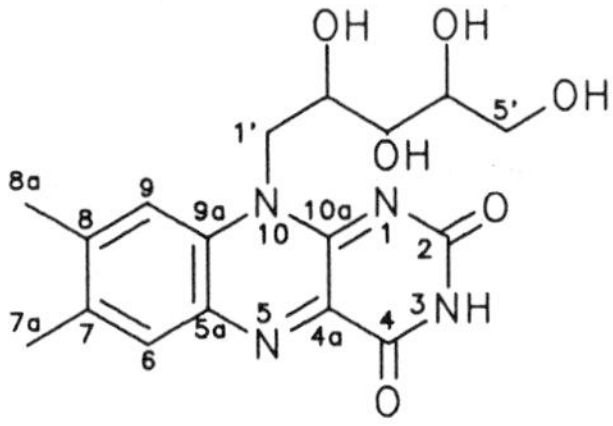

1

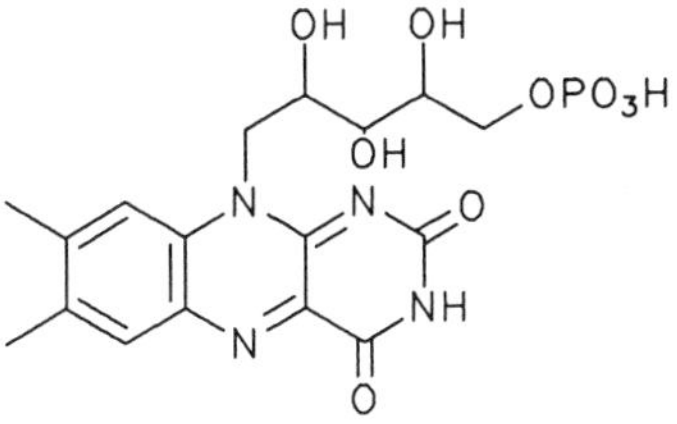

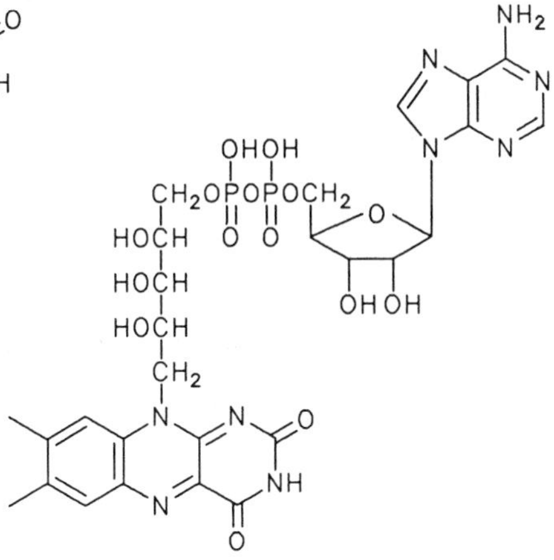

2 3

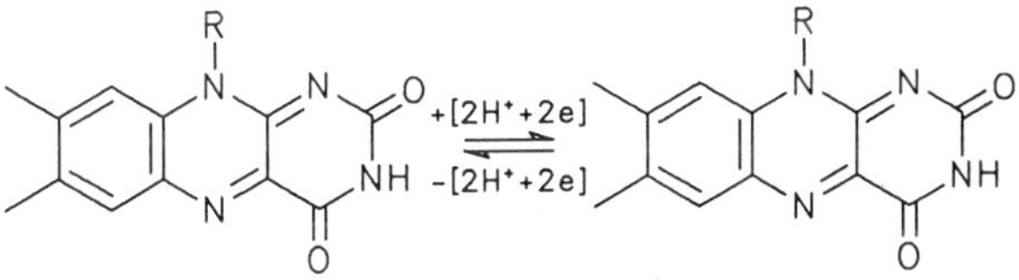

$1\,Fl_{ox}$ $1\,Fl_{red}$

Figure 1 Structural formulae of riboflavin, FMN, and FAD: 1, riboflavin in oxidized (FL_{ox}) or reduced form (FL_{red}); 2, FMN, flavin mononucleotide; 3, FAD, flavin adenine dinucleotide.

4′-, 3′-, and 2′-phosphate (6). In addition, the phosphoric ester group of FMN is hydrolyzed in acidic solution with a pH-maximum at about pH 4.0 (7).

The spectral properties of flavins in different oxidized and reduced states have been studied in detail (8,9). In the oxidized state (Fl_{ox}), flavins and flavoproteins are yellow pigments with two characteristic absorption bands at about 370 nm and 450 nm (Fig. 3).

Table 1 Physicochemical Properties of Riboflavin, FMN, and FAD

Compound	Structure	Relative molecular mass	Melting point (°C)	Solubility (g/liter)
Riboflavin	$C_{17}H_{20}N_4O_6$	376.4	278–282 dec.	Water: 0.10–0.13 Ethanol: 0.045 Insoluble: ether, CHCl$_3$, acetone
FMN(Na-salt)	$C_{17}H_{20}N_4NaO_9P$	478.4	>280–290 dec.	Water:30
FAD(Na$_2$-salt)	$C_{27}H_{31}N_9Na_2O_{15}P$	829.5	>280–290 dec.	Soluble in water

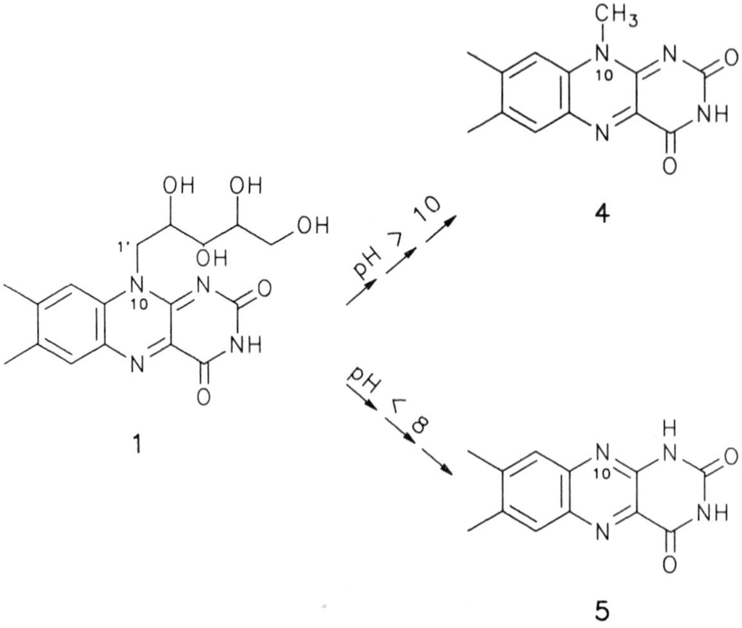

Figure 2 Photolysis of riboflavin: 1, riboflavin; 4, lumiflavin; 5, lumichrome.

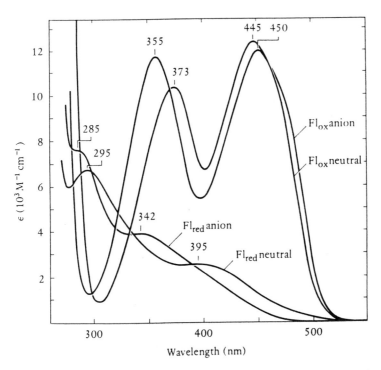

Figure 3 Absorption spectrum of FMN in water in the oxidized (FL_{ox}), reduced (FL_{red}), neutral, and anionic states, according to Ghisla (9).

In solution, flavins show a green-yellow fluorescence with an emission maximum around 520–530 nm. Due to interactions with the protein shell, the emission of flavins may be quenched in flavoproteins. The fluorescence of riboflavin and FMN occurs with the same quantum yield, whereas the quantum yield is about 10 times less in FAD. Chemical modifications of the ring structure can change the emission spectrum drastically.

1.3 Biochemistry

Based on their tricyclic structure, flavin coenzymes are the most versatile catalysts in biological redox systems. As they can participate both in two- and one-electron processes, flavins can act as a redox switch between two-electron donors (NADH, succinate) and one-electron acceptors (heme proteins, iron-sulfur proteins). In addition, flavins can react with molecular oxygen. As a consequence, flavoproteins catalyze a large number of different chemical reactions (for a recent review see Ref. 3).

The specific catalytic function of a given flavoprotein is based on and regulated by the interaction between coenzyme and apoprotein. A simplified classification of the biological function of flavoproteins according to the different reaction types was given by Müller et al. (Table 2) (3). The problem of this and some earlier proposals of flavoprotein classification is the fact that a given flavoprotein can catalyze quite different redox reactions.

1.4   Physiological Function

Riboflavin is synthesized in plants and various microorganisms (for a review, see Ref. 10). The biosynthesis starts from guanosine 5′-triphosphate (compound 6) by the removal of C-8 from the purine ring and pyrophosphate from the ribosyl side chain (Fig. 4).

In yeasts, the next steps are rearrangement and reduction of the sugar residue followed by a deamination in position 2 of the pyrimidine ring. The 5-amino-6-ribitylamino-2,4(1H,3H)-pyrimidinedione (compound 7) formed, reacts with 3,4-dihydroxybutanone 5′-phosphate (compound 8, derived from ribulose 5′-phosphate) to form 6,7-dimethyl-8-ribityllumazine (compound 9). Dismutation of two molecules of the lumazine results in the formation of riboflavin by the action of riboflavin synthase. In bacteria, the deamination in position 2 of the pyrimidine precedes the reduction of the ribosyl side chain.

Table 2   Functions of Flavoproteins[a]

Function	Typical reaction	Typical enzyme
I Dehydrogenation	$-CXH \rightarrow C=X + 2H^+ + 2e^-$ $(X = CH_2, NH, O)$	Acyl-CoA dehydrogenase
II O_2 activation (hydroxylation, monoxygenation)	$O_2 + 4e^- + 4H^+ \rightarrow 2H_2O$	P-Hydroxybenzoate hydroxylase
III Electron transfer	$+ e^-, - e^- \rightarrow 2e^- \rightarrow 1e^- + 1e^-$	Flavodoxin transhydrogenases
IV Light emission		Bacterial luciferase
V Photo(bio)chemistry	Phototropism	"Bluelight receptors"
VI Regulation (?)		Oxynitrilase Carboligase

[a] According to Müller et al. (3).

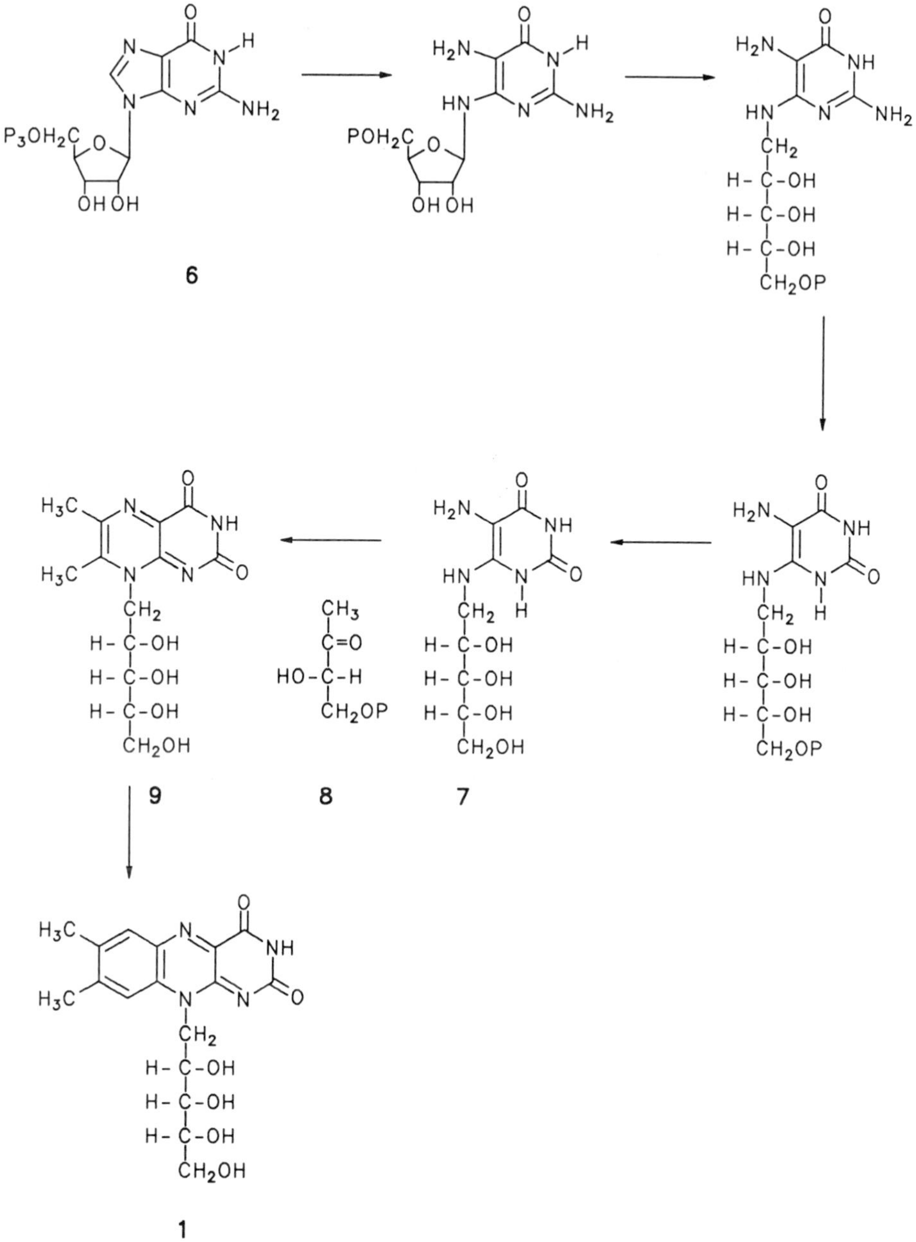

Figure 4 Biosynthesis of riboflavin in yeasts: 6, GTP; 7, 5-amino-6-ribitylamino-2,4(1*H*,3*H*)pyrimidine dione; 8, 3,4-dihydroxy-2-butanone 4-phosphate; 9, 6,7-dimethyl-8-ribityllumazine; 1, riboflavin.

According to the *Recommended Dietary Allowances*, 9th ed. (1980), a daily intake of 0.6 mg vitamin B_2/1000 kcal is desirable for an adult (11). Animal proteins (i.e., milk) and some vegetables (broccoli) are good sources of riboflavin, even when cooked. However, exposure to daylight, for example of milk, can destroy most of the riboflavin (70% loss in 4 h).

In humans, riboflavin is absorbed in the upper jejunum by a fast and saturable mechanism (12). FMN and FAD are hydrolyzed prior to intestinal absorption by the action of an FMN phosphatase and an FAD pyrophosphatase (13). Proteolytic digestion of food proteins containing covalently bound flavins results in the liberation of S-cysteinylriboflavin and N-histidylriboflavin. These compounds are absorbed in rats but seem to have no vitamin activity (14). In plasma, most of the riboflavin is weakly bound to albumin and more tightly bound to a subclass of immunoglobulins (12). A class of riboflavin-binding proteins has been found in liver, blood, and eggs of hens (15). These proteins are induced by estrogens and have a function in riboflavin storage and its transports to the ovarial follicles. Similar transport proteins have been found in pregnant mammals including humans (16).

Within the mammalian cells, most of the riboflavin is converted to FAD and FMN (Fig. 5).

Flavins are mainly excreted in human urine in the form of riboflavin and some catabolites (17).

Riboflavin deficiency causes a disease with pellagralike symptoms ("pellagra sine pellagra") (18). Lesions around the corner of the mouth (stomatitis angularis), cheilosis, glossitis, and seborrhoic changes at the nose and ears are the main symptoms of vitamin B2 deficiency. Insufficient dietary intake is the main cause of riboflavin deficiency in undeveloed countries, whereas alcoholism accounts for vitamin B_2 deficiency in economically strong countries. Besides the general malnu-

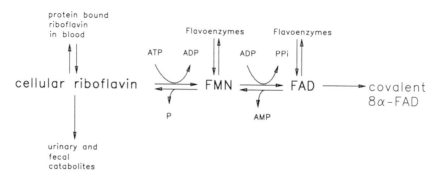

Figure 5   Metabolic pathways of riboflavin in mammals.

trition in alcoholics, ethanol seems to reduce the utilization of the vitamin, especially from FAD-containing sources (19).

Furthermore, riboflavin deficiency is found in newborn infants with hyperbilirubinemia, which were treated with phototherapy (20).

1.5 Pharmacological Function

Riboflavin and synthetic FMN are used in numerous pharmaceutical preparations for the prophylaxis and therapy of riboflavin deficiency. However, in western countries a clear indication for vitamin B2-treatment is rare. When newborn infants are given 0.5 mg FMN/day during phototherapy, a decrease in riboflavin status can be avoided. In some cases of inborn errors in the flavoprotein dependent metabolism of carboxylic acids, treatment with high doses of riboflavin alleviated some symptoms (21).

2. PAPER, THIN-LAYER, AND CONVENTIONAL COLUMN CHROMATOGRAPHY

2.1 Introduction

For the analytic determination of flavins in different matrices, paper chromatography has only historical interest, mainly due to its rather qualitative character. To a lesser degree, the same is true for thin-layer chromatography. However, when based on modern equipment, including a TLC densitometer, TLC may have some advantages in the field of flavin analysis even when compared with HPLC methods.

For preparative applications, conventional column chromatography (ion-exchange, gel, affinity chromatography) and paper and TLC chromatography are still valuable tools for isolation and purification of flavin compounds.

2.2 Paper Chromatography

Paper chromatography has been used for the separation and isolation of new flavin metabolites in rat urine. Ohkawa et al. orally administered a high dose (0.25 mg/kg) of [2-^{14}C]riboflavin to rats and isolated new catabolites from rat urine (22). Flavins were extracted from 20 ml of acidified rat urine with phenol. After paper chromatography using paper Toyo no. 50 (Toyo Kagaku Co., Ltd., Tokyo) and a solvent mixture of n-butanol-glacial acetic acid-water (4:1:5, v/v, upper phase) two clearly separated radioactive peaks (accounting for 46% of total urinary activity) were observed in the radiochromatogram and were subsequently identified as 7-carboxylumichrome and 8-carboxylumichrome.

2.3   Thin-Layer Chromatography

As compared to paper chromatography, thin-layer chromatography (TLC) and its advanced form HPTLC (high-performance thin-layer chromatography) are more modern analytical methods. The benefit of TLC for identification of unknown flavin compounds by comparing R_f values of the unknown flavins with authentic material is beyond doubt (23). The quantification of the separated flavin compounds can be performed by the use of a modern densitometry. Various high-quality precoated plates with low and uniform particle diameters are available for HPTLC, including stationary phases of silica gel, cellulose, or various reversed phases (TLC-RP). For special applications, TLC may have some advantage, for example, in separation capability (multidimensional development), even when compared with HPLC.

Depending on the mobile phase, TLC can clearly differentiate riboflavin from FMN and some flavin analogs (Table 3) (7). In addition, riboflavin phosphates are separated from riboflavin bisphosphates,

Table 3   Thin-Layer Chromatography of Flavins[a]

Compound	Rf							
	I	II	III	IV	V	VI	VII	VIII
Riboflavin	0.42	0.54	0.41	0.81	0.74	0.93	0.57	0.53
5'-FMN	0.27	0.11	0.62	0.55	0.14	0.82	0.34	0.28
4'-FMN	0.30	0.12	0.64	0.56	0.21	0.82	0.39	0.29
3'-FMN	0.28	0.10	0.62	0.55	0.21	0.84	0.36	0.29
2'-FMN	0.31	0.11	0.68	0.55	0.12	0.82	0.36	0.31
4',5'-RBP[b]	0.16	0.04	0.67	0.52	0.05	0.46	0.27	0.09
3',5'-RBP	0.15	0.04	0.61	0.52	0.04	0.39	0.23	0.05
2',5'-RBP	0.16	0.04	0.62	0.52	0.04	0.32	0.25	0.14
3',4'-RBP	0.15	0.04	0.65	0.52	0.04	0.37	0.16	0.10
5-Deaza-FMN	0.36	0.27		0.54		0.85	0.43	0.36
5-Deaza-3',5'-RBP		0.15		0.42		0.18		0.10
Hexafluoro-5'-FMN	0.51	0.14		0.68			0.39	0.45

[a] Precoated cellulose or silica gel plates (Cellulose $\pm_{254}$, kiesel gel $60\pm_{254}$), (Merck AG, Darmstadt, West Germany) were developed with the solvent systems indicated: I, n-butanol/ethanol/water (50:15:35, v/v)/cellulose; II, n-butanol/ethanol/water (50:15:35, v/v)/silica gel; III, tert-butanol/water (60:40, v/v)/cellulose; IV, tert-butanol/water (60:40, v/v)/silica gel; V, collidine/water (75:25, v/v)/cellulose; VI, collidine/water (75:25, v/v) silica gel; VII, n-butanol/acetic acid/water (50:20:30, v/v)/cellulose; and VIII, n-butanol/acetic acid/water (50:20:30, v/v)/silica gel (from Ref. 7).

[b] RBP, riboflavin bisphosphate.

whereas the isomeric riboflavin phosphates comigrate in all systems under study.

TLC was used for both qualitative (24–27) and quantitative analysis (28–30) of riboflavin in different matrices (Table 4). The separation and identification of vitamin B_2 from other water-soluble vitamins (B_1, B_6, B_{12}) (27) or fat-soluble vitamins (A, D_2, and E) (24) in multivitamin preparations can be performed by TLC methods. The sensitive determination of riboflavin from pollen and vitamin B complexes by scanning densitometry or spectrophotometry after elution of the compounds from the TLC plate was demonstrated (29,30).

An interesting application of TLC was reported by Bochner and Ames (31). These authors described a complete analysis of cellular nucleotides (including FMN and FAD) from $^{32}P_i$-labeled cells of *Salmonella typhimurium* by two-dimensional thin-layer chromatography. Nucleotides were extracted from appropriate cell cultures with cold formic acid (pH 2.0). After centrifugation, the supernatant was neutralized and applied to precoated polyethyleneimine cellulose TLC plates (anion-exchange PEI-cellulose). In the first dimension the nucleotides (including FMN and FAD) were separated based on the negative charge of their phosphate groups (i.e., cyclic, mono-, di-, triphosphates) by the use of aqueous solutions of amine chlorides (i.e., Tris-HCl) at pH 8.0. In the second dimension, the use of saturated ammonium sulfate as mobile phase resulted in a separation due to the presence of different nucleobases. This analytical technique provides a metabolic fingerprint of the intracellular nucleotide pools.

It should be mentioned that similar results were achieved by HPLC and included quantitative determination of nucleotides (see section 3.4).

2.4 Ion-Exchange Chromatography

Conventional ion-exchange chromatography is a useful technique for the preparation of substantial amounts of purified FMN and FAD.

The separation of FMN from riboflavin and riboflavin bisphosphates can be achieved efficiently on DEAE-Sephacel (acetate form) with a discontinuous gradient of triethylammonium acetate pH 7.0 in 30% 2-propanol as mobile phase (7). This has some practical relevance because commercial preparations of FMN contain significant amounts of riboflavin and riboflavin bisphosphates (6). The riboflavin monophosphate fraction obtained by this chromatographic technique still consists of an isomeric mixture of riboflavin 5'-, 4'-, and 3'-phosphate. Milligram amounts of almost pure FMN can be obtained by ion-exchange chromatography on DEAE-cellulose (chloride form) eluted with ammonium

Table 4 Determination of Riboflavin by Thin-Layer Chromatography

Reference	Source	Stationary phase	Mobile phase	Detection
			Qualitative determination	
Thielemann (1981) (24)	Multivitamin preparation	UV-254 (CSSR)	Water	Chlorine-tolidine staining
Airaudo (1983) (25)	Natural dyes	Silica gel	Butanol/ethanol/water (2:1:1, v/v/v)	
Kawanabe (1985) (26)	Multivitamin preparation	Cellulose Wakogel HEC-LR250	Chloroform/ethanol/acetic acid (100:50:1, v/v/v)	UV-detection sensitivity: 1μg
Bhushan (1987) (27)	Multivitamin preparation	Silica gel	(a) Butanol/acetic acid/water (9:4:5, v/v/v) (b) Butanol/benzene/acetic acid/water (8:7:5:3, v/v/v/v)	
			Quantitative determination	
Ni (1985) (28)	Multivitamin preparation	Silica gel HF$_{254}$	Chloroform/ethanol/acetic acid/water (54:27:9:4, v/v/v/v)	Reflectance densitometry 444 nm
Chen (1986) (29)	Pollen	Silica gel HF$_{254}$	Chloroform/ethanol/acetic acid/water (53:20:25:2, v/v/v/v)	Densitometry 445 nm Detection limit 0.1 μg
Chen (1986) (30)	Liquid vitamin B complex	Silica gel HF$_{254}$	Chloroform/ethanol/acetic acid/water (54:27:9:4, v/v/v/v)	Elution with acetate buffer, followed by spectrophotometry at 444 nm

carbonate, pH 7.8 (7,32), or by preparative HPLC (6,7). Pure FAD in 500-mg amounts (98%) were prepared from the culture broth of *Sarcina lutea* by the method of Chibata et al. (33). This method involves adsorption of the crude FAD on Florisil followed by ion-exchange chromatography on Amberlite IRA-401 and a final purification step on *p*-acetoxymercurianiline-agarose. A biosynthetic method for the preparation of labeled FMN and FAD ([^{14}C]riboflavin, [^{14}C- or ^{3}H]adenine, or [^{32}P]phosphate labeling) using *Clostridium kluyveri* was described by Decker and Hamm (34). The separation of labeled FMN and FAD was achieved by ion-exchange chromatography on a DEAE-cellulose column. FMN was eluted with 3 mM HCl containing 15 mM LiCl. Subsequently, FAD was eluted with 3 mM HCl containing 30 mM LiCl.

2.5 Affinity Chromatography

It has been shown earlier that pure FMN can be obtained by chromatography on immobilized apoflavodoxin from *Megaspaera elsdenii* (35). An analogous purification technique has been presented for FAD using immobilized glucose oxidase and D-amino acid oxidase (36). The use of affinity chromatography on immobilized egg white riboflavin-binding apo-protein for separation of different flavin compounds was demonstrated by Kozik and Zak (37). A solution containing riboflavin, isoriboflavin, FAD, and FMN was applied to a column containing Bio-Gel P-150 coupled with riboflavin-binding apoprotein. The column was eluted with a linear gradient of pH (3.8 to 3.0) and ionic strength (0.5–1.0 M NaCl). This procedure resulted in a fair separation of the flavin coenzymes from isoriboflavin and riboflavin, whereas FMN and FAD coeluted.

2.6 Gel Chromatography

Using a two-column gel chromatographic system with the tightly cross-linked gels Sephadex G-15 and Bio-Gel P-2, Nagy et al. described the separation of very complex mixtures of flavins and flavin peptides (38). Besides the molecular sieving action of the gels, specific gel-solute interactions supposedly play an important role in this chromatographic system. As pointed out by the authors, an important application of this gel chromatographic system could be the purification of flavin coenzymes and flavin peptide adducts obtained by proteolytic digestion of flavoproteins.

3. HIGH-PERFORMANCE LIQUID CHROMATOGRAPHY

3.1 Introduction

With the development of high-performance (high-pressure) liquid chromatography (HPLC), the classical column chromatography technique has undergone a renaissance. In the field of flavin (bio)chemistry, HPLC is the analytical method of choice and has superseded other chromatographic methods more or less completely. The determination of riboflavin and flavin coenzyme as well as flavin degradation products, catabolites, or analogs from various sources, including pharmaceutical preparations, foods, and blood, have been described (see below).

Analytical Systems

STATIONARY PHASES.   Many different kinds of stationary phases are available for HPLC. Among these, reversed-phase columns (i.e., 18-C or 8-C alkyl chain length) are frequently used for chromatography of the water-soluble, ionic or nonionic flavin compounds.

MOBILE PHASE.   For reversed-phase HPLC, mixtures of methanol (or acetonitrile) and aqueous buffer solution are preferred for the chromatography of flavin compounds. Addition of ion-pair compounds (such as triethylammonium chloride or hexanesulfonates) can modify the retention behavior of ionic compounds (riboflavin phosphates, FAD) significantly (ion-pair HPLC).

DETECTION.   For routine HPLC analysis, the detection of flavins is carried out either spectrophotometrically, using variable-or fixed-wave length HPLC detectors in the ultraviolet (e.g., 254 nm) or visible (e.g., 405 nm) region, or fluorimetrically. For riboflavin, the excitation wavelength for fluorimetric detection is usually 440–450 nm, and the emission wavelength 530 nm. The detection limit for fluorescence detectors is better than 1 pmol (0.38 ng) riboflavin, whereas less than 30 pmol (11 ng) can be detected spectrophotometrically at 254 nm.

Photodiode array detectors have been applied to the determination of flavins in goat milk (39) and multivitamin preparations (40). However, these detectors are significantly less sensitive as compared to normal HPLC spectrophotometers (40). In the case of isomeric impurities (riboflavin phosphates) their use may lead to an erroneous conclusion of peak purity (41).

In combination with liquid chromatography, a number of new ("prototype") detectors have been described that offer more selectivity and sensitivity for flavin analysis as compared to the photometric of fluorimetric detectors.

A laser-based FDCD (fluorescence-detected circular dichroism) detector combines the selectivity of fluorescence and optical activity for the analysis of riboflavin (42). Using a common reversed-phase HPLC system, the detection limit for riboflavin is 170 pg. Further refinements in the laser sources and the modulation systems as well as extension of the detector principle to microbore HPLC may improve the sensitivity in the future.

A true on-column, laser-based fluorescence detector, which utilizes a portion of the capillary column as the detector cell, was constructed by Guthrie et al. (43). Using a 3 m × 25 μm (ID) fused silica capillary column without any stationary phase and acetonitrile/water (65:35, v/v) as the mobile phase, the minimum detectable amount of riboflavin injected on the column (excitation wavelength 442 nm) was found to be 35 fg. The detector linearity was demonstrated over 4.5 orders of magnitude. In principle, riboflavin can be detected by liquid chromatography mass spectrometry (LC-MS coupling) (44,45). The main problem for HPLC-MS coupling is the interface technique, which has to handle large volumes of effluents containing low-volatility compounds. Using thermospray ionization as an interface technique, the whole effluent of a standard 4.6-mm ID column with aqueous 0.1 M ammonium acetate solution as mobile phase and riboflavin as test compound was introduced into the mass spectrometer (44). In addition, the performance of a moving-belt interface for LC/MS was evaluated for the determination of riboflavin (45).

However, all these new detection principles described above have in common that their practical benefit for the determination of flavin compounds from different matrices is not yet obvious.

INTERNAL STANDARD. Theobromine (46), p-hydroxybenzoic acid (47), and nicotinamide (48) have been used as internal standards in HPLC determination of riboflavin. These compounds have solubilities in water similar to riboflavin; however, their chemical structures are quite different. Lambert et al. suggested isoriboflavin as a better internal standard for liquid-chromatographic determination of riboflavin in human urine because of its closer structural similarity (49).

3.2 Riboflavin

Numerous methods for the determination of riboflavin in pharmaceutical multivitamin preparations and food have been described. In biological samples, significant amounts of free (non-coenzymic) riboflavin are found only in the urine and in the retina of the eye, whereas protein-bound FAD and FMN are the predominant flavin species.

Pharmaceutical Preparations

Riboflavin is an ingredient of many pharmaceutical multivitamin preparations. Methods have been described for the determination of riboflavin and of other water-soluble vitamins (B_1, B_6, B_{12}, niacin, niacinamide, folic acid, ascorbic acid). For an efficient separation of the different compounds, ion-pair HPLC seems to be favored because this technique results in better peak shapes, especially of thiamine, pyridoxine, and folic acid, as compared to classical reversed-phase HPLC. Details of some methods are outlined in Table 5. No special pretreatment procedure is necessary. The finely powdered material is dissolved directly in the mobile phase (containing internal standard). After centrifugation or filtration, appropriate aliquots are injected directly onto the column. Reversed-phase C_8 or C_{18} columns and mixtures of methanol/acetonitrile with aqueous buffer solutions (containing different ion-pairing reagents) are used as stationary and mobile phases, respectively.

Walker et al. analyzed four vitamins (B_2, B_1, B_6, and niacinamide) in 12 multivitamin products and found a good correlation between the HPLC method and the results of non chromatographic assays (fluorimetric assay for riboflavin) (47). A typical baseline separation of water-soluble vitamins by ion-pair HPLC is given in Fig. 6 (51).

Dong et al. studied the factors affecting the ion-pair chromatography of water-soluble vitamins in some detail (55). Following comparison of six different reversed-phase columns (C_8 and C_{18}), it was found that the influence of the stationary phase on the separation quality is only limited. Riboflavin and folic acid have significantly higher k' values on C_{18} bonded phases, but baseline separation was obtained on all the column studied. Smaller particle size (3 and 5 μm) generated a higher resolution of the seven water-soluble vitamins. According to the authors, the mobile phase should contain 12.5–20% methanol as an organic modifier for optimum separation. Acetonitrile gave slightly sharper peaks but yielded inadequate separation of ascorbic acid and niacin. A concentration of 4–7 mM of 1-hexanesulfonate as ion-pairing reagent and a pH of 2.8–3.2 gave the best separation of all seven compounds. At 0.10–0.13%, triethylamine as an additive resulted in symmetrical peaks and the best separation of thiamine from riboflavin.

Foods

A review of different methods for the HPLC determination of riboflavin, thiamine, and niacin in foods was published in 1987 (56). From 1980 onward, numerous HPLC methods for the determination of riboflavin alone (59–64,66,71,73,78,79,82,83) or riboflavin together with other water-soluble vitamins such as thiamine (39,57,58,65,67–70,72,74–77,84,86) and/or niacin (58,67,86), ascorbic acid (39), or pyridoxine (75,81,84,86) in foods have been described (Table 6). Isocratic classical reversed-phase chromatography or ion-pair chromatography was used by all of the authors for the determination of vitamin B_2 in meat or meat

Table 5 HPLC determination of Riboflavin in Pharmaceutical Preparations

Reference	Column	Mobile phase	Detection	Other compounds detected simultaneously	Detection limit (d.l.) and linear range (l.r.)
Amin (1987) (50)	RP18-5μm LiChrosorb Vertex 25 × 0.4 cm	Methanol/water (50:50, v/v)	UV spectrometry, 254 nm	B_2, B_1, B_6, B_{12}	10 ng (d.l.) 20–100 ng (l.r.)
Vandemark (1981) (51)	RP8-10μm Perkin-Elmer 25 × 0.46 cm	Acetonitrile/water (10–90% gradient), 5 mM hexanesulfonic acid, pH 2.8	UV spectrometry, 246–293 nm	B_2, B_1, C, B_6 Niacin, niacinamide Folic acid	
Walker (1981) (47)	RP18 μBondapak Waters Associates	Methanol/water (25:75, v/v), 1% acetic acid, 3–8 mM Na-hexanesulfonate	UV spectrometry, 254, 280 nm	B_2, B_1, B_6 Niacinamide	360–840 ng (l.r.)
Vandemark (1981) (52)	RP8-10μm Perkin-Elmer 25 × 0.46 cm	A, methanol; B, 1% ammonium carbonate solution (gradient 0–100% A)	UV spectrometry, 272 nm	B_2, B_1, C, B_6 Niacinamide	
Jenkins (1982) (53)	RP18 μBondapak Waters Associates	Methanol/water/acetic acid (20:79:1, v/v/v) + 5 mM hexanesulfonic acid	UV spectrometry, 280 nm	B_2, B_1, C, B_6 Niacin, niacinamide Folic acid	150–750 ng (l.r.)
Amin (1987) (54)	RP18-10μm LiChrosorb Vertex 25 × 0.4 cm	Methanol/water/ phosphoric acid (85%) (55:45:1, v/v/v) + octane sulfonic acid, 650 mg/liter	UV spectrometry, 254 nm	B_2, B_1, B_6, B_{12} Nicotinamide, folic acid	5–10 ng (d.l.) (for all 7 vitamins)
Dong (1988) (55)	RP8-3μm Pecosphere-3CR 8.3 × 0.46 cm	Methanol/water (15:85), 5 mM Na-hexane sulfonate/1% acetic acid/ 0.10–0.13% triethylamine, pH 3.2	UV spectrometry, photodiode array	B_2, B_1, C, B_6 Niacin, niacinamide Folic acid	0.2 ng (?) (d.l.)

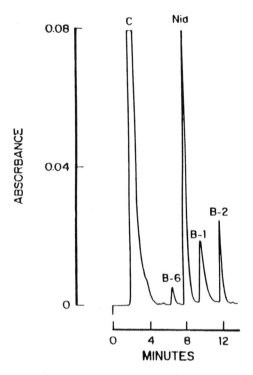

Figure 6 HPLC of water-soluble vitamins from a multivitamin preparation. C, ascorbic acid; B-1, thiamine; B-2, riboflavin; B-6, pyridoxine; Nia, niacinamide. Column, RP-8-10μm; eluant, methanol/1% ammonium carbonate (4ml/min); UV detection 272 nm (from Ref. 51).

products (57,58,67,68,72,73,76), cow milk (59–62,63,66,67), human milk (60), cereals (72,74–76), fruits and vegetables (68–70,72,79,80), and beverages (82–87).

As far as the chromatographic conditions are concerned (column, mobile phase), the variations between the different methods are only small (Table 6).

It should be mentioned that some methods have been applied only to selected foods and their general validity has not been demonstrated, whereas other methods were successfully used with a wide variety of different food matrices (63,66–73,76).

For simultaneous determination of riboflavin *and* thiamine in food, various workers have proposed HPLC methods, which analyze riboflavin either as riboflavin or lumiflavin and thiamine as thiochrome by fluorescence detection. The thiochrome was formed either before (57,65,67–

Table 6 HPLC Determination of Riboflavin in Foods

Reference	Source	Pretreatment	Column	Mobile phase	Detection	Detection limit	Results (mg B_2/100 g)
Ang (1980) (57)	Meat	Acid hydrolysis Enzymic hydrolysis Lumiflavin method	Silica-20μm Spherisorb 50 × 0.21 cm	Chloroform/methanol (90:10, v/v)	Fluorescence ex:270 nm em:418 nm	0.02 ng	0.14–0.22
Dawson (1988) (58)	Meat	Acid hydrolysis Enzymic hydrolysis	RP10-10μm Alltech	Methanol/0.02 M phosphate buffer, pH 7.0 (30:70, v/v)	Fluorescence ex: 464 nm em:540 nm	0.25 ng	0.16–0.22
Kneifel (1986) (59)	Cow milk	Acid hydrolysis Enzymic hydrolysis	RP18-10μm Nucleosil Macherey 25 × 0.4 cm	Methanol/0.1% NaH_2PO_4 (35:65 v/v), pH 3.0, + 5 mM heptanesulfonic acid	Fluorescence ex:375 nm em:525 nm	10μg/liter	0.22
Toyosaki (1986) (60)	Cow milk Human milk	Acidification centrifugation, filtration	RP18-5μm Cosmosil Nakari Chem. 15 × 0.46 cm	Methanol/water/acetic acid (45:65:0.1 v/v/v)	UV spectroscopy 254 nm	0.11–0.13 0.13 ±0.24	
Roughead (1990) (61)	Cow milk	Phenol extract	RP18 μBondapak Waters Associates 30 × 0.39 cm	Methanol/50 mM ammonium acetate buffer, pH 6.0, linear gradient	Fluorescence ex: 305–395 nm em:475–650 nm	0.54 B2 0.23 FAD	
Ribarova (1987) (62)	Cow milk Yogurt	Acid hydrolysis Filtration	RP-5μm Spherisorb 5ODS 25 × 0.45 cm	Acetonitrile/water (20:80 v/v)	Fluorescence ex:453 nm em:580 nm	0.5 ng	0.13–0.16 0.11–0.13
Lavigne (1987) (39)	Goat milk	Acid hydrolysis Enzymic hydrolysis	RP18-5μm Nova-Pak cartridge Sep-Pak cartridge	Methanol/water (30:70, v/v) + 5mM radial compress.	Photodiode array, hexanesulfonic acid	0.17 ± 0.01 200–400 nm	

Table 6 Continued

Reference	Source	Pretreatment	Column	Mobile phase	Detection	Detection limit	Results (mg B_2/100 g)
Ashoor (1983) (63)	Cow milk Yogurt Eggs Cheese	Water/MeOH suspension, acidification, centrifugation	RP18 μBondapak Water Assoc. 30 × 0.39 cm	Methanol/water/acetic acid (32:68:0.1 v/v)	UV spectroscopy 270 nm	10 ng	0.10–0.11 0.12 ± 0.10 0.32 ± 0.21 0.06–0.29
Stancher (1986) (64)	Italian cheese	Water/MeOH suspension, acidified, centrifuged	RP18-5μm LiChrosorb E. Merck 25 × 0.4 cm	Acetonitrile/water (20:80 v/v)	UV spectroscopy 267, 446 nm	2.5 ng	0.11–0.38
Kamman (1980) (65)	Fortified foods	Acid hydrolysis Enzymic hydrolysis	RP18-10μm μBondapak Waters Associates	Acetonitrile/10 mM phosphate Bufer (12.5:85.5, v/v) 5 mM Heptanesulfonic acid	UV spectroscopy 254 nm	5 ng	
Lumley (1981) (66)	Cow milk Flour Eggs Bread	Acid hydrolysis Enzymic hyrolysis	RP22 Magnusil Magnus Science 15 × 0.4 cm	Methanol/water/0.1 M Na₃-citrate/ 0.1M citric acid (40:10:38:12), pH 5.8	Fluorescence ex:449 nm em:520 nm		0.15 0.07 1.4 0.03–0.08
Skurray (1981) (67)	Cow milk Meat Bread Corn flakes	Acid hydrolysis Enzymic hydrolysis	RP18-10μm μBondapak Waters Associates 30 × 0.39 cm	0.2 M Acetate buffer (43:56:1 v/v), 5 mM heptanesulfonic acid	Fluorescence ex:450 nm em:510 nm		
Bognar (1981) (68)	Meat Rice Bread	Acid hydrolysis Enzymic hydrolysis	Amino-10μm LichrosorbNH₂ 25 × 0.46 cm	Methanol/2 M sodium acetate buffer, pH 4.5 (50:50)	Fluorescence ex:467 nm em: 525 nm	5 μg/100 g	0.25 ± 0.004 0.02 ± 0.001 0.29 ± 0.005
Fellman (1982) (69)	Milk powder Flour Vegetable powder	Acid hydrolysis Enzymic hydrolysis Sep-Pak C18	RP8-10μm Radial-PAK Waters Associates 10 × 0.18 cm	Methanol/0.01 M phosphate buffer, pH 7.0 (37:63 v/v)	Fluorescence ex:450 nm em: 530 nm	1.0 ng	1.68 ± 0.16 0.24 ± 0.04 0.29 ± 0.03

Reference	Sample	Cleanup/Method	Column	Mobile phase	Detection	Detection limit	Results
Augustin (1984) (70)	Milk powder, Flour, Vegetable powder	?	RP18-5μm Ultrasphere 25 × 0.46 cm	Methanol/water (20:80 v/v) +5 mM tetrabutylammonium phosphate, pH 7.5	Fluorescence ex: 450 nm em: 530 nm	0.1–1 ng	
Johnsson (1987) (71)	Baby food, Flours, Cow milk, Corn flakes	Acid hyrolysis, Enzymic hydrolysis	RP-5μm Hypersil Shandon 25 × 0.46 cm	Methanol/water (2:3) + acetic acid, pH 4.5	Fluorescence ex:440 nm em: 520 nm	50 pg	0.50–1.3, 0.13–0.22, 0.15, 1.1
Wills (1985) (72)	Meat, Cereals, Vegetables	Acid hydrolysis, Enzymic hydrolysis, Sep-Pak C_{18}	RP18 Radial-Pak μBondapak Waters Associates	Methanol/water (40:60 v/v), 5 mM PIC B_6	Fluorescence ex:360 nm em:500 nm		0.18–0.23, 0.09–0.53, 0.04–0.29
Reyes (1988) (73)	Meat products, Cow milk, Flour	Acid hydrolysis	RP8-10μm Lichrosorb E. Merck 25 × 0.4 cm	Methanol/5 mM aqueous 1-hexanesulfonic acid (40:60, v/v)	Fluorescence ex:440 nm em:565 nm	1 ng	0.03–0.04, 0.12–0.13, 0.21
Mauro (1984) (74)	Cereals	Acid hydrolysis, Enzymic hydrolysis	RP18 μBondapak Waters Associates 30 × 0.41 cm	Methanol/water/acetic acid (36:64:1, v/v/v) + 5 mM hexanesulfonic acid	Fluorescence 400–700 nm	13 ng/g	
Wehling (1984) (75)	Cereals, Products	Acid hydrolysis, Enzymic hydrolysis	RP18-10μm μBondapak Waters Associates 25 × 0.46 cm	Methanol/water/acetic acid (30:69:1, v/v/v) + 5 mM hexanesulfonic acid	Fluorescence ex:288 nm em:418 nm	1 μg/g	2.77 ± 0.41
Wimalasiri (1985) (76)	Cereals, Milk, Meat	Acid hydrolysis, Enzymic hydrolysis, Sep-Pak	RP18-10μm μBondapak Radial-Pak Waters Associates	Methanol/water (40:60, v/v), 5 mM Pic B_6	Fluorescence ex:360 nm em:500 nm	3 ng	
Fernando (1990) (77)	Soy products	Acid hydrolysis, Centrifugation	RP18-5 μm Ultrasphere Beckman 15 × 0.46 cm	Acetonitrile/0.01 M acetate buffer pH 5.5 (13:87, v/v)	Fluorescence ex:436 nm em:535 nm	2 ng/ml	soy flour, 0.9–1.1 μg/g ww Tofu, 0.1 μg/g ww

Table 6 Continued

Reference	Source	Pretreatment	Column	Mobile phase	Detection	Detection limit	Results (mg B$_2$/100 g)
Woodcock (1982) (78)	Pasta	Acid hydrolysis Centrifugation Filtration	RP18 μBondapak Waters Assoc. 30 × 0.39 cm	Methanol/water/acetic acid (43:56:1 v/v/v)	Fluorescence ex: 450 nm em:510 nm	0.01 ng	0.56 ± 0.012
Watada (1985) (79)	Fruits Vegetables	Acid hydrolysis Enzymic hydrolysis	RP-5μm Ultrasphere Altex 25 × 0.46 cm	Methanol/water (40:60 v/v) + 5 mM heptane sulfonic acid pH 4.5	Fluorescence ex: 450 nm em: 530 nm	0.2 ng	0.04–0.16
Finglas (1987) (80)	Potatoes	Acid hydrolysis Enzymic hydrolysis	RP18 μBondapak Waters Associates 25 × 0.46 cm	Methanol/water (30:70, v/v)	Fluorescence ex:450 nm em:510 nm	0.1 ng	0.01–0.02
Ayi (1986) (81)	Infant formula	Distilled water Extraction	RP18-5μm Spherisorb-ODS1 Phase Sep. 15 × 0.46 cm	Methanol/acetonitrile/40 mM triethylammonium phosphate (10:5:85, v/v), pH 3.0 + 1.63 g/liter Na-octanesulfonate	Fluorescence ex:285 nm em:546 nm		0.57–1.0
Jaumann	Beer	Liquid extraction	RP18	Methanol/5 mM Na-pentanesulfo-	UV spectroscopy		

Reference	Sample	Pretreatment	Column	Mobile phase	Detection	
(1985) (82)	Chocolate drink Grape mix	Precolumn RP8(2 × 0.41 cm)	LiChrosorb 25 × 0.41 cm	nate/5 mM Na-heptanesulfonate (20:55:25, v/v/v) + 1 g phosphoric acid	280 nm	
Metschies (1985) (83)	Fruit juice	Acid hydrolysis RP8-cartridge (Baker)	RP8-7μm Nucleosil Knauer 25 × 0.4 mm	Methanol/water/acetic acid (39:60:1, v/v/v)	Fluorescence ex:370 nm em:418 nm	0.95
Maeda (1989) (84)	Oral liquid tonics	No	RP18-7μm Nucleosil Gasukurokogyo 25 × 0.46 cm	Acetonitrile/0.01 M phosphate buffer/triethylamine (80:91.5:5, v/v), 5 mM octanesulfonic acid, pH 2.8	UV spectroscopy 254 nm	2.1–13.7
Moll (1988) (85)	Alcoholic beverages		RP18-10μm μBondapak Waters Associates	Methanol/water (40:60, v/v)	Fluorescence ex:450 nm em:525 nm	
Kitada (1988) (86)	Beverages	No	RP18-7μm Nucleosil 25 × 0.46 cm	Acetonitrile/water/triethylamine (9:90.5:0.5, v/v)	UV spectroscopy 210 nm	
Anan (1988) (87)	Tea	Acid hydrolysis Enzymic hydrolysis	ODS-120A	Acetonitrile/water/acetic Acid (11:88.5:0.5, v/v)	Fluorescence ex:360 nm em:500 nm	

70,77,80) or after column separation (72,74–76), while lumiflavin was formed precolumn (57). A strong argument against the precolumn oxidation of thiamine to thiochrome is the fact that some of the riboflavin may be destroyed during the oxidation step in alkaline solution. Therefore, a state-of-the-art procedure for this special separation is the postcolumn derivatization of thiamine (see Chapter 8 on vitamin B_1). Most of the methods involve a pretreatment procedure to remove the protein-bound coenzymes from the respective flavoproteins and to hydrolyze phosphoric ester bonds. The total flavin content is determined in these methods in the form of riboflavin, and no information is available about the concentrations of FMN and FAD. Usually, homogenized samples in 0.1 N HCl are first autoclaved for 30 min followed by an enzymatic treatment (Taka-diastase or papain) to obtain a complete cleavage of the phosphate esters. Additional precipitation of proteins by the addition of trichloroacetic acid can be performed to extend the lifetime of the HPLC column. After pH adjustment and filtration or centrifugation, the resulting riboflavin solution is chromatographed. In order to concentrate the samples and to remove some of the interfering materials, the riboflavin-containing solution can be passed through reversed-phase cartridges (C_{18} Sep-Pak or RP-8 Baker) (39,69,72,76,83). Usually, an aliquot (2-10 ml) of the respective solution is placed onto one of these short disposable columns. After washing the column with water or a water/methanol mixture to remove salts and some impurities, the vitamins are eluted with a small volume of pure methanol.

SENSITIVITY. It has been pointed out by different authors that UV detection techniques suffer from a lack of sensitivity and from UV-absorbing interferences, especially when low amounts of riboflavin in some nonenriched foods have to be determined (60,63–65).

VALIDITY. The HPLC results for the riboflavin content in foods have been found to agree well with those obtained by the Association of Official Analytical Chemists (AOAC) microbiological assay (66,71,73) and fluorimetric assay (63,65,67–69,72,73,75,80,81). However, lower values for the HPLC method compared to the AOAC method have also been reported in some foods (63,67). This might indicate the presence of interfering material in the AOAC fluorimetric assay and the higher selectivity of the HPLC method.

STABILITY OF RIBOFLAVIN IN FOODS. Very little is known about the degradation of vitamins in different foodstuffs that are stored under adverse environmental conditions or that are processed.

The photochemical degradation of riboflavin in pasta was studied by Woodcock et al. in some detail (78). Riboflavin and lumichrome were extracted from light-exposed macaroni and assayed by reversed-phase

HPLC. The light intensity was the rate-determining factor for riboflavin loss, whereas increased temperatures had only little effect. Under the experimental conditions used in this study more than 50% of the riboflavin content was lost within 1 day.

An HPLC method for the simultaneous determination of riboflavin and its decomposition products in cow milk and human milk was described by Toyosaki et al. (60). As shown in Fig. 7, three peaks with close retention times were observed. Peak 2 was identified as riboflavin, and peak 1 and 3 represent decomposition products that account for more than 26% of the total flavin content in cow milk. In contrast, only a slight or no decomposition due to photolysis reactions was observed in human milk (60) and in goat milk (39).

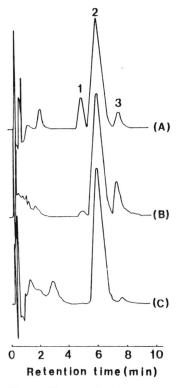

Figure 7   HPLC of homogenized milk (A), cow milk (B), and human milk (C). Peak 2, riboflavin; peaks 1 and 3 represent photolysis decomposition products. Column, Cosmosil C_{18}-5μm; eluant, methanol/water/acetic acid (45:65:0.1, v/v/v) (from Ref. 60).

The quantitative assessment of flavins in cow milk and the effect of pasteurization on these compounds were studied by Roughead and McCormick (61) (see Table 6) using the phenol extraction technique and reversed-phase HPLC. Riboflavin (61%), FAD (26%), and 10-(2'-hydroxyethyl) flavin (11%) were the predominant flavin compounds in all milk samples studied. The distribution of flavins in raw and pasteurized milk reveals little difference, with the exception of a decrease in the FAD content with pasteurization.

The influence of different heat-processing methods on the riboflavin content in meat was investigated by HPLC (58). It was found that in contrast to thiamine, riboflavin was stable in meat under all the heat-processing methods studied.

Biosamples

As compared with the concentration of FAD and FMN in most biological materials (blood, tissue, organs), a significant amount of riboflavin is found only in urine.

URINE. Besides riboflavin (26% of total flavin), small amounts of catabolites such as lumichrome and lumiflavin (photodegradation) and 7,8-dimethyl-10-(2'-hydroxyethyl)isoalloxazine (formed by intestinal microflora) were detected in urine (88), whereas FMN and FAD are apparently absent. More recently, 7α-hydroxyriboflavin (31% of the total flavin concentration) and 8α-hydroxyriboflavin (5%) were found in human urine, indicating that the oxidations of the 7- and 8-methyl groups of riboflavin in the liver are new metabolic pathways for flavins in mammals (17,22). These hydroxylated metabolites were shown to arise from tissue oxidation of riboflavin (17).

The sensitive determination of riboflavin excreted into urine is of some interest because it seems to be a good means for monitoring dietary intake of the vitamin. It can establish the vitamin B_2 status of an individual and it can be used as an index of the relative bioavailability of vitamin formulations. About 200 μg/day riboflavin are renally excreted by a normal person. Excretion of 40–70 μg/d (or <17 μg/g creatinine) indicates a riboflavin deficiency (89).

No special pretreatment procedure is necessary for HPLC of urine samples. Fresh urine samples (15–200 μl) are either injected directly or after centrifugation, to remove most of the sediment. For special investigations, flavin compounds can be concentrated from large volumes of urine by extraction procedures. According to Chastain et al. (90), a phenol extraction is performed by saturating urine samples with ammonium sulfate followed by centrifugation to remove solids. The supernatant fluid is shaken twice with 0.1 volume of 80% aqueous phenol, centrifuged, and the upper phenolic layers are combined. An equal volume of distilled water is added and the solution is extracted with diethyl ether to remove the phenol from the aqueous flavin-containing solution. Lumichrome-type compounds can be extracted from acidified urine samples (pH 2.0) with chloroform (90). A typical HPLC profile (phenol extract) of human urine is shown in Fig. 8.

The stability of riboflavin in fresh urine is limited. According to Smith (91), no change in riboflavin peak response was observed in urine samples protected from light and stored at room temperature for 24 h and at 5°C for at least 2 weeks. However, as pointed out by Lambert et al. (49), a considerable loss of riboflavin is caused by bacterial degradation at room temperature even in the dark. Consequently, all flavin-containing urine samples should be stabilized by acidification (acetic or oxalic acid) and/or adding a small amount of toluene (90).

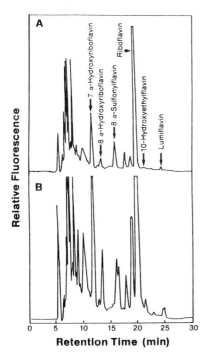

Figure 8 HPLC pattern of phenol extracts from human urine. (A) Typical chromatogram for a subject who received no supplemental riboflavin. (B) Chromatogram for a subject who received a dietary supplement of 3.4 mg riboflavin. Column, μBondapak C_{18}; eluant, 5 mM ammonium acetate, pH 6.0, methanol (gradient 0–70 methanol) (from Ref. 90).

High-pressure liquid chromatography has been shown to be a fast, sensitive, simple, and reproducible analytical method for urinary flavins (Table 7) (85–91). Unlike the observations of Seki et al. (95), who demonstrated a good separation of riboflavin from fluorescent compounds on a hydrophilic gel column, most authors use the more common C-18 reversed-phase HPLC columns. A baseline separation of riboflavin from FMN, FAD and nonflavin fluorescent compounds was achieved by all methods. Using fluorimetric detection, all these methods are rather sensitive (detection limit: 0.05–0.30 µg/ml riboflavin), and concentrations up to 2–12 µg/ml can be measured without dilution. Analytical recovery of added riboflavin was >95%. The normal reference interval 36–349 µg/g of creatinine (n = 50) (49) or 22–907 µg/g (n = 38) (92) of endogenous riboflavin in adults, measured by HPLC, confirmed earlier results obtained by other analytical methods.

MISCELLANEOUS.   Riboflavin in serum was determined by Lambert et al. using a reversed-phase technique (see Table 7) (49). Proteins were denatured by trichloroacetic acid. Contaminating interferents were removed by a simple Sep-Pak pretreatment resulting in a long lifetime of the analytical column (more than 650 samples on one column). The normal reference value for riboflavin detected by HPLC in serum was 15–38 (mean 23.4) nM (n = 50).

A method for simultaneous determination of total flavin, B_1, and B_6 vitamers in whole blood and serum was described (96). Protein-bound FAD and FMN were converted to free riboflavin by an acidic and subsequent enzymatic hydrolysis. Total riboflavin in serum (13.1 ±2.7 nM) and whole blood (185 ±56 nM) from normal volunteers was determined by ion-pair chromatography (Table 7).

The presence of protein-bound riboflavin in rat hepatocyte plasma membranes has recently been reported (97). The fluorophore was quantitatively extracted with water at 80°C and identified by analytical reversed-phase HPLC. FMN and FAD were not detectable in the plasma membrane. It is assumed that the presence of reduced riboflavin in the plasma membrane may represent a sort of defense mechanism against OH free radical attack.

The cellular flavin content (riboflavin, FAD, and FMN) or *Neurospora crassa* was determined by reversed-phase HPLC (98) (Table 7). It was found that free cellular riboflavin (not FAD or FMN) is involved in phase shifting by light of the circadian clock of *N. crassa*.

The sensitive determination of picomolar levels of flavins in seawater by solid-phase extraction and reversed-phase (99) or ion-pair HPLC with fluorescence detection (100) was described. According to Vastano et al., 500-ml samples of seawater were concentrated by solid-phase extraction on Sep-Pak C18 cartridges (100). The chromatographic system (Table 7)

Table 7 Determination of Flavins in Biosamples by HPLC

Reference	Source	Pretreatment	Column	Mobile phase	Detection	Detection limit (d.l.) and linear range (l.r.)
Smith (1980) (91)	Urine	Centrifugation	RP18-10μm μBondapak 30 × 0.4 cm	0.01 M KH_2PO_4/methanol (65:35), pH 5.0	Fluorescence ex:320–400 nm em:400–700 nm	0.05–0.07 μg/ml (d.l.) >12 μg/ml (l.r.)
Gatautis (1981) (92)	Urine	Centrifugation	RP18 μBondapak Waters Associates 30 × 0.39 cm	Methanol/water (34:66)	Fluorescence ex:450 nm em:530 nm	0.01 μg/ml (d.l.) >2 μg/ml (l.r.)
Ohkawa (1983) (93)	Urine	No	PRAZ-5μm DevosilODS-5 25 × 0.4 cm Nomura Inc.	0.01 M NaH_2PO_4/methanol, pH 5.5 (gradient) (30–40% methanol)	Fluorescence ex:440 nm em:530 nm	
Lambert (1985) (49)	Urine	Centrifugation	RP18-5μm ROSIL C18 HL All tech 15 × 0.32 cm	Methanol/water/CH_3COOH (36:63:1)	Fluorescence ex:450 nm em:500 nm	0.01 μg/ml (d.l.) >1.5 μg/ml (l.r.)
Chastain (1987) (90)	Urine	Phenol extract	RP18-10μm μBondapak Waters Associates		Fluorescence ex:305–395 nm em:475–650 nm	
Lopez-Anaya (1987) (94)	Urine	No	RP18-10μm PRP-1 Hamilton 25 cm × 4.6 mm	CH_3CN/water/CF_3COOH (10%)/H_3PO_4 (14:84:1.5:0.09)	Fluorescence ex:470 nm em:525 nm	0.015 μg/ml (d.l.)

Table 7 Continued

Reference	Source	Pretreatment	Column	Mobile phase	Detection	Detection limit (d.l.) and linear range (l.r.)
Seki (1987) (95)	Urine	Urine + meta-phosphoric acid (5%), β-thioglycol (0.5%)	Hydrophilic gel Asahipak CS32OH Asahi Chemical 25 × 0.76 cm	1 M Proportionate buffer, pH 4.4	Fluorescence ex:450 nm em:525 nm	0.04 μg/ml (d.l.)
Bötticher (1987) (96)	Serum, whole blood	Enzymatic hydrolysis TCA-precipitation Baker-10-SPE	RP18-5μm Nova Pak Waters Associates 12.5 × 0.46 cm	Methanol/1% acetic acid 3 mM 1-hexanesulfonic acid (20:80)	Fluorescence ex:290 nm em:395 nm	2 ng/ml (d.l.)
Nokubo (1989) (97)	Rat liver Plasma Membrane	Hot-water extract from subcellular fractions	Bilepak-II Jasco	Methanol/acetonitrile/ 0.1 M sodium acetate buffer, pH 5.0 (1:1:8, v/v)	Fluorescence ex:468 nm em:525 nm	
Fritz (1989) (98)	Neurospora grassa cells	Water/methanol (1:1) extract	RP18-5μm Lichrosorb Merck 25 × 0.45 cm	Pyridine (5 g/kg)/ethanol (70 g/kg) in 25 mM phosphate buffer, pH 6.25	UV absorption 450 nm	1 pmol
Vastano (1987) (100)	Seawater	Solid-phase extraction, Sep-Pak C18	RP18-10μm Hypersil Hewlett-Pack. 10 × 0.46 cm	Methanol/10 mM Na acetate, pH 5.8 (30:70, v/v), 4.5 mM TBA acetate	Fluorescence ex:305–395 nm em:435–650 nm	0.32 nM B$_2$ 4.50 nM FMN 28.6 nM FAD
Speek (1982) (108)	Whole blood	TCA precipitation Centrifugation	RP18-5μm Hypersil Shandon 25 × 0.46 cm	Methanol/0.3 M KH$_2$PO$_4$ (16.7:83.3, v/v), pH 2.9	Fluorescence ex:470 nm em:525 nm	

Reference	Sample	Sample preparation	Column	Mobile phase	Detection	Detection limits
Floridi (1985) (109)	Whole blood	TCA precipitation in 20% acetonitrile Centrifugation	Amino-5 μm Spherisorb-NH$_2$ 15 × 0.4 cm	CH$_3$CN/0.1 M Na phosphate buffer, pH 2.9 (30:70, v/v)	Fluorescence ex:436 nm em:530 nm	0.5 μg/ml (d.l.) 0.6–20 μg/ml (l.r.)
Pietta (1982) (48)	Plasma	No	RP18-10μm μBondpak Waters Associates 25 × 0.46 cm	CH$_3$CN/10 mM (NH$_4$)$_2$HPO$_4$, pH 5.5 (12:100)	UV absorption 254 nm	
Ichinose (1985) (110)	Fish serum	TCA precipitation Centrifugation	Amino-10μm Zorbax-NH$_2$ 15 × 0.46 cm	Methanol/20 mM NaH$_2$PO$_4$, pH 3 (10:90)	Fluorescence ex:328 nm em:526 nm	B$_2$ 4.9 ng/ml (d.l.) FMN 9.1 ng/ml (d.l.) FAD 73.1 ng/ml (d.l.)
Yagi (1981) (111)	Rat liver, kidney	Hot-water extraction	Ion-exchange IEX-540-10μm Toyo Soda 25 × 0.4 cm	Water/0.5 M KH$_2$PO$_4$, linear gradient	Fluorescence ex:450 nm em:530 nm	B$_2$ 0.25 pmol (d.l.) FMN 0.37 pmol (d.l.) FAD 4.9 pmol (d.l.)
Cann-Moisan (1988) (112)	Fish liver, brain, muscle	TCA precipitation Centrifugation	Amino-5μm Hypersil-APS Interchim 15 × 0.46 cm	CH$_3$CN/0.1 M NaH$_2$PO$_4$ pH 3.05 (30:70, v/v)	Electrochemical detection; LC4B amperometry TL4 glassy carbon electrode	1.25 pmol FAD
Payne (1982) (113)	Bacterial cells	Formic acid extract	(a) RP18-5μm Ultrasphere 25 × 0.46 cm (b) RP18-5μm Ultrasphere 25 × 0.46 cm	Methanol/0.25 m ammonium acetate, pH 6.0 (0–40:100–60) CH$_3$CN/4% CH$_3$CN, 30 mM KH$_2$PO$_4$, pH 6.0, 5 mM TBA phosphate (0–40:100–60)		
Batey (1990) (115)	Retina tissue, rats	Hot-water extraction TCA precipitation Centrifugation	RP-5μm Sepralyte CH Analytichem 15 × 0.46 cm	CH$_3$CN/ M (NH$_4$)$_2$HPO$_4$, pH 5.5 (10:90, v/v)	Fluorescence ex:447 nm em:530 nm	2 pmol FAD (d.l.) 2 pmol FMN (d.l.) 2 pmol B$_2$ (d.l.)

was able to separate riboflavin from lumiflavin, lumichrome, FMN, and FAD. Riboflavin concentrations of 2 to 20 pM were present throughout the water column, whereas lumiflavin (2–20 pM) and lumichrome (20–200 pM) were generally confined to the photic zone. FMN and FAD, excreted by several organisms, were only occasionally observed.

3.3   Flavin Mononucleotide and Riboflavin Phosphates

Riboflavin 5′-phosphate (FMN) is synthetically prepared on a large scale for use in pharmaceutical preparations, especially for parenteral administration. It has been demonstrated by reversed-phase HPLC that the chemical phosphorylation of riboflavin invariably yields a complex mixture of various riboflavin phosphates besides FMN (6). The HPLC chromatogram of a commercial FMN sample is shown in Fig. 9. 5′-FMN

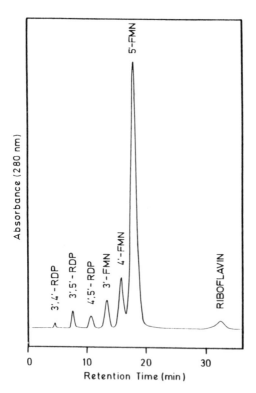

Figure 9   HPLC of commercial FMN (Sigma). Column, Nucleosil 100–10 C$_{18}$, 25 × 0.4 cm; injection volume, 3 µl (40 µg); eluant, 100 mM ammonium formate and 100 mM formic acid in 17% methanol. 3′,4′-RDP, riboflavin 3′,4′-bisphosphate (from Ref. 7).

accounts only for 75% of the total flavin content. Significant amounts of isomeric monophosphates (4'-FMN, 3'-FMN) and riboflavin bisphosphates (3', 5'-RBP, 4', 5'-RBP, and 3, 4'-RBP) are detectable in all commercial FMN samples analyzed (6,7).

The isomeric riboflavin phosphates can also be separated by ion-pair chromatography on reversed-phase HPLC columns (7,101). However, the reversed-phase technique was found to be more reproducible (7). Milligram amounts of pure 5'-FMN ($>95\%$) can be obtained by preparative HPLC, which may be significant in work with rare riboflavin analogs and with isotope-labeled samples (6). HPLC methods for the detection of FMN in pharmaceutical preparations have to take into account that about 25% of the total flavin content is present in the form of isomeric riboflavin phosphates.

A second remark concerns the rapid isomerization of riboflavin phosphates in acid solution (pH <2), especially at elevated temperature. The thermodynamic equilibrium is characterized by the presence of about 65% 5'-FMN, 11% 4'-FMN, 8% 3'-FMN, and 15% 2'-FMN (102). The rate constants for the various isomerization reactions under a variety of experimental conditions have been determined by reversed-phase HPLC (102). According to the official method of the Amercan Association of Analytical Chemists, protein-bound flavins are extracted from biological samples by treatment with 0.1 M HCl at 121°C for 15–30 min. It is known that this treatment leads to hydrolysis of FAD. As shown in Fig. 10, it should also be noted that a substantial fraction of 5'-FMN is converted to other isomeric phosphates under these conditions.

Pharmaceutical Preparations

Synthetic FMN (containing isomeric riboflavin mono- and bisphosphate impurities) is an ingredient of many liquid multivitamin preparations for intravenous application (103). Several methods for simultaneous determination of FMN and other water-soluble vitamins by reversed-phase or ion-pair HPLC are available (103–107). A typical HPLC separation is demonstrated in Fig. 11.

Foods

The determination of riboflavin and FMN in foods has been described by Lumley and Wiggins (66) using reversed-phase HPLC and Reyes et al. (73) using ion-pair HPLC (see Table 6). Samples were prepared by acid hydrolysis but without enzymatic hydrolysis step in order not to convert FMN into free riboflavin. Relatively high amounts of FMN were found in raw beef, corned beef, fresh and cooked liver, and canned mushrooms (73). Summation of riboflavin and FMN determined by HPLC gave a good correlation with standard analytical AOAC procedures.

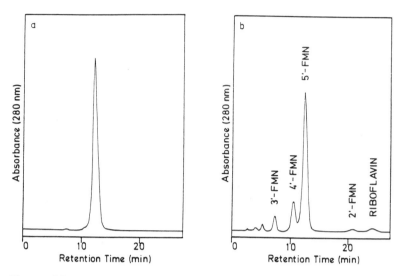

Figure 10 HPLC of (a) pure 5'-FMN and (b) a 5'-FMN sample heated at 121°C for 15 min in 0.1 *M* HCl. Column, Nucleosil, 100–10 C$_{18}$; eluant, 100 m*M* ammonium formate in 20% methanol, pH 6.3 (from Ref. 7).

Biosamples

The HPLC-determination of FMN in biological samples is described together with that of FAD (section 3.4).

3.4 Flavin Adenine Dinucleotide

In most tissues and organs, protein-bound FAD is the predominant flavin species. HPLC methods have been developed for the determination of FAD in whole blood, plasma, and organs. A significant hydrolysis of FAD due to (a) the pretreatment procedure (i.e., acid hydrolysis) and (b) an enzymatic degradation (e.g., in plasma) has to be considered.

Biosamples

WHOLE BLOOD AND SERUM.   The first reliable HPLC method for the analysis of FAD in whole blood of humans was described by Speek et al. (108). For preparation of the sample extract, 1 ml of whole blood or plasma was mixed with 3 ml of 10% trichloroacetic acid (TCA). After standing at 4°C for 30 min, the reaction mixture is neutralized by the addition of 2 ml of 4.5 *M* sodium acetate buffer, pH 6.2, and centrifuged. The supernatant was injected onto the reversed-phase HPLC column (Table 7). The detection limit (fluorescence detection) was found to correspond to blood concentrations of 20 n*M* FAD, 15 n*M* FMN, and

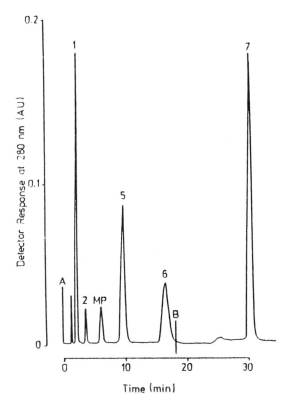

Figure 11 HPLC of a multivitamin intravenous injection solution: 1, FMN; 2, riboflavin; MP, methylparaben (preservative used in the formulation); 5, niacinamide; 6, pyridoxine; 7, thiamine. Column, μBondapak RP18-10 μm; eluant, methanol/water/formic acid containing 1 g/liter Na-dioctyl sulfosuccinate, pH 4.6; A, 17:82:1; B, 45:54:1, UV detection 280 nm (from Ref. 104).

10 nM riboflavin, respectively. From the analysis of FAD in a group of 70 normal volunteers, a total range of FAD of 240–460 nM (mean value 310 nM) was found.

Using the procedure of Speek et al., Floridi et al. found a premature loss in column efficiency, probably due to the presence of organic material in the samples that was irreversibly adsorbed onto the column (109). To overcome these difficulties, the TCA extraction was carried out without subsequent sample neutralization, which resulted in a prolonged lifetime of the column. Using a Spherisorb-NH$_2$ column (reversed-phase and ion-exchange properties) (Fig. 12), a mean concentration ($\pm$SD) of 280 $\pm$21 nM FAD was found in whole blood of normal humans.

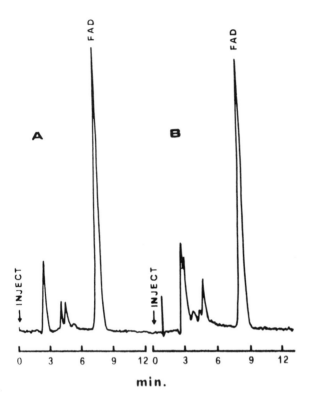

Figure 12 HPLC of FAD in whole blood: (A) standard FAD; (B) blood sample extract. Column, Spherisorb NH_2-5 μm; eluant, acetonitrile/0.1 M Na phosphate buffer, pH 2.9 (30:70, v/v); fluorescent detection 435/500 nm (from Ref. 109).

The hydrolysis of FAD and FMN in human blood plasma was monitored by reversed-phase HPLC (48). One milliliter of blood plasma was mixed with 100 μl stock solution, containing 15 μg FAD or FMN. After appropriate time intervals, the hydrolysis was stopped by injecting aliquots of the supplemented plasma directly onto the HPLC precolumn. It was found that FAD added to the plasma was hydrolyzed to FMN almost completely within 60 min at 37°C in the dark, whereas added FMN was hydrolyzed only to a very small extent.

Ichinose et al. modified the method of Speek et al. for the determination of flavins in serum of different fish (110). A Zorbax-NH_2 column that has both reversed-phase and ion-exchange properties was used for the separation of riboflavin (RF) and its coenzyme forms [mobile phase, methanol/0.2 M NaH_2PO_4 (10:90), pH 3.0]. Using fluorimetric detection, the detection limits of RF, FMN, and FAD in serum were 13,19 and 88 nM. The concentration of B$_2$ vitamers was found to be 0.54–0.99 (RF), 0.08 (FMN), and 0.70–0.87 (FAD) μM, respectively.

MISCELLANEOUS. Yagi and Sato determined the flavin content in various tissues of rat by HPLC (111). For a careful extraction of flavins, small pieces of tissue were heated in water at 80°C for 3–5 min. After homogenization in a Potter-Elvehjem glass homogenizer, the homogenate was heated to 80°C for 15 min. After centrifugation, the supernatant was directly injected onto the HPLC column. The chromatographic separation of riboflavin, FAD, and FMN was performed on an anion-exchange column with linear gradient elution from 0 to 0.5 M KH$_2$PO$_4$ (Table 7). A typical chromatographic flavin profile from rat liver is shown in Fig. 13. From appropriate standard curves, the amount of each flavin in various rat tissues was determined (Table 8). The HPLC data were in good agreement with the results determined by lumiflavin fluorescence method using paper chromatography.

A method for the determination of FAD in animal tissues by HPLC with electrochemical detection was described by Cann-Moisan et al. (112). Frozen tissues (fish liver, brain, or muscle) were mixed with cold TCA-diethyl ether solution 30 min before homogenization. FAD was detected by an LC4B amperometric detector equipped with a TL5 glassy carbon electrode and a silver-silver chloride electrode at a potential of −280 mV. With this detection principle, a calibration graph was linear over the range of 2–500 pmol FAD injected. The detection limit for FAD was found to be 1.25 pmol, which makes the technique as sensitive as fluorimetric detection. For fish liver, a concentration of 16.9 nmol/g wet weight FAD was found.

A procedure for the rapid extraction and HPLC separation of nucleotides (including FMN and FAD) from bacterial cells was described by Payne and Ames (113). Ribonucleotides were extracted from the cells with formic acid separated by boronate affinity chromatography and subsequently by reversed-phase HPLC or ion-pair reversed-phase chromatography. The complete separation reveals approximately 170 peaks in four chromatographic runs. A similar investigation for the determination of purine and pyrimidine nucleotides from rat liver was reported by Reiss et al. (114). Very recently, Batey and Eckhert analyzed the flavin content in rat retinal tissue (115). Retinas from two to three rats were isolated and homogenized. Flavins were extracted by a hot-water treatment and analyzed by reversed-phase HPLC (Table 7). The flavin content in retina (FAD, 46.5 ±2.8; FMN, 17.6 ±0.7; riboflavin, 4.80 ±0.34 pmol/mg protein) was found 5–10 times smaller than in liver but 1–2 orders of magnitude higher than in plasma. In liver and retina FAD was the predominant flavin, followed by FMN and riboflavin.

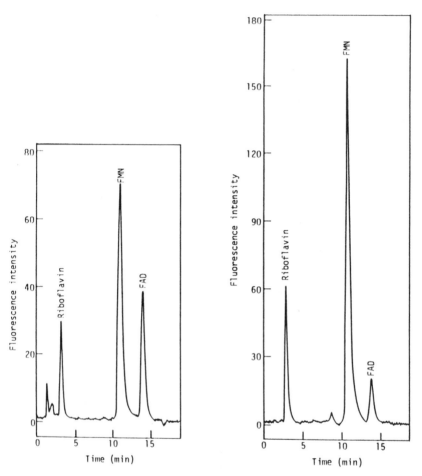

Figure 13 HPLC elution pattern of flavins of rat liver. Column, anion exchange IEX-540-10μm, 25 × 0.4 cm; eluant, linear gradient between water and 0.5 M KH_2PO_4, 0.05 M/min; fluorescent detection 450/530 nm (from Ref. 111).

3.5 Flavin Analogs

A variety of flavin analogs at the riboflavin, FMN, and FAD levels was separated, quantitated, or isolated by HPLC, including 5-deazaflavin (7,116,117), 1-deazaflavin (116–118), and malonylriboflavin (119).

Light et al. (116) and Hausinger et al. (117) described HPLC methods for the purification of flavin analogs at the FAD level. The reversed-phase HPLC separation of different flavin analogs is demonstrated in Fig. 14.

Table 8 Flavins in Rat Tissues as Determined by HPLC [a]

Organ	FAD µg/g	FAD %	FMN µg/g	FMN %	Riboflavin µg/g	Riboflavin %	Total flavin µg/g
Liver	23.9	89.0	2.7	9.9	0.30	1.1	26.9
	(23.2)	(86.6)	(3.1)	(11.1)	(0.51)	(1.9)	(26.8)
Kidney	23.2	61.9	13.7	36.5	0.60	1.6	37.5
	(21.9)	(58.4)	(15.3)	(40.8)	(0.30)	(0.8)	(37.5)
Heart	19.6	94.9	1.0	4.9	0.05	0.2	20.7
	(18.4)	(94.2)	(1.1)	(5.7)	(0.02)	(0.1)	(19.5)
Brain	2.2	87.4	0.29	11.4	0.03	1.2	2.5
	(2.9)	(85.8)	(0.45)	(13.6)	(0.02)	(0.6)	(3.3)
Spleen	3.0	91.6	0.22	6.6	0.06	1.8	3.3
	(3.3)	(92.2)	(0.24)	(6.7)	(0.04)	(1.1)	(3.6)

[a] Values in parentheses were measured with paper chromatography (from Ref. 111).

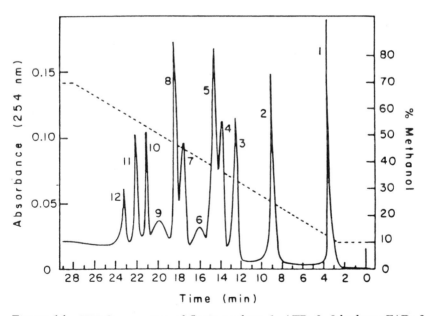

Figure 14 HPLC separation of flavin analogs: 1, ATP; 2, 8-hydroxy-FAD; 3, FAD; 4, 1-deaza-FAD; 5, 5-deaza-FAD; 6, FMN; 7, 1-deaza-FMN; 8, riboflavin; 9, 5-deaza-FMN; 10, 1-deazariboflavin; 11, methylriboflavin; 12, 5-deazaflavin. Column, Lichrosorb RP18, 25 × 1 cm; linear gradient between 5 mM ammonium acetate buffer, pH 6.0, and methanol (from Ref. 116).

HPLC was used for the study of naturally occurring flavin analogs in methanogenic bacteria (117,119–121). The 5-deazaflavins from *Methanobacterium thermoautotrophicum* (117,120,121) and *Methanosarcina barkeri* (122) were readily separated and isolated on the preparative-scale by reversed-phase HPLC.

4. GAS CHROMATOGRAPHY

As indicated by the lack of appropriate references in the literature, gas chromatography has no practical relevance for the analysis of flavin compounds.

5. FUTURE TRENDS

High-performance liquid chromatography is a tremendously versatile tool that can be used for the determination and the small-scale isolation of various flavin compounds. In the analytical field, HPLC has already superseded paper chromatography completely and thin-layer chromatography more or less completely. This trend will undoubtedly go on in the future, although the efficiency of high-performance thin-layer chromatography coupled with TLC densitometry is comparable to that of HPLC.

A modern HPLC apparatus, including a fluorescence detector, leaves little to be desired in regard to sensitivity, reliability, and reproducibility. Various reversed-phase or ion-pair HPLC systems are available that allow the separation and determination of riboflavin in different matrices. However, future work has to optimize the pretreatment procedures for the careful extraction and the reliable determination of flavin coenzymes, FAD, and FMN, especially from biological materials.

REFERENCES

1. T. Wagner-Jauregg, in *The Vitamins*, Vol. 5 (W. H. Sebrell and R. S. Harris, eds.), Academicx Press, New York, p. 3 (1972).
2. P. Hemmerich, *Fortschr. Chem. Org. Naturst.* 33:451 (1971).
3. F. Müller, S. Ghisla, and A. Bacher, in *Vitamine II* (O. Isler, C. Brubacher, S. Ghisla, and B. Kräutler, eds.), Thieme Stuttgart, New York (1988).
4. W. L. Chairns and D. E. Metzler, *J. Am. Chem. Soc.*, 93:2772 (1971).
5. A. R. Surrey, *J. Am. Chem. Soc.*, 73:2336 (1951).
6. P. Nielsen, P. Rauschenbach, and A. Bacher, *Anal. Biochem.* 130:359 (1983).
7. P. Nielsen, P. Rauschenbach, and A. Bacher, *Methods Enzymol.*, 122:209 (1986).

8. H. Beinert, *The Enzymes*, 2:339 (1963).

9. S. Ghisla, V. Massey, J. M. Lhoste, and S. G. Mayhew, *Biochemistry*, 13:589 (1974).

10. A. Bacher, in Chemistry and Biochemistry of Flavoproteins (F. Miller ed.), CRC Press, Boca Raton, p. 245 (1990).

11. National Academy of Science, *Recommended Dietary Allowances*, National Academy of Sciences, Washington, DC (1980).

12. W. J. Jusko and G. Levy, in *Riboflavin* (R. S. Rivlin, ed.), Plenum Press, New York, p. 99 (1975).

13. T. Akiyama, J. Selhub, and I. H. Rosenberg, *J. Nutr.*, 112:263 (1982).

14. C. P. Chia, R. Addison, and D. B. McCormick, *J. Nutr.*, 108:373 (1978).

15. W. Ostrowski, B. Skarzynski, and Z. Zak, *Biochim. Biophys. Acta*, 59:515 (1962).

16. C. V. R. Murthy and P. R. Adiga, *Biochem. Int.*, 5:289 (1982).

17. H. Ohkawa, N. Ohishi, and K. Yagi, *J. Biol. Chem.*, 258:5629 (1983).

18. G. A. Goldsmith, in *Riboflavin* (R. S. Rivlin, ed.), Plenum Press, New York, p. 279 (1975).

19. J. Pinto, Y. P. Huang, and R. S. Rivlin, *Clin. Res.*, 30:634A (1982).

20. R. S. Rivlin, *Nutr. Rev.*, 37:241 (1979).

21. A. Green, T. G. Marshall, M. J. Bennett, R. G. F. Gray, and R. J. Pollitt, *J. Inher. Metab. Dis.*, 8:67 (1985).

22. H. Ohkawa, N. Ohishi, and K. Yagi, *Biochem. Int.*, 6:239 (1983).

23. M. S. Jorns, G. B. Sancar, and A. Sancar, *Biochemistry* 23:2673 (1984).

24. H. Thielemann, *Pharmazie*, 35:125 (1980); 36:574, 783 (1981).

25. C. B. Airaudo, V. Cerri, A. Gayte-Sorbier, and J. Andrianjafiniony, *J. Chromatogr.*, 261:273 (1983).

26. J. Kawanabe, *J. Chromatogr.*, 333:115 (1985).

27. R. Bhushan and I. Ali, *Arch. Pharm.*, 320:1186 (1987).

28. Q. Ni, X. Song, X. Yu, Y. Chen, and R. Yu, *Nanjing Yaoxueyuan Xuebao*, 16:27 (1985); *Chem. Abstr.*, 104:24241w (1985).

29. Y. Chen, C. Jiang, Q. Yang, and R. Yu, *Nanjing Yaoxueyuan Xuebao*, 17:208 (1986); *Chem. Abstr.*, 106:46653a (1986).

30. Q. Chen, *Yaoxue Tongbao*, 21:202 (1986); *Chem. Abst.*, 105: 232512h (1986).

31. B. R. Bochner and B. N. Ames, *J. Biol. Chem.*, 257:9759 (1982).

32. C. G. van Schagen and F. Müller, *Eur. J. Biochem.*, 120:33 (1981).

33. I. Chibata, T. Tosa, and Y. Matuo, *Methods Enzymol.*, 66:221 (1980).

34. K. Decker and H.-H. Hamm, *Methods Enzymol.*, 66:227 (1980).

35. S. G. Mayhew and M. J. J. Strating, *Eur. J. Biochem.*, 59:539 (1975).

36. V. Massey and L. D. Mendelsohn, *Anal. Biochem.*, 95:156 (1979).

37. A. Kozik and Z. Zak, *Anal. Biochem.*, 121:224 (1982).

38. J. Nagy, J. Knoll, W. C. Kenney, and T. P. Singer, in *Flavins and Flavoproteins* (V. Massey and C. H. Williams, eds.), Elsevier North Holland, Amsterdam, p. 573 (1982).

39. C. Lavigne, J. A. Zee, R. E. Simard, and C. Gosselin, *J. Chromatogr.*, 410:201 (1987).

40. Y. Arai and T. Hanai, *J. Liq. Chromatogr.*, 11:2409 (1988).

41. G. W. Schieffer, *J. Chromatogr.*, *319*:387 (1985).
42. R. E. Synovec and E. S. Yeung, *J. Chromatogr.*, *368*:85 (1986).
43. E. J. Guthrie, J. W. Jorgenson, and P. R. Dluzneski, *J. Chromatogr. Sci.*, *22*:171 (1984).
44. J. R. Chapman, *J. Chromatogr.*, *323*:153 (1985).
45. D. E. Games, M. A. McDowall, K. Levsen, K. H. Schafer, P. Dobberstein, and J. L. Gower, *Biomed. Mass Spectrosc.*, *11*:87 (1984).
46. F. L. Vandemark and G. J. Schmidt, *J. Liq. Chromatogr.*, *4*:1157 (1981).
47. M. C. Walker, B. E. Carpenter, and E. L. Cooper, *J. Pharm. Sci.*, *70*:99 (1981).
48. P. Pietta and A. Calatroni, *J. Chromatogr.*, *229*:445 (1982).
49. W. E. Lambert, P. M. Cammaert, and A. P. De Leenheer, *Clin. Chem.*, *31*:1371 (1985).
50. M. Amin and J. Reusch, *J. Chromatogr.*, *390*:448 (1987).
51. F. L. Vandemark and G. J. Schmidt, *J. Liq. Chromatogr.*, *4*:1157 (1981).
52. F. L. Vandemark, *Chromatogr. Newslett.*, *8*:27 (1980).
53. C. Jenkins, *Pharm. Technol.*, *March*:53 (1982).
54. M. Amin and J. Reusch, *Analyst*, *112*:989 (1987).
55. M. W. Dong, J. Lepore, and T. Tarumoto, *J. Chromatogr.*, *442*:81 (1988).
56. P. M. Finglas and R. M. Faulks, *J. Micronutr. Anal.*, *3*:251 (1987).
57. C. Y. W. Ang and F. A. Moseley, *J. Agric. Food. Chem.*, *28*:483 (1980).
58. K. R. Dawson, N. F. Unklesbay, and H. B. Hedrick, *J. Agric. Food. Chem.*, *36*:1176 (1988).
59. W. Kneifel, *Dtsch. Molkereiz.*, *9*:212 (1986).
60. T. Toyosaki, A. Yamamoto, and T. Mineshita, *J. Micronutr. Anal.*, *2*:117 (1986).
61. Z. K. Roughead and D. B. McCormick, *J. Nutr.*, *120*:382 (1990).
62. F. Ribarova, S. Shishkov, N. Obretenova, and L. Metchkufva, *Die Nahrung*, *31*:77 (1987).
63. S. H. Ashoor, G. J. Seperich, W. C. Monte, and J. Welty, *J. Food Sci.*, *48*:92 (1983).
64. B. Stancher and F. Zonta, *J. Food Sci.*, *51*:857 (1986).
65. J. F. Kamman, T. P. Labuza, and J. J. Warthesen, *J. Food. Sci.*, *45*:1497 (1980).
66. I. D. Lumley and R. A. Wiggins, *Analyst*, *106*:1103 (1981).
67. G. R. Skurray, *Food Chem.*, *7*:77 (1981).
68. A. Bognar, *Dtsch. Lebensm. Rundschau*, *77*:431 (1981).
69. J. K. Fellman, W. E. Artz, P. D. Tassinari, C. L. Cole, and J. Augustin, *J. Food. Sci.*, *47*:2048 (1982).
70. J. Augustin, *J. Assoc. Off. Anal. Chem.*, *67*:1012 (1984).
71. H. Johnsson and C. Branzell, *Int. J. Vitam. Nutr. Res.*, *57*:53 (1987).
72. R. B. H. Wills, P. Wimalasiri, and H. Greenfield, *J. Micronutr. Anal.*, *1*:23 (1985).
73. E. S. P. Reyes, K. M. Norris, C. Taylor, and D. Potts, *J. Assoc. Off. Anal. Chem.*, *71*:16 (1988).
74. D. J. Mauro and D. L. Wetzel, *J. Chromatogr.*, *299*:281 (1984).

75. R. L. Wehling and D. L. Wetzel, *J. Agric. Food. Chem.*, *32*:1326 (1984).
76. P. Wimalasiri and R. B. H. Wills, *J. Chromatogr.*, *318*:412 (1985).
77. S. M. Fernando and P. A. Murphy, *J. Agric. Food. Chem.*, *38*:163 (1990).
78. E. A. Woodcock, J. J. Warthesen, and T. P. Labuza, *J. Food. Sci.*, *47*:545 (1982).
79. A. E. Watada and T. T. Tran, *J. Liq. Chromatogr.*, *8*:1651 (1985).
80. P. M. Finglas and R. M. Faulks, *Food Chem.*, *15*:37 (1984).
81. B. K. Ayi, D. A. Yuhas, and N. J. Deangelis, *J. Assoc. Off. Anal. Chem.*, *69*:56 (1986).
82. G. Jaumann and H. Engelhardt, *Chromatographia*, *20*:615 (1985).
83. M. Metschies und G. Schwedt, *Dtsch. Lebensm. Rundschau*, *81*:385 (1985).
84. Y. Maeda, M. Yamamoto, K. Owada, S. Sato, T. Masui, and H. Nakazawa, *J. Assoc. Off. Anal. Chem.*, *72*:244 (1989).
85. N. Moll, *Dev. Food Sci.*, *17*:753 (1988).
86. Y. Kitada, M. Sasaki, Y. Yamazoe, Y. Maeda, M. Yamamoto, H. Nakazawa, *Bunseki Kagaku*, *37*:561 (1988); *Chem. Abstr.*, *110*:22375t (1988).
87. T. Anan, H. Takayanagi, and K. Ikegaya, *Nippon Shokuhin Kogyo Gakkaishi*, *35*:396 (1988); *Chem. Abstr.*, *110*:6451j (1988).
88. M. Oka and D. B. McCormick, *J. Nutr.*, *115*:496 (1985).
89. C. J. Bates, *Nutr. Diet.*, *50*:215 (1987).
90. J. L. Chastain and D. B. McCormick, *Am. J. Clin. Nutr.*, *46*:830 (1987).
91. M. D. Smith, *J. Chromatogr.*, *182*:285 (1980).
92. V. J. Gatautis and H. K. Naito, *Clin. Chem.*, *27*:1672 (1981).
93. H. Ohkawa, N. Ohishi, and K. Yagi, *J. Biol. Chem.*, *258*:5623 (1983).
94. A. Lopez-Anaya and M. Mayersohn, *J. Chromatogr.*, *423*:105 (1987).
95. T. Seki, K. Noguchi, and Y. Yanagihara, *J. Chromatogr.*, *385*:283 (1987).
96. B. Bötticher and D. Bötticher, *Int. J. Vitam. Nutr. Res.*, *57*: 273 (1987).
97. M. Nokubo, M. Ohta, K. Kitani, and I. Zs.-Nagy, *Biochim. Biophys. Acta*, *981*:303 (1989).
98. B. J. Fritz, S. Kasai, and K. Matsui, *Plant Cell. Physiol.*, *30*:557 (1989).
99. W. C. Dunlop and M. Susic, *Mar. Chem.*, *17*:185 (1985).
100. S. E. Vastano, P. J. Milne, W. L. Stahovec, and K. Mopper, *Anal. Chim. Acta*, *201*:127 (1987).
101. B. Entsch and R. G. Sim, *Anal. Biochem.*, *133*:401 (1983).
102. P. Nielsen, J. Harksen, and A. Bacher, *Eur. J. Biochem.*, *152*:465 (1985).
103. A. van der Horst, H. J. M. Martens, and P. N. F. C de Goede, *Pharm. Weekbl. [Sci.]* *11*:169–174 (1989).
104. D. C. Woollard, *J. Chromatogr.*, *301*:470 (1984).
105. F. L. Lam and A. Lowande, *J. Pharm. Biomed. Anal.*, *6*:87 (1988).
106. N. Akimoto, *Gijutso Joho*, *5*:4 (1987); *Chem. Abstr.*, *107*:161771v.
107. K. Shimura, T. Yamada, K. Sakurai, Y. Mori, N. Masuda, and T. Shiomi, *Mie-ken Eisei Kenkyusho Nenpo*, *32*:105 (1987); *Chem. Abstr.*, *110*:121509w.
108. A. J. Speek, F. van Schaik, J. Schrijver, and W. H. P. Schreurs, *J. Chromatogr.*, *228*: 311 (1982).

109. A. Floridi, C. A. Palmerini, C. Fini, M. Pupita, and F. Fidanza, *Int. J. Vitam. Nutr. Res.*, *55*:187 (1985).
110. N. Ichinose, K. Adachi, and G. Schwedt, *Analyst*, *110*:1505 (1985).
111. K. Yagi and M. Sato, *Biochem. Int.* 2:327 (1981).
112. C. Cann-Moisan, J. Caroff, and E. Girin, *J. Chromatogr.*, *442*:441 (1988).
113. S. M. Payne and B. N. Ames, *Anal. Biochem.*, *123*:151 (1982).
114. P. D. Reiss, P. F. Zuurendonk, and R. L. Veech, *Anal. Biochem.*, *140*:162 (1984).
115. D. W. Batey and C. D. Eckhert, *Anal. Biochem.*, *188*:164 (1990).
116. D. R. Light, C. Walsh, and M. A. Marletta, *Anal. Biochem.*, *109*:87 (1980).
117. R. P. Hausinger, J. F. Honek, and C. Walsh, *Methods Enzymol.*, *122*:199 (1986).
118. M. Kurfürst, P. Macheroux, S. Ghisla, and J. W. Hastings, *Eur. J. Biochem.*, *181*:453 (1989).
119. S. Ghisla, R. Mack, G. Blankenhorn, P. Hemmerich, E. Krienitz, and T. Kuster, *Eur. J. Biochem.*, *138*:339 (1984).
120. R. Kern, P. J. Keller, G. Smith, and A. Bacher, *Arch. Microbiol.*, *136*:191 (1983).
121. R. P. Hausinger, W. H. Orme-Johnson, and C. Walsh, *Biochemistry*, *24*:1629 (1985).
122. P. van Beelen, W. J. Geerts, A. Pol, and G. D. Vogels, *Anal. Biochem.*, *131*:285 (1983).

10

VITAMIN B$_6$

Johan B. Ubbink

University of Pretoria, Pretoria, South Africa

1. INTRODUCTION

1.1 History

Vitamin B$_6$ was first identified as an essential nutritional component to prevent a florid dermatitis called acrodynia in rats (1). In 1938, a crystalline substance having vitamin B$_6$ activity was isolated and identified (2,3). This component, named pyridoxine, was required for growth of several lactic acid bacteria (4). However, Snell and co-workers found that extraordinarily large amounts of pyridoxine were required to support growth of *Lactobacillus casei* or *Streptococcus faecalis* (5). Heat sterilization of the pyridoxine-containing growth medium reduced the amount of vitamin required for growth of the above-mentioned bacteria (5). These results indicated that heat treatment altered pyridoxine to form growth factors more potent than pyridoxine; subsequently, pyridoxal and pyridoxamine were discovered in 1944 (6).

1.2 Chemical Properties

The generic term vitamin B$_6$ refers to all 3-hydroxy-2-methylpyridine derivatives that exhibit the biological activity of pyridoxine in rats (7). Pyridoxine [3-hydroxy-4,5-bis(hydroxymethyl)-2-methyl pyridine] should not be used as generic term synonymous with vitamin B$_6$. Two other

399

forms of vitamin B_6, pyridoxal (PL) and pyridoxamine (PM), differ from pyridoxine (PN) in the respective location of an aldehyde and amine group at the 4-position of the pyridine ring structure (Fig. 1). The 5'-phosphoric ester of pyridoxal, pyridoxal-5'-phosphate (PLP), is the metabolically active form of vitamin B_6. Pyridoxamine-5'-phosphate (PMP) and pyridoxine-5'-phosphate (PNP) are also widely distributed in animal and plant tissue. The oxidized metabolites of pyridoxal, 3-hydroxy-5-hydroxymethyl-2-methylpyridine-4-carboxylic acid and the corresponding lactone, are designated 4-pyridoxic acid (4-PA) and 4-pyridoxolactone, respectively. The abbreviations for the B_6 vitamers and 4-pyridoxic acid, as listed in Fig. 1, are often encountered in the vitamin B_6 literature and will also be used in this review.

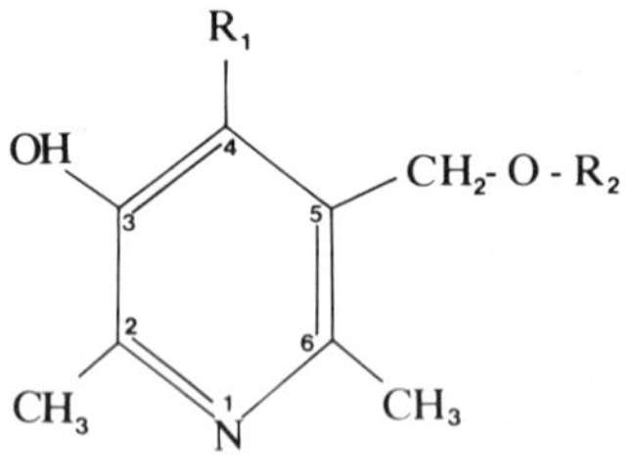

NAME	R_1	R_2
PYRIDOXINE (PN)	CH_2OH	H
PYRIDOXINE-5'-PHOSPHATE (PNP)	CH_2OH	$HO-\overset{\overset{O}{\|\|}}{P}-OH$
PYRIDOXAL (PL)	CHO	H
PYRIDOXAL-5'-PHOSPHATE (PLP)	CHO	$HO-\overset{\overset{O}{\|\|}}{P}-OH$
PYRIDOXAMINE (PM)	CH_2NH_2	H
PYRIDOXAMINE-5'-PHOSPHATE (PMP)	CH_2NH_2	$HO-\overset{\overset{O}{\|\|}}{P}-OH$
4-PYRIDOXIC ACID (4-PA)	COOH	H

Figure 1 Structural formulas of pyridoxine derivatives.

1.3 Biochemistry

The different forms of vitamin B$_6$ as found in animal tissues are interconvertible. Intracellular PLP is derived by phosphorylation of PL (8); the reaction requires ATP (9,10) and is catalyzed by pyridoxal kinase (EC 2.7.1.35). Some tissues (liver, brain, erythrocytes) may utilize PN or PM as precursors for PLP; these vitamers are first phosphorylated by pyridoxal kinase and then oxidized (11–13) to PLP by PM(PN)-5'-phosphate oxidase (EC 1.4.3.5). Synthesis of PLP is balanced by dephosphorylation (14) to PL in a reaction catalyzed by PLP phosphatase. PL may then be oxidized to 4-PA, the end product of vitamin B$_6$ metabolism.

Vitamin B$_6$ is absorbed from the jejunum as PL, PM, and PN; phosphorylated B$_6$ vitamers are first hydrolyzed before absorption can occur (15,16). The liver plays a major role in the metabolism of vitamin B$_6$ (17,18). Liver uptake of PN, PM, and PL occurs by diffusion followed by 5'-phosphorylation catalyzed by PL kinase, which results in effective metabolic trapping of the B$_6$ vitamers (19). In humans, the liver releases PLP, PL, and 4-PA into the circulation (17,18). Circulating PL presumably serves as transport form of vitamin B$_6$, which crosses into extrahepatic tissues to be phosphorylated to the active coenzyme PLP (20,21). Circulating PLP, which is predominantly albumin bound (22,23), does not cross cellular membranes (20,22); the function of circulating PLP is therefore still uncertain.

1.4 Physiological Function

Intracellular PLP, which is derived from extracellular PL, functions as a very versatile coenzyme. Various reactions in α-amino acid metabolism, including transaminations, α decarboxylations, α, β eliminations, β, γ eliminations, aldolizations, and racemizations are PLP dependent.

Decarboxylases function in the synthesis of major neurotransmitters (24); adequate PLP supply in brain tissue is therefore essential for normal brain function. Aminotransferases have a key function in both amino acid biosynthesis and catabolism. PLP also has a structural function (25) in glycogen phosphorylase (EC 2.4.1.1), and a role for PLP in lipid metabolism has been proposed (26).

1.5 Pharmacological Function

The use of pyridoxine therapy in a whole spectrum of diseases was reviewed recently (27). It is noteworthy that several apparently unrelated diseases, ranging from asthma (28) and autistic syndrome (29) to cancer (30) and gestational diabetes (31), have been reported to respond to pyridoxine therapy. Although it is not the purpose of this review to comment on the claims made for PN therapy in the literature, the reason for this "cure-all" effect of PN may simply be the varied and broad metabolic function of B_6. It is thought that increased saturation of enzymes with the cofactor, PLP, may explain most of the pharmacological effects of pyridoxine therapy.

In certain cases, such as carpal tunnel syndrome (32) or Down's syndrome (33), very large PN dosages are required before clinical improvements are observed. This may indicate that pyridoxine has a direct pharmacological effect that is not necessarily related to the normal cofactor function of PLP.

1.6   Different Approaches to Vitamin B_6 Analysis

The measurement of vitamin B_6 in biological material is complicated by (a) the natural occurrence of vitamin B_6 in six different forms (Fig. 1), (b) the relatively low levels of vitamin B_6 in most biological samples, (c) the water solubility of vitamin B_6, which excludes the use of organic solvent extraction procedures for purification and enrichment prior to analysis, and (d) the photosensitivity of vitamin B_6, which requires the availability of darkroom facilities.

Various methods specifically designed to satisfy different requirements in vitamin B_6 analysis have been developed, but few are suitable for the simultaneous analysis of all six natural forms of vitamin B_6 at the low concentrations encountered in biological material. Enzymatic methods, however sensitive, are only suitable for PLP quantification (34–37). Microbiological assay of different forms of vitamin B_6 is cumbersome, indirect, and very time-consuming. These methods employ either different microorganisms sensitive to the different forms of vitamin B_6 (38), or the PL-sensitive *Lactobacillus casei* with sequential conversion of PN and PM to PL by treatment with manganese dioxide and glyoxylic acid (39). Furthermore, growth-promoting and/or growth-inhibitory substances in blood and plasma may render microbiological assays in these samples invalid (40–42).

Direct fluorimetric quantification of PLP and PL has been described (43–46), but these methods are either unreliable due to interfering fluorescent compounds (43), or tedious due to the prior requirement for sample cleanup procedures.

Immunoassays for the different B_6 vitamers have been reported (47,48). However, the need to develop different antibodies against the various B_6 vitamers and the possibility of cross-reactivity are serious practical limitations that prohibit the use of immunoassay in vitamin B_6 analysis.

Compared to the methods mentioned above, chromatographic methods are superior since separation and quantification of the different B$_6$ vitamers can be achieved simultaneously. Especially HPLC, and to a lesser extent GLC, has been exploited to develop various methods suitable for different applications in vitamin B$_6$ analysis.

2. THIN-LAYER CHROMATOGRAPHY

Due to the advent of HPLC, thin-layer chromatography is today seldom used as a quantitative technique in vitamin B$_6$ analysis. However, it remains a convenient qualitative method to study vitamin B$_6$ metabolism. A recent example is provided by the study of Coburn and Mahuren, who investigated vitamin B$_6$ metabolism in cats (49). Coburn and Mahuren found that although about 70% of the ingested [^{14}C]PN dose appeared in the urine, only 2–3% of the excreted dose was 4-pyridoxic acid. Cation-exchange liquid chromatography revealed that two unknown radioactive components were excreted in cat urine. Using thin-layer chromatography, pyridoxine 3-sulfate and pyridoxal 3-sulfate were identified as the major urinary metabolites of ingested pyridoxine; this result was confirmed by infrared spectroscopy of the vitamin B$_6$ metabolites isolated from cat urine.

3. HIGH-PERFORMANCE LIQUID CHROMATOGRAPHY

3.1 Introduction

Before the introduction of HPLC, several different liquid column chromatographic procedures to separate mixtures of B$_6$ vitamers from each other had been developed. Resolution of mixtures of pure vitamins was found to be quite simple. However, application to analysis of food and biological material was difficult, mainly due to low concentrations of the vitamers encountered and unsatisfactory means of detection. Quantification often involved laborious microbiological determination for the different B$_6$ vitamers in column eluate fractions (50).

Several chromatographic procedures published before 1980 relied on UV detection for B$_6$ vitamer quantification; these methods lacked sensitivity for B$_6$ analysis in food and biological fluids (51). Yet these methods, recently reviewed by Coburn (51), form the foundation of modern vitamin B$_6$ analysis by HPLC. The challenge of the 1980s was to develop HPLC methods sensitive enough to allow reliable vitamin B$_6$ determination in biological tissues and food. A wide variety of methods, suitable for different applications has been developed.

1. HPLC methods designed to separate and quantify the six major forms of vitamin B_6 and 4-PA in biological material are termed comprehensive methods in this review. These methods were usually applied in studies of human vitamin B_6 metabolism or pharmacokinetics of pyridoxine supplementation.

2. Comprehensive methods usually require sophisticated HPLC equipment and/or long analysis times per sample, which handicapped the use of these methods in large-scale population studies on vitamin B_6 nutritional status. For nutrition survey studies, sensitive methods for determination of plasma/whole-blood PLP, and preferably including PL, are required.

3. Food analysis also requires comprehensive vitamin B_6 analysis, although differentiation between unphosphorylated vitamers and the 5'-phosphoric acid esters usually is not required. Recent research has shown that certain plant foods may contain considerable amounts of conjugated forms of pyridoxine (52–54), that is, 5'-O-(β-D-glucopyranosyl) pyridoxine (PN-glucoside), which has a much lower bioavailability than pyridoxine (55,56). Methods have therefore been developed for the specific assay of PN-glucoside.

4. Analysis of pharmaceutical preparations is relatively simple when compared to analysis of biological material, because only PN is used as supplementary B_6 vitamer. Methods for PN determination are usually optimized to include determination of other vitamins of the B group.

It has already been pointed out that earlier attempts to use HPLC for B_6 vitamer quantification were hampered by either laborious (microbiological) or insensitive (UV) detection procedures. Modern HPLC analysis of the different B_6 vitamers now exploits the fluorescence characteristics of these vitamers, which allows quantification in the nanomolar range. Modern fluorescence detectors for HPLC are easy to use and are unrivaled as far as both sensitivity and selectivity for vitamin B_6 analysis are concerned. A thorough understanding of the fluorescence characteristics of the different B_6 vitamers is therefore essential before different published HPLC methods can be evaluated.

3.2 Spectral Characteristics of B_6 Vitamers

Ultraviolet Absorption

The UV absorption spectra of PL, PN, PM, and their phosphorylated derivatives dissolved in 0.1 M HCl are similar and the absorption maximum for each B_6 vitamer is about 290 nm (57). At pH 7.0, PN, PM, PNP, and PMP have absorption maxima at 253 and 325 nm. The spectra for PL and PLP at pH 7.0 differ from the other B_6 vitamers in displaying an absorption maximum at about 390 nm, which relates to the aldehyde group on the 4-position of the pyridine ring structure (57). Table 1 compares the molar extinction coefficients of the different B$_6$ vitamers at their respective absorption maxima as determined by pH 7.0.

Fluorescence

The fluorescence characteristics of hydroxypyridines, including the different B$_6$ vitamers, were thoroughly studied by Bridges and co-workers (58). Table 2 summarizes information on vitamin B$_6$ fluorescence that may be useful in development or application of HPLC methods for vitamin B$_6$ analyses. PL, PN, and PM show strong fluorescence in both slightly acidic to neutral and strongly alkaline conditions (Table 2). PNP and PMP show fluorescence characteristics similar to the respective dephosphorylated vitamers.

It should be noted that PL can exist in solution as a cyclic hemiacetal, aldehyde hydrate, or free aldehyde. The cyclic hemiacetal form is predominantly found in solution (59); the fluorescence characteristics of PL listed in Table 2 therefore refer to the cyclic hemiacetal form of the vitamer. If pyridoxal occurred in the aldehyde form, the fluorescence observed should be considerably less, since the aldehyde group tends to diminish the fluorescence of aromatic systems due to its tendency to withdraw electrons from the ring structure (58,60).

Table 1   Molar Extinction Coefficients of B$_6$ Vitamers[a]

Vitamer	Absorbance maximum (nm)	Molar extinction coefficient
PN	253	3700
	325	7100
PNP	253	3700
	325	7400
PL	318	8200
	390	200
PLP	330	2500
	388	4900
PM	253	4600
	325	7700
PMP	253	4700
	325	8300

[a] Data derived from Peterson and Sober (57). Absorption spectra were obtained at pH 7.0 with 0.1 M sodium phosphate buffer as solvent.

Table 2 Fluorescence Characteristics of B$_6$ Vitamers[a]

Vitamer	Excitation/ emission wavelengths (nm)	Observed fluorescence intensity	pH range of maximum fluorescence
PN	332/400	238	6.5–7.5
	320/380	168	12.0–14.0
PL (hemiacetal)	330/382	207	6.0
	310/365	283	12.0
PLP	330/410	11	6.0
	315/370	17.5	12.0–14.0
PM	337/400	370	4.0–5.5
	320/370	410	14.0
4-PA	320/420	770	1.5–4.0
	315/425	650	6.1–9.4
4-Pyridoxolactone	365/423	32	2.5–4.8
	360/430	2150	8.7–13.0

[a] Data derived from Bridges et al. (58). Fluorescence intensity is expressed relative to the fluorescence intensity of the 3-hydroxypyridine anion at pH = 11.0, which was arbitrarily chosen as 100.

Unfortunately, PLP is only weakly fluorescent when compared to PL, PN, or PM, presumably due to withdrawal of electrons from the aromatic ring structure as discussed above. For PLP, however, the phosphoric acid ester on the 5-position of the pyridine ring structure prohibits hemiacetal formation. The natural fluorescence shown by PLP is therefore much lower and inadequate for accurate quantification of this vitamer in biological samples. Several methods, however, have been described to enhance PLP fluorescence: Bonavita and Scardi reported in 1959 that PLP reacts with potassium cyanide in presence of a phosphate buffer, resulting in characteristic changes in the absorption and fluorescence spectra of the coenzyme (61). Except for pyridoxal, none of the other B$_6$ vitamers was able to react with potassium cyanide. The cyanide reaction greatly enhanced the fluorescence of both PL and PLP. The spectral changes of PL and PLP treated with potassium cyanide were initially thought to be the result of cyanohydrin derivative formation of these vitamers (62). However, it was later discovered that cyanide acts as catalyst in the oxidation (by air) of PL and PLP to 4-pyridoxolactone and 4-pyridoxic acid 5′-phosphate, respectively (63).

Reagents that attack the aldehyde group usually enhance PLP fluorescence, presumably by elimination of the electron-withdrawing effect of the aldehyde group. Aldehydes are known to react on sodium bisulfite to form hydroxysulfonic acid salts (64). The hydroxysulfonate derivative of PLP is much more fluorescent than native PLP; fluorescence shown by the hydroxysulfonate derivative at pH 7.5 is strong enough to allow PLP quantification in the nanomolar range (65).

Ammonia derivatives may react with carbonyl groups, resulting in products containing a carbon-nitrogen double bond and elimination of a molecule of water. PLP has thus been shown to react with semicarbazide to form PLP-semicarbazone, which is not very fluorescent in slightly acid to neutral solutions (66) but shows strong fluorescence at pH 12 (67). Pyridoxal semicarbazone is also very fluorescent at alkaline pH (Fig. 2). The semicarbazone reaction has been shown by Conant et al. (68) to be a general acid-catalyzed reaction with a slightly acidic pH optimum. The correct acidity of the reaction medium is important, because addition involves nucleophilic attack by the basic semicarbazide on the carbonyl carbon (Fig. 3). When the carbonyl oxygen is protonated, the carbonyl carbon becomes more susceptible to nucleophilic attack, indicating that addition will be favored by high acidity. However, semicarbazide (: NH$_2$NHCONH$_2$) might also undergo protonation to form an ion ($^+$NH$_3$NHCONH$_2$), which lacks unshared electrons and is no longer nucleophilic. As far as semicarbazide is concerned, addition will be favored by lower acidity.

We therefore studied PLP-semicarbazone formation under various pH conditions and found that semicarbazone formation was quantitative even in the presence of a 3.3% solution of trichloroacetic acid (pH < 2.0) if semicarbazide was present in concentrations 4000-fold more than the PLP concentrations (69). This implied that trichloroacetic acid-protein precipitation and the semicarbazide reaction could be performed in a single step, a possibility that has been exploited in the development of a HPLC method for PLP and PL quantification in biological material (69). An attractive, additional feature of the semicarbazide reaction is that semicarbazone derivatives of PLP and PL are stable under ordinary laboratory light conditions, thus eliminating the need for light-protective precautions (70).

Attaching of fluorescent probes to PLP has also been used to determine PLP. Chauhan and Dakshinamurti employed reductive amination of PLP with methyl anthranilate and sodium cyanoborohydride to form a highly fluorescent amine (71). Durko et al. (44) prepared diphenyl-isobenzofurane derivatives of B$_6$ vitamers to enable fluorometric measurement of vitamin B$_6$. However, the use of fluorescent probes is generally not suitable for routine analytical work, mainly because the unreacted fluorescent probe may interfere in B$_6$ vitamer quantification (71).

408 UBBINK

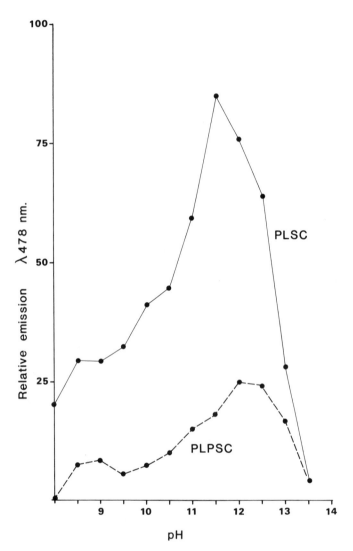

Figure 2 The pH-dependent fluorescence of the semicarbazone derivatives of PLP (40 nmol/liter ------) and PL (60 nmol/liter _____). A stock solution of PLP (40 μmol/liter) and of PL (60 μmol/liter) were separately made up in 0.025 mol/liter semicarbazide. A blank solution containing only semicarbazide was also prepared. All three solutions were heated to 37°C in a water bath for 30 min to effect semicarbazone formation. Each solution was diluted 1000-fold in the following buffers: (a) 0.1 M Na$_2$HPO$_4$/NaH$_2$PO$_4$ at pH 8.0, 8.5, and 9.0; (b) 0.1 M NaHCO$_3$/Na$_2$CO$_3$ at pH 9.5, 10.0, and 10.5; (c) 0.1 M Na$_2$HPO$_4$/NaOH at pH 11.0, 11.5, and 12.0; (d) 0.1 M KCl/NaOH at pH 12.5, 13.0, and 13.5. Fluorescence emission intensity at 478 nm, after excitation at 367 nm, was determined for PLP semicarbazone (PLPSC) and PL semicarbazone (PLSC) at the above-mentioned pH values, using the different solutions as indicated.

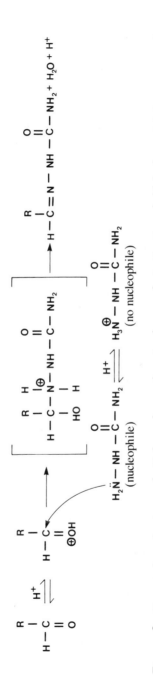

Figure 3 Proposed mechanism and pH dependency of semicarbazone derivatization of aldehyde-containing compounds.

3.3 Pharmaceutical Preparations

Analysis of vitamins in multivitamin preparations is essential to ensure quality control and to establish the shelf life of the multivitamin product. The form of vitamin B_6 usually present in pharmaceutical preparations is PN; this vitamer is noteably more stable than the aldehyde derivative, PL (72,73). Compared to biological matrixes, vitamin B_6 analysis in pharmaceutical preparations is relatively simple, because PN is the only B_6 vitamer present and analysis of the complete B_6 vitamer profile is therefore not required. Moreover, PN concentrations in multivitamin products are usually high enough to allow UV detection. A summary of available methods is given in Table 3.

Table 3   HPLC Determination of Pyridoxine in Pharmaceutical Preparations

Vitamins determined	Chromatographic conditions[a]	Detection	Reference
PN, thiamine, niacinamide, riboflavin, niacin	μBondapak C18; 5 mM S6S in 1% acetic acid : methanol (75:25)	UV (270 nm)	74
PN, thiamine, riboflavin, niacinamide	μBondapak C18; 5 mM S6S in 1% acetic acid : methanol (75:25)	UV (254/280 nm)	75
PN	Zorbax C8; 5 mM $NaClO_4$, 5 mM S6S, pH to 2.5 with $HClO_4$, containing 10–20% methanol	Colorimetric[c] (650 nm)	76
PN, thiamine, riboflavin vitamin B_{12}	Lichrosorb RP-18; methanol : water (50:50).	UV, 254 nm	77
PN, thiamine, riboflavin, vitamin B_{12}, folate, nicotinamide	μBondapak C18; binary SP 0.2 M ammoniumphosphate, pH 5.1 (solvent A); 30% methanol in water (solvent B)[b]	UV, 254 nm	78

[a] Only the most pertinent characteristics of the chromatographic separation are listed. Separations were achieved isocratically, unless indicated otherwise. Abbreviations: S6S = sodium hexanesulfonate, SP = solvent program.

[b] Solvent program: 100% solvent A for 21 min, change to 100% solvent B. Flow rate: 2.0 ml/min.

[c] Pyridoxine is reacted with 2.6 dibromoquinone-4-chlorimide.

Kirchmeier and Upton (74) developed an ion-pair HPLC procedure with UV detection for the simultaneous determination of niacin, niacinamide, pyridoxine, thiamine, and riboflavin extracted from multivitamin preparations (Table 3). Minimal interference from other vitamins, dyes, or preservatives was experienced; the use of sodium hexanesulfonate as an ion-pair agent allowed use of a mobile phase containing 25% methanol, and vitamins A, D, and E, folic acid, and calcium pantothenate were reported either to be insoluble in the aqueous portion of the mobile phase or to elute at the solvent front (74).

Walker et al. (75), using essentially the same chromatographic conditions as Kirchmeier and Upton (74), optimized pyridoxine detection by dual-wavelength UV detection. Pyridoxine elution was monitored at 280 nm, while other vitamins (thiamine, riboflavin, and niacinamide) were measured at 254 nm.

Kawamoto and co-workers used HPLC and postcolumn derivatization with 2,6-dibromoquinone-4-clorimide to quantify PN in pharmaceutical products (76). The condensation product shows strong absorption in the visible spectrum (650 nm); detection has been reported to be almost seven times more sensitive when compared to UV (250 nm) detection of PN. The main advantage of this method is selectivity; other B vitamins or caffeine (often present in vitamin preparations) were shown not to interfere in PN quantification. The disadvantage of the method is that two postcolumn reaction pumps with reaction coils are required to deliver reagents to the column eluate. Furthermore, only PN can be analyzed by this method, while most modern quality control programs tend to optimize vitamin analyses by simultaneous analysis of several vitamin compounds.

Amin and Reusch (77) described a rapid HPLC separation of pyridoxine, riboflavin, thiamine, and vitamin B$_{12}$. Separation has been reported to be complete within 3 min of injection. The work of Kothari and Taylor (78) provides yet another example of the use of HPLC in vitamin analysis for the pharmaceutical industry. This method is suitable for simultaneous analysis of PN, thiamine, riboflavin, nicotinamide, and folic acid. This comprehensive vitamin analysis was possible by using a binary solvent program, which distinguishes this method from the above isocratic ones (Table 3).

It seems that HPLC analysis of multivitamin preparations today is widely accepted to ensure quality control. Colorimetric, fluorometric, and microbiological methods have often been replaced by HPLC analysis. The main advantage of HPLC analysis is perhaps its versatility and flexibility; published vitamin analysis methods are usually easily adapted to suit different requirements of the pharmaceutical industry.

3.4 Analysis of Food

Comprehensive Food Analysis

Vitamin B_6 analysis in foods is a difficult analytical problem, because all six vitamers occur in relatively low concentrations in complex, organic matrices. Due to the complicated composition of food, it is clear that reliable vitamin B_6 determinations require high chromatographic efficiency and detection sensitivity, as well as excellent detection specificity. Fluorescence detection fulfills these requirements. This mode of detection is therefore virtually exclusively used in modern chromatographic vitamin B_6 analysis of food. Several methods suitable for food analysis, summarized in Table 4, have been described in the literature.

Using anion-exchange HPLC, Vanderslice and co-workers were able to separate the six nutritionally active B_6 vitamers from each other within 70 min (79). Two fluorescence detectors were connected in series to monitor the column eluate; the second detector was optimized for PLP quantification, for which a lower detection limit of 100 ng was reported. Application of this method to food required prior extraction of B_6 vitamers using sulfosalicylic acid (80). As sulfosalicylic acid binds strongly to the analytical anion-exchange column used, an additional ion-exchange purification step was introduced to remove sulfosalicylic acid from the sample.

Although this method has been applied to pyridoxine determination in vitamin B_6 fortified cereals (81), the method was not suitable for general vitamin B_6 analysis in food due to the low fluorescence exhibited by PLP. A modification of this method was therefore described to increase sensitivity for PLP (82). Two anion-exchange columns were connected by a six-way valve; the first column was thermostated at 50° C and semicarbazide was added to the mobile phase to a final concentration of 0.005 M. It was assumed that semicarbazide derivatives of PLP and PL would be formed on column, resulting in increased sensitivity. Although increased sensitivity was obtained, it resulted in excessive peak broadening for PLP and PL. This necessitated the sophisticated dual-column setup; after elution of PMP, PM, PNP, and PN from the first column, the six-way valve was activated to direct first-column eluate through the second column to facilitate separation of PLP from 3-hydroxypyridine, the internal standard. After elution of 3-hydroxypyridine, the six-way valve was activated again to bypass the second column and PL was eluted from the first column. In addition to column switching, the fluorescence detector wavelengths had to be changed to allow optimum detection of the semicarbazide derivatives of PLP and PL. This complicated, relatively long procedure severely limited the number of specimens that could be analyzed per day. However, this was partially offset by automation of the vitamin B$_6$ analysis system (83,84). Vanderslice and co-workers used this method for analysis of a wide variety of foods, ranging from powdered milk to hamburgers (80).

The method of Vanderslice and co-workers was time-consuming and the anion-exchange resin used was not commercially available in prepacked HPLC columns. This prompted other investigators to develop simpler HPLC methods suitable for vitamin B$_6$ food analysis. Based on their reversed-phase HPLC method for the determination of PLP and PL in animal tissues as semicarbazone derivatives (66), Gregory and co-workers modified this technique to analyze selected foods from animal origin (85). In animal tissues, vitamin B$_6$ activity is almost entirely due to PL, PM, and their 5'-phosphorylated derivatives (85). Glyoxylate treatment of processed food samples before semicarbazone derivatization has been shown to deaminate PMP to PM and PLP and PL, respectively (85); analysis of food samples with and without glyoxylate treatment thus allowed calculation of the PMP and PM content of the sample. Although this method was not suitable for plant foods that usually contain PN, Gregory et al. pointed out that manganese dioxide could possibly be used to oxidize PN and PNP to PL and PLP, respectively (85). This would allow measurement of PN and PNP as semicarbazone derivatives of PL and PLP. However, this possibility was not further pursued, presumably due to later developments that allowed direct HPLC determination of the different B$_6$ vitamers (86–88).

The work of the groups of Vanderslice (79–84) and Gregory (66,85), as discussed above, could be regarded as pioneering efforts to establish reliable HPLC analysis of vitamin B$_6$ in food. Later reports on food vitamin B$_6$ analysis are usually based on reversed-phase HPLC with or without ion pairing and can be divided into two groups: (a) methods for direct determination of all six nutritionally active B$_6$ vitamers (86–88), and (b) methods for PL, PN and PM determination after dephosphorylation of the 5'-phosphorylated vitamers (89–92). Gregory and Feldstein (86) developed an ion-paired, reversed-phase HPLC method for individual B$_6$ vitamers in foods. Vitamer extraction from food was accomplished using the sulfosalicylic acid extraction method of Vanderslice et al. (80). Using a ternary solvent program, elution of nutritionally active B$_6$ vitamers from the analytical column was complete within 30 min. PLP was determined as its hydroxysulfonate derivative, following postcolumn introduction of a buffered solution of sodium bisulfite. This method was found suitable for vitamin B$_6$ analysis in foods of both plant and animal origin. Recoveries for PLP and PL from pork loin were less than 90%; it was suggested that these vitamers were not completely released from muscle proteins, even in the presence of 5% sulfosalicylic acid.

Table 4 HPLC Determination of B_6 Vitamers in Food

Vitamers determined	Chromatographic conditions[b]	Detection[f]	PLP derivative	Foods analyzed	Reference
PL, PLP, PM, PMP, PN, PNP	Aminex-A25; 0.4 M sodium chloride, 0.01 M glycine, 0.005 M semicarbazide (pH 10)[c]	Fl(310/380 and 280/487)[g]	SC On-C	Broiled pork, carp, powdered milk, fresh hamburgers	80
PL, PLP, PM, PMP	Ultrasphere IP; 0.033 M potassium phosphate (pH 2.2) with 2.5% acetonitrile	Fl (365/400)	SC Pre-C	Cow milk, raw and cooked beef liver	85
PL, PLP, PM, PMP, PN, PN glucoside	Perkin-Elmer, 3 µM ODS; ternary SP with 0.033 M potassium phosphate (pH 2.2), 8mM S8S and propanol[d]	Fl (330/400)	Bisulfite Post-C	Frozen broccoli, pork chops, cows' milk	86,94
PL, PLP, PM, PMP, PN, 4-PA	LiChrospher RP-18; binary SP with: methanol (solvent A) and 0.03 M potassium phosphate (pH 2.2) + 4 mM S8S (solvent B)[e]	Fl (330/400)	Bisulfite Post-C	Pork liver, cows' milk	87

All[a]	TSK-gel, ODS-120A; 0.1 M sodium perchlorate, 0.1 M potassium phosphate, 1% acetonitrile (pH 3.5)	Fl (305/390)	KCN Pre-C	Fruit juice, wheat flour, asparagus, eggs, milk, cheese, rice bran	88
PL, PM, PN	Spherisorb-ODS; 0.08 M sulfuric acid	Fl (290/395)	—	Pork, beef, eggs, milk, potatoes, frozen peas	92

[a] "All" refers to the six nutritionally active B_6 vitamers and 4-PA. Abbreviations: SC = semicarbazide; SP = solvent program; on-C = on-column; post-C = post-column; pre-C = precolumn; Fl = fluorescence; NS = not specified; S6S = sodium hexanesulfonate, S7S = sodium heptanesulfonate, S8S = sodium octanesulfonate; solv = solvent.

[b] Columns and eluants used are tabled. Separations were achieved isocratically, unless indicated otherwise.

[c] A dual-column setup with column switching is required.

[d] Solvent program: Linear gradient from 100% solvent A to 100% solvent B over 12 min (1.8 ml/min flow rate), followed by a programmed switch to 100% solvent C 15 min after injection. Solvent A = 0.033 M potassium phosphate, 8 mM S8S (pH 2.2); solvent B = 0.033 potassium phosphate, 8 mM S8S, 2.5% propanol (pH 2.2); solvent C = 0.033 M potassium phosphate, 6.5% 2-propanol (pH 2.2).

[e] Solvent program: 90% B and 10% A from 0 to 2 min, linear gradient from 90% B at 2 min to 60% B at 12 min, 60% B and 40% A from 12 to 17 min, 60% B from 17 min to 90% B at 19 min. Flow rate: 1.5 ml/min.

[f] Figures in brackets indicate excitation and emission wavelengths used for fluorescence detection.

[g] Switching of excitation and emission wavelengths is required for detection of PLP semicarbazone and PL semicarbazone.

415

Bitsch and Möller (87) modified the method of Gregory and Feld-stein by changing the mode of elution to a binary gradient. A further modification included the use of perchloric acid for B_6 vitamer extraction from food and omission of the preparative anion exchange chromatography step for purification of food samples. Recovery for PLP and PL from liver was better than that obtained by Gregory and Feldstein on pork loin, presumably indicating that perchloric acid is a more efficient B_6 vitamer extraction agent from animal tissues than sulfosalicylic acid. This view is supported by Toukairin-Oda et al. (88), who found that extraction with 1 M perchloric acid gave most reliable data. Neither the method of Bitsch and Möller (87) nor the method of Gregory and Feld-stein (86) was able to quantify PNP. However, the exclusion of PNP is of little importance, as this vitamer occurs only in minute amounts in food.

Toukairin-Oda reported an isocratic, reversed-phase HPLC method for determination of all six nutritionally active B_6 vitamers in food (88). PLP fluorescence was enhanced by precolumn potassium cyanide treatment to convert PLP to the highly fluorescent 4-pyridoxic acid 5′-phosphate. Although the isocratic solvent system is simpler to use than the gradient elution programs discussed above, this method suffers from the drawback that each sample has to be analyzed twice: with and without prior potassium cyanide treatment. Potassium cyanide causes oxidation of PL to 4-pyridoxic acid lactone, which shows little fluorescence at the acid pH (pH = 3.5) of the mobile phase used (Table 2). This problem is circumvented by duplicate analysis: (a) without prior potassium cyanide treatment to determine all the B_6 vitamers except PLP, and (b) after potassium cyanide treatment to determine PLP as 4-pyridoxic acid 5-phosphate. This method has been applied to fruit juices, wheat flour, cream cheese, eggs, and baker's yeast.

A major advantage of the HPLC procedures discussed above is that PN-glucoside is not included in the determination of food vitamin B_6 content. These glucosides appear to be largely unavailable in humans (55). Microbiological assay procedures rely on autoclaving in the presence of HCl for B_6 vitamer extraction (39). These harsh, acid conditions result in hydrolysis of both phosphate esters and glycoside conjugates, thus resulting in an overestimation of the biologically available vitamin B_6 content of food.

The phosphorylated B_6 vitamers are dephosphorylated in the gastrointestinal tract before absorption (15,16); from a nutritional viewpoint there is little or no difference in the bioavailability of phosphorylated versus unphosphorylated B_6 vitamers. Therefore, phosphorylated and unphosphorylated B_6 vitamers could be measured together, provided that a suitable dephosphorylation step is included in the assay procedure. HPLC separation of PL, PN, and PM is simple and can usually be achieved with an isocratic solvent system (89–92). This principle has been utilized by Bognar (92), who used sulfuric acid treatment at 120°C to hydrolyze phosphoric acid esters of PL, PN, and PM. Quantification of PL, PN, and PM using reversed-phase HPLC and fluorescence detection was then easily accomplished. The advantage of this method is that derivatization steps to enhance PLP fluorescence become redundant. A possible disadvantage of this procedure is that hydrolysis of B$_6$ vitamerglycosides may also occur, resulting in an overestimation of the biologically available vitamin B$_6$ content of food, as discussed above. This problem may be circumvented by enzymatic hydrolysis of the phosphorylated B$_6$ vitamers in the food extract prior to HPLC analysis; this principle has already been applied to analysis of several food products (85,93).

PN-glucosides in plant foods may be determined by direct or indirect methods. The indirect method utilizes β-glucosidase treatment of homogenized food samples. The vitamin B$_6$ content of the sample is determined before and after enzyme treatment, and the increase in pyridoxine concentration after β-glucosidase treatment reflects the PN-glucoside concentration in the food sample (54). In the direct method, PN-glucoside is quantitated by ion-pair, reversed-phase HPLC separation and fluorescence detection (94). The latter method could become the method of choice in food analysis because information on the concentration of the other B$_6$ vitamers is also obtained (Fig. 4).

Determination of Pyridoxine in Fortified Food Products

The majority of breakfast cereals in the United States are fortified to contain one-fourth of the recommended daily allowance of vitamin B$_6$ per serving (81), while additional PN is also added to infant formula products to ensure adequate vitamin B$_6$ supply to the infant. Both Vanderslice et al. (81) and Gregory (89) reported isocratic HPLC methods for the determination of PN in breakfast cereals (Table 5). Other investigators attempted simultaneous determination of PN and other vitamins used in food fortification. Wehling and Wetzel used ion-pair HPLC to separate pyridoxine, riboflavin and thiamine from each other after acid extraction of the vitamins from cereals (96). Using a dual fluorescence detector setup, pyridoxine and riboflavin were monitored by the first detector. After the column eluate had passed the first detector, an alkaline ferricyanide solution was introduced, resulting in the formation of a fluorescent thiochrome derivative of thiamine, which was detected by the second fluorescence detector. A similar method for simultaneous determination of pyridoxine and riboflavin in infant formula products has also been described (97). Methods for the determination of pyridoxine in fortified food products are summarized in Table 5.

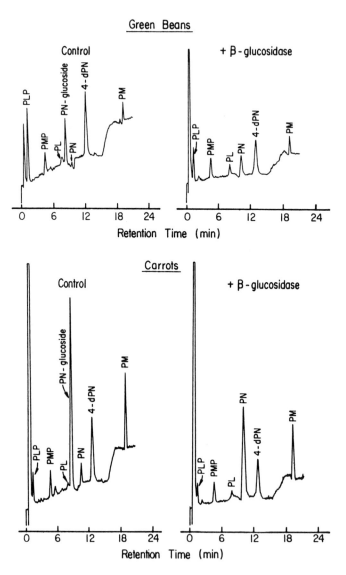

Figure 4   HPLC analysis for vitamin B_6 in green beans and carrots. Note the presence of PN glucoside, which disappears after treatment with β-glucosidase (refer also to Table 4). Reprinted from Gregory and Ink (94) with permission.

Table 5 Determination of Pyridoxine in Fortified Food Products

Vitamins determined	Chromatographic conditions[a]	Detection[b]	Foods analyzed	Reference
PN	Aminex A-25; 0.04 M NaCl, 0.01 M glycine, 5 mM semicarbazide (pH 10)	Fl (310/380)	Breakfast cereal	81
PN	μBondapak C18; 0.033 M potassium phosphate (pH 2.2)	Fl (295/405)	Breakfast cereal	95
PN, riboflavin, thiamine	μBondapak C18; methanol : water : acetic acid (30:69:1); containing 5 mM S7S	Fl (288/418)	Breakfast cereal	96
PN, PL, riboflavin	Spherisorb ODS-1; 7.5 mM S8S in 0.04 M triethylamine (pH to 3 with H_3PO_4): acetonitrile : methanol (85:5:10)	Fl (285/546)	Infant formula products	97

[a] Methods cited used isocratic elution. Abbreviations: refer to Table 4.

[b] Figures in brackets indicate excitation and emission wavelengths used for fluorescence detection.

3.5 Biological Materials

Comprehensive Vitamin B$_6$ Analysis

Vitamin B$_6$ quantification should be comprehensive enough to allow detailed metabolic studies in humans, yet also simple enough to allow large-scale population studies on vitamin B$_6$ nutritional status. From studies on the vitamin B$_6$ composition of food, it is clear that separation of the six nutritionally active vitamers in a single run needs either binary or ternary solvent programs (86,87) or a dual-column system (80). In biological material, vitamin B$_6$ analysis is further complicated because (a) determination of 4-PA, the end-product of vitamin B$_6$ metabolism, is now also required, and (b) levels of individual B$_6$ vitamers in certain biological matrices (e.g., human plasma) are lower than those encountered in food samples.

Table 6 summarizes several methods for vitamin B$_6$ analysis in biological materials. Vanderslice et al. adapted their dual-column HPLC method (originally developed for food analysis) to include the analysis of human plasma (98) and human milk samples (99). These workers used a glycine buffer (pH = 10) as mobile phase for their dual-column system,

Table 6 Comprehensive Measurement of B_6 Vitamers in Biological Tissues

Vitamers determined	Chromatographic conditions[b]	Detection[f]	PLP derivative	Matrix	Reference
All[a]	AminexA-25; binary SP with 0.01 M glycine buffers containing 0.4 M NaCl and 0.005 M semicarbazide[c]	Fl (310/380 and 280/487)[g]	SC On-C	Human plasma and milk	98,99
All	Vydac 401 TP-B; ternary SP with 0.02 M HCl (solvent A), 0.1 M sodium phosphate, pH 3.3 (solvent B), 0.1 M sodium phosphate, pH 5.9 (solvent C)[d]	Fl (330/400)	Bisulfite Post-C	Human plasma, plasma of domestic animals, different organs	65,102,103,104
PL, PLP, PM, PMP, PN, PNP	Partisil 10 SCX; 0.1 M ammonium phosphate, pH 4.0	Fl (290/389)	Bisulfite Pre-C	Cell-free yeast culture media	106
All	μBondapak C18; binary SP with 4 mM S7S and 4m M S8S in 0.09 % acetic acid (solvent A), 20 % acetonitrile in 0.9 % acetic acid (solvent B)[e]	Fl (330/400)	Bisulfite Post-C	Human blood and plasma	108,109

PL, PM PN	μBondapk C18; binary SP with water : methanol (85:15) (solvent A), 5 mM S7S in 1% acetic acid (solvent B)[h]	Fl (300/375)	—	Plasma, brain, kidney, liver from rats	89,90
PL, PLP, PM, PMP, PN	Biosphere ODS; 0.033 M potassium phosphate (pH 2.9) containing 3% methanol	Fl (NS)	Bisulfite Post-C	Human milk	110
All	TSK ODS-120 T (LKB); 0.075 M sodium phosphate containing 0.075 M sodium perchlorate, 0.85% acetonitrile, 0.05% triethanolamine (pH 3.38)	Fl (325/400)	Bisulfite Post-C	Human plasma	111

[a,b,f,g] Refer to footnotes to Table 4. Abbreviations: Refer to Table 4.

[c] Two glycine buffers are required: one is adjusted to pH = 10 with an NaOH solution (solvent A), and the other is adjusted to pH 2.5 with HCl (solvent B). Solvent program: Elute with 100% A for 80 min, change to 100% B for 40 min. Flow rate: 1.25 ml/min.

[d] Solvent program: 100% A from 0 to 13 min, 100% B from 13 to 17 min, linear gradient from 100% B at 17 min to 88% B and 12% C at 25 min, linear gradient from 25 min to 100% C at 30 min, maintaining 100% C until 40 min. Flow rate: 1.5 ml/min.

[e] Solvent program: Linear gradient from 100% A to 50% A and 50% B over 10 min, linear gradient from 10 min to 30% A and 70% B at 20 min, isocratic elution at 30% A and 70% B until 40 min. Flow rate: 1.0 ml/min.

[h] Solvent program: Concave gradient from 100% B to 60% B and 40% A over 11 min, isocratic elution at 60% B and 40% A from 11 to 17 min. Flow rate 1.5 ml/min.

which eluted the nutritionally active B_6 vitamers from the column(s) within 70 min. By changing the pH to 2.5 after elution of the nutritionally active B_6 vitamers, 4-PA could be eluted from the column. However, the drawback of this method is that preparative anion exchange chromatography is required to remove sulfosalicylic acid from the sample. The nutritionally active B_6 vitamers were found to elute close to the void volume of the preparative anion exchange column, but 4-PA eluted later from the column (86), implying that 4-PA levels would be underestimated if the complete elution volume from the preparative column was not recovered. It should be pointed out that analytical losses might not be sufficiently covered by the internal standard (3-hydroxypyridine), because the elution pattern of the internal standard from the preparative column resembled that of the active B_6 vitamers and was thus distinctly different from 4-PA's elution pattern.

In the discussion on food analysis, it has been pointed out that the method of Vanderslice et al. used on-column semicarbazone formation of PLP and PL to enhance fluorescence of the aldehyde B_6 derivatives. Although increased sensitivity was obtained, both PLP and PL showed excessive peak broadening. Excessive peak broadening is presumably the reason why Vanderslice et al. were unable to detect PL in plasma from unsupplemented volunteers (98). The peak broadening could be related to incomplete in situ semicarbazone formation. Since a glycine buffer was used (82), the possibility is not excluded that Schiff base formation between glycine and PLP or PL could compete with semicarbazone formation. Finally, the high pyridoxine levels in plasma reported by Vanderslice and co-workers (98) seem to be spurious; others have shown that pyridoxine is rapidly cleared from the circulation (100), resulting in low to undetectable (100,101) plasma PN concentrations.

Difficulties experienced in reproducing the anion exchange method of Vanderslice and co-workers led Coburn and Mahuren to develop cation-exchange HPLC for comprehensive vitamin B_6 analysis (65,102). The cation-exchange method is based on a ternary solvent program to separate the B_6 vitamers. PLP, PNP, and 4-PA were eluted from the column using 0.02 M HCl as mobile phase; subsequently, a gradient program using 0.1 M NaH_2PO_4 (pH = 3.3) and 0.5 M NaH_2PO_4 (pH = 5.9) was used to elute the remaining B_6 vitamers and the internal standard. A sodium bisulfite solution in 1 M phosphate buffer (pH = 7.5) was introduced as postcolumn reagent. This served two functions: (a) the bisulfite ion reacts with PLP to form a hydroxysulfonate derivative with enhanced fluorescence, and (b) the pH of the column eluate is raised to about 7, which further enhances the fluorescence of the other vitamers. PNP, which elutes with the 0.02 M HCl solution, would not have been detected without increasing the pH.

The elution of PLP and 4-PA has been reported to be sensitive to both ionic strength and pH of the sample. With increasing pH or ionic strength, PLP retention will be diminished resulting in faster elution and possible interference by nonspecific, early-eluting compounds (65). Column ageing also resulted in a considerable decrease in the retention times for PLP and 4-PA, and in a deterioration of the resolution of early eluting vitamers and impurities (103).

Coburn and Mahuren used 5-chloroanthranilic acid as internal standard, which was only suitable to monitor HPLC analysis and could not be left to stand in the sample for an extended period of time (65). Deoxypyridoxine was not used as internal standard because it eluted after PM (the last vitamer to be eluted from the column) and would have increased total analyses time. Shephard et al. suggested the use of deoxy-pyridoxine 5'-phosphate as internal standard, which was shown to elute from the cation-exchange column between PLP and 4-PA (103).

The method of Coburn and Mahuren has been applied to plasma samples of several animal species (104) and to a variety of biological tissues (101). This method has been reproduced and established in other laboratories (103,105). PLP measurement by this method has been shown to correlate well with the apo-tyrosine decarboxylase enzymatic method of PLP quantification (103). Results obtained with the cation-exchange HPLC method also correlated well with total vitamin B$_6$ determinations determined by a radiometric microbiological assay (104). A good correlation between the cation-exchange HPLC method and the open-column chromatography method of Lui et al. (105) was also reported. It may be concluded that the cation-exchange HPLC method of Coburn and Mahuren is reproducible and correlates well with other established procedures for B$_6$ vitamer quantification.

Argoudelis reported an isocratic cation-exchange HPLC method for separation of the six biologically active B$_6$ vitamers (106). Using a Whatman Partisil 10 SCX analytical column, separation was completed within 20 min. Precolumn derivatization of PLP with sodium bisulfite was used to improve PLP fluorescence. Up to now the method has only been applied to cell-free yeast culture media, and it is not yet known whether the method will allow sufficient resolution between B$_6$ vitamers and impurities often encountered in biological material.

Tryfiates and Sattsangi described an ion-paired, reversed-phase HPLC separation of all the B$_6$ vitamers (including 4-PA) within 40 min (107). The separation is accomplished by using a binary solvent program. However, since a UV detector was used, this method was not directly applicable for analysis of biological samples. Using a fluorescence detector and postcolumn sodium bisulfite addition to enhance PLP fluorescence, Henderson and co-workers applied the method of Tryfiates and Sattsangi to analysis of biological samples (108,109). Greater column stability renders reversed-phase ion-pair chromatography preferable to ion-exchange chromatography. However, more laborious sample preparation is required to avoid interference in ion pairing. The supernatant obtained after trichloroacetic acid protein precipitation had to be washed extensively with diethyl ether to remove residual trichloroacetic acid, which could interfere in ion pairing (108,109). Subsequently, the aqueous phase was dried under nitrogen; the extracts were then reconstituted in the mobile phase prior to injection. The sample preparation is time-consuming, and only a limited number of samples could therefore be analyzed daily.

Ordinary reversed-phase HPLC has also been reported to yield promising results in biological tissue analysis. Hamaker et al. used an isocratic method for analysis of human milk (110), while Edwards and coworkers reported an isocratic method suitable for determination of the six B_6 vitamers and 4-PA in human plasma (111).

Pierotti et al. (90) used perchloric acid to extract B_6 vitamers from selected rat tissues; after alkalinization to remove perchloric acid as potassium perchlorate, the supernatant was acidified with hydrochloric acid and autoclaved to hydrolyze the phosphorylated B_6 vitamers. A binary solvent program and ion-pair reversed-phase HPLC was used to separate PL, PM, and PN. A later modification of this method, applied to rat plasma, omitted acid protein hydrolysis and used potato acid phosphatase to hydrolyze phosphate esters (91). The advantage of the latter procedure is its simplicity. However, since PLP is tightly protein bound, incomplete hydrolysis of PLP to PL might occur with this method. While albumin-bound PLP is hydrolyzable by phophatases (22), PLP binds to liver proteins with widely different affinities; in fact, PLP from dialyzed rat liver cytosol could hardly be hydrolyzed by alkaline phosphatase treatment (112). As far as could be established, the enzymatic procedure has not yet been applied to other biological tissues. If this is attempted, rigid recovery studies, especially for PLP, should be performed to demonstrate complete PLP hydrolysis.

A major drawback of the method of Pierotti et al. is that the phosphorylated B_6 vitamers are not determined separately; this renders the method unsuitable for metabolic studies in which information on the active co-enzyme forms of vitamin B_6 (PLP and PMP) is essential.

Methods for the determination of PLP and/or PL

The comprehensive methods described above are generally unsuitable for clinical studies, which may require analysis of many blood samples to define vitamin B_6 status in (different) population groups. Studies on large population groups preferably require rapid and reliable HPLC methods to measure vitamin B$_6$ status. The plasma PLP level has been thought to be a sensitive parameter for vitamin B$_6$ nutritional status (113), and several methods suitable for plasma/erythrocyte PLP determination have been developed.

Several methods to measure PLP by HPLC are complementary enzymatic determinations of PLP (Table 7). An often-used enzymatic method (36) for assaying plasma PLP is based on the coenzyme-dependent decarboxylation of tyrosine catalyzed by L-tyrosine decarboxylase (EC 4.1.1.25). By using a well-resolved apo-enzyme preparation, it was shown that the reaction rate is directly proportional to the amount of PLP added to the reaction mixture. Conventionally, the reaction is monitored by $^{14}CO_2$ liberation from L-tyrosine-$^{14}C_1$; the liberated $^{14}CO_2$ is trapped in a potassium hydroxide solution and subsequently quantitated by liquid scintillation counting.

The enzymatic method described above has two disadvantages: (a) trapping of $^{14}CO_2$ is a cumbersome procedure, and (b) the use of a radioactive substrate requires special precautions for use and disposal of reagents. Measurement of the primary amine formed by decarboxylation of the amino acid can also be exploited to monitor the PLP-dependent, enzyme-catalyzed reaction. This principle has been applied by Allenmark et al. (114), who used L-3,4 dihydroxyphenylalanine (L-DOPA) as substrate for tyrosine decarboxylase; the dopamine produced by the decarboxylation reaction was determined by HPLC followed by amperometric detection. Both Hamfelt (115) and Lequeu et al. (116) utilized apo-tyrosine decarboxylase with tyrosine as substrate. The tyramine produced by the decarboxylation reaction was separated from the substrate (tyrosine) by HPLC and quantitated by either amperometric (116) or fluorometric (115) detection. The procedures discussed above are still subject to the main disadvantage of enzymatic methods: possible interference by other materials present in the PLP-containing extract that could either inhibit reconstitution of the holoenzyme or alter the reaction rate of enzyme catalysis. Moreover, HPLC with amperometric detection can hardly be described as less cumbersome than $^{14}CO_2$ trapping; difficulties in baseline stabilization encountered with these detectors are well known.

Dissatisfaction with enzymatic procedures prompted several investigators to develop HPLC methods for the direct quantification of PLP. The detection of PLP as its semicarbazone derivative, already used in paper chromatography in 1964 (117), seemed a viable alternative to enzymatic methods. Gregory described an isocratic HPLC procedure for determination of semicarbazone derivatives of PLP and PL after perchloric acid extraction from animal tissues (66). The low pH (pH = 2.2) of the mobile phase resulted in excellent chromatographic efficiency,

Table 7 Methods for the Determination of Plasma PLP and PL

Vitamers determined	Chromatographic conditions[a]	PLP derivative	Detection	Reference
PLP	Nucleosil SA; 0.05 M sodium acetate, 0.03 M citric acid, 0.06 M NaOH, 0.017 M acetic acid, pH 5.2	Enzymatic conversion[b]	Amperometric (+0.55 V)	114
PLP	MPLC RP-18; 0.07 M sodium acetate, pH 3.75	Enzymatic conversion[c]	Fl (280/353)	115
PLP	Lichrosorb RP-18; 0.1 M sodium phosphate, containing 2 mM S8S and 10% acetonitrile, pH 4.9	Enzymatic conversion[c,d]	Amperometric (+0.85V)	116
PL, PLP	ODS-Hypersil; 0.05 M potassium phosphate, pH 2.9	SC Post-C	Fl (367/478)[e]	67
PL, PLP	Partisil 10 ODS-3; 0.05 M potassium phosphate, containing 7% acetonitrile, pH 2.9	SC Pre-C	Fl (367/478)[e]	69,70
PLP	Shimadzu STR ODS-H; 2 M potassium acetate containing 1 mM S7S, pH 2.9	KCN Pre-C	Fl (318/418)	128
PLP	μBondapak TM C-18; 0.033 M potassium phosphate containing 0.05 M semicarbazide and 3% acetonitrile, pH 2.5	KCN Pre-C	Fl (284/470)	129

[a] All the reported methods used isocratic elution. See also footnotes to Table 4. Abbreviations: Refer to Table 4.

[b] Based on the measurement of PLP in deproteinized plasma by addition of L-3,4-dihydroxyphenylalanine and apo-tyrosine decarboxylase; the dopamine formed is measured by HPLC and the concentration found is directly proportional to the PLP level in the sample.

[c] Based on measurement of PLP in deproteinized plasma by addition of tyrosine (substrate) and apo-tyrosine decarboxylase; the tyramine formed is measured by HPLC and the concentration found is directly proportional to the PLP level of the sample.

[d] Plasma samples were not deproteinized.

[e] For optimum detection, the pH of the column eluate was adjusted to 12.

but also in relatively low fluorescence intensity of the semicarbazone derivatives.

Schrijver et al. (67) described an isocratic HPLC separation for PLP and PL, followed by postcolumn semicarbazone derivatization. The pH of the column eluate was increased to 12–13 by introduction of a 8% NaOH solution to the column eluate before it passed through the fluorometer; in this way much higher fluorescence intensities of the semicarbazone derivatives of PLP and PL were obtained. The increased fluorescence obtained by postcolumn alkalinization resulted in adequate sensitivity required for reliable PLP and PL quantification in human whole blood (67). The method could be easily automated, and has been used in several clinical studies (118–121).

Ubbink et al. demonstrated that extraction of human plasma with trichloroacetic acid and semicarbazone derivatization could be performed simultaneously (69). The semicarbazone derivatives of PLP and PL were then separated by reversed-phase HPLC, using an acidic (pH = 2.8) mobile phase in order to achieve optimum chromatographic efficiency as described by Gregory (66). Postcolumn alkalinization before fluorometric detection resulted in excellent sensitivity, and the method has been applied in analysis of human plasma (69,122,123), whole blood (124), erythrocytes (122), and lymphocytes (Fig. 5).

The simultaneous determination of PLP and PL proved to be an important feature of methods based on semicarbazone derivatization. Determination of PL may sometimes offer an explanation for depressed PLP levels in various physiological or clinical conditions. Using semicarbazone derivatization and HPLC analysis, Barnard et al. found that declining plasma PLP levels during human pregnancy (125) or starvation of beagle dogs (126) could be explained by elevated plasma PL levels, thus indicating altered vitamin B$_6$ homeostasis. Similarly, a study on asthmatics revealed severely depressed plasma PLP levels, but normal PL levels (127), indicating that PL phosphorylation could be impaired during asthma.

Quantification of PLP and PL as semicarbazone derivatives was also utilized for analysis of PL kinase (EC 2.7.1.35), PM (PN)-5'-phosphate oxidase (EC 1.4.3.5), and PLP phosphatase activities (Fig. 6). The enzymes mentioned above are expressed in human erythrocytes, which renders the erythrocyte a valuable cell system to study vitamin B$_6$ metabolism in relation to disease (128). As detection of semicarbazone derivatives of both PLP and PL is very sensitive, enzyme-kinetic studies may be done directly in hemolysates. For example, kinetic studies in human hemolysates have shown that the depressed vitamin B$_6$ status of asthmatics could be explained by inhibition of PL kinase by theophylline, a

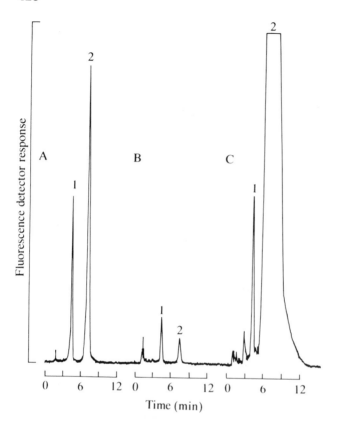

Figure 5 Application of HPLC to study vitamin B_6 metabolism in human lymphocytes. HPLC conditions: Column, Partisil 10 ODS-3 (Whatman, Clifton, NJ). Mobile phase, isocratic elution with 0.05 mol/liter KH_2PO_4 buffer, pH = 2.9, containing 3% acetonitrile, at flow rate 1.1 ml/min. Detection, fluorescence, excitation 367 nm, emission 478 nm. Postcolumn alkalinization of mobile phase to pH 12.0 was achieved by addition of 4% NaOH solution. Peaks: 1 = PLP semicarbazone; 2 = PL semicarbazone. PLP and/or PL concentrations were determined using an external standard (A: 300 nmol/liter of PLP and PL, respectively) and are expressed per milligram of lymphocyte protein: (A) standards, (B) lymphocyte extract, and (C) quantitation of PL kinase activity using added PL as a substrate.

bronchodilator very often used in asthma treatment (122). However, a word of caution should be voiced here: the strong binding of both PLP and PL to hemoglobin may affect the kinetics of the enzyme catalyzed reaction (129). It is therefore essential to confirm results obtained in hemolysates by kinetic experiments with purified enzyme. Nevertheless, HPLC analysis of enzyme activities involved in vitamin B_6 metabolism

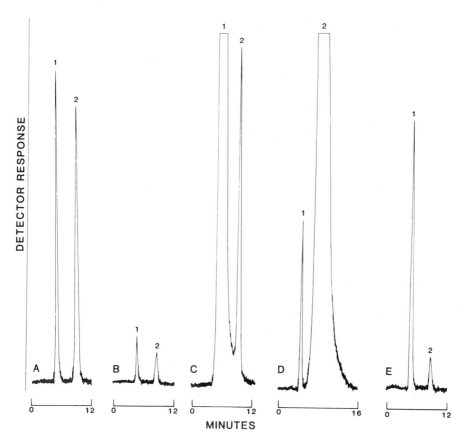

Figure 6 HPLC assay of enzymes involved in vitamin B$_6$ metabolism. (A) Standard solution, containing PLP (226 nmol/liter) and PL (147 nmol/liter); (B) hemolysate; (C-E) the same hemolysate, to which PLP (C), PL (D), and PMP (E) were added to measure PLP phosphatase, PL kinase, and PM (PN)-5'-phosphate oxidase activities, respectively. Peaks: 1 = PLP; 2 = PL. Reprinted from Ubbink et al. (128) with permission of the publisher.

may become an important tool for future investigation of the relationship between depressed vitamin B$_6$ status and disease.

The sensitivity of semicarbazone derivatization in PLP and PL analysis is illustrated by the application of HPLC to study vitamin B$_6$ metabolism in human lymphocytes. Lymphocytes were isolated from 10 ml of blood; 5 μl of packed lymphocytes was diluted to 100 μl using a 10 mM triethanolamine buffer (pH = 7.4) containing 0.1% Triton X-100. After homogenization (MSE ultrasound homogenizer), 60 μl of the homogenized suspension were diluted to 400 μl in buffer A (10 mmol/

liter triethanolamine, 90 mmol/liter K_2HPO_4, 2 mmol/liter $MgCl_2$, 2.6 mmol/liter ATP; pH = 7.4). To a 100-μl aliquot, 50 μl of 10% trichloroacetic acid and 30 μl of 0.5 mol/liter semicarbazide were simultaneously added; the mixture was incubated at 37°C for 30 min and the supernatant obtained after low-speed centrifugation was used for HPLC analysis of PLP semicarbazone and PL semicarbazone (Fig. 5B). Figure 5C depicts analyses of lymphocyte pyridoxal kinase activity. A 100-μl aliquot of homogenized cell suspension diluted in buffer A was incubated at 30°C for 10 min; subsequently, 10 μl of a 1.8 mmol/liter pyridoxal (substrate) solution was added. The reaction was terminated after 1 h by simultaneous addition of 50 μl of 10% trichloracetic acid and 30 μl of 0.5 mol/liter semicarbazide. HPLC was used to quantify PLP production from PL.

Potassium cyanide-catalyzed oxidation of PLP with subsequent quantification of the highly fluorescent oxidation product, 4-pyridoxic acid 5′-phosphate, has been used to determine PLP levels in human plasma, brain tissue, and cell cultures (130,131). The sensitivity of this method has been reported to be even better than methods based on PLP semicarbazone formation (131). PL is not determined by these methods; this vitamer is oxidized to 4-pyridoxic acid lactone, which shows little fluorescence at pH 2.5–3.8 of the mobile phases used (Table 2). However, it should be possible to adapt methods based on potassium cyanide catalyzed oxidation to include PL. Postcolumn alkalinization of the mobile phase results in strong fluorescence of 4-pyridoxic acid lactone (Table 2), thus enabling PL quantification.

Urine

Vitamin B_6 is predominantly excreted in urine as 4-pyridoxic acid (132). The relatively high urinary concentration and strong fluorescence of 4-PA enable the direct determination of 4-PA in urine after deproteinization (132,133). However, spontaneous lactonization of 4-PA in acid medium may create an analytical problem (132); a separate determination of recovery is therefore needed to account for 4-PA lactonization. This could be circumvented by precolumn lactonization of 4-PA with subsequent HPLC analysis of 4-PA lactone (134). Figure 7 illustrates the determination of urinary 4-PA levels as 4-PA lactone.

Analysis of urine samples for the other B_6 vitamers is difficult due to high concentrations of other interfering compounds present in urine. Ubbink et al. (123) demonstrated that the anion-exchange column cleanup procedure originally described by Vanderslice et al. (80) was effective in removing interfering urinary compounds. The purified urine extract was then analyzed by cation-exchange HPLC and fluorescence detection. Urinary B_6 vitamer excretion in a fasting person was below

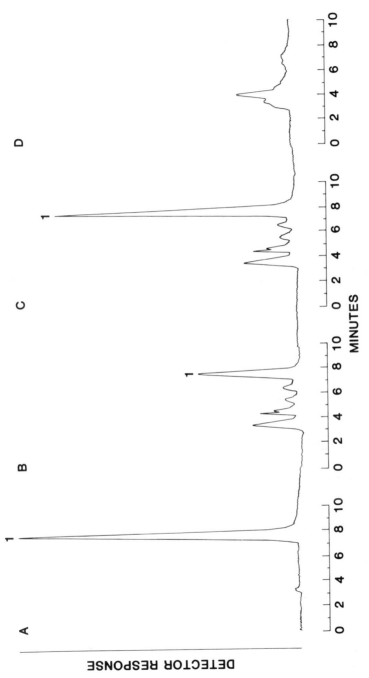

Figure 7 The determination of urinary 4-pyridoxic acid levels as 4-pyridoxic acid lactone: (A) standard of 11 μmol/liter 4-PA; (B) urine sample from a normal, fasting person; (C) the same urine sample spiked with 5.5 μmol/liter 4-PA, and (D) the same urine sample without lactonization. Each sample was injected at time = 0 min. Peaks: 1 = 4-pyridoxolactone, unmarked peaks were unidentified background components. HPLC conditions: Column, Partisil 10 SCX (Whatman). Mobile phase, isocratic elution with 0.025 M ammonium dihydrogen phosphate (pH 2.8). Detection, fluorescence, excitation 360 nm, emission 430 nm. Postcolumn alkalinization of mobile phase to pH 12.0 was achieved by addition of a 4% NaOH solution. Reprinted from Ubbink et al. (134) with permission.

the sensitivity limit of the HPLC procedure used. However, the method was suitable to study urinary B_6 vitamer excretion in pharmacokinetic studies of pyridoxine supplementation (123).

4. GAS-LIQUID CHROMATOGRAPHY

Although gas-liquid chromatography is one of the most widely used separation techniques to date, its application in B_6 vitamer analysis has been hampered by the high polarity of these compounds. Nevertheless, GLC of a variety of B_6 vitamer derivatives has been reported. Analysis of PL, PM, and PN as trimethylsilyl (135,136), trifluoroacetyl (137), acetyl (138), and heptafluorobutyryl derivatives (139) have been reported. These techniques have recently been reviewed by Coburn (49). However, the GLC techniques mentioned above suffer from lack of sensitivity, poor peak shapes, and excessive tailing, as well as inconsistent derivatization of certain vitamers (i.e., pyridoxine), which often resulted in appearance of more than one peak per vitamer on the chromatogram. The inadequate sensitivity of the flame-ionization detector could be improved by using an electron-capture detector. Lim et al. recently employed GLC separation of N-methyl-bistrifluoroacetamide derivatives of PN, PM, and PL with subsequent electron-capture detection to quantify levels of these vitamers in food (140). Double peaks were observed for PN, but the sum of peak heights reportedly gave satisfactory linear calibration plots.

Compared to HPLC, GLC is much less used for routine vitamin B_6 analysis. However, combined with mass spectrometry, GLC might become the ultimate reference method in B_6 vitamer analysis. Hachey et al. (141) described analysis of B_6 vitamers in biological samples by isotope dilution mass spectrometry. Deuterated forms of the different B_6 vitamers were added in the early stages of the sample preparation procedure; these deuterated vitamers were effectively used as internal standards to compensate for analytical losses during the isolation and derivatization steps. The B_6 vitamers in the homogenized tissue sample were separated by cation-exchange HPLC as described previously (65). Acetylation was chosen as derivatization procedure for GLC. However, prior to acetylation, the 5'-phosphoric esters (PLP, PMP) were hydrolyzed in acid and PL was reduced to PN with sodium borohydride. Results obtained by GC/MS analysis of actylated B_6 vitamers compared well with those of the cation-exchange HPLC method previously reported by Coburn and Mahuren (65). Samples with a vitamin B_6 content as low as 0.02 nmol/ ml could be analyzed with this method. However, this method is laborintensive and requires expensive instrumentation, excluding its use in routine analysis of biological samples. Due to its high sensitivity and accurate compensation for analytical losses, the method might become a valuable reference method to verify results obtained by other analytical techniques.

The combination of GC with mass spectrometry has been used to study pyridoxine metabolism in tumor cells. Using radiolabeled PN and paired-ion, reversed-phase HPLC (107), Tryfiates and co-workers (142) demonstrated that about 30% of the radiolabel was associated with a product showing a retention time different from any of the known B$_6$ vitamers. Using mass spectrometry, with and without prior GLC separation, the product was eventually identified as adenosine-N^6-methyl propyl thioether N-pyridoximine 5'-phosphate (143,144).

To summarize, HPLC has replaced GLC for routine B$_6$ vitamer analysis in both food and biological samples. However, the latter technique, in combination with mass spectrometry, is used as a reference analytical method or as an advanced research tool to elucidate vitamin B$_6$ metabolism.

5. FUTURE TRENDS

In view of the low concentrations encountered in biological material, accurate B$_6$ vitamer analysis has always been a formidable challenge. Chromatography, especially HPLC, has perhaps become the method of choice in vitamin B$_6$ analysis, because this technique allows the combination of efficient separation with sensitive detection. However, application of chromatographic techniques in B$_6$ vitamer analysis is not without problems. Coburn and Mahuren have underlined the importance of peak identity and purity verification (65,102,104). These authors have published examples where background components were shown to interfere in vitamin B$_6$ analysis (64,103). Fluorescence quenching is a further problem that may be encountered in B$_6$ vitamer analysis. We have encountered this problem in analysis of urine for PL and for PN and PM (123). Further research will therefore be directed at improving present HPLC methods in vitamin B$_6$ analysis.

More efficient columns for HPLC will contribute significantly toward maintaining a high standard in B$_6$ vitamer analysis. Peak verification is much easier when efficient separation of the B$_6$ vitamers is achieved. In addition, the use of highly efficient columns may simplify comprehensive B$_6$ vitamer analysis. Modern developments in column technology will presumably allow simple, isocratic separation of B$_6$ vitamers encountered in biological material. This trend is already visible in the literature. In 1983, Coburn and Mahuren utilized cation-exchange HPLC that required a ternary solvent program to separate the B$_6$ vitamers (including 4-PA) encountered in biological samples (65). Using a modern, efficient Partisphere (Whatman, Clifton, NJ) strong cation-exchange column, which reportedly has an efficiency in excess of 75,000 theoretical plates per meter, Argoudelis (1988) managed the separation of the six biologically active B_6 vitamers by an isocratic method (106). A similar trend is observed with methods based on reversed-phase HPLC, where earlier methods depended on binary solvent programs to separate the B_6 vitamers from each other (107–109). Recently, Edwards and co-workers reported that isocratic separation of the B_6 vitamers (including 4-PA) was not only possible but also applicable to analysis of human plasma (111). The use of modern, efficient HPLC columns and sensitive fluorescence detectors will eventually result in simple isocratic B_6 vitamer analysis of biological samples. This may eventually replace current relatively simple methods for measurement of only PLP and/or PL.

Methods based on semicarbazone derivatization of PLP and PL allow extremely sensitive quantitation of these two vitamers (67,69,70). However, postcolumn alkalinization is needed because the semicarbazone derivatives show strong fluorescence at pH 12–13. Recently, silica-based pH stable packing materials have become commercially available in prepacked columns. The possible use of these columns with a pH 12 phosphate buffer as mobile phase will eliminate the need for postcolumn alkalinization. This possibility is currently investigated in our laboratory.

In conclusion, current advancements in column technology will presumably enable the chromatographer to employ a simple, isocratic HPLC method for simultaneous analysis of the six nutritionally active B_6 vitamers and 4-PA. The high sensitivity of certain methods for PLP/PL analyses may be improved further by using columns compatible with alkaline buffers. Furthermore, these methods allow enzyme studies in small amounts of biological material, which will contribute to our current understanding of vitamin B_6 metabolism in health and disease.

REFERENCES

1. P. Gyorgy, *Nature, 133*:489 (1934).
2. S. Lepkovsky, *Science, 87*:169 (1938).
3. P. Gyorgy, *J. Am. Chem. Soc., 60*:1267 (1938).
4. E. F. Müller, *Z. Physiol. Chem, 254*:285 (1938).
5. E. E. Snell, *Proc. Soc. Exp. Biol. Med., 51*:356 (1939).
6. E. E. Snell, *J. Biol. Chem., 154*:313 (1944).
7. IUPAC-IUB Commission on Biochemical Nomenclature, *Eur. J. Biochem, 2*:1 (1967).
8. J. E. Leklem, in *Current Topics in Nutrition and Disease, Vol 19, Clinical and Physical Applications of Vitamin B_6* (J. E. Leklem and R. D. Reynolds, eds.), Alan R. Liss, New York, p. 3 (1988).

9. D. B. McCormick, M. E. Gregory, and E. E. Snell, *J. Biol. Chem*, *236*:2076 (1961).

10. A. Hamfelt, *Clin. Chim. Acta*, *16*:7 (1967).

11. B. M. Pogell, *J. Biol. Chem.*, *232*:761 (1961).

12. H. Wada and E. E. Snell, *J. Biol. Chem.*, *236*:2089 (1961).

13. D. B. McCormick and A. H. Merril, in *Vitamin B$_6$ Metabolism in Growth* (G. P. Tryfiates, ed.), Food & Nutrition Press, Westport, CN, p. 1 (1980).

14. M. Ebadi, in *Coenzymes and Cofactors, Vol. 1. Vitamin B$_6$-Pyridoxal Phosphate; Chemical, Biochemical and Medical Aspects, Part B*. (D. Dolphin, R. Poulson, and O. Avramovic, eds.), John Wiley & Sons, New York, p. 449 (1986).

15. H. A. Serebro, H. M. Solomon, J. H. Johnson, and T. R. Hendrix, *Bulletin: John Hopkins Hospital*, *119*:166 (1966).

16. H. M. Middleton, *J. Nutr.*, *115*:1079 (1985).

17. L. Lumeng and T. K. Li, in *Current Topics in Nutrition and Disease, Vol. 13, Vitamin B-6: Its Role in Health and Disease* (R. D. Reynolds and J. E. Leklem, eds.), Alan R. Liss, New York, p. 35 (1985).

18. L. Lumeng, A. Lui, and T.-.K. Li, *J. Clin. Invest.*, *66*:688 (1980).

19. H. Mehansho, D. D. Buss, M. W. Hamm, and L. M. Henderson, *Biochim. Biophys. Acta*, *631*:112 (1980).

20. B. B. Anderson, C. E. Fulford-Jones, J. A. Child, M. E. J. Beard, and C. J. T. Bateman, *J. Clin. Invest.*, *50*:1901 (1971).

21. H. Mehansho and L. M. Henderson, *J. Biol. Chem.*, *255*:11901 (1980).

22. L. Lumeng, R. E. Brashear, and T. Li, *J. Lab. Clin. Med.*, *84*:334 (1974).

23. B. B. Anderson, P. A. Newmark, M. Rawlins, and R. Green, *Nature*, *250*:502 (1974).

24. M. Ebadi and P. Govitrapong, in *Vitamin B-6 and Role in Growth* (G. P. Tryfiates, ed.), Food & Nutrition Press, Westport, CT, p. 223 (1980).

25. Y. C. Chang, R. D. Scott, and D. J. Graves, *Biochemistry*, *25*:1932 (1986).

26. S. C. Cunnane, M. S. Manku and D. F. Horrobin, *J. Nutr.*, *114*:1754 (1984).

27. R. G. Wilson and R. E. Davis, *Adv. Clin. Chem.*, *23*:1 (1983).

28. R. D. Reynolds and C. L. Natta, *Am. J. Clin. Nutr.*, *41*:684 (1985).

29. B. Rimland, E. Calloway, and P. Dreyfus, *Am. J. Psychiatr.*, *135*:472 (1978).

30. D. Byar, and C. Blackard, *Urology*, *10*:556 (1977).

31. H. J. T. C. Bennink and W. H. P. Schreurs, *Br. Med. J.*, *3*:13 (1975).

32. F. J. L. Guzman, J. M. Gonzalez-Buitrago, F. de Arriba, F. Mateos, J. C. Moyano, and T. Lopez, *Klin. Wochenschr.*, *67*:38 (1989).

33. M. Coleman, in *Current Topics in Nutrition and Disease, Vol. 19, Clinical and Physiological Applications of Vitamin B-6* (J. E. Leklem and R. D. Reynolds, eds.), Alan R. Liss, New York, p. 317 (1988).

34. B. Chabner and D. Livingston, *Anal. Biochem.*, *34*:413 (1970).

35. B. E. Haskell and E. E. Snell, *Anal. Biochem.*, *45*:567 (1972).
36. A. Hamfelt, *Clin. Chim. Acta*, *7*:746 (1962).
37. C. Plese, W. Fox, and K. Williams, *Clin. Chem.*, *29*:407 (1983).
38. E. M. Benson, J. M. Peters, M. A. Edwards, M. R. Malinow, and C. A. Storvick, *J. Nutr.*, *96*:83 (1968).
39. C. A. Storvick and J. M. Peters, in *Vitamins and Hormones, Vol. 22* (R. S. Harris, I. G. Wool, and J. A. Lorraine, eds.), Academic Press, New York, p. 833 (1964).
40. J. C. Rabinowitz and E. E. Snell, *Proc. Soc. Exp. Biol. Med.*, *70*:235 (1949).
41. E. I. Short and G. Fairbairn, *Tubercle*, *43*:11 (1962).
42. B. E. Haskell and U. Wallnofer, *Anal. Biochem.*, *19*:569 (1967).
43. S. F. Contractor and B. Shane, *Clin. Chim. Acta*, *21*:71 (1968).
44. I. Durko, Y. Vladovska-Yukhnovska, and C. P. Ivanov, *Clin. Chim. Acta*, *49*:407 (1973).
45. M. S. Chauhan and K. Dakshinamurti, *Anal. Biochem.*, *96*:426 (1979).
46. G. P. Smith, D. Samson, and T. J. Peters, *J. Clin. Pathol.*, *36*:701 (1983).
47. J. W. Thanassi and J. A. Cidlowski, *J. Immunol. Methods*, *33*:261 (1980).
48. D. L. Bandon, J. W. Corse, J. J. Windle, and L. C. Layton, *J. Immunol. Methods*, *78*:87 (1985).
49. S. P. Coburn and J. D. Mahuren, *J. Biol. Chem.*, *262*:2642 (1987).
50. M. M. Polansky and E. W. Toepfer, *J. Agric. Food Chem.*, *17*:1394 (1969).
51. S. P. Coburn, in *Coenzymes and Cofactors, Vol. 1, part A. Vitamin B-6-Pyridoxal Phosphate: Chemical, Biochemical and Medical Aspects* (D. Dolphin, R. Poulson, and O. Avramovic, eds.), John Wiley & Sons, New York, p. 497 (1986).
52. E. W. Nelson, C. W. Burgin, and J. J. Cerda, *J. Nutr.*, *107*:2128 (1977).
53. K. Yasumoto, H. Tsuji, K. Iwami, and H. Mitsuda, *Agric. Biol. Chem.*, *6*:1061 (1977).
54. H. Kabir, J. Leklem, and L. T. Miller, *J. Food Sci.*, *48*:1422 (1983).
55. H. Kabir, J. E. Leklem, and L. T. Miller, *Nutr. Rep. Int.*, *28*:709 (1983).
56. P. R. Trumbo, J. F. Gregory, and D. B. Sartain, *J. Nutr.*, *118*:170 (1988).
57. J. W. Bridges, D. S. Davies, and R. T. Williams, *Biochem. J.*, *98*:451 (1966).
58. E. A. Peterson and H. A. Sober, *J. Am. Chem. Soc.*, *76*:169 (1954).
59. D. E. Metzler and E. E. Snell, *J. Am. Chem. Soc.*, *77*:2431 (1955).
60. J. W. Bridges and R. T. Williams, *Nature*, *196*:59 (1962).
61. V. Bonavita and V. Scardi, *Anal. Chim. Acta*, *20*:47 (1959).
62. V. Bonavita, *Arch. Biochem. Biophys.*, *88*:366 (1960).
63. N. Ohishi and S. Fukui, *Arch. Biochem. Biophys.*, *128*:606 (1968).
64. I. L. Finar, *Organic Chemistry*, Vol. 1, 5th ed., Longmans, Green, London, p. 176 (1967).
65. S. P. Coburn and J. D. Mahuren, *Anal. Biochem.*, *129*:310 (1983).

66. J. F. Gregory III, *Anal. Biochem.*, *102*:374 (1980).
67. J. Schrijver, A. J. Speek, and W. H. P. Schreurs, *Int. J. Vit. Nutr. Res.*, *51*:216 (1981).
68. J. B. Conant and P. D. Bartlett, *J. Am. Chem. Soc.*, *54*:2881 (1932).
69. J. B. Ubbink, W. J. Serfontein, and L. S. de Villiers, *J. Chromatogr.*, *375*:399 (1986).
70. J. B. Ubbink, W. J. Serfontein, and L. S. de Villiers, *J. Chromatogr.*, *342*:277 (1985).
71. M. S. Chauhan and K. Dakshinamurti, *Clin. Chim. Acta.*, *109*:159 (1981).
72. C. Y. W. Ang, *J. Assoc. Off. Anal. Chem.*, *62*:1170 (1979).
73. B. Saidi and J. J. Warthesen, *J. Agric. Food Chem.*, *31*:876 (1983).
74. R. L. Kirchmeier and R. P. Upton, *J. Pharm. Sci.*, *67*:1444 (1979).
75. M. C. Walker, B. E. Carpenter, and E. L. Cooper, *J. Pharm. Sci.*, *70*:99 (1981).
76. T. Kawamoto, E. Okada, and T. Fujita, *J. Chromatogr.*, *267*:413 (1983).
77. M. Amin and J. Reusch, *J. Chromatogr.*, *390*:448 (1987).
78. R. M. Kothari and M. W. Taylor, *J. Chromatogr.*, *247*:187 (1982).
79. J. T. Vanderslice, K. K. Stewart, and M. M. Yarmas, *J. Chromatogr.*, *176*:281 (1979).
80. J. T. Vanderslice, C. E. Maire, R. F. Doherty, and G. R. Beecher, *J. Agric. Food Chem.*, *28*:1145 (1980).
81. J. T. Vanderslice, C. E. Maire, and J. E. Yakupkovic, *J. Food. Sci.*, *46*:943 (1981).
82. J. T. Vanderslice and C. Maire, *J. Chromatogr.*, *196*:176 (1980).
83. J. T. Vanderslice, J. Brown, G. Beecher, C. Maire, and S. G. Brownlee, *J. Chromatogr.*, *216*:338 (1981).
84. J. F. Brown, J. T. Vanderslice, C. Maire, S. G. Brownlee, and K. K. Stewart, *J. Auto Chem.*, *3*:187 (1981).
85. J. F. Gregory, D. B. Manley, and J. R. Kirk, *J. Agric. Food Chem.*, *29*:921 (1981).
86. J. F. Gregory and D. Feldstein, *J. Agric. Food Chem.*, *33*:359 (1985).
87. R. Bitsch and J. Möller, *J. Chromatogr.*, *463*:207 (1989).
88. T. Toukairin-Oda, E. Sakamoto, N. Hirose, M. Moiri, T. Itoh, and H. Tsuge, *J. Nutr. Sci. Vitamin.*, *35*:171 (1989).
89. K. L. Lim, R. W. Young, and J. A. Driskell, *J. Chromatogr.*, *188*:285 (1980).
90. J. A. Pierotti, A. G. Dickinson, J. K. Palmer, and J. A. Driskell, *J. Chromatogr.*, *306*:377 (1984).
91. T. E. Hefferan, B. M. Chrisley, and J. A. Driskell, *J. Chromatogr.*, *374*:155 (1986).
92. A. Bognar, Z. *Lebensm. Unters. Forsch.*, *181*:200 (1985).
93. J. F. Gregory and J. R. Kirk, *J. Food Sci.*, *43*:1585 (1978).
94. J. F. Gregory and S. L. Ink, *J. Agric. Food Chem.*, *35*:76 (1987).
95. J. F. Gregory, *J. Agric. Food Chem.*, *28*:486 (1980).

96. R. L. Wehling and D. L. Wetzel, *J. Agric. Food Chem.*, *32*:1326 (1984).
97. B. K. Ayi, D. A. Yuhas and N. J. Deangelis, *J. Assoc. Off. Anal. Chem.*, 69:56 (1986).
98. J. T. Vanderslice, C. E. Maire, and G. R. Beecher, *Am. J. Clin. Nutr.*, 34:947 (1981).
99. J. T. Vanderslice, S. G. Brownlee, C. E. Maire, R. D. Reynolds, and M. Polansky, *Am. J. Clin. Nutr.*, 37:867 (1983).
100. J. B. Ubbink and W. J. Serfontein, in *Current Topics in Nutrition and Disease, Vol. 19, Clinical and Physiological Applications of Vitamin B-6* (J. E. Leklem and R. D. Reynolds, eds.), Alan R. Liss, New York, p. 29 (1988).
101. A. Lui, L. Lumeng, G. R. Aronoff, and T. Li, *J. Lab. Clin. Med.*, 106:491 (1985).
102. S. P. Coburn and J. D. Mahuren, *Methods Enzymol.*, *122*:102 (1986).
103. G. S. Shephard, M. E. J. Louw, and D. Labadarios, *J. Chromatogr.*, 416:138 (1987).
104. S. P. Coburn, J. D. Mahuren, and T. R. Guilarte, *J. Nutr.*, 114:2269 (1984).
105. A. Lui, L. Lumeng, and T. K. Li, *Am. J. Clin. Nutr.*, 41:1236 (1985).
106. C. J. Argoudelis, *J. Chromatogr.*, 424:315 (1988).
107. G. P. Tryfiates and S. Sattsangi, *J. Chromatogr.*, 227:181 (1982).
108. B. Hollins and J. M. Henderson, *J. Chromatogr.*, 380:67 (1986).
109. J. M. Henderson, M. A. Codner, B. Hollins, M. H. Kutner, and A. H. Merril, *Hepatology*, 6:464 (1986).
110. B. Hamaker, A. Kirksey, A. Ekanayake, and M. Borschel, *Am. J. Clin. Nutr.*, 42:650 (1985).
111. P. Edwards, P. K. S. Liu, and G. A. Rose, *Clin. Chem.*, 35:241 (1989).
112. L. Lumeng and T. K. Li, in *Vitamin B-6 Metabolism and Role in Growth* (G. P. Tryfiates, ed.), Food & Nutrition Press, Westport, CT, p. 27 (1980).
113. J. E. Leklem and R. D. Reynolds, in *Current topics in Nutrition and Disease, Vol. 19, Clinical and Physiological Applications of Vitamin B-6* (J. E. Leklem and R. D. Reynolds, eds.), Alan R. Liss, New York, p. 437 (1988).
114. S. Allenmark, E. Hjelm, and U. Larsson-Cohn, *J. Chromatogr.*, 146:485 (1978).
115. A. Hamfelt, *Upsala J. Med. Sci.*, 91:105 (1986).
116. B. Lequeu, J. Guilland, and J. Klepping, *Anal. Biochem.*, 149:296 (1985).
117. R. Hakanson, *J. Chromatogr.*, 13:263 (1964).
118. H. van den Berg, E. S. Louwerse, H. W. Bruinse, J. T. N. M. Thissen, and J. Schrijver, *Hum. Nutr. Clin. Nutr.*, 40:441 (1986).
119. J. Schrijver, J. Alexieva-Figusch, N. Van Breederode, and H. A. van Gilse, *Nutr. Cancer*, 10:231 (1987).
120. E. J. van der Beek, W. van Dokkum, J. Schrijver, M. Wedel, A. W. K. Gaillard, A. Wesstra, H. van de Weerd, and R. J. J. Hermus, *Am. J. Clin. Nutr.*, 48:1451 (1988).

121. F. J. Kok, J. Schrijver, A. Hofman, J. C. M. Witteman, D. A. C. Kruyssen, W. J. Remme, and H. A. Valkenburg, *Am. J. Cardiol.*, 63:513 (1989).
122. J. B. Ubbink, R. Delport, P. J. Becker, and S. Bissbort, *J. Lab. Clin. Med.*, 113:15 (1989).
123. J. B. Ubbink, W. J. Serfontein, P. J. Becker, and L. de Villiers, *Am. J. Clin. Nutr.*, 46:78 (1987).
124. W. J. Vermaak, H. C. Barnard, E. M. S. P. Van Dalen, and G. M. Potgieter, *Enzyme*, 35:215 (1986).
125. H. C. Barnard, J. J. de Kock, W. J. H. Vermaak, and G. M. Potgieter, *J. Nutr.*, 117:1303 (1987).
126. H. C. Barnard, W. J. H. Vermaak, and G. M. Potgieter, *Int. J. Vitam. Nutr. Res.*, 56:351 (1986).
127. R. Delport, J. B. Ubbink, W. J. Serfontein, P. J. Becker, and L. Walters, *Int. J. Vitam. Nutr. Res.*, 58:67 (1988).
128. J. B. Ubbink and A. M. Schnell, *J. Chromatogr.*, 431:406 (1988).
129. J. B. Ubbink, S. Bissbort, W. J. H. Vermaak, and R. Delport, *Enzyme*, 43:72 (1990).
130. M. Naoi, H. Ichinose, T. Takahashi, and T. Nagatsu, *J. Chromatogr.*, 434:209 (1988).
131. H. Millart and D. Lamiable, *Analyst*, 114:1225 (1989).
132. J. F. Gregory III and J. R. Kirk, *Am. J. Clin. Nutr.*, 32:879 (1979).
133. K. Schuster, L. B. Bailey, J. J. Cerda, and J. F. Gregory, *Am. J. Clin. Nutr.*, 39:466 (1984).
134. J. B. Ubbink, W. J. Serfontein, P. J. Becker, and L. de Villiers, *Am. J. Clin. Nutr.*, 44:698 (1986).
135. W. Korytnyk, G. Fricke, and B. Paul, *Anal. Biochem.*, 17:66 (1966).
136. W. Richter, M. Vecchi, W. Vetter, and W. Walther, *Helv. Chim. Acta*, 50:364 (1967).
137. T. Imanari and Z. Tamura, *Chem. Pharm. Bull.*, 15:896 (1967).
138. W. Korytnyk, *Methods Enzymol.*, 18:500 (1970).
139. A. K. Williams, *J. Agric. Food Chem.*, 22:107 (1974).
140. K. L. Lim, R. W. Young, and J. A. Driskell, *J. Chromatogr.*, 250:86 (1982).
141. D. L. Hachey, S. P. Coburn, L. T. Brown, W. Erbelding, B. Demark, and P. D. Klein, *Anal. Biochem.*, 151:159 (1985).
142. G. P. Tryfiates, *Anticancer Res.*, 3:53 (1983).
143. G. P. Tryfiates, R. Bishop, and R. Smith, in *Chemical and Biological Aspects of Vitamin B-6 Catalysis* (A. E. Evangelopoulos, ed.), Alan R. Liss, New York, p. 21 (1984).
144. G. P. Tryfiates and R. E. Bishop, *Prog. Clin. Biol. Res.*, 259:295 (1988).

11

BIOTIN

Michel Gaudry and Olivier Ploux

Université Pierre et Marie Curie, Paris, France

1. INTRODUCTION

Biotin (*cis*-tetrahydro-2-oxothienol[3,4-*d*]imidazoline-4-valeric acid) (Fig. 1) has been isolated from egg yolk in crystalline form by Kögl (1), with Tönnis (2). The structure of that vitamin, named also bios II, factor X, coenzyme R, anti-egg white injury, or vitamin H, was established in 1942 by Melville et al. (3) and its synthesis was achieved by Harris et al. a year later (4,5). The absolute configuration of biotin was elucidated by x-ray determination on biotin by Traub (6,7) and confirmed by Bonnemere et al. (8) and Trotter and Hamilton (9), who worked on an N_1'-carboxy derivative of biotin. These determinations have been confirmed and extended by De Titta et al. (10,11). NMR studies by Gasel (12) and by Lett and Marquet (13), demonstrated that the conformation of the thiophane ring is the same in the solid state and in solution: the sulfur atom lies above the thiophane ring and the valeric chain adopts a quasi-equatorial position (Fig. 1). The same conformation is encountered in the biotin sulfoxides (Fig. 2) (13). Numerous total syntheses of biotin have been published till recently (14 and references included); but the bulk of biotin is produced industrially according to the original Hoffmann-La Roche process (15).

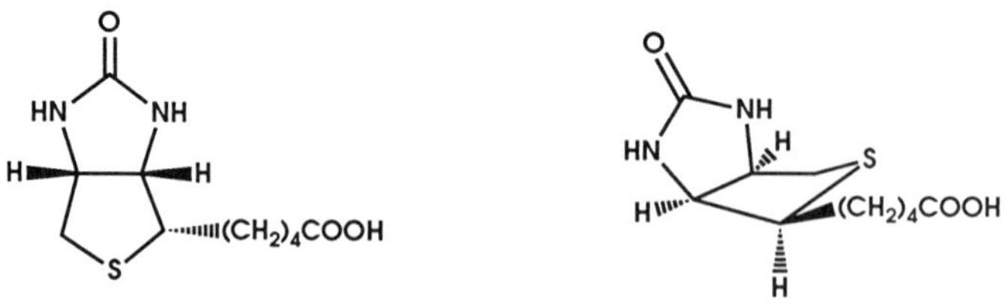

Figure 1 Structure and conformation of biotin.

2. CHEMICAL PROPERTIES

2.1 Stability

In contrast to the reputation of lability of vitamins, biotin is very stable and can be autoclaved without being affected. This molecule even resists autoclaving in concentrated sulfuric acid (4 M, 120°C, 2 h), conditions commonly used to extract biotin from biological samples (16,17). However, biotin can be easily oxidized into biotin sulfoxides (Fig. 2). This process, which is negligible in concentrated solutions, can become predominant in very dilute solutions, for instance, during anion-exchange column or thin-layer chromatography purification of small amounts of material derived from biosynthesis experiments or even during purification of radiolabeled biotin (18). This can be prevented by use of carefully degassed solvents (18). In addition to this oxidation process, microbial growth can drastically lower the concentration of nonsterile dilute solutions of the vitamin.

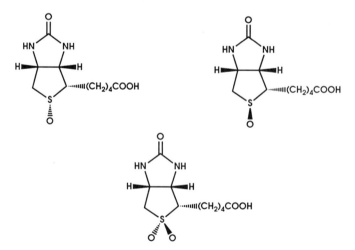

Figure 2 Structure of d-biotin sulfoxide, l-biotin sulfoxide, and biotin sulfone.

2.2   Chemical Reactivity

Biotin exhibits normal reactivity at the potentially reactive centers of the molecule. The carboxyl group of "free" biotin has a pK around 4.5 and can be esterified without problem by classical methods. Several methods for the titation of biotin take advantage of the reaction of biotin with diazo derivatives (vide infra). The sulfur atom can be easily oxidized with various reagents (hydrogen peroxide, sodium periodate) yielding a mixture of isometric d- and l-biotin sulfoxides (13,19,20), which can further react, leading to biotin sulfone (Fig. 2) (21). Reactions of the ureido ring occur almost exclusively at the N_1' atom upon nitrosation (22) or methoxycarboxylation (23), whereas both N_1' and N_3' atoms are methylated by a mixture of formaldehyde and formic acid (22) (Fig. 3).

3.   BIOCHEMICAL PROPERTIES

Biotin is required by all living cells and is biosynthesized only by some plants, fungi, and the majority of microorganisms. Sources of exogenous biotin are for instance liver, cereals, rice, egg yolks, chocolate, tomatoes, and yeast extracts.

3.1   Biotin Biosynthesis

Biotin is biosynthesized by microorganisms starting from pimelic acid according to Fig. 4. This pathway has been well established in *Escherichia coli* and *Bacillus sphaericus* (24–26). All the intermediates have been identified, all the activities have been elucidated, and some of the enzymes involved have been purified and characterized. However our knowledge concerning the last step of the biosynthesis, that is, the introduction of the sulfur atom in dethiobiotin, is still very elusive. The metabolic genes in *E. coli* are clustered at 17 min in a divergent operon, which is negatively controlled (27) (Fig. 5). This operon has now been entirely sequenced (28). The repressor, which supports also the holocarboxylase synthetase activity, has been cloned, sequenced, overproduced,

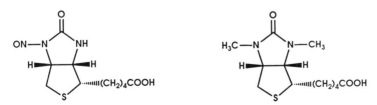

Figure 3   Structure of nitrosobiotin and N,N'-dimethylbiotin.

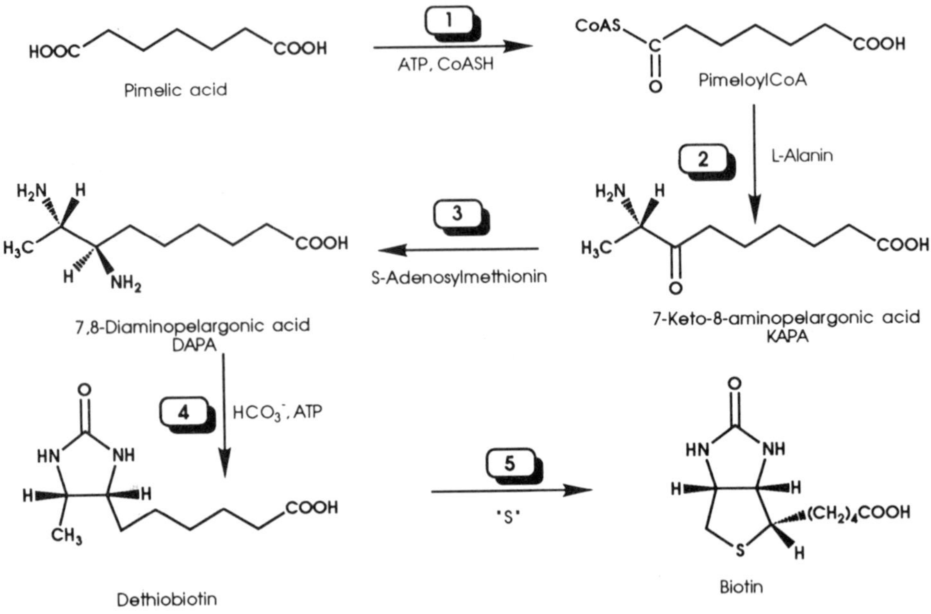

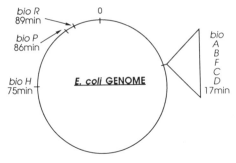

Figure 4   Biosynthesis of biotin.

STEP	ENZYME	E.coli GENE
1	PIMELOYL-CoA SYNTHETASE	bio C
2	KAPA SYNTHETASE	bio F
3	DAPA SYNTHETASE	bio A
4	DTB SYNTHETASE	bio D
5	BIOTINE SYNTHETASE	bio B

Figure 5   Genes involved in biotin biosynthesis.

and crystallized (29). Another gene named *bioH*, whose function has to be established, has been mapped at 75 min (30). This analysis has now been extended to gram-positive bacteria by the elucidation, cloning, and sequencing of the *bio* genes of *B. sphaericus* (31,32). Recently, the interest for microbiological production of biotin has driven several companies to develop genetically engineered strains. This will certainly renew the interest for the study of this metabolic pathway.

3.2 Biotin Transport

The biotin transport has been extensively studied with microorganisms: *Lactobacillus plantarum* (33), *Saccharomyces cerevisiae* (34,35), and *Escherichia coli* (36–39). The microorganisms are able to recover biotin from the medium and to concentrate it intracellularly by an active process, that is, against a concentration gradient, mediated by a specialized protein and dependent on an energy source. The biosynthesis of the transport system is regulated by the level of external biotin in *S. cerevisiae* (40) and in *E. coli* (37,39).

The transport of biotin by animal cells has been studied more recently in mice 3T3-L1 cells (41) and human skin fibroblasts (42). Here again the transport is mediated through a specific protein but is not apparently dependent on an energy source (42). Unexpectedly Dakshinamurti et al. observed that the avidin-biotin complex enters animal cells more efficiently than biotin itself (43–46). In relationship with the problems of biotin deficiency (vide infra) several groups studied the absorption of biotin by culture rat hepatocytes (47). Attention has been focused on the intestinal absorption of biotin. Several techniques— cultured hamster enterocytes (48), everted sac technique (49), intestinal brush border membrane vesicles (50,51), basolateral membrane (52)— led to the conclusion that biotin was absorbed more efficiently in the proximal part of the small intestine (52) via a carrier-mediated process.

3.3 Attachment of Biotin to the Apoenzymes

After entering the cell, biotin becomes covalently bound to the apoenzymes of biotin-dependent enzymes during the last step of their biosynthesis (53). In all the enzymes examined so far, biotin has been shown to be linked through an amide bond of the ϵ-amino group of a lysin (Fig. 6). This reaction occurs in two steps, an activation step yielding biotinyl AMP (Eq. 1), which reacts with the lysine ϵ-amino group, yielding the active holoenzyme (Eq. 2):

$$ATP + biotin \rightarrow biotinyl-AMP + PPi \tag{1}$$

$$Biotinyl-AMP + apoenzyme \rightarrow holoenzyme + AMP \tag{2}$$

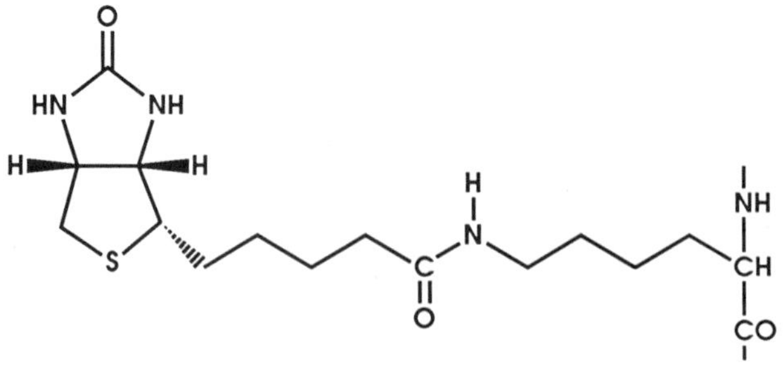

Figure 6   Structure of biotin covalently linked to its apoprotein.

The holocarboxylase synthetases (HCS), which do not seem to be very specific of the apoenyzme, and HCS from different sources (microorganisms or animals) are able to link biotin to apoenzymes from heterologous sources. The location of HCS in rat liver has been elucidated recently (54). One is mitochondrial and the other is cytoplasmic.

The sequence surrounding the lysine to which biotin is linked is highly preserved among the different carboxylases (55) with a common Ala-Met-Lys-Met sequence. The effect of mutations on the biotinyl subunits of carboxylases is now under investigation (56).

3.4   Biotin-Dependent Enzymes

The biotin-dependent enzyme group includes three classes of enzymes: carboxylases, transcarboxylase, and decarboxylases (57,58). In all the reactions catalyzed by these enzymes, biotin acts as a CO_2 carrier either to activate CO_2 and transfer it to a substrate, as in carboxylases, or to transfer a CO_2 moiety between two substrates, as in transcarboxylase, or to abstract the CO_2 from a substrate as in decarboxylases. In the three cases, N-carboxybiotin (Fig. 7) is an intermediate.

The evolutionary conservation among biotin enzymes has been reviewed recently (59).

Carboxylases

The carbon dioxide ligase group comprises six enzymes. Acetyl-CoA carboxylase (EC 6.4.1.2) catalyzes the formation of malonyl-CoA from acetyl-CoA and is involved in fatty acid synthesis (Eq. 3) (60).

$$CH_3COSCoA + ATP + HCO_3^- \rightarrow {}^-O_2CCH_2COSCoA + ADP + Pi \quad (3)$$

The mechanism of the regulation of the activity of the enzyme from animal tissues by phosphorylation (61,62) or by ADP ribosylation (63) is actively studied.

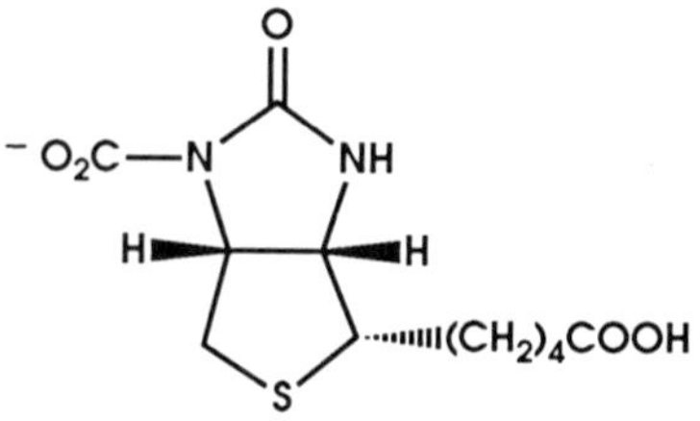

Figure 7 Structure of *N*-carboxybiotin.

Propionyl-CoA carboxylase (EC 6.4.1.2) converts propionyl-CoA into methylmalonyl-CoA (64). This enzyme is essential in isoleucine degradation (Eq. 4):

$$CH_3CH_2COSCoA + ATP + HCO_3^- \rightarrow CH_3(CO_2^-)CHCOSCoA + ADP + Pi \quad (4)$$

β-Methylcrotonyl-CoA carboxylase (EC 6.4.1.4), which transforms β-methylcrotonyl-CoA into β-methylglutaconyl-CoA (Eq. 5), is a key enzyme in leucine degradation (65).

$$(CH_3)_2C = CHCOSCoA + ATP + HCO_3^- \rightarrow$$
$$^-O_2CCH_2(CH_3)C = CHCOSCoA + ADP + Pi \quad (5)$$

Pyruvate carboxylase (EC 6.4.1.1) is an important regulatory enzyme since it converts pyruvate into oxaloacetate (Eq. 6) (66):

$$CH_3COCOOH + ATP + HCO_3^- \rightarrow {}^-O_2CCH_2COCOOH + ADP + Pi \quad (6)$$

These four carboxylases are found in animals, and a deficiency in one or all of these activities leads to serious metabolic troubles.

Urea carboxylase (EC 6.3.4.6) is induced in microorganisms growing on urea as nitrogen source (67). It catalyzes the transformation of urea in allophanate, which is further hydrolyzed to carbon dioxide and ammonia by an allophanate hydrolase.

Geranyl-CoA carboxylase (EC 6.4.1.5) is found in microorganisms and is involved in the degradation of isoprenoid compounds (68).

Transcarboxylase

The carboxyltransferase group contains only one enzyme, the methylmalonyl-CoA transcarboxylase (EC 2.1.3.1), which is induced in *Propionibacterium shermanii* and catalyzes the transcarboxylation between methylmalonyl-CoA and pyruvate (69,70) (Eq. 7). This enzyme is important in the metabolism of propionate:

$$CH_3(CO_2^-)CHCOSCoA + CH_3COCOOH \rightarrow$$
$$CH_3CH_2COSCoA + {}^-O_2CCH_2COCOOH \quad (7)$$

Decarboxylases

Two enzymes, the methylmalonyl-CoA decarboxylase (EC 4.1.1.41) (71) and the oxaloacetate decarboxylase (EC 4.1.1.3) (72), are encountered in microorganisms.

3.5 Biotin Deficiency

Daily requirements are very low, and biotin deficiency can be induced in animals by feeding them with raw egg whites, which contain avidin, a glycoprotein that has a very high affinity for biotin. Cases of spontaneous biotin deficiency in humans were not detected before 1976, but since that time several cases of this deficiency have been diagnosed (73–75). The clinical symptoms (alopecia, skin rashes, and presence of metabolites in urine), linked to low or even absent carboxylase activities, can be eliminated by biotin absorption. The multiple carboxylase deficiency has been reviewed recently (76). Two forms of the deficiency have been described so far: the neonatal and the late-onset forms (77). The neonatal form, which affects patients in the first days of their life, is due to a very low holocarboxylase synthetase activity (78–80), resulting from an altered affinity for biotin. The late-onset form [currently 1 in 60,000 births (76)] is characterized by a very low level of plasmatic biotin resulting from an absence of biotinidase activity (81,82). The patient is unable to use bound biotin, that is, biotin linked to lysine through a peptidic bond. This prevents the patient's absorbing most of biotin from food and presumably recycling the biotin pool present in the patient's liver as holocarboxylases.

3.6 Biotin Binding Proteins

Antibodies to Biotin

The first antibodies to biotin were developed in the late 1970s by Berger (83,84). Several monoclonal antibodies have now been produced and characterized (85,86).

Biotin Binding Proteins

EGG YOLK AND CHICKEN PLASMA BIOTIN BINDING PROTEINS. Egg yolk of chicken contains a very acidic protein that binds biotin, although with a lower affinity than avidin (vide infra) (87,88). Its role is to transport and store biotin for the developing embryo. A closely related biotin binding protein is found in the plasma of young chickens (88).

AVIDIN. Avidin, a glycoprotein from egg white, is composed of four identical subunits (MW = 18,000) and exhibits a very high affinity for biotin ($K_D = 10^{-15}M$) (89). Each unit contains a biotin binding site (90) where tryptophan residues 70 and 110 are essential for binding biotin. Isolation of nonglycosylated avidin reveals that the presence of carbohydrate (10% of total weight) is not necessary for binding (91). Streptavidin, a tetrameric protein from yeast strains *Streptomyces avidinii* (92,93), has almost the same properties. It has been recently crystallized and analyzed by x-ray diffraction (94,95). In contrast with avidin, the binding of biotin to streptavidin seems to be cooperative (96).

The high affinity of avidin or streptavidin for biotin has been extensively used to induce biotin deficiencies, in affinity chromatography (97), and as a tool in molecular biology, in biotin determinations, or in bioanalytical application (98).

4. BIOTIN DETERMINATIONS

The classical methods for biotin determination are not chromatographic techniques but take advantage of the biochemical properties of the vitamin. Depending on whether avidin is used, they can be classified into two categories.

4.1 Methods without Avidin

Reaction with Paradimethylaminocinnamaldehyde

Upon reaction with this compound (99,100) in acidic medium, a pink color develops, which is characteristic of the ureido ring and can be used to determine the biotin concentration spectrophotometrically at 533 nm. This method is easy to use but its sensitivity is low, in the microgram range.

Enzymatic Determination

This assay is based on the formation of holopyruvate carboxylase from apopyruvate carboxylase and biotin followed by the determination of the pyruvate carboxylase activity, the activity being proportional to the amount of biotin available to form the active holoenzyme (101). This method is not very easy to use, but its sensitivity is very good (as low as 0.5 ng).

Microbiological Determinations

These determinations have been used from the beginning and are among the most sensitive assays for biotin (0.1 ng). Several microorganisms have been tested (102), but the more commonly used are *Saccharomyces cerevisiae* (Fleischmann strain 139 ATCC 9896), whose growth allows the determination of "total biotin," that is, biotin, biotin sulfoxides, biocytine, dethiobiotin, KAPA, and DAPA (103), and *Lactobacillus plantarum* 17.5 (ATCC 8014), which responds to "true biotin," that is, biotin and biotin sulfoxides (104). Recently attention has been drawn to interferences of dethiobiotin (Fig. 8), the precursor of biotin, in the *L. plantarum* assay (105). This interference, that is, an enhancement of growth of the microorganisms due to biotin in the presence of large amounts of diethiobiotin, can be eliminated by coupling with the yeast growth method of Snell et al. (103).

Two different techniques have been designed: measurements of growth response in liquid media or on agar diffusion plates (106). Both techniques are very sensitive (0.1 ng/assay) and easy to set up for routine analysis.

This is exemplified by the following experimental part (107) (see Fig. 9):

> *L. plantarum* is grown in *Lactobacilli* MRS broth (108) at 37°C (shaking is not required) and kept at −80°C in 25% glycerol, 50% reconstituted milk (12% milk powder) in MRS. Plates (245 × 245 mm² petri dishes) are prepared daily (2% agar in Biotin Assay Medium from DIFCO) autoclaved at 0.8 atm for 15 minutes and inoculated with 1% of a fresh overnight culture of *L. plantarum* previously washed twice with sterile water. The plate is then dried and 5 μl of biotin standards (0.01 to 1 μg/ml) and 5 μl of unknowns are applied to 6 mm paperdiscs. After an overnight incubation at 37°C the diameters of the circles corresponding to growth are measured and plotted against the logarithm of the biotin concentration. The standard curves are linear and determination of unknowns is easy.

4.2 Methods Involving Avidin

2-(4′-Hydroxyazobenzene)benzoic Acid (HABA) Method

This method (89,109,110) takes advantage of the formation of a complex between avidin and HABA. Biotin, which has a higher affinity for the avidin than HABA, quantitatively displaces the dye from the complex.

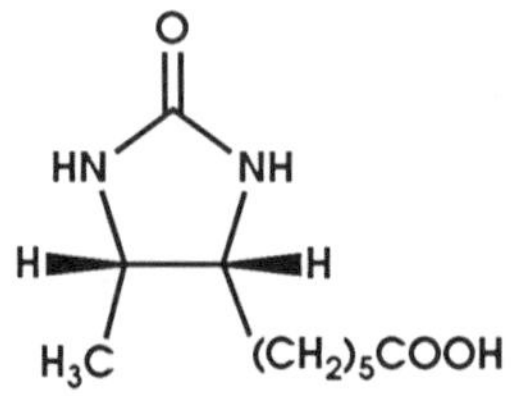

Figure 8 Structure of dethiobiotin.

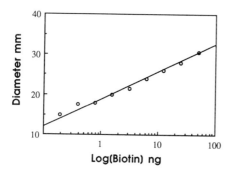

Figure 9 Typical standard curve for the determination of biotin by the agar diffusion plate technique.

The titration is generally monitored spectrophotometrically at 500 nm. This method is easy to use, but its sensitivity is low (around 1 μg).

Spectral Shift Method

Upon complexation with biotin, the avidin absorbance at 233 nm is modified (89,109,110). The sensitivity of this method is similar to that of the HABA method.

Fluorescence Determinations

Two methods have been described so far that monitor the titration of biotin with avidin using fluorescence. The first one measures the quenching of the avidin tryptophan fluorescence by biotin (111,112), whereas the second involves the increase of fluorescence of a fluorescently labeled avidin upon addition of biotin (113). The sensitivities are, respectively, 20 and 0.5 ng. More recently, an assay based on the variation of the fluorescence polarization of a biotin fluorescein upon interaction with avidin (114) has been applied to avidin or to biotin determinations. Minimal detectable concentrations reported are 5 ng/ml avidin and 100 pg/ml biotin (114). Mock et al. reported another technique relying on the displacement of the fluorescent probe 2-anilinoaphthalene-6-sulfonic acid or 2,6-ANS (Fig. 10) by biotin (115). The advantage of this method is obviously the very low fluorescence of 2,6-ANS in water solution compared to the fluorescence of avidin-bound ANS.

Chemiluminescence

This method (116) is based on the competition between biotin and a biotin luminol derivative for avidin. The titration is monitored using the chemiluminescence of the luminol derivative (Fig. 11). More recently, Williams and Campbell improved the sensitivity of this kind of assay

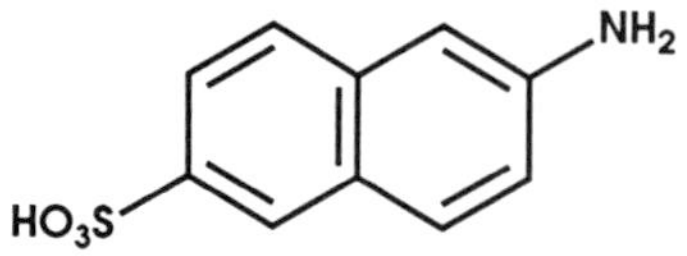

Figure 10   Structure of 2,6-ANS.

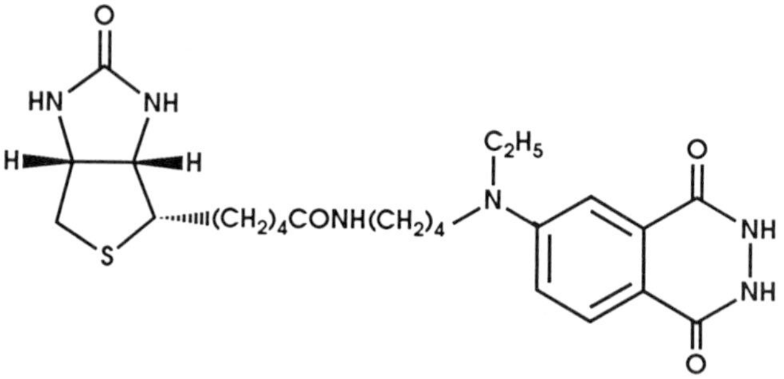

Figure 11   Structure of chemiluminescent derivative of biotin.

by quenching the chemiluminescence of the biotin luminol with fluorescein-labeled avidin (117). The detection limit reported seems to be below 10 μg per sample (117).

Isotope dilution methods

These methods, which depend on the availability of labeled biotin, have been developed recently and are based on the dilution of the biotin to be estimated by a known amount of labeled biotin, followed by the determination of the specific activity of the avidin complexed and/or the free biotin after thorough separation of both species. [^{14}C]Biotin (118–121), [^{3}H]biotin (122), and even a ^{125}I-labeled derivative of biotin (123) have been used. The separation of free and avidin-complexed biotin has been achieved with bentonite (122), zinc hydroxide (118–120), or dextran-coated charcoal (121). The sensitivity depends on the specific activity of the labeled biotin and can range from 20 ng with [^{14}C]biotin, to 1 ng with [^{3}H] biotin, down to less than 0.1 ng with the ^{125}I-labeled derivative.

    The use of readily available ^{125}I-avidin allowed a significant improvement of the sensitivity of that method (124) down to the plasma concentrations met during severe biotin deficiency experiments.

Enzymatic Activity Coupled Detection Methods

The general goal of all these methods that have been developed in the past few years is to use an enzymatic activity, most of the time easy for detection and for quantification. The enzyme can be either linked to the avidin or streptavidin or to biotin. Bayer et al. designed a sensitive assay that does not require the use of radiolabeled compounds (125). The coupling of biotin with alkaline phophatase (but other enzymes can be used instead) allowed use of hydrolysis of *p*-nitrophenyl phosphate to monitor the reaction. Sensitivities of 2 pg of biotin per sample are described (125). The use of a natural biotin enzyme such as pyruvate carboxylase has been suggested (126), although in that case the enzyme is not commercially available or stable. Labeling biotin with adenosine deaminase allowed Kjellström and Bachas to use potentiometric determination (127) for biotin concentration in the 10^{-8} M range. Terouanne et al. recommended the use of glucose-6-phosphate dehydrogenase conjugates that can be detected by colorimetry or by bioluminescence (128), and that lead to detection of 0.1 pg of biotin.

Bioaffinity Sensors

This technique has been developed during the last 5 years by Aizawa and co-workers. The goal is to build a convenient and specific detector using an enzymatic activity as signal. In the case of biotin determination, avidin coupled with catalase is bound to a membrane bearing covalently linked HABA residues. Addition of biotin destroys quantitatively the HABA-avidin-catalase complex. Washing the membrane and measurement of the catalase activity remaining afford a sensitive and convenient titration of biotin (129,130).

5.   CHROMATOGRAPHIC STUDIES

5.1   Ion-Exchange Chromatography

Since anion-exchange resins are available with high chemical purity, ion-exchange chromatography can be used for the purification and concentration of traces of weakly acidic materials such as biotin. This technique has been applied to isolate and purify biotin and biotin vitamers from the culture filtrate of many microorganisms, including molds, yeasts, and bacteria.

Ogata (17,131) used a Dowex 1×2 fomate column. After washing with deionized water, the biotin vitamers [biotin, biotin sulfoxide (Fig. 2), and dethiobiotin (Fig. 8)] were eluted with formic acid (0.012 M). This has also been achieved on a Dowex 1-acetate column (132). After

washing with water, the column was developed with increasing concentrations of acetic acid (0.5-2 M). The biotin, biotin sulfoxide, and
dethiobiotin were eluted together with acetic acid (1.5 M).

In order to purify biotin and its sulfoxides extracted from the culture
medium of *Aspergillus niger*, Tepper et al. (133) and Im et al. (134) converted them to biotin sulfone by treatment with hydrogen peroxide in
excess and chromatographed them on a Dowex 1×8 formate column.
Biotin sulfone was eluted with a linear gradient of ammonium sulfate
(0-1 M). The ammonium ion has been removed on Dowex 50, a sulfonic
acid cation-exchange resin.

The same Dowex 1×2 chromatography technique proved to be a
very good technique to monitor and titrate biotin and vitamers in biological medium during an investigation of the biosynthesis of biotin (135–
137). The elution pattern in Fig. 12 illustrates, for instance, the chromatographic separation of a mixture of [^{3}H]dethiobiotin and [^{14}C]biotin.

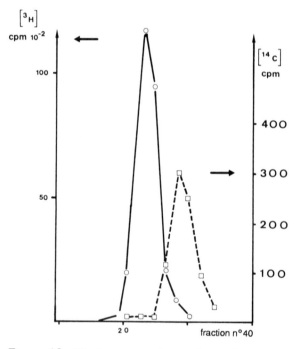

Figure 12 Elution pattern from column chromatography of [^{3}H] dethiobiotin
(50 µg, SA = 200 mCi/mmol) and [^{14}C]biotin (5 µg, SA = 31 mCi/mmol). The
mixture was poured over a column 1.5 × 16.5 cm of Dowex 1 × 2 (formate)
and eluted with a linear gradient of formic acid (0–1 M, 600 ml). Fractions (12
ml) were collected.

5.2 Paper Chromatography

So far, few examples of identification of biotin by paper chromatography have been described in the literature. Ascending paper chromatography has been carried out with n-butanol-HCl, 1M (6:1) (138), n-butanol-acetic acid-water (60:15:25) (132), n-butanol-acetic acid-water (2:1:1) (139), or n-butanol-formic acid-water (4:1:1) as developing solvents. More recently, Shrift (140) compared biotin and selenobiotin by descending paper chromatography using Whatman 1 filter paper with the solvent system ethanol-t-butanol-formic acid-water (24:8:2:6).

5.3 Thin-Layer Chromatography

TLC and Visualization Conditions

Thin-layer chromatography (TLC) has been applied to analyze biotin in biotin vitamers or multivitamin mixtures. This technique is more convenient and gives better results than paper chromatography. Silica-gel plates have been generally used as support, but cellulose powder has also been proposed. The developing solvents are listed in Table 1.

Several detection reagents have been proposed to detect biotin (142): 1% potassium permangante, 1% dimethylaminobenzaldehyde in HCl (1 M), or iodine vapor. The detection limits obtained with such agents are relatively high, about 5 μg. Better results have been obtained by spraying with mixtures of o-toluidine-potassium iodide (141) or o-toluidine-chlorine (143); biotin is revealed as a deep blue spot. The detection limit was found to be 0.3 μg (141).

However, the best detection agent is p-dimethylaminocinnamaldehyde (p-DACA). Shimada et al. observed that upon reaction with p-DACA in sulfuric acid-methanol mixtures, biotin yielded an intense reddish orange color with maximal absorbance at 533 nm (145). This reagent is quite specific for biotin, since the uriedo ring is a prerequisite

Table 1 TLC Developing Solvents

Solvents	Proportions (v/v)	References
Acetone-acetic acid-benzene-methanol	1 : 1 : 14 : 4	141–143
Acetone-acetic acid-benzene-methanol	1 : 1 : 11 : 11	143
Butanol-water	1 : 1	142
Butanol-water-acetic acid	4 : 5 : 1	142
Chloroform-methanol-4% formic acid	10 : 1 : 1	142
Chloroform-methanol-formic acid	70 : 40 : 2	144
Butanol-water-benzene-methanol	2 : 1 : 1 : 1.1	136, 137

for suitable color response. The reaction proceeds by formation of the conjugate imine (Schiff's base) with cyclic compounds (93). A spray reagent composed of equal volumes of 2% sulfuric acid in ethanol and 0.2% p-DACA has been used by McCormick to develop chromatograms (99).

Another very convenient visualization technique for TLC plates is bioautography: the TLC plate is inverted on the surface of an agar plate seeded with *L. plantarum* or *S. cerevisiae*, allowing the diffusion of the chromatographed compounds (biotin or its vitamers, for instance). The selectivity and sensitivity have already been discussed (section 4.1).

Analysis of Multivitamin Mixtures

Nuttall and Bush (141) described a chromatographic method for the analysis of multivitamin preparations. After extraction of fat-soluble vitamins, water-soluble vitamins and water-soluble materials were separated in three TLC systems. Biotin was resolved with acetone-acetic acid-benzene-methanol (1:1:14:4) as solvent and visualized by spraying *o*-toluidine-potassium iodide. Addition of standard samples could be included if quantitative results are required. However, the reproducibility of the technique has not been tested.

Groningsson and Jansson (144) worked out a method for the determination of biotin in the presence of other water-soluble vitamins. After dissolution of the lyophilized preparation and addition of the internal standard (2-imidazolidone), the sample was applied on a silica-gel plate and eluted with chloroform-methanol-formic acid (70:40:2). Biotin was visualized by spraying with p-DACA and determined in situ by reflectance measurements. The sensitivity of the method could be increased by spraying with paraffin after the coloring procedure. Under these conditions, the detection limit was 10 ng.

5.4 Gas-Liquid Chromatography Techniques

GLC

Biotin is not volatile enough for direct GLC analysis, but it is possible to use this technique after substitution of the active hydrogen of the carboxyl group. While developing a general method for the analysis of urinary acids Horning et al. (146) observed that trimethylsilyl ester and trimethylsilyl ether were the most attractive derivatives for GLC separation of hydroxy acids and water-soluble vitamin acids. They used bis-trimethylsilyl acetamide (BSA) as silylating agent.

Using this procedure, Viswanathan et al. (147) described the quantitative determination of biotin after its conversion into silyl ester. The column was a 2% OV17 on diatomite (chromosorb G, AW/HMDS treated). *n*-Octosane was added as internal standard, and detection was achieved with a flame ionization detector. The detection limit for biotin trimethylsilyl (TMS) ester was approximately 3 μg. Viswanathan et al. observed that BSA was suitable for complete silylation, whereas the hexamethyldisilazane-trimethylchlorosilane (2:1) mixture was not. Furthermore, they assumed that the reaction occurred exclusively at the carboxyl group and no reaction took place on the two amido NH groups (Fig. 13).

More recently, Johnson and Boyden (148) proved that the proposed structure (Fig. 13) was incorrect. In fact, the silyl derivative prepared according to reference 147 was not the silyl ester but the trisilyl derivative (Fig. 14).

This trisilyl derivative can be formed upon heating biotin with a solution of BSA and pyridine (1:1). The same silylating procedure can be applied to the biotin methyl ester in order to prepare the N-silylated methyl ester.

In an earlier study, Janecke and Voege (149) attempted to determine biotin and its oxidation products in commercial multivitamin preparations using the silylation technique. However, the separation of biotin, biotin sulfone, and sulfoxides from a multivitamin mixture was not thorough, and the two isomeric sulfoxides could not be separated.

GC-MS

Johnson and Boyden (148) analyzed biotin with gas chromatography-mass spectrometry (GC-MS) using a 3% OV17 column. They characterized the trisilylated biotin derivative (Fig. 14) and the corresponding methyl ester. The mass spectra consisted of the molecular ion and a base peak at m/z = 73, probably corresponding to the loss of one trimethysilyl group.

In conclusion, the silylation derivatization seems to give the best results for analysis of biotin by GLC. However, this reaction is hardly reproducible, and no direct application to the identification or estimation of biotin in biological mixture has been described in literature so far.

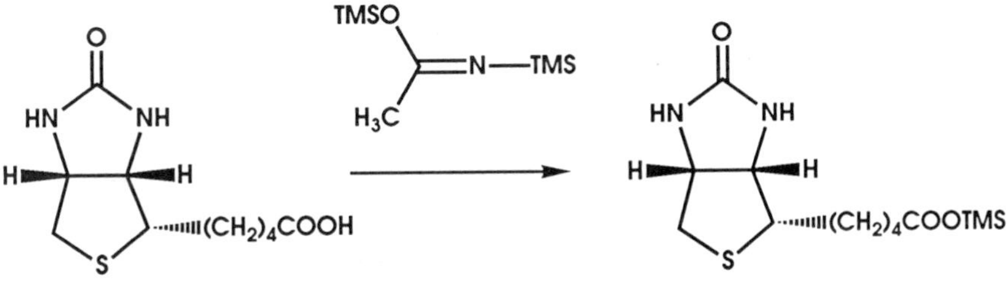

Figure 13 TMS esterification of biotin.

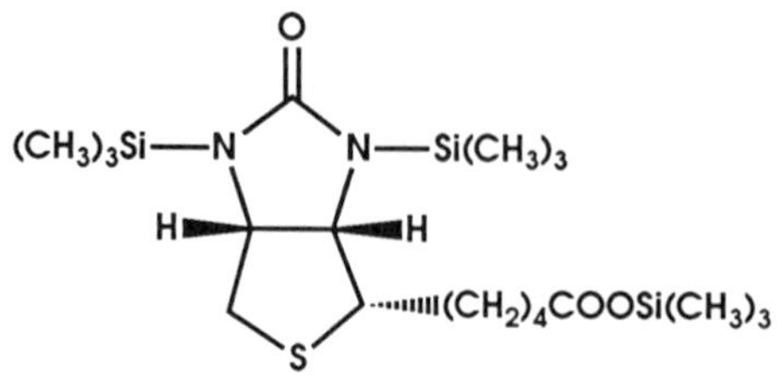

Figure 14   Trisilyl derivative of biotin.

5.5   Liquid Chromatography Techniques

LC

In the case of thermostable and nonvolatile compounds such as biotin, LC is a very valuable technique of analysis. However, the limitation lies in the availability of a suitable detection system.

Biotin does not absorb in the UV region, and only refractometer detection can be applied to direct analysis. Biotin methyl ester has been easily identified and separated from its metabolic precursor dethiobiotin methyl ester using reversed-phase chromatography (C18) with a methanol-water mixture in isocratic mode (4:6) (150). Satisfactory results, although with the usual low sensitivity due to the detector, have been obtained.

In order to facilitate the analysis of small quantities of biotin and its analogs, a convenient derivatization of UV or fluorimetric detection has been described (151). Biotin has been converted to UV-absorbing bromoacetophenone (BAP) esters by reaction with 4-dibromoacetophenone (DBAP) and to fluorescent methoxycoumarin (Mmc) esters by reaction with 4-bromomethoxycoumarin (Br-Mmc) (Fig. 15). Biotin and dethiobiotin are easily separated using a reversed-phase C18 bonded system with methanol-water or tetrahydrofuran (THF)-water as mobile phase. A continuous THF-water gradient is the best system to achieve a good chromatographic separation of the BAP or Mmc esters of dethiobiotin, biotin, and its oxydative derivatives, sulfone and sulfoxides (Fig. 16). With the UV technique ($\lambda = 254$ nm), the detection limit was approximately 50 ng, whereas it fell to 5 ng with fluorescence detection.

These LC methods are helpful in qualitative and quantitative analysis. In each case the regressions between the detection response and the injected samples are linear for the concentration range usually seen in biological samples (from 0.15 to 4 nmol for BAP esters and 0.015 to 1 nmol for Mmc esters).

This detection technique has been greatly improved recently by use of 9-anthryl or 1-pyrenyl esters (Fig. 15) for the separation by reversed-phase HPLC (152).

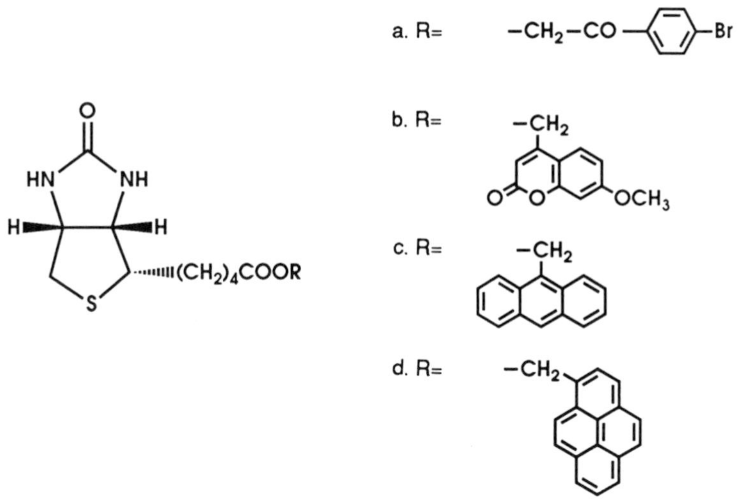

Figure 15 Structure of (a) BAP, (b) Mmc, (c) anthryl and (d) pyrenyl esters of biotin.

LC-MS

Recently interesting results were obtained by using the combined LS-MS technique (153). Mass spectrometry is very specific and appeared as sensitive as UV detection (Table 2). After treatment with diazomethane (136,137), biotin has been identified in biological medium as methyl ester (153), using a reversed-phase C8 bonded column and an isocratic system of methanol-water (4:6) as the mobile phase. The mass spectrometer was operated in positive-ion chemical ionization mode, and the limit of detection was lower than 10 ng. The regression between the detector response and the injected sample was found to be linear up to 300 ng.

6. CONCLUSION

It appears that in order to meet the standards of molecular biology the sensitivity of detection of biotin or of avidin has been greatly improved.

The choice of the detection method is highly dependent on the biotin concentration range. At high levels, the HABA methods remain the more convenient ones, since they require no radioactive materials or sophisticated detection. For the "normal biotin concentration range" in tissues (blood, yeast extracts, etc.) the microbiological method appears well adapted when it is run routinely.

Titration with fluorescent esters implies an extra HPLC column step but avoids the use of avidin. It can be very sensitive and overcomes the formation of artefacts.

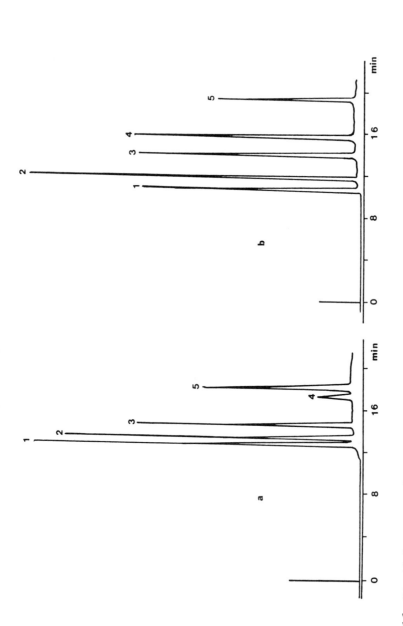

Figure 16 Liquid chromatographic separation of (a) BAP esters and (b) Mmc esters of biotin and some analogs. Peak 1, *l*-biotin sulfoxide; peak 2, *d*-biotin sulfoxide; peak 3, biotin sulfone; peak 4, biotin; peak 5, dethiobiotin. Conditions: 0.2 × 33 cm C18 bonded column; gradient, THF–water from 30:70 to 60:40; flow rate, 1 ml/min. (From Ref. 151.)

Table 2 Comparison of the Detection Limits of Biotin Determination Methods

Method	Detection limit (ng)	References
p-DACA	10^3	99–100
Enzymatic	0.5	101
Microbiological	0.1	102–108
Avidin, HABA	10^3	89,109,110
Avidin spectral shift	10^3	89,109,110
Fluorescence	20	111,112
	0.5	113,115
Chemiluminescence	1–2	116,117
Isotope dilution		
^{14}C	20	118–121
^{3}H	1	122
^{125}I	0.1	123,124
TLC	3×10^2	141
	10	144
GLC	3×10^3	147
LC		
UV	50	151,152
Fluorescence	5	151,152
LC-MS	10	153
Enzyme-coupled detection	2×10^{-3}	125–128
Bioaffinity sensors	0.5	129,130

The amplification methods through avidin-enzyme-linked activity are obviously the more sensitive methods, and in the next few years the biosensor techniques will definitely improve the simplicity of the biotin or avidin concentration determinations.

However, it must be kept in mind that in all cases involving the biotin-avidin interaction, it is important for determinations that the equilibrium has been already achieved. Although the interaction is very tight, the time required to reach a "quasi stoichiometry" can become very long (Table 3) (42).

This obviously precludes accurate and reproducible determinations in the picomolar range, especially for techniques involving modified avidin or streptavidin, whose affinity for biotin can be significantly lowered.

Table 3 Influence of Avidin and Biotin Concentrations on the Time Required to Bind 90% of the Biotin ([Biotin] = [Avidin Monomer])[a]

[Avidin] (monomer, mol/liter) or [biotin](ng/ml)		Time to achieve 90% binding
M	ng/ml	
10^{-7}	2.4410^3	0.13 s
10^{-8}	244	1.3 s
10^{-9}	24.4	12.8 s
10^{-10}	2.44	2.13 min
10^{-11}	0.24	21.3 min
10^{-12}	0.024	3.6 h
10^{-13}	0.0024	36 h

[a] From Ref. 42.

REFERENCES

1. F. Kögl, *Chem. Ber.*, *68*, A16 (1935).
2. F. Kögl and B. Tönnis, *Z. Physiol. Chem.*, *242*, 43 (1936).
3. D. B. Melville, A. W. Meyer, K. Hofmann, and V. Du Vigneaud, *J. Biol. Chem.*, *146*, 487 (1942).
4. S. A. Harris, D. E. Wolf, R. Mozingo, and K. Folkers, *Science*, *97*, 447 (1943).
5. S. A. Harris, D. E. Wolf, R. Mozingo, G. E. Arth, R. C. Anderson, N. R. Easton, and K. Folkers, *J. Am. Chem. Soc.*, *67*, 2096 (1945).
6. W. Traub, *Nature*, *178*, 649 (1956).
7. W. Traub, *Science*, *129*, 210 (1959).
8. C. Bonnemere, J. A. Hamilton, L. K. Steinrauf, and J. Knappe, *Biochemistry*, *4*, 240 (1965).
9. J. Trotter and J. A. Hamilton, *Biochemistry*, *5*, 713 (1966).
10. G. T. De Titta, J. W. Edmonds, W. Stallings, and J. Donohue, *J. Am. Chem. Soc.*, *98*, 1920 (1976).
11. G. T. De Titta, R. Parthasarathy, R. H. Blesing, and W. Stallings, *Proc. Natl. Acad. Sci. USA*, *77*, 333 (1980).
12. J. A. Glasel, *Biochemistry*, *5*, 1851 (1966).
13. R. Lett and A. Marquet, *Tetrahedron*, *30*, 3365 (1974).
14. V. Alcazar, I. Tapia, and J. R. Moran, *Tetrahedron*, *46*, 1057 (1990), and references cited.
15. M. Goldberg and L. H. Sternback, US Patents 2,489,232 and 2,489,238 (1949); *Chem. Abst.*, *45*, 184b, 186a (1951).
16. C. H. Pai and H. C. Lichstein, *Biochim. Biophys. Acta*, *100*, 28 (1965).
17. K. Ogata, *Methods Enzymol.*, *18A*, 390 (1970).
18. F. Frappier, M. Gaudry, and S. Lavielle, unpublished results (1983).

19. D. B. Melville, *J. Biol. Chem.*, *208*, 495 (1954).

20. R. Lett and A. Marquet, *Tetrahedron*, *30*, 3379 (1974).

21. K. Hofmann, D. B. Melville, and V. Du Vigneaud, *J. Biol. Chem.*, *141*, 207 (1941).

22. A. B. A. Jansen and P. J. Stokes, *J. Chem. Soc.*, 4909 (1962).

23. J. Knappe, E. Ringelmann, and F. Lynen, *Biochem. Z.*, *335*, 168 (1961).

24. Y. Izumi and H. Yamada, in *Biotechnology of Vitamins Pigments and Growth Factors* (I. E. Vandamme, ed.), Elsevier Science, Essex, p. 231 (1989).

25. M. A. Eisenberg, in *Escherichia coli and Salmonella typhimurium: Cellular and Molecular Biology* (F. C. Neidhart, ed.), vol. 1, American Society for Microbiology, Washington, DC, p. 544 (1989).

26. M. A. Eisenberg, *Adv. Enzymol. Relat. Areas Mol. Biol.*, *38*, 317 (1973).

27. M. A. Eisenberg, *Ann. N.Y. Acad. Sci.*, *447*, 335 (1985) and literature cited.

28. A. J. Otsuka, M. R. Buoncristiani, P. K. Howard, J. Flamm, C. Johnson, R. Yamamoto, K. Uchida, C. Cook, J. Ruppert, and J. Matsuzaki, *J. Biol. Chem.*, *263*, 19577 (1988).

29. R. G. Brennan, S. Vasu, B. W. Matthews, and A. J. Otsuka, *J. Biol. Chem.*, *264*, 5 (1989).

30. M. O'regan, R. Gloeckler, S. Bernard, C. Ledoux, I. Ohsawa, and Y. Lemoine, *Nucleic Acid Res.*, *17*, 8004 (1989).

31. I. Ohsawa, D. Speck, K. Kisou, K. Hayakawa, M. Zinsuis, R. Gloeckler, Y. Lemoine, and K. Kamogawa, *Gene*, *80*, 39 (1989).

32. R. Gloeckler, I. Ohsawa, D. Speck, C. Ledoux, S. Bernard, M. Zinsuis, D. Villeval, T. Kisou, K. Kamogawa, and Y. Lemoine, *Gene*, *87*, 63 (1990).

33. J. R. Waller and H. C. Lichstein, *J. Bacteriol.*, *90*, 853 (1965).

34. T. O. Rogers and H. C. Lichstein, *J. Bacteriol.*, *100*, 587 (1969).

35. J. M. Becker, M. Wilchek, and E. Katchalski, *Proc. Natl. Acad. Sci. USA*, *68*, 2604 (1971).

36. C. H. Pai, *J. Bacteriol.*, *112*, 1280 (1972).

37. O. M. Prakash and M. A. Eisenberg, *J. Bacteriol.*, *120*, 785 (1974).

38. A. Piffeteau, M. Zamboni, and M. Gaudry, *Biochim. Biophys. Acta*, *688*, 29 (1982).

39. A. Piffeteau and M. Gaudry, *Biochim. Biophys. Acta*, *816*, 77 (1985).

40. J. F. Cicmanec and H. C. Lichstein, *J. Bacteriol.*, *119*, 718 (1974).

41. N. Cohen and M. Thomas, *Biochem. Biophys. Res. Commun.*, *108*, 1508 (1982).

42. M. Zamboni, Thesis, Paris VII (1981).

43. K. Dakshinamurti and L. E. Chalifour, *J. Cell. Physiol.*, *107*, 427 (1981).

44. L. E. Chalifour and K. Dakshinamurti, *Biochim. Biophys. Acta*, *721*, 64 (1982).

45. L. E. Chalifour and K. Dakshinamurti, *Biochem. Biophys. Res. Commun.*, *104*, 1047 (1982).

46. L. E. Chalifour and K. Dakshinamurti, *Biochem. J.*, *210*, 121 (1983).

47. D. L. Weiner and B. Wolf, *Ann. N.Y. Acad. Sci.*, *447*, 435 (1985).

48. J. Gore and C. Huinard, *J. Nutr.*, *117*, 527 (1987).
49. H. M. Said and R. Redha, *Am. J. Physiol.*, *252*, 52 (1987).
50. H. M. Said and R. Redha, *Biochim. Biophys. Acta*, *945*, 195 (1988).
51. H. M. Said, D. M. Mock, and J. C. Collins, *Am. J. Physiol.*, *256*, 306 (1989).
52. H. M. Said, R. Redha, and W. Nylander, *Gastroenterology*, *95*, 1312 (1988).
53. P. N. A. Murthy and S. P. Mistry, *Biochem. Rev.*, *43*, 1 (1972).
54. N. D. Cohen, M. Thomas, and M. Stack, *Ann. N.Y. Acad. Sci.*, *447*, 393 (1985).
55. H. G. Wood and R. E. Barden, *Annu. Rev. Biochem.*, *46*, 385 (1977).
56. V. L. Murtif and D. Samols, *J. Biol. Chem.*, *262*, 11813 (1987).
57. J. Moss and M. D. Lane, *Adv. Enzymol.*, *35*, 321 (1971).
58. H. G. Wood, *TIBS*, *1*, 4 (1976).
59. D. Samols, C. G. Thorton, V. L. Murtif, G. K. Kumar, F. C. Haase, and H. G. Wood, *J. Biol. Chem.*, *263*, 6461 (1988).
60. A. W. Alberts and P. R. Vagelos, *Enzymes*, *6*, 37 (1972).
61. K. G. Thampy and S. Wakil, *J. Biol. Chem.*, *263*, 6447 (1988).
62. K. G. Thampy and S. Wakil, *J. Biol. Chem.*, *263*, 6454 (1988).
63. L. A. Witters and J. M. McDermott, *Biochemistry*, *25*, 7216 (1986).
64. F. Kalousek, M. D. Darigo, and L. E. Rosenberg, *J. Biol. Chem.*, *255*, 60 (1980).
65. F. Lynen, *Methods Enzymol.*, *71*, 781 (1981).
66. M. C. Scrutton and M. R. Young, *Enzymes*, *6*, 1 (1972).
67. P. A. Whitney and T. G. Cooper, *J. Biol. Chem.*, *247*, 1349 (1972).
68. W. Seubert, E. Fass, and U. Remberger, *Biochem. Z*, *338*, 265 (1963).
69. H. G. Wood, *Enzymes*, *6*, 83 (1972).
70. H. G. Wood, *CRC Crit. Rev. Biochem.*, *7*, 143 (1979).
71. J. H. Galivan and S. G. H. Allen, *Arch. Biochem. Biophys.*, *126*, 838 (1969).
72. J. R. Stern, *Biochemistry*, *6*, 3545 (1967).
73. A. Munnich, J. M. Saudubray, A. Cotisson, F. X. Coudé, H. Ogier, C. Charpentier, C. Marsac, G. Carré, M. Bourgeay-Causse, and J. Frezal, *Eur. J. Pediatr.*, *137*, 203 (1981).
74. B. M. Charles, G. Hosking, A. Green, R. Pollitt, K. Bartlett, and L. S. Taitz, *Lancet*, *2*, 118 (1979).
75. M. J. Cowan, D. W. Wara, S. Packman, A. J. Ammann, H. Yishino, L. Sweetman, and W. L. Nyhan, *Lancet*, *2*, 115 (1979).
76. W. L. Nyhan, *Int. J. Biochem.*, *20*, 363 (1988).
77. L. Sweetman, *J. Interit. Metab. Dis.*, *4*, 53 (1981).
78. B. J. Burri, L. Sweetman, and W. L. Nyhan, *J. Clin. Invest.*, *68*, 1491 (1981).
79. H. K. Ghneim and K. Bartlett, *Lancet*, *2*, 1187 (1982).
80. M. Zamboni, M. Gaudry, A. Marquet, A. Munnich, J. M. Saudubray, and C. Marsac, *Clin. Chim. Acta.*, *122*, 241 (1982).
81. B. Wolf, R. E. Grier, R. J. Allen, S. I. Goodman, and C. L. Kien, *Clin. Chim. Acta*, *131*, 273 (1983).

82. M. Gaudry, A. Munnich, J. M. Saudubray, H. Ogier, G. Mitchell, C. Marsac, M. Causse, A. Marquet, and J. Frezal, *Lancet, i,* 297 (1983).

83. M. Berger, *Biochemistry, 14,* 2338 (1975).

84. M. Berger, *Methods Enzymol., 62,* 319 (1979).

85. A. Scoot, K. Dakshinamurti, E. Rector, G. Delespesse, and A. Sehon, *Ann. N.Y. Acad. Sci., 447,* 423 (1985).

86. K. Dakshinamurti, R. P. Bhullar, A. Scoot, E. Rector, G. Delespesse, and A. Sehon, *Biochem. J., 237,* 447 (1986).

87. H. B. White, *Ann. N.Y. Acad. Sci., 447,* 202 (1985).

88. H. B. White and C. C. Whitehead, *Biochem. J., 241,* 677 (1987).

89. N. M. Green, *Adv. Prot. Chem., 29,* 85 (1975).

90. G. Gitlin, E. A. Bayer, and M. Wilchek, *Biochem. J., 250,* 291 (1988).

91. Y. Hiller, J. M. Gershoni, E. A. Bayer, and M. Wilchek, *Biochem. J., 248,* 167 (1987).

92. F. Tausig and F. Wolf, *Biochem. Biophys. Res. Commun., 14,* 205 (1964).

93. H. C. Lichstein and J. Birnbaum, *Biochem. Biophys. Res. Commun., 20,* 41 (1965).

94. P. C. Weber, M. J. Cox, F. R. Salemme, and D. H. Ohlendorf, *J. Biol. Chem., 262,* 12718 (1987).

95. A. Pähler, W. A. Hendrickson, M. A. Gawinowiczkolks, C. E. Argaña, and C. R. Cantor, *J. Biol. Chem., 262,* 13933 (1987).

96. T. Sano and C. R. Cantor, *J. Biol. Chem., 265,* 3369 (1990).

97. E. A. Bayer and M. Wilchek, *Methods Biochem. Anal., 26,* 1 (1980).

98. M. Wilchek and E. A. Bayer, *Anal. Biochem., 171,* 1 (1988).

99. D. B. McCormick and J. A. Roth, *Anal. Biochem., 34,* 226 (1970).

100. D. B. McCormick and J. A. Roth, *Methods Enzymol., 18A,* 383 (1970).

101. S. Haarasilta, *Anal. Biochem., 87,* 306 (1978).

102. R. B. Ferguson and H. C. Lichstein, *J. Bacteriol., 75,* 366 (1958).

103. E. E. Snell, R. E. Eakin, and R. J. Williams, *J. Am. Chem. Soc., 62,* 175 (1940).

104. H. R. Skeggs, in *Analytical Microbiology* (F. Kavanagh ed.), Academic Press, New York, p. 421 (1963) and references cited therein.

105. E. DeMoll and W. Shive, *Anal. Biochem., 158,* 55 (1986).

106. D. S. Genghof, C. W. H. Partridge, and F. H. Carpenter, *Arch. Biochem., 17,* 413 (1948).

107. O. Ploux, unpublished results.

108. DIFCO Manual, 3rd ed., p. 1076.

109. N. M. Green, *Methods Enzymol., 18A,* 418 (1970).

110. N. M. Green, *Biochem., J., 94,* 23c (1965).

111. H. J. Lin and J. C. Kirsch, *Anal. Biochem., 81,* 442 (1977).

112. H. J. Lin and J. C. Kirsch, *Methods Enzymol., 62D,* 287 (1979).

113. M. H. H. Al-Hakeim, J. Landen, D. S. Smith, and R. D. Nargessi, *Anal. Biochem., 116,* 264 (1981).

114. K. J. Schray, P. G. Artz, and R. C. Hevey, *Anal. Biochem., 60,* 853 (1988).

115. D. L. Mock, G. Langford, D. B. Dubois, N. Criscimagna, and P.

Horowitz, *Anal. Biochem.*, *151*, 178 (1985).

116. H. R. Schroeder, P. O. Vogelhut, R. J. Carris, R. C. Bogulaski, and R. T. Buckler, *Anal. Chem.*, *48*, 1933 (1976).
117. E. J. Williams and A. K. Campbell, *Anal. Biochem.*, *155*, 249 (1986).
118. R. L. Hood, *J. Sci. Food Agric.*, *26*, 1847 (1975).
119. R. L. Hood, *Methods Enzymol*, *62D*, 179 (1979).
120. R. L. Hood, *Anal. Biochem.*, *79*, 635 (1977).
121. R. Rettenmaier, *Anal. Chim. Acta*, *113*, 107 (1980).
122. K. Dakshinamurti and R. Allan, *Methods Enzymol.*, *62D*, 284 (1979).
123. T. Horsburg and D. Gompertz, *Clin. Chim. Acta.*, *82*, 215 (1978).
124. D. M. Mock and D. B. Dubois, *Anal. Biochem.*, *153*, 272 (1986).
125. E. A. Bayer, H. Ben-Hur, and M. Wilchek, *Anal. Biochem.*, *154*, 367 (1986).
126. S. Daunert, B. R. Payne, and L. Bachas, *Anal. Chem.*, *61*, 2160 (1989).
127. T. L. Kjellström and L. Bachas, *Anal. Chem.*, *61*, 1728 (1989).
128. B. Terouanne, M. Bencheick, P. Balaguer, A. M. Boussioux, and J. C. Nicolas, *Anal. Biochem.*, *180*, 43 (1989).
129. Y. Ikariyama, M. Furuki, and M. Aizawa, *Anal. Chem.*, *57*, 496 (1985).
130. Y. Ikariyama and M. Aizawa, *Methods Enzymol.*, *137*, 111 (1988).
131. K. Ogata, T. Tochikura, S. Inaura, K. Irushima, S. Takasawa, M. Kikuchi, and A. Nishimura, *Agric. Biol. Chem. (Tokyo)*, *29*, 895 (1965).
132. M. A. Eisenberg, *Biochem. Biophys. Res. Commun.*, *8*, 437 (1962).
133. J. P. Tepper, D. B. McCormick, and L. D. Wright, *J. Biol. Chem.*, *241*, 5734 (1966).
134. W. B. Im, D. B. McCormick, and L. D. Wright, *Methods Enzymol.*, *62D*, 385 (1979).
135. G. Guillerm, F. Frappier, M. Gaudry, and A. Marquet, *Biochimie*, *59*, 119 (1977).
136. A. G. Salib, F. Frappier, G. Guillerm, and A. Marquet, *Biochem. Biophys. Res. Commun.*, *88*, 312 (1979).
137. F. Frappier and A. Marquet, *Biochem. Biophys. Res. Commun.*, *103*, 1288 (1981).
138. K. Ogata, Y. Izumi, K. Aoike, and Y. Tani, *Agric. Biol. Chem. (Tokyo)*, *37*, 1093 (1973).
139. S. Iwahara, D. B. McCormick, and L. D. Wright, *Methods Enzymol.*, *18A*, 404 (1970).
140. C. Lindblow Kull, F. J. Kull, and A. Schrift, *Biochem. Biophys. Res. Commun.*, *93*, 572 (1980).
141. R. T. Nuttall and B. Bush, *Analyst*, *96*, 875 (1971).
142. V. M. Svetlaeva, D. S. Danilova, and M. T. Yanotovskii, *Khim. Farm. Zh.*, *12*, 140 (1978); *Chem. Abstr.*, *90*, 12365 u (1979).
143. H. Thieleman, *Sci. Pharm.*, *42*, 221 (1974).
144. K. Groningsson and L. Jansson, *J. Pharm. Sci.*, *68*, 364 (1979).
145. K. Shimada, Y. Nagase, and U. Matsumoto, *Yakugaku Zasshi*, *89*, 436 (1969).
146. M. G. Horning, E. A. Boucher, and A. M. Moss, *J. Gas Chromatogr.*, 5 297 (1967).

147. V. Viswanathan, F. P. Mahn, V. S. Venturella, and B. Z. Senkowski, *J. Pharm. Sci.*, *59*, 400 (1970).
148. R. N. Johnson and G. R. Boyden, *J. Pharm. Sci.*, *66*, 1212 (1977).
149. H. Janecke and H. Voege, *Z. Anal. Chem.*, *254*, 355 (1971).
150. M. Jouany, A. Olesker, P. L. Desbene, and F. Frappier, unpublished results (1982).
151. P. L. Desbene, S. Coustal, and F. Frappier, *Anal. Biochem.*, *128*, 359 (1983).
152. T. Yoshida, A. Uetake, C. Nakai, N. Nimura, and T. Kinoshita, *J. Chromatogr.*, *456*, 421 (1988).
153. M. Azoulay, P. L. Desbene, F. Frappier, and Y. Georges, unpublished results.

12

COBALAMINS

Jan Lindemans

*University Hospital Rotterdam Dijkzigt
and Sophia Children's Hospital, Rotterdam,
The Netherlands*

1. INTRODUCTION

1.1 History

In 1926 Whipple et al. (1) described the successful treatment of dogs suffering from an experimental form of anemia by feeding them with large amounts of raw liver. In the same year Minot and Murphy (2) showed that this treatment was equally effective in patients with pernicious anemia. However, it took another 20 years of research to isolate and identify the active substance: vitamin B_{12} or cyanocobalamin. The red-colored material was isolated from liver in crystalline form almost simultaneously by Folkers and co-workers (3) in the United States and by Smith in Great Britain (4). Its corrinoid structure was defined by chemical analysis (5) and by X-ray crystallography (6) in 1956. Once it was recognized that the biologically active forms of vitamin B_{12} were highly photosensitive, Barker et al. (7–9) were able to isolate coenzyme B_{12} (adenosylcobalamin) from *Clostridium tetanomorphum* and from liver. A second biologically active form of vitamin B_{12} was detected in extracts of human plasma by Lindstrand and Ståhlberg and proved to be identical with already synthetically prepared methylcobalamin (10,11).

From the very beginning chromatographic techniques have enabled researchers to separate and isolate specific cobalamin compounds from natural substances and preparative mixtures. Today these techniques contribute to the expansion of our detailed knowledge of cobalamin biosynthesis in microorganisms and the reaction mechanisms in cabalamin-dependent metabolic pathways.

It is the aim of this chapter to summarize established and modern techniques for the chromatographic separation and identification of cobalamins and to evaluate their value in present biochemical, pharmaceutical, and clinical investigations.

1.2 Chemical Properties

Structure

Vitamin B_{12} or cyanocobalamin belongs to the corrinoids. This is a group of compounds having in common a corrin nucleus, that is, a partially hydrogenated tetrapyrrole of which two pyrroles are joined directly rather than through methene bridges, and with a central cobalt atom bound by coordinate linkages to the nitrogen atoms of the four pyrroles. Vitamin B_{12} is further characterized by a specific number of methyl, propionamide, and acetamide side chains attached to the pyrroles, and one side chain on ring D in which the propionic acid is amidated with 1-amino-2-propanol. The latter, in turn, is esterified with α-D-ribofuranosyl-(5,6-dimethylbenzimidazole) 3'-phosphate. The second N atom of the 5,6-dimethylbenzimidazole forms the fifth coordinate linkage with the cobalt atom in the α-position (Fig. 1). The β position in the naturally occurring cobalamins is occupied by a CN^- (cyanocobalamin), OH^- (hydroxycobalamin), H_2O (aquocobalamin), CH_3 (methylcobalamin), or deoxyadenosyl group (adenosylcobalamin or coenzyme B_{12}). Other members of the corrinoid group, described in the section on biosynthesis, are depicted in Fig. 2. For an extensive treatise on corrinoid nomenclature the reader is referred to the IUPAC-IUB reports on this subject (12,13).

Stability

At room temperature cyanocobalamin is fairly soluble in water (12 g/liter), lower alcohols, and phenol, but almost insoluble in acetone, ether, and chloroform. The molecular weight is 1355.4 ($C_{63}H_{88}O_{14}N_{14}PCo$) and the molecule is neutral in water. Between pH 4 and 7 cyanocobalamin is stable in aqueous solution and can be heated at 120°C without significant loss.

Alkaline hydrolysis (0.1 M) at 100°C induces the formulation of "dehydrovitamin B_{12}," a biologically inactive form with a lactam ring fused to ring B of the cobamide nucleus (14). Cyanide can be split off on exposure to light with the production of hydroxocobalamin. This process

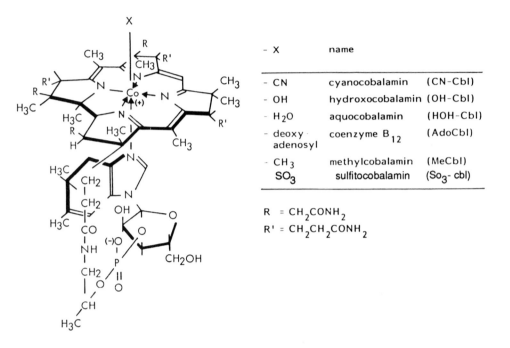

- X	name
- CN	cyanocobalamin (CN-Cbl)
- OH	hydroxocobalamin (OH-Cbl)
- H_2O	aquocobalamin (HOH-Cbl)
- deoxy adenosyl	coenzyme B_{12} (AdoCbl)
- CH_3	methylcobalamin (MeCbl)
SO_3	sulfitocobalamin (SO_3- cbl)

R = CH_2CONH_2
R' = $CH_2CH_2CONH_2$

Figure 1   Structural formula of cobalamin.

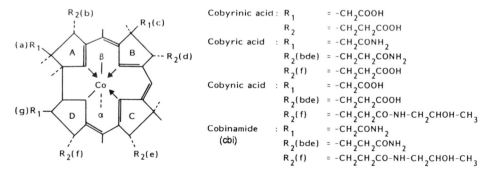

Cobyrinic acid : R_1 = -CH_2COOH
R_2 = -CH_2CH_2COOH
Cobyric acid : R_1 = -CH_2CONH_2
R_2(bde) = -$CH_2CH_2CONH_2$
R_2(f) = -CH_2CH_2COOH
Cobynic acid : R_1 = -CH_2COOH
R_2(bde) = -CH_2CH_2COOH
R_2(f) = -$CH_2CH_2CO-NH-CH_2CHOH-CH_3$
Cobinamide : R_1 = -CH_2CONH_2
(cbi) R_2(bde) = -$CH_2CH_2CONH_2$
R_2(f) = -$CH_2CH_2CO-NH-CH_2CHOH-CH_3$

Figure 2   Structural formulas of cobalamin percursors.

is stimulated by the addition of acid (15). Hydroxocobalamin occurs in neutral or acid solution as aquocobalamin. Hydroxocobalamin can be converted to cyano-, sulfito-, chloro-, cyanato-, nitrito-, bromo-, thiocyanato-, and azidocobalamin by the addition of the respective reactants under the appropriate conditions (16). At alkaline pH and excess of cyanide the stable dicyanocobalamin is formed. Mild acid hydrolysis of corrinoids causes the loss of the peripheral amides from the propionamide side chains, forming mono-, di-, and tricarboxylic acids (17). The most vulnerable is the propionamide in the e position. Deamidation of the more stable acetamide side chains requires more drastic conditions, in which the nucleotide moiety is also released together with the isopropylamine group at position f. The susceptibility to acid hydrolysis is influenced by the ligands in α and β position. Cyanocobinamide, 1-α-D-ribofuranosyl-5,6-dimethylbenzimidazole, and phosphate are formed during alkaline hydrolysis of cyanocobalamin in a suspension of cerous hydroxide, pH 8–9, at 100°C for 2 h (18).

In cyano- and hydroxocobalamin the cobalt atom is in the 3+ state. Reduction to the Co^{2+}, and even the Co^{1+}, state can be brought about by electrochemical and purely chemical means (19). The color then changes from red (Co^{3+}) to brown (Co^{2+}) and gray-green (Co^{+1}). Co^{2+}-cobalamin is also formed when aquocobalamin is treated with monothiols (20,21).

The naturally occurring organocorrinoids AdoCbl and MeCbl share extreme photosensitivity with most other artificially synthesized organocorrinoids. This makes it necessary to perform all analytical work with these compounds in the dark or under dim red light.

In the absence of oxygen the photodecomposition of adenosylcobalamin leads to the formation of Co^{3+}-cobalamin (22) and a 5'-deoxyadenosyl that cyclizes to 8,5-cyclic-adenosine (23). In the presence of oxygen, aquocobalamin and adenosine-5'-carboxaldehyde are formed (24). Photolysis of methylcobalamin occurs very rapidly in aqueous solution, with formation of formaldehyde and aquocobalamin as the major products. In the absence of oxygen the reaction is rather slow and gives rise to the formation of Co^{2+}-cobalamin and methane (25,26). Remarkably, photolysis of methylcobalamin in the presence of homocysteine yields methionine, a methylation reaction that under aerobic, intracellular conditions occurs only in an enzyme-catalyzed reaction with reductive activity (27).

The carbon-cobalt bond in methyl- and adenosylcobalamin is stable in neutral aqueous solution in the dark and withstands even heating for 20 min at 100°C (28). By heating in 0.1 M HCl the carbon-cobalt bond of adenosylcobalamin is cleaved; the alkylcobalamins are relatively stable in dilute acid or alkali. Cyanide forms another threat to the adenosyl-cobalt bond, in particular at alkaline pH and at elevated temperature, by inducing dicyanocobalamin. The alkylcorrinoids are more resistant to the effect of cyanide, but are cleaved through electrophilic attacks on the methyl group, for instance by ionic mercury or thallium, into aquocobalamin and the methylmercury cation or the methylthallic dication (29).

Treatment of Co^{3+}-corrinoids with sodium bisulfite yields sulfito-corrinoids, which behave very similarly to the alkyl corrinoids with respect to photodecomposition and reactions with various compounds (30,31).

Spectroscopy

All corrinoids have distinct colors, varying from yellow, red, and purple to brown-green and blue (28), which can be utilized advantageously to identify the various compounds. The most reliable standard for the determination of the extinction coefficient of a corrinoid is the γ band of the compounds dicyanocobalamin or dicyanocobinamide, which are readily formed from all other forms of cobalamin and cobinamide by cyanide, alkaline pH, and light. The molar extinction coefficient of the sharp γ band at 367–368 nm amounts to $30.8 \times 10^3 \, M^{-1} \, cm^{-1}$ (28,32).

The absorption spectra of some representative corrinoids are presented in Fig. 3.

1.3 Biochemistry

Biosynthesis of Cobalamin

The biosynthesis of cobalamin (Fig. 4) is restricted to specific microorganisms, and most of our knowledge on the biosynthetic pathways stems from studies with cultures of *Streptomyces griseus*, *Propionibacterium shermanii*, and *Clostridium tetanomorphum*. The process has been extensively reviewed by Friedman (33,34) and Battersby and McDonald (35). The first steps in cobalamin biosynthesis follow those of porphyrin biosynthesis. At the stage of uroporphyrinogen III, seven methyl groups, derived from S-adenosylmethionine, are attached and a hydrolytic ring contraction takes place by which the methene bridge between rings A and D is lost. Subsequently, the cobalt atom is inserted and several side-chain modifications take place. The acetate side chain of ring C is decarboxylated to become a methyl group (Fig. 2). At this stage the intermediate is called cobyrinic acid. By amidation of the remaining carboxylic groups, with exception of the propionic acid side chain of ring D, cobyric acid is formed, which is converted to cobinamide by the attach-

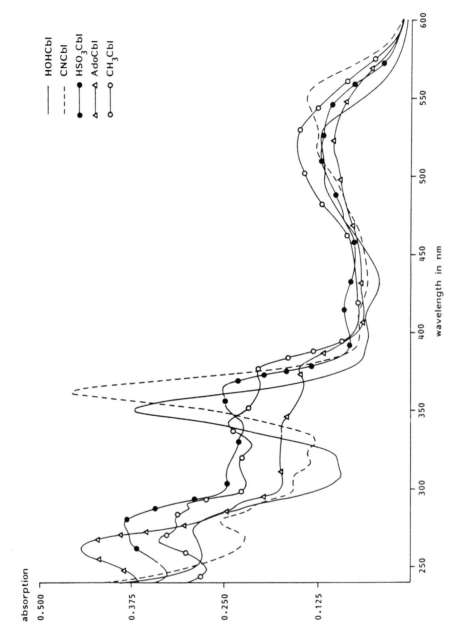

Figure 3 Absorption spectra of the naturally occurring cobalamins.

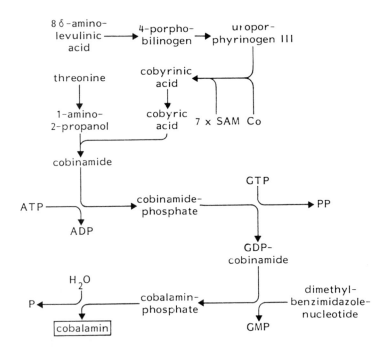

Figure 4 Biosynthesis of cobalamin.

ment of 1-amino-2-propanol to the last propionic acid side chain. Cobinamide phosphate is formed at the expense of ATP through a cobinamide kinase activity. The next step in the biosynthesis is the formation of an anhydride linkage between the N-β-glycosidic ribonucleoside 5′-phosphate of GTP and the phosphate of cobinamide phosphate to form GDP-cobinamide. The GMP moiety is subsequently exchanged for 5,6-dimethylbenzimidazole-N-α-ribose 5′-phosphate. The latter compound, with its rather unique N-α-glycosidic bond, is synthesized by the action of trans-N-glycosidase or nicotinate nucleotide phosphoribosyltransferase (EC 2.4.2.21). This enzyme has very little base specificity, and it is possible to induce the formation of different corrinoids by feeding the growing bacteria all kinds of different bases. The final product of the base-exchange reaction, cobalamin phosphate, is ultimately dephosphorylated to cobalamin, preferentially in the "base-off" condition.

Cobalamin-Dependent Reactions

The natural, metabolically active forms of vitamin B_{12} are adenosylcobalamin and methylcobalamin (AdoCbl and MeCbl), both of which can be formed from hydroxocobalamin. The conversion of hydroxo- and cyanocobalamin into the active coenzyme forms has mainly been studied in bacterial systems (36,37), but there is evidence that it is representative for the mammalian system as well (15,38,39). The first step in the conversion of hydroxocobalamin is the two-step reduction of the Co^{3+} atom to the Co^{1+} state by two different but cooperative reductases at the expense of NADH. After this reduction an adenosylating enzyme catalyzes the transfer of the adenosyl moiety from ATP to the Co^{1+}-cobalamin, yielding deoxyadenosylcobalamin and tripolyphosphate. The formation of methylcobalamin probably occurs in the process of the complex methyltransferase reaction catalyzed by N^5-methyltetrahydrofolate homocysteine methyltransferase (EC 2.1.1.13) (40), which will be described later.

Adenosylcobalamin-dependent reactions always involve the exchange of a hydrogen atom from one carbon atom with another group (R) from an adjacent carbon atom. The only exception is the Adocbl-dependent ribonucleotide reductase reaction in bacteria and the eukaryotic flagellate *Euglena gracilis*. An overview of Adocbl-dependent reactions is presented in Table 1 (41). Of these only the methylmalonyl-CoA mutase (EC 5.4.99.2) reaction takes place in mammalian metabolism and forms the link between the metabolism of odd-chain fatty acids, cholesterol, isoleucine, valine, threonine, methionine, and propionic acid on the one hand, and the tricarboxylic acid cycle through succinyl-CoA on the other (Fig. 5). The reaction is of special importance for ruminants in which propionate, arising from cellulose degradation, forms a major source of

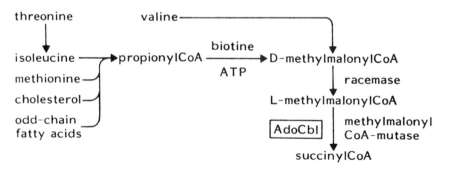

Figure 5   Propionic acid pathway.

Table 1 Adenosylcobalamin-Dependent Reactions

Enzyme	Substrate	Transferred group (R)	Product
Glutamate mutase	L-Glutamate	Glycine	L-*threo*-β-Methyl aspartate
Methylmalonyl CoA mutase	L-Methylmalonyl CoA	-COSCoA	Succinyl CoA
α-Methyleneglutarate mutase	α-Methyleneglutarate	-C($=CH_2$)COOH	Methylitaconate
Dioldehydrase	Ethylene glycol 1,2-Propanediol	OH	Acetaldehyde Propionaldehyde
Glycerol dehydrase	Glycerol	OH	β-Hydroxypropionaldehyde
Ethanolamine ammonia lyase	Ethanolamine	NH_2	Acetaldehyde + NH_3
β-Lysine mutase	L-β-Lysine	NH_2	L-Erythro-3,5-diamino-hexanoic acid
α-Lysine mutase	D-Lysine	NH_2	D-2,5-Diaminohexanoic acid
α-Leucine 2,3-aminomutase	α-Leucine	NH_2	β-leucine
Ornithine mutase	D-Ornithine	NH_2	D-*threo*-2,4-Diaminovaleric acid
Ribonucleotide reductase	Ribonucleotide	—	2'-Deoxyribonucleotide

energy. The enzyme involved is located in the mitochondria and is composed of two nonidentical subunits, one of which binds adenosylcobalamin. A deficiency of adenosylcobalamin or the apoenzyme results in the accumulation of methylmalonic acid, which is secreted by the kidneys and gives rise to methylmalonic aciduria (42).

Methylcobalamin-dependent reactions, involved in the synthesis of methionine in animals and microorganisms and in the formation of acetate and methane in bacteria, have been reviewed by Poston and Stadtman (43) and more recently by Taylor (40). As stated before, methylcobalamin is formed from reduced Co^{2+}-cobalamin in the course of the methyltetrahydrofolate homocysteine methyltransferase reaction (Fig. 6). Presumably, the Co^{2+}-cobalamin is bound by the apoenzyme, further reduced to Co^{1+}-cobalamin in a $FADH_2$-requiring process, and methylated by 5′-methyltetrahydrofolate in the presence of catalytic amounts of S-adenosylmethionine. Further transfer of methyl groups from methyltetrahydrofolate to homocysteine occurs independently of S-adenosylmethionine. Through this reaction, cobalamin is involved in the regeneration of tetrahydrofolate, an indispensible folate intermediate in the de novo biosynthesis of purines and thymidilate and in the regeneration of methionine.

Various bacteria from sewage sludge use methanol and acetate as major sources of energy. The methyl group is first transferred to cobalamin and then released as methane as a result of reductive cleavage (43). In *Clostridium thermoaceticum* acetate is synthesized from CO_2 in a folate- and MeCbl-dependent pathway. CO_2 is first reduced to formate, which is used to form 10-formyltetrahydrofolate. After further reduction to 5-methyltetrahydrofolate, the methyl group is transferred to cobala-

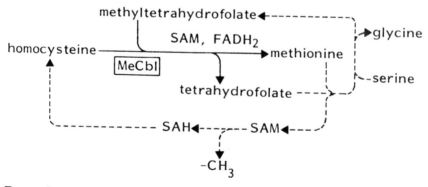

Figure 6 MeCbl-dependent regeneration of methionine and tetrahydrofolate.

min, thus forming methylcobalamin. Subsequently, two molecules of acetate arise from a reaction between methylcobalamin and pyruvate, with carboxymethyl-Cbl as a likely intermediate (44).

1.4 Physiology

The ultimate source of cobalamin for mammalian metabolism is microbial synthesis. The cobalamins from the microbial flora in the gastro intestinal system of herbivorous animals are absorbed by the host and stored by their tissues. From there cobalamin is passed on to other animals in the food chain. A normal daily adult human diet contains about 5 μg of cobalamin, which is about three times the minimum daily requirement to maintain cobalamin homeostasis. The total amount of cobalamin in the human body is about 3 mg.

The hydrophilic cobalamin molecule has to be transported from the intestine to the blood by an elaborate transfer system. Cobalamin is first released from binding substances in the food by peptic activity at low pH in the stomach and becomes bound to so-called R-binders present in saliva and gastric juice. In the ileum pancreatic proteolytic enzymes dissociate the cobalamins from the R-binders and in this way facilitate their binding to intrinsic factor, a glycoprotein that in humans is synthesized and released by the gastric parietal cells. The cobalamin-intrinsic factor complex becomes attached to specific receptors on the mucosal surface of the distal part of the ileum (45). Through an incompletely defined mechanism, cobalamin enters the mucosal cell and is passed on to the plasma transport protein transcobalamin II (46). This 38,000 MW polypeptide carries cobalamin through the portal circulation first to the liver and distributes it from there to the other tissues.

Transcobalamin II-bound cobalamin is taken up by those tissues through receptor-mediated endocytosis in which the protein-moiety is degraded in the lysosomes (47). The daily turnover of transcobalamin II-bound cobalamin is 5–10 μg per day. The transport of cobalamin from peripheral tissues to the central storage organ, the liver, is assured by R-type cobalamin-binding proteins, which are a group of glycoproteins occurring in almost all body fluids, produced mainly by granulocytes.

The most frequent cause of cobalamin deficiency is insufficient absorption due to a lack of intrinsic factor. This condition is more generally known as pernicious anemia and is caused by the occurrence of auto-antibodies against parietal cells and intrinsic factor, blocking its capacity to bind cobalamin and preventing its absorption. Less frequent causes are abnormal intestinal flora, partial or total gastrectomy, tropical sprue, fish tapeworm infestation, and the congenital intrinsic factor abnormality and intrinsic factor receptor dysfunction (Imerslund-Gräsbeck disease).

1.5 Pharmacology of Cobalamin

Pure nutritional cobalamin deficiency being extremely rare, most other causes of cobalamin deficiency require lifelong treatment with parenteral, mainly intramuscular, administration of cobalamin. Both cyano- and hydroxocobalamin are being used for this purpose. Unbound cobalamin in the circulation cannot be retained by the kidney and is excreted. As hydroxocobalamin binds more strongly to plasma proteins other than the specific cobalamin binders, it is better retained by the body and thus more effective. After replenishment of the cobalamin stores by about 5 doses of at least 250 μg hydroxocobalamin on alternate days, cobalamin homeostasis can be maintained by bimonthly injections of 1000 μg cobalamin.

A particular application of hydroxocobalamin is its use in the treatment of cyanide-poisoning. Large and frequent doses can be given without significant side effects to scavenge the cyanide from the circulation.

Allergic and anaphylactic reactions to cobalamin are extremely rare. Several reports have appeared on patients having developed circulating immunoglobulin (IgG) antibodies against cobalamin or against the cobalamin-transcobalamin II complex (48,49). This leads to an accumulation of cobalamin in the circulation but seems of no clinical consequence.

Oral treatment of cobalamin deficiency due to malabsorption can only be successful when a dose of at least 500–1000 μg is given to allow the passive absorption of about 5–10 μg per day.

Specific treatment schedules are devised for patients with one of the various forms of congenital metabolic disturbance of cobalamin metabolism. In general these conditions require daily injections, sometimes in combination with folic acid, carnitine, betaine, or choline (50).

2. THIN-LAYER CHROMATOGRAPHY

2.1 Extraction Procedures

In living organisms cobalamin is for the greater part bound with high affinity to the enzymes for which it functions as cofactor. Chromatographic analysis therefore has to be preceded by liberation and extraction from these complexes. An overview of established extraction methods has been given by Pawelkiewicz (51) and Friedrich (52). In summary, cell material is homogenized in either dilute buffer, 1% acetic acid, 75, 80, or 90% ethanol and heated for 20–30 min at 80 or 100°C. The extraction efficiency improves by adding 0.01% cyanide, but then only cyano forms of the different corrinoids are recovered. For extraction of organocorrinoids, such as AdoCbl and MeCbl, the whole procedure must be carried out under dim red illumination to avoid photodecomposition.

After the heating, particulate matter is removed by filtration or centrifugation. The corrinoids are recovered from the solution by adsorption onto Amberlite IRC-50-H cation-exchanger with ammonia or, after washing with dilute acid, with 0.1 M HCl in 75% acetone (53) or 0.1% H_2SO_4 in 50% acetone (54). Further purification of the cobalamins is generally performed with phenol extraction (55,56). Similar extraction procedures have been found applicable to the isolation of the rhodium analogs of methylcobalamin and coenzyme B_{12} (57). Ford and Friedman have extracted various forms of cobyric acid, cobinamide, cobinamide phosphate, and GDP-cobinamide from *P. shermanii* using aqueous 75% acetone at room temperature in the dark. Further purification was obtained by phenol extraction (58). The use of phenol has been largely replaced by the nonpolar adsorbent Amberlite XAD or silanized silica gel 60 H (59). *Colums* are prepared in Pasteur pipettes plugged with glass wool or in 5- to 10-ml syringes filled with a few milliliters of Amberlite XAD in methanol.

The mesh size of the Amberlite must be reduced by crushing in a mortar to obtain a suitable flow rate. The silica gel 60 H is ready for use. The column has to be pretreated by subsequent elution with degassed ethanol, methanol/water/acetic acid (50:50:5, v/v), and water/acetic acid (100:5). An evaporated ethanol extract is dissolved in a small volume of 1% acetic acid and applied to the adsorbent column. Salts and other polar substances are washed away with 1% acetic acid, whereas corrinoids are eluted with degassed water/methanol/acetic acid (50:50:5). Recoveries of 90–98%, as reported for OHCbl, SO_3Cbl, and AdoCbl, are about 10% higher than achieved by phenol extraction. Elution of cobalamin from Amberlite XAD can also be carried out with alkaline solvents such as methanolic 1% ammonium hydroxide. However, under these conditions OHCbl is strongly retained by silanized silica gel (60).

Amberlite XAD adsorption has been applied by Koppenhagen et al. (57) for the isolation of rhodium analogs of cobalamin cofactors. Gimsing et al. (61) used it for the desalting of chemically prepared radioactive cobalamin forms and Stupperich et al. (62) extracted cobamides from various bacterial species with this material. The latter authors also introduced a neutral aluminum oxide column for further purification but did not indicate its specific advantages.

The reversed-phase cartridge Sep-Pak C18 (Waters) has been found applicable by Jacobson et al. (63) for the desalting of an extract from L1210 lymphoblasts. Elution of cobalamins from this type of column is brought about by 50% acetonitrile.

In all presented studies little attention has been paid to the recovery of individual cobalamin forms in extracts. Frenkel et al. (64) reported a variably decreased recovery of OHCbl in comparison with the other cobalamin forms and proposed a tentative correction for the apparent loss of OHCbl on the basis of the difference between total tissue cobalamin content and the sum of the collected cobalamin fractions after separation.

In many studies on plasma cobalamin forms, the method initially described by Lindstrand and Ståhlberg in 1963 (10) is still being used. One volume of plasma is poured into 4 volumes of absolute alcohol and heated for 20 min at 80°C. After removal of the precipitate by filtration the alcohol in the filtrate is evaporated under vacuum at 30°C. The residual water phase is extracted three to six times with ether to remove lipid material. In the next step cobalamins are extracted from the water phase into phenol by shaking with four volumes of phenol containing 15% water. The phenol phase is shaken with one part of acetone, three parts of ether, and a small amount of water. Phenol in the resulting water phase is further removed with ether. The water phase containing the cobalamin is evaporated to remove residual ether. Linnell et al. (65,66) used essentially the same procedure with smaller volumes of blood plasma.

Unsatisfactory extraction recoveries of cobalamin from plasma were first mentioned by Gimsing et al. (67). By adding cyano [^{57}Co] cobalamin as an internal standard they showed that a loss of 30–50% of the original amount of cobalamin occurred during the ethanol and phenol extractions. At first they reported equally low extraction recoveries for all cobalamin forms present in plasma, while later a selective underestimation of OHCbl, due to inadequate extraction, was reported (68). Similar observations had been published by Mahoney and Rosenberg (69) and by Frenkel et al. (64). Inadequate extraction of one component obviously invalidates the values of the concentrations of all other individual forms when calculated on the basis of their relative amounts in a chromatographed extract and the total amount of cobalamin in the original sample.

Gimsing et al. (70) attributed the loss of hydroxo- and sulfitocobalamin during ethanol extraction to binding onto histidine residues of plasma proteins, a phenomenon already described by Bauriedel et al. (71), Taylor and Hanna (72), and Lien and Wood (73). This binding process is optimal at pH 7.3, has specificity for aquocobalamin but not for sulfitocobalamin, increases in the presence of 5 M urea, and is competitively inhibited by Cd^{2+} ions. In the histidine-bound form, Co^{3+}-cobalamin should be more resistant to reducing agents than in the free form.

By utilizing the inhibiting effect of cadmium, Gimsing et al. (70) were able to improve the extraction recovery of OHCbl as well as sulfito-Cbl to levels comparable to the extraction of CN-, Ado-, and MeCbl, as calculated from recoveries of added radioactive cobalamin forms.

Studies in our laboratory by Van Kapel et al. (74) confirmed the selective loss of OHCbl during plasma extraction in either hot ethanol or 1% acetic acid by showing an extraction recovery of 83–93% for added CN-, Ado-, and MeCbl, but only 30–40% for added OHCbl and SO_3Cbl. In this study silanized silica gel 60H, according to the method of Fenton and Rosenberg (60), was used to adsorb cobalamins from the extraction medium. The extraction efficiency could be improved by selective conversion of OHCbl into SO_3-, NO_2-, or N_3-cobalamin by adding $Na_2S_2O_5$, $NaNO_2$, or NaN_3, but this made it impossible to separate the individual cobalamin forms thereafter. In the course of these studies it was noticed that during the heating step in ethanol as well as in dilute acid a color change from red to brown occurred in plasma spiked with about 100 pmol OHCbl/liter. Since thiols reduce Co^{3+}-corrinoids to brown Co^{2+}-corrinoid-thiol complexes (20,21), it was assumed that this reduction might originate from thiol groups of proteins that had become more accessible by denaturation during heating (75). Protein-thiol in plasma occurs in a concentration of 0.4–0.6 mmol/liter (76), which is in large excess to OHCbl. Various thiol-blocking agents were therefore investigated with respect to their ability to prevent the loss of OH- and SO_3Cbl. In this respect chloroacetophenone, β-hydroxomercuribenzoate, ethylacrylate, N-ethylmaleimide, and iodoacetamide indeed improved the OHCbl recovery to the level of the other cobalamins, but only ethylacrylate and N-ethylmaleimide did not alter the distribution of the individual cobalamin forms during subsequent chromatography.

The extraction efficiencies of added cobalamins under the influence of N-ethylmaleimide, using silanized silica 60 H for desalting, are presented in Table 2.

Comparing the two proposed mechanisms for OHCbl-binding to plasma proteins (70,74), various arguments favor the concept of SH-binding. Incomplete OHCbl extraction has been observed both at pH 4.3

Table 2 Influence of N-Ethylmaleimide on the Extraction Efficiency of Exogenously Added Cobalamins

Cobalamin[a]	Control[b]	NEM[b]
OHCbl	19.5	77.2
SO$_3$Cbl	23.1	73.6
CNCbl	78.4	86.8
AdoCbl	78.6	86.8
MeCbl	79.6	82.6

[a] Plasma enriched with about 800 pmol/liter of each individual cobalamin.

[b] Extraction with 4 volumes of 1% acetic acid (+12.5 mmol/liter N-ethylmaleimide) followed by desalting on silanized silica gel 60H. Recovery is expressed as a percentage of the amount added, determined by radioisotope dilution assay.

in acetate buffer and at neutral pH during hot ethanol extraction, whereas histidine binding apparently occurs only above pH 5.0 (72). Moreover, OHCbl binding to plasma proteins can be prevented by N-ethylmaleimide, p-hydroxomercuribenzoate, or iodoacetamide, which are all SH-directed agents. In addition, Cd^{2+} ions not only bind to histidine in proteins, but can also block SH groups (77). This observation has been confirmed in our laboratory in 1% acetic acid and hot ethanol extracts of human plasma using protein-SH-group detection within 5, 5'-dithio-bis-(2-nitrobenzoic acid, DTNB) according to Sedlak and Lindsay (78).

2.2 Paper Chromatography

Paper chromatography is one of the earlier techniques for the separation of cobalamins and corrinoids. Whatman number 2 paper in combination with sec-butanol/glacial acetic acid/water (100:3:50) (10) or n-butanol/isopropanol/water (10:7:10) (11) is most frequently used. Whatman 3MM paper has been found useful for the separation of acid hydrolysis products of cyanocobalamin using 2-butanol/glacial acetic acid/water (440:4.1:150) with 0.07% KCN as the ascending solvent (79). A similar system was applied by Kolhouse and Allen (80) for the preparation of various cobalamin analogs and by Kondo et al. (81) for the analytical separation of analogs from animal tissues.

2.3 Thin-Layer Chromatography

The separation of a large number of different organocobalamins by thin-layer chromatography (TLC) on cellulose with four different solvent

COBALAMINS

485

systems has been described by Firth et al. (82) and is presented in Table 3. These systems have been found applicable also for the analysis of fluoroalkylcobalamins (56) and formylmethyl derivatives of cobalamin (83).

Two-dimensional TLC separation of cobalamins from blood plasma has been introduced by Linnell et al. (65,84). The cobalamins in the chromatogram were made visible by a bioautography technique. This

Table 3 Thin-Layer Chromatography of Vitamin B_{12} Derivatives on Cellulose[a]

Axial ligands	Solvent I	Solvent II	Solvent III	Solvent IV
		Cobalamins		
H_2O	0.15–0.75[b]	0.25–0.75[b]	0.30	0.55–0.75[b]
$N \equiv C-$	1.00[(0.25)]	1.00[(0.25)]	1.00[(0.31)]	1.00[(0.37)]
$CH \equiv C-$	1.50	1.45	1.40	1.15
$CH_2=$	1.75	1.85	1.60	1.20
$CHBrCH=$	1.80	1.85	1.60	1.20
CH_2OHCH_2	0.90	1.00	0.90	1.05
CF_3CH_2-	1.95	2.10	1.60	1.20
$-SO_3CH_2-$	0.25	0.30	0.25	0.55
$HOOCCH_2$	1.10	1.15	0.65[d]	1.10
CH_3-	1.80	1.80	1.50	1.20
CH_3CH_2-	1.90	1.80	1.60	1.20
$CH_3CH_2CH_2-$	2.05	2.15	1.70	1.20
C5'-deoxyadenosyl	0.65	0.70	0.65	0.95
		Cobinamides		
H_2O	0.20–0.50[b]	0.35–0.50[b]	0.20[b]	0.80–1.00[b]
$N \equiv C-$	0.60,110[c]	0.80,1.20[c]	0.50,0.80[c]	0.95,1.05[c]
$CH_2=CH-$	1.45	1.65	1.35	1.15
CH_3-	1.35	1.55	1.25	1.15
CH_3CH_2-	1.40	1.55	1.30	1.15
$CH_3CH_2CH_2$	1.60	1.75	1.50	1.20
SO_3^{2-}	0.75	0.74	0.59	0.83

[a] Solvent I, *sec*-butanol/water, 9.5:4; Solvent II, *sec*-butanol/glacial acetic acid/water, 100:1:50; Solvent III, *sec*-butanol/0.88 ammonia/water, 9.5:0.675:4; Solvent IV, *n*-butanol/glacial acetic acid/water, 4:1:5. Retention values relative to the R_f value of cyanocobalamin (in parenthesis). From Ref. 82.

[b] Elongated spots due to equilibration between aquo and hydroxo form on the plate.

[c] Double spots due to the existence of stereoisomers involving the axial ligands.

[d] Ionized carboxylic acid.

technique was first described by Lindstrand and Ståhlberg (10). They placed a paper chromatogram on an agar plate, which was inoculated with the cobalamin-dependent *E. coli* strain 113-3 (ATCC 105ĉ6). After 16 h at 37°C the chromatograms were removed and the plates were further incubated. The presence of bacterial growth indicated the location of cobalamin subfractions. Linnell et al. (65) improved the sensitivity by incorporating the growth indicator 2,3,5-triphenyltetrazolium chloride in the medium. The color intensity of the growth spots could be quantified by light-reflection measurement (85). The growth response of the bacteria was found to be equal for OHCbl, CNCbl, and AdoCbl, but a little lower for MeCbl. Gimsing et al. (67,70) estimated the growth response by photometric measurement of the indicator in an ethanol extract of the culture plate and have found that in the range between 10 and 80 fmol an almost identical and linear response could be achieved for OH-, CN-, Ado-, and MeCbl, if the chromatograms were exposed to light and a bisulfite-soaked filter paper was placed between culture plate and chromatogram.

The ascending solvent for silica gel TLC was butanol/ammonia/water (75:2:25) in the first dimension and water-saturated benzyl alcohol in the second. A representative separation is shown in Figure 7. A one-dimensional separation on silica-gel TLC with *sec*-butanol/isopropanol/water/ammonia (30:45:25:2) was developed by Nexo and Anderson (86). In this solvent R_f values for the different cobalamins were as follows: MeCbl, 0.40; AdoCbl, 0.23; CNCbl, 0.35; OHCbl, 0.00; sulfito-Cbl, 0.58; (Ad0)CNCba (7-adenylcobamide cyamide) 0.22; and $(CN)_2$Cbi, 0.03.

Fenton and Rosenberg (60) introduced the principle of nonpolar adsorption chromatography to the field of TLC separation of cobalamins. The R_f values for various cobalamins on silanized silica gel TLC with different solvents are presented in Table 4. It shows that complete separation of all cobalamins found in human plasma, and in particular Ado- and CNCbl, still requires two-dimensional chromatography.

Cobalamins in Tissues

Linnell et al. (85) and Dillon et al. (87) have analyzed the cobalamin distribution in the tissues of normal humans, pernicious anemia patients, and patients with various congenital disorders of cobalamin metabolism, using TLC with bioautographic detection. The results for normal tissues, summarized in Table 5, show that AdoCbl is the most abundant cobalamin form, the concentration of MeCbl is quite variable, and CNCbl is hardly present except in blood cells. In pernicious anemia the distribution of cobalamins remains quite normal in liver and kidney, but in leu-

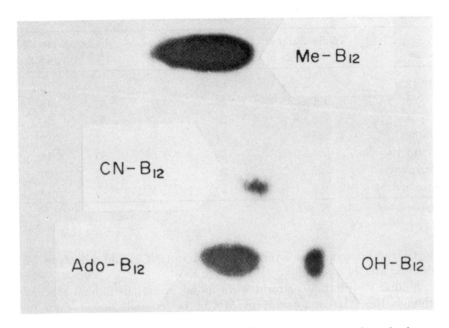

Figure 7 Two-dimensional chromatography and bioautography of plasma cobalamins from a normal subject, the origin marked at the left-hand corner. (From Ref. 85.)

Table 4 R$_f$ Values for Cobalamins on Reversed- and Normal-Phase TLC

	R$_f$				
	OHCbl	MeCbl	AdoCbl	SO$_3$Cbl	CNCbl
Reversed phase[a]					
1:60:140	0.10	0.16	0.40	0.71	0.42
1:80:120	0.11	0.40	0.63	0.83	0.66
1:100:100	0.25–0.45	0.64	0.80	0.89	0.80
5:30:65	0.37	0.21	0.19	0.65	0.46
10:30:60	0.46	0.35	0.40	0.63	0.56
Normal phase[b]	0.02	0.52	0.27	0.61	0.45

[a] Prepoured silanized silica gel plates developed for 1–2 h with acetic acid/methanol/water in the indicated proportions.

[b] Prepoured silica gel plates (IB 2) developed for 10 h with ammonium hydroxide/2-propanol/2-butanol/water (1:50:50:50).

Source: From Ref. 60.

Table 5 Tissue Cobalamins in Normal Human Subjects

Tissue	Total cobalamin (nmol/g)	OHCbl (%)	CNCbl (%)	AdoCbl (%)	MeCbl (%)
Liver	615 ± 122	44	2.0	45	9.0
Kidney	170 ± 30	28	0.6	53	18
Spleen	24 ± 3	24	0.8	50	26
Brain	38 ± 7	24	0.5	63	13
Erytrocytes	0.15 ± 0.02	26	6	53	15
Leukocytes	2.90 ± 0.32	28	4	48	20
Bone marrow	9.6 ± 1.1	30	2	55	13

Source: data from Refs. 85 and 87.

kocytes and bone marrow a remarkable rise in CNCbl and a decrease in Ado- and MeCbl is found.

Similar distribution patterns were found in various animal species, although the relative amount of MeCbl is generally lower than in humans (88). In 50% of rat tissues and 60% of guinea pig tissues unidentified corrinoids were detected. In erythrocytes of rats, cats, and guinea pigs the levels of OH- and MeCbl were higher than in plasma, in contrast to human red blood cells. Cobalamin deprivation led to lower cobalamin levels in the tissues of rats without effect on the cobalamin distribution (68). Choline-deficient food caused a relative decrease of MeCbl in the liver, whereas a methionine-deficient diet exerted the opposite effect (89).

Cobalamins in Plasma

The concentrations of the different cobalamin forms found with TLC/bioautography in human plasma are presented in Table 6. The difference between the two quoted papers may be the result of the differences in extraction techniques and/or the difference in quantitation of the growth response.

2.4 Nonpolar Adsorption Chromatography

As already mentioned in the section on corrinoid extraction, the nonpolar adsorbent Amberlite XAD-2 has proven valuable for batch separation of cobalamins from polar materials (60). This technique is based on the work of Vogelmann and Wagner (90), who collected a vast amount of data on the chromatographic behavior of 50 different corrinoids, includ-

Table 6 Distribution of Cobalamins in Human Plasma[a]

Cobalamin	Linnell et al. (85)[b]	Gimsing et al. (61,67)[c]	
		− CdAc	+ CdAc
OH- + SO$_3$Cbl	47 (35–145)	(0–30)	38 (10–104)
CNCbl	2 (0–40)	(0–70)	13 (2–48)
AdoCbl	60 (22–185)	(6–90)	20 (2–77)
MeCbl	276 (117–458)	(212–512)	250 (135–427)

[a] Mean concentrations in pmol/liter, ranges in parentheses.

[b] Extraction with hot ethanol and phenol, TLC and bioautography.

[c] Extraction with hot ethanol and XAD-2, TLC and bioautography.

ing rhodibamides and hydrogenobamides, and on the influence of C8, C10, and C13 substitutions, the axial ligands, and nucleotides on retention times. Elution was generally performed with 3–20 vol% *tert*-butanol at various pH and cyanide concentrations. The method was used successfully in the isolation of descobaltocobalamin from a crude extract of chromatium by Koppenhagen et al. (91). An aqueous ethanol/acetic acid extract from 500 g wet cells was applied on an Amberlite XAD-2 column (4.0 × 7.0 cm) and sequentially eluted with: 0, 2, 10, 20, and 50% *tert*-butanol (v/v) in water. Hydrogenobyric acid eluted at 10%, descobaltocobalamin at 20%, and uroporphyrins at 50% butanol. After insertion of the rhodium atom in the descobaltocobalamin, the reaction mixture was subjected to desalting on an XAD-2 column, followed by further purification on CM- and DEAE-cellulose and once more on an XAD-2 column to obtain the pure mono- and dicyanorhodibalamins, which eluted at 8 and 10% *tert*-butanol respectively.

2.5 Ion-Exchange Chromatography

Ion-exchange chromatography has been used mainly in preparative separations of cobalamin forms and their precursors. The use of Amberlite resins and cellulose derivatives has been reviewed by Pawelkiewicz (51). With these materials it was impossible to separate methyl-, cyano-, ado-, and hydroxocobalamin in one step. Tortolani et al. (92) first described a combination of CM-cellulose and Dowex 50W-X2, but later a one-step separation on SP-Sephadex (93). Subsequently, Gams et al. (94,95) and Gimsing and Hippe (96) used this procedure to separate the various coenzyme forms in L1210 cells, mitochondria, and plasma. Begley and

Hall (97) measured the conversion of CN [^{57}Co]Cbl into coenzyme forms in cells in tissue culture with this technique. They found that a fifth form of cobalamin, later identified as sulfitocobalamin, almost coeluted with the CNCbl peak, but by a small modification of the fraction collection procedure the SO$_3$Cbl peak was recovered separately from the CNCbl peak (Fig. 8).

Separation of adenosyl forms of cobyric acid and various cobinamide and corrinoid intermediates in the biosynthesis of cobalamin in *P. shermanii* on Dowex 50W-X8 (200–400 mesh) by stepwise increase in pH of the eluting 0.05 *M* acetate buffer, was carried out by Ford and Friedman (59). Ion-exchange paper chromatography on Whatman CM-82 paper was applied by Lee (98) for the separation of biosynthetic intermediates of cobyrinic acid, isolated from *P. shermanii*. Ion-exchange chromatography seems particularly suitable for the separation of the different carboxylic acid derivatives obtained by mild acid hydrolysis of cyanocobalamin. Each additional hydrolysis of an amide group on the corrin side chain results in longer retention on a QAE-Sephadex-column eluted with an acetic acid gradient in 0.4 *M* pyridine (79). Katada et al. (99) described a novel isomeric form of vitamin B$_{12}$ and its derivatives that could be separated from native cobalamin by DEAE-Sephadex chromatography, on which the isomeric form is retained, unlike the native cobalamin, or by SP-Sephadex chromatography, in which the isomeric form always moves just a little faster than its normal counterpart.

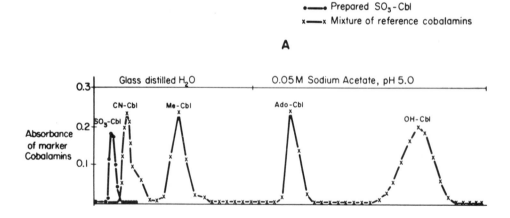

Figure 8   SP-Sephadex C-25 column chromatography of marker cobalamins at approximately 100 μg each. (From Ref. 97.)

3. HIGH-PERFORMANCE LIQUID CHROMATOGRAPHY

3.1 Introduction

An overview of methods and applications of high-performance liquid chromatography is presented in Table 7. They can be divided in methods for separation of multivitamin mixtures, preparative separation of cobalamin coenzymes and analogs, and the analytical separation of biosynthetic intermediates, food cobalamins, and serum and tissue cobalamins.

3.2 Multivitamin Mixtures

For the separation of vitamin B_{12} from the vitamins B_2, K_3, C_1, D_2, E, and A in a multivitamin preparation, Schmit et al. (100) proposed a gradient elution on a Zibax ODS "Permaphase" column with a gradient changing from 0 to 100% methanol in water at 3% per minute and a flow rate of 0.9 ml/min. The separation of vitamin B_{12} from vitamin B_2 on the one side and vitamin K_3 on the other was not impressive, but as the authors stated, chromatographic conditions can be adjusted to meet the specific requirements of a particular vitamin. Optimal conditions for the separation of a mixture of seven water-soluble vitamins on μBondapak C18 and μBondapak NH_2 have been thoroughly investigated by Wills et al. (101), as demonstrated in the Figs. 9 and 10. The best eluent combination for each of the individual vitamins in the preparation can be chosen from these data. Maeda et al. (102) reported the simultaneous determination of nicotinamide, thiamine, riboflavin (phosphate), pyridoxine, caffeine, benzoate, cyanocobalamin, and folic acid using a reversed-phase C18 column eluted with acetonitrile/0.01 M potassium phosphate/triethylamine (8:91.5:0.5), containing 5 mM sodium octanesulfonate, adjusted to pH 2.8.

3.3 Preparative Separation of Cobalamin Coenzymes and Analogs

Partial separation of OH- from CN- and MeCbl on a Partisil ODS 10 μm column was described by Pellerin et al. (103) who used methanol/0.2% ammonia (90:10) at a flow rate of 2.6 ml/min. Complete separation of OH-, CN-, Ado-, and MeCbl was achieved by Mourot et al. (104) using gradient elution from 15 to 45% methanol in 0.05% sulfuric acid with an increase of 5% per minute at 80 ml/h on a Lichrosorb RP8 10 μm column. For the quantitative analysis of cyanocobalamin in veterinary drugs these authors proposed isocratic elution with 0.05% sulfuric acid/acetonitrile (85:15) at 1 ml/min on a 10-cm Lichrosorb RP8 column. With UV monitoring at 350 nm, a lower detection limit of about 100 ng was reached.

Table 7 HPLC Separation of Cobalamins and Related Corrinoids

Column	Column dimensions	Mobile phase	Flow rate	Separated compounds	Reference
Partisil ODS 10 μm	250 × 4.5 mm	Methanol/0.2% ammonia (90:10 v/v)	2.6 ml/min	OHCbl and methyl-/CNCbl	103
Lichrosorb RP8 10 μm	250 × 4.6 mm	Acetonitrile/water (30:70 v/v); or 10 min linear gradient from 10 to 25% acetonitrile in 0.083 M phosphoric acid/triethanolamine, pH 3.3	2.0 ml/min	OH-, CN-, Ado-, and MeCbl	106
Lichrosorb RP8 10 μm	150 × 4.7 mm	6 min linear gradient from 15 to 45% methanol in 0.05% sulfuric acid	1.33 ml/min	OH-, CN-, Ado-, and MeCbl from other water-soluble vitamins	104
Lichrosorb RP8 10 μm	250 × 4.6 mm	Acetonitrile/1 mM ammonium acetate, pH 4.4 (30:70 v/v); or 10 min linear gradient from 5 to 30% acetonitrile in 0.05 M sodium phosphate, pH 3.0	2.0 ml/min — 2.0 ml/min	OH-, CN-, Ado-, and MeCbl — Cbl and Cbi analogues	63
Lichrosorb RP8 10 μm	250 × 4.6 mm	17 min linear gradient from 0 to 25% acetonitrile in 0.085 M phosphoric acid/triethanolamine, pH 3.3	2.0 ml/min	OH-, CN-, Ado-, and MeCbl from human plasma	74
Lichrosorb Si-60 5 μm	250 × 4.6 mm	Methanol/0.01% sodium cyanide (40:60 v/v)	0.8 ml/min	diCN-Cbl in human plasma	111
Zibax ODS "Permaphase"	100 × 2.1 mm	33 min linear gradient from 100% water to 100% methanol (50°C)	0.9 ml/min	Multivitamin preparation (B_2, B_{12}, K_3, C, D_2, E, A)	100

Column	Dimensions	Mobile phase	Flow rate	Compounds	Ref.
μBondapak C18	300×3.9 mm	Methanol/1% KCl (20:80% v/v)	1.0 ml/min	Multivitamin preparation (B_1, B_2, B_6, B_{12}, C, folic acid, niacine, niacinamide)	101
		Methanol/1.5% tetrabutylammonium phosphate (30:70% v/v)	1.0 ml/min		101
μBondapak NH_2	300×3.9 mm	Methanol/0.125% citrate, pH 2.4 (80:20 v/v)	1.0 ml/min	Multivitamin preparation (B_1, B_2, B_6, B_{12}, C, folic acid, niacine, niacinamide)	101
μBondapak C18 Zorbax ODS 6 μm	300×3.9 mm 250×4.6 mm	10 min concave gradient from 23 to 70% methanol in 0.05 M NaH_2PO_4 (40°C)	1.8 ml/min	OH-, CN-, Ado-, MeCbl, cobalamin analogs, SO_3Cbl, monobasic acids of CNCbl, alkanolamine analogues, anilide derivative of monobasic acids	105
μBondapak C18	300×3.9 mm	H_2O/acetic acid/isopropanol (90:1:9 v/v); or 10 min linear gradient from 3 to 21% isopropanol in 0.005 M 1-heptane sulfonic acid	0.3 ml/min	CNCbl and analogs of CNCbl and CNCba	107
			1.0 ml/min	SO_3^-, CN-, OH-, Ado-, MeCbl	107
μBondapak NH_2	300×3.9 mm	58 mM Pyridine acetate pH 4.4/ tetrahydrofuran (96:4: v/v)	0.3 ml/min	Cbl and Cbl monocarboxylic acids	107
μBondapak RP18	300×3.9 mm	Methanol/0.1% acetic acid (24:76), or methanol/0.1% acetic acid (5 min 25:75 followed by a gradient of 25 min to 65:35)	1.0 ml/min	Bacterial cobamides	62

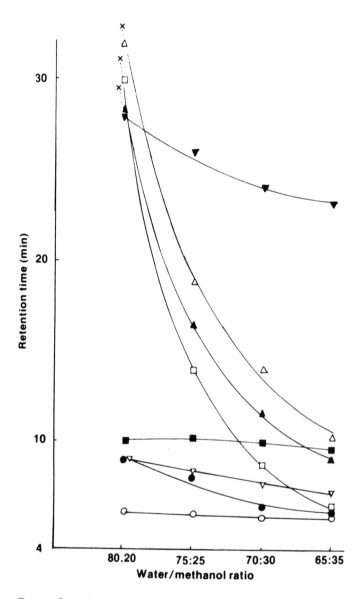

Figure 9 Effect of water/methanol ratio with tetrabutyl ammonium phosphate reagent on retention times of water-soluble vitamins on μBondapak C18: ascorbic acid ($\bigcirc$), niacin ($\bullet$), folic acid ($\square$), pyridoxin ($\blacksquare$), riboflavin ($\triangle$), vitamin B_{12} ($\blacktriangle$), niacinamide ($\triangledown$), thiamine ($\blacktriangledown$), $\times$-not eluted from column. (From Ref. 101.)

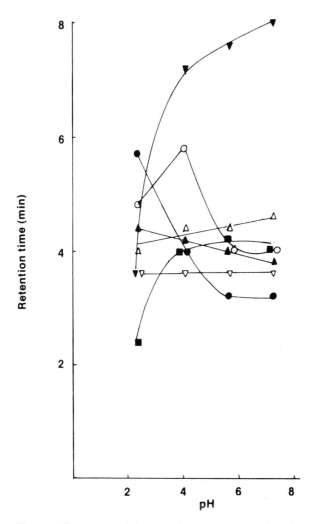

Figure 10 Effect of the pH of 1% citrate/methanol (20:80) on retention times of water-soluble vitamins on Bondapak NH$_2$. See Fig. 9 for explanation of symbols. (From Ref. 101.)

A similar gradient elution system for the separation of different cobalamin forms and various synthetic cobalamin analogs was described by Frenkel et al. (64,105). The detection was linear between 100 ng and 50 μg of injected cobalamin. Jacobsen and Green (106) achieved complete separation of the four cobalamin forms by isocratic elution on a C8 reversed-phase column using acetonitrile/water (30:70) at 2 ml/min, but separation was improved by elution at 2 ml/min with a 10-min gradient from 10 to 25% acetonitrile in 0.083 mol/liter phosphoric acid, titrated to pH 3.3 with triethanolamine. In a later report, Jacobsen et al. (63) have compared the separation of the naturally occurring cobalamins, coenzyme analogs, aminoalkylcobalamins, and various cobinamide forms by gradient elution and isocratic elution (Table 8). In both elution systems a 10 μm Lichrosorb C8 column was used. Isocratic elution was carried out with 30% acetonitrile in 1 mM ammonium acetate, pH 4.4; the gradient system consisted of 0.05 M phosphoric acid titrated to pH 3.0 with concentrated ammonia and acetonitrile from 5 to 30% or 50% (as required) at a rate of 2.5% per minute and a flow rate of 2.0 ml/min (Fig. 11). In general, separation in the isocratic system was satisfactory despite minor disadvantages of small pH-dependent mobility changes of some cobalamin forms (Ado- and H_2OCbl) and prolonged retention of some analogs. The elution methods also proved excellently suitable for the analysis of the conversion of radioactive cyanocobalamin into other cobalamin forms after uptake by either *Lactobacillus leichmanii* or L1210 lymphoblasts. The retention of an even larger number of cobalamin analogs was investigated on either μBondapak C18 columns or μBondapak NH_2 columns by Binder et al. (107) (Table 9). The elution solvent on C18 columns was H_2O/acetic acid/isopropanol (90:1:9), and the flow rate was 0.3 ml/min. NH_2 columns were eluted with 58 mM pyridine acetate (pH 4.4) tetrahydrofuran (96:4) at a flow rate of 0.3 ml/min. The latter column was used to separate different monocarboxylic derivatives of cyanocobalamin (Fig. 12). For the separation of the five naturally occurring cobalamins the authors used elution of a C18 column with a 10-min linear gradient from 3 to 21% isopropanol in 5 mM 1-heptane sulfonic acid. Cobalamins were monitored at 254 nm (Fig. 13). Stupperich et al. (62) published a list of retention times for still another series of cobamides from bacterial origin, obtained with a μBondapak RP18 column, 3.9 $\times$ 300 mm, eluted with a gradient of methanol in 0.1% acetic acid (5 min 25% methanol, followed by a linear gradient to 65% methanol in 20 min) at 1 ml/min. The system has been used in several other studies (108,109).

3.4 Analytical Separation of Plasma and Tissue Cobalamin

Chromatography of only 25 pg CN(^{57}Co)Cbl on a Lichrosorb RP8 column, according to Jacobsen and Green (106), demonstrated that this small amount could be recovered in a sharp peak for more than 99% (74). Consequently, it also proved possible to separate cobalamins in

Table 8 Retention Times of Cobalamin Coenzymes and Related Corrinoid
Analogs on a LiChrosorb C8 Column

Corrinoid	Gradient elution (min)	Isocratic elution (min)
Naturally occurring		
AqCbl	9.0	4.6–4.8[a]
HSO$_3$Cbl	9.7	1.1
CNCbl	10.2	1.6
AdoCbl	11.4	2.8–3.0[a]
MeCbl	12.8	2.2
Coenzyme analogs		
CNCbl	10.9	5.2
TubCbl	11.1	9.6
AraACbl	11.2	3.3
ForCbl	11.1	4.3
ε-AdoCbl	11.7	3.5
PrCbl	14.5	9.1[b]
DapCbl	16.8	27.1[b]
Aminoalkylcobalamins		
AC$_2$Cbl	9.8	5.9
AC$_3$Cbl	10.5	10.4[b]
AC$_5$Cbl	11.2	nd
AC$_8$Cbl	12.8	nd
AC$_{11}$Cbl	14.9	nd
Cobinamides		
(Aq)$_2$Cbl	7.8	33.8
(CN)$_2$Cbi	—[c]	1.6
CNCbi	9.0,10.5[d]	4.9,5.7[d]
AC$_3$Cbi	9.2	nd
AdoCbi	10.2	6.1
MeCbi	12.7	9.6
DapCbi	17.0	23.9

[a] Sharp peaks but positions somewhat variable.

[b] Spreading.

[c] Compounds unstable at pH 3.0; monocyano isomers observed

[d] Isomeric forms.

Source: From Ref. 63.

Table 9 Separation of Cobalamin Analogs by HPLC[a]

Cobalamin	Retention time	
	Min	Relative to CNCbl
	30.0	1.00
Alterations adjacent to corrin ring		
CN-Cbl[C_8-OH,c-OH]	22.0	0.73
CN-Cbl[c-lactam]	24.0	0.80
CN-Cbl[c-lactone]	35.0	1.17
CN-Cbl[10-Cl,c-lactone]	68.3	2.28
CN-Cbl[13-epi]	21.1	0.72
CN-Cbl[b-OH]	38.5	1.30
CN-Cbl[d-OH]	41.8	1.38
CN-Cbl[e-OH]	45.8	1.53
CN-Cbl[C_8-OH,dc-OH]	23.7	0.79
CN-Cbl[C_8-OH,ec-OH]	27.7	0.92
CN-Cbl[C_8-OH,bc-OH]	26.7	0.89
CN-Cbl[de-OH]	61.4	2.04
CN-Cbl[bd-OH]	52.3	1.74
CN-Cbl[be-OH]	53.2	1.77
CN-Cbl[bde-OH]	90.2	3.01
CN-Cbl[13-epi.d-OH]	29.4	0.97
CN-Cbl[13-epi.e-OH]	42.3	1.38
CN-Cbl[13-epi.h-OH]	27.2	0.92

CN-Cbl[c-lactam.d-OH]	27.8	0.93
CN-Cbl[c-lactam.e-OH]	24.2	0.81
CN-Cbl[c-lactam.b-OH]	20.9	0.70
CN-Cbl[c-lactone.d-OH]	52.3	1.74
CN-Cbl[c-lactone.e-OH]	46.6	1.55
CN-Cbl[c-lactone.b-OH]	38.4	1.28
Alterations in nucleotide		
[5,6-Cl$_2$BZA]CN-Cba	43.1	1.44
[NZA]CN-Cba	34.8	1.16
[5,(6)-MeBZA]CN-Cba	25.7	0.86
[5,(6)-ClBZA]CN-Cba	28.8	0.96
[5,(6)-NO$_2$BZA]CN-Cba	19.5	0.65
[5,(6)-OCH$_3$BZA]CN-Cba	23.4	0.78
[5,(6)-COOH BZA]CN-Cba	19.5	0.65
[5,(6)-OH BZA]CN-Cba	21.1	0.70
[BZA]CN-Cba	23.6	0.79
[3,5,6-Me$_3$BZA](CN,OH)Cba	36.4;121.7[b]	1.21;4.06
[CN,OH]Cbi	22.7;14.0[b]	0.76;0.47
[2-MeAde]CN-Cba	20.4	0.68
[Ade]CN-Cba	21.0	0.70

[a] Separation was performed on a Waters μBondapak C18 reversed-phase column (10 μm particle size, 300 × 3.9 mm ID) using H$_2$O-acetic acid-isopropanol (90:1:9) at a flow rate of 0.3 ml/min. Samples of 0.1–1.0 nmol were injected in a volume of 10 μl and detected based on absorbance at 365 nm. From Ref. 107.

[b] Two peaks are seen with these analogs in which the base is absent or cannot coordinate as the lower axial ligand; thus, the CN can be present as either the upper or the lower axial ligand.

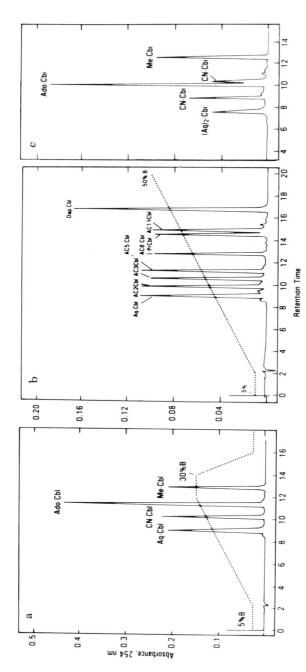

Figure 11 Gradient separation of cobalamin and cobinamide standards on a Lichrosorb C8 column. The gradient profile is indicated in (a) and (b) by the dotted line. (a) Separation of the naturally occurring cobalamins, 5 nmol each. (b) Separation of a mixture of cobalamins containing different upper-axional ligands. (c) Separation of cobinamide analogs, 5 nmol each, with a gradient identical to that in (a). (From Ref. 63.)

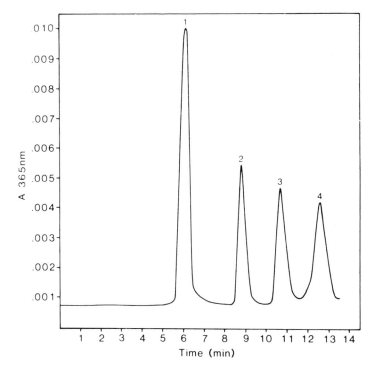

Figure 12 HPLC separation of Cbl (20 pmol) and Cbl-monocarboxylic acids (10 pmol each) on μBondapak NH₂. (1) CNCbl, (2) CNCbl {d-OH}, (3) CNCbl {b-OH}, and (4) CNCbl {e-OH}. (From Ref. 107.)

extracts from human plasma by HPLC with a sensitive radioisotope dilution assay for the detection of cobalamins in the column fractions. In the search for a solution of the specific problems of cobalamins extraction, Van Kapel et al. (74) investigated the effects of NaN_3, $Na_2S_2O_5$, $NaNO_2$, chloroacetophenone, *p*-hydroxomercuribenzoate, iodoacetamide, and *N*-ethylmaleimide on the separation of a mixture of reference cobalamins (Fig. 14 and 15). Only *N*-ethylmaleimide left the separation pattern unchanged. A typical distribution of cobalamin and cobalamin analogs extracted from human plasma in the presence of SH-blocking *N*-ethymaleimide is presented in Fig. 16. Recovery of injected cobalamins (about 1 pmol) in the eluate fractions varied from 97 to 100%. Day-to-day variations of retention time for individual cobalamins were less than 10 s. Table 10 contains the data for the normal distribution of cobalamin forms in human plasma as found with this method.

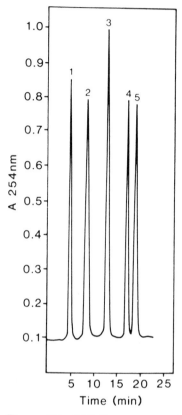

Figure 13   HPLC separation of the naturally occurring cobalamins on μBondapak C18 with an isopropanol gradient from 3 to 21% in 5 mmol/liter 1-heptane sulfonic acid: (1) SO₃Cbl, (2) CNCbl, (3) OHCbl, (4) MeCbl, and (5) AdoCbl. (From Ref. 107.)

This procedure has proven its value in the analysis of two patients with congenital homocystinuria. In the plasma of both we found an almost complete deficiency of methylcobalamin with a compensatory rise in adenosylcobalamin (publication submitted).

The same separation technique was used to measure specifically the distribution of transcobalamin II-bound cobalamins in human plasma. For that purpose 10 ml plasma was incubated with 15 mg CM-Sephadex C50 in 5 ml 0.4 M glycine buffer, pH 3.0. After an overnight rotation at room temperature the Sephadex was collected by centrifugation and washed twice with 15 ml 25 mM phosphate/175 mM NaCl, pH 5.6. The supernatant was kept for later analysis of R-binder-bound cobalamin

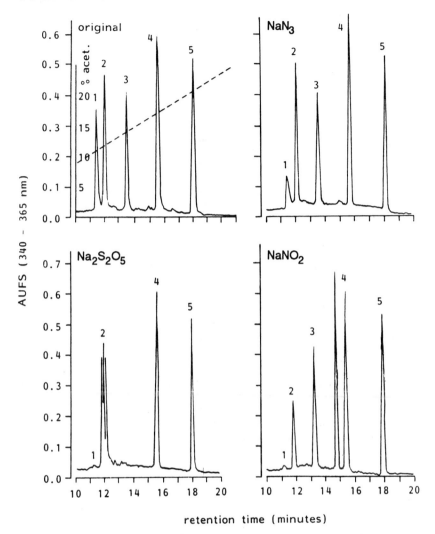

Figure 14 HPLC separation of a mixture of reference cobalamins (1.4 nmol each) on Lichrosorb RP8 with an 8–25% acetonitrile gradient in 85 mmol/liter phosphate/triethanolamine buffer, pH 3.3, after extraction from plasma without (original) or with additives NaN_3 (10 mmol/liter), $Na_2S_2O_5$ (1 mmol/liter) or $NaNO_2$ (5 mmol/liter): (1) OHCbl, (2) SO_3Cbl, (3) CNCbl, (4) AdoCbl, (5) MeCbl. (From Ref. 74.)

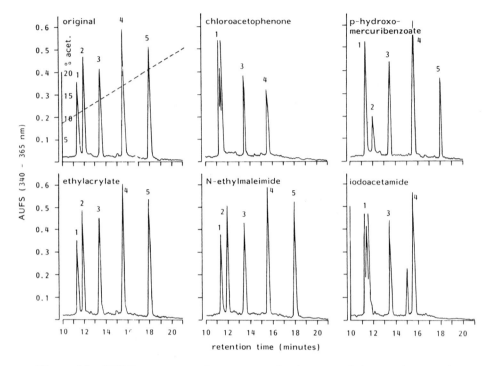

Figure 15 HPLC separation of a mixture of reference cobalamins (1.4 nmol each) on Lichrosorb RP8 with an 8–25% acetonitrile gradient in 85 mmol/liter phosphate/triethanolamine buffer, pH 3.3, after extraction from plasma without (original) or with thiol-blocking agents (5 mmol/liter each): (1) OHCbl, (2) SO₃Cbl, (3) CNCbl, (4) AdoCbl, (5) MeCbl. (From Ref. 74.)

Table 10 Distribution of Cobalamins in Human Plasma Measured with HPLC and RIDA[a]

Cobalamin	−NEM	+NEM
OH-+SO₃Cbl	47 (0–95)	161 (45–280)
CNCbl	35 (0–90)	15 (0–30)
AdoCbl	55 (25–85)	32 (10–52)
MeCbl	252 (80–428)	182 (80–282)

[a] Mean concentrations in pmol/liter ranges in parentheses. Extraction with 1% acetic acid and silanized silica 60 H.

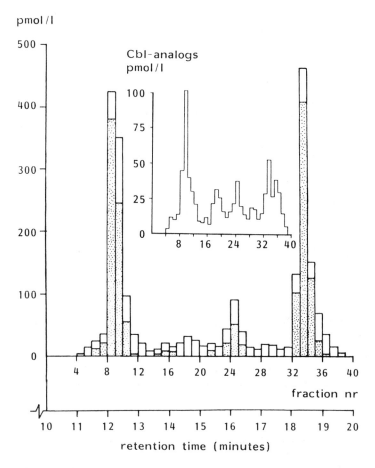

Figure 16 Distribution pattern of cobalamins and cobalamin analogs (insert) in normal human plasma, measured in the HPLC eluate by radioisotope dilution assay using R-binder (□) or "R-binder blocked" intrinsic factor (▨): OH/SO₃Cbl (fractions 7–12), CNCbl (fractions 15–17), AdoCbl (fractions 22–26), MeCbl (fractions 33–36), fraction volume 0.5 ml. (From Ref. 74.)

coenzymes; 50 μl 30% acetic acid and 10 μl N-ethylmaleimide (final concentration 10 mM) were added to the pellet and the mixture was heated in a boiling water bath for 15 min. After cooling, 150 mg sodium acetate was added and the Sephadex was removed by centrifugation, and 300 μl of the supernatant was used for injection on the HPLC column. The remainder was used to measure the total amount of cobalamin in the transcobalamin II extract.

The transcobalamin II-free plasma was mixed with 4 volumes of 1% acetic acid and N-ethylmaleimide to a concentration of 10 mM and treated further as a normal plasma sample. The results of the analyses are presented in Table 11 and confirm earlier semiquantitative observations by Nexo (110) that transcobalamin II carries relatively less MeCbl and more AdoCbl, but the differences are considerably less impressive than suggested by Nexo. The interesting point of this method is that now the more rapidly changing ($T_{1/2}$ ±1 h) pool of TCII-Cbl can be analyzed separately from the slowly ($T_{1/2}$ ±10 days) exchanging pool of R-binder-Cbl.

Butte et al. (111) used HPLC for the quantitative separation of CNCbl as a tool in the estimation of the glomerular filtration rate. CNCbl (2 mg) is injected intravenously to saturate binding sites in blood and cells. Then 5 mg CNCbl is administered intravenously 8–14 h later, and blood samples are taken at various time invervals, up to 90 min. The plasma is extracted with trichloroacetic acid (TCA), and bromocresyl green is added as an internal standard. Desalting is carried out on Sep-pak C18. After elution from the Sep-Pak with methanol, a sample is injected on a Lichrosorb Si60 column and eluted with methanol-sodium cyanide, 0.1 g/liter (40:60), at a flow rate of 0.8 ml/min. The relative peak area is taken as a measure for the amount of cobalamin in the sample in comparison with a series of standard CNCbl concentrations in plasma. The analytical recovery of the procedure is about 65%. Precision varies from 4% at 500 μg/liter to 7% at 200 μg/liter cobalamin in plasma.

4.   GAS CHROMATOGRAPHY-MASS SPECTROMETRY

4.1   Introduction

Corrinoids lend themselves very poorly to gas chromatographic separations due to their low volatility and thermal instability. These properties have also been an obstacle for mass spectrometric analysis. Still, in the last 10 years considerable progress has been made in finding new mild methods for ionization of these complex molecules. Siebel and Schulten (112) have written an excellent review on the subject of soft ionization of biomolecules, in which they describe the results of 10 different methods with corrins and vitamin B_{12}. In fact, vitamin B_{12} has become a model compound for the development of new mass spectrometric methods. Mass spectrometry has contributed and no doubt will contribute in the future to our knowledge of the biosynthesis and biological activity of corrins, vitamin B_{12}, and their synthetically prepared analogs.

Table 11 Distribution of Transcobalamin-II and R-Binder-Associated
Cobalamin

Cbl-coenzyme	Percentage(%)			Concentration (pmol/liter)		
	Range	Mean	SD	Range	Mean	SD
Transcobalamin II-bound						
OHCbl	30–62	49	9	13–74	30	19
CNCbl	0.7–10.5	4.6	3.2	1–4	2.4	1.3
AdoCbl	4.3–17.1	12.2	4.1	1–13	7.6	4.2
MeCbl	20–53	34	8	6–41	20	11
R-binder-bound						
OHCbl	28–56	38	9	14–196	86	56
CNCbl	2–18	6.1	4.7	1–30	11	7
AdoCbl	2–12	6.6	2.9	2–37	20	15
MeCbl	31–61	49	10	17–319	147	105

4.2 Soft Ionization Methods

The first systematic mass spectrometric investigations on corrins were
carried out by Seibl (113) on methyl-substituted corrin complexes and
were published in 1968. He used electron-impact ionization, but this
technique led to massive thermal and ionization-induced degradation of
the molecule. Less destructive but still unsuitable was electron capture
ionization as reported by Von Ardenne et al. (114). The experiences with
chemical ionization, heavy-ion-induced desorption, and field ionization
have not been much better, and it was the technique of field desorption
that turned out to be a breakthrough in that it yielded abundant molecular ions of all types of corrins and even of intact vitamin B_{12} (115). The
essential difference from the earlier mentioned technique is that the ionization process in field desorption takes place when the substance is
adsorbed on the emitter surface, thereby reducing the thermal stress on
the molecule before ionization (soft ionization). The much higher sensitivity of the method makes it possible to detect substance amounts even
in the nanogram range and allows experiments using stable-isotope-
labeled corrins.

Field desorption has more recently been extended with several
specific ionization techniques, such as secondary ion mass spectrometry
or SIMS. When the latter method is applied to samples taken up in a
liquid matrix such as glycerol, it is known as fast atom bombardment or

FABMS. An advantage of FABMS in corrin research is the high amount of structural information that arises from the particular fragment patterns. Stupperich et al. (108) used FABMS for the identification of various corrinoids occurring in acetogenic bacteria. Kräutler et al. (109) did the same for the various forms of cobamides, differing in their nucleotide bases, in some sulfate-reducing and sulfur-metabolizing bacteria.

One of the later developments in mass spectrometry of corrins is the online coupling with high-performance liquid chromatography using a Thermospray interface (116).

5. FUTURE TRENDS

In the last 10 years HPLC has become the method of choice for the separation of cobalamin metabolites and coenzyme forms from all sources. Thin-layer chromatography, in combination with bioautography, still has the advantage of a very high sensitivity and thus requires only small quantities of tissue and plasma for a full analysis. Nevertheless, more detailed knowledge of cobalamin biosynthesis and reaction mechanisms of cobalamin-mediated enzymatic reactions has been gained thanks to the application of HPLC. This is particularly true for the investigations concerning the corrins from acetogenic, methanogenic, and sulfur-metabolizing bacteria, which are of special significance due to their role in the environment.

So far little progress has been made in defining the nature of the cobalamin analogs in human plasma, but this may not be as much the result of insufficient separation power as of the inability to obtain enough material for molecular analysis. Following this trail, it might be worthwhile to develop a reference method for the measurement of cobalamin in human plasma, based on HPLC separation. Such a development might end the discussion on the true value of the cobalamin concentration in human plasma and might provide us with established serum standards with assayed values to be used in less specific radioisotope dilution assays.

The latest developments in mass spectrometry with respect to soft ionization of nonvolatile and thermolabile compounds have brought this technique up to the level where it may open new ways in cobalamin research, especially when integrated with HPLC.

REFERENCES

1. G. H. Whipple, F. S. Robscheit, and C. N. Hooper, *Am. J. Physiol.*, *3*, 236 (1920).

2. G. R. Minot and W. P. Murphy, *J. Am. Med. Assoc.*, *87*, 470 (1926).
3. E. L. Rickes, N. G. Brink, F. R. Koiuszy, T. R. Wood, and F. Folkers, *Science*, *107*, 396 (1948).
4. E. L. Smith, *Nature*, *161*, 638 (1948).
5. R. Bonnett, J. R. Cannon, V. M. Clark, A. W. Johnson, L. F. J. Parker, E. L. Smith, and A. R. Todd, *J. Chem. Soc.*, *1*, 1158 (1957).
6. D. C. Hodgkin, J. Kamper, M. Mackay, J. W. Pickworth, K. N. Trueblood, and J. G. White, *Nature*, *178*, 64 (1956).
7. H. A. Barker, H. Weissbach, and R. D. Smyth, *Proc. Natl. Acad. Sci. USA 44*, 1093 (1958).
8. H. Weissbach, J. I. Toohey, and H. A. Barker, *Proc. Natl. Acad. Sci., USA 45*, 521 (1959).
9. J. I. Toohey and H. A. Barker, *J. Biol. Chem.*, *236*, 560 (1961).
10. K. Lindstrand and K.-G. Ståhlberg, *Acta Med. Scand.*, *174*, 665 (1963).
11. K.-G. Ståhlberg, *Scand. J. Haematol.*, *1*, 220 (1964).
12. IUPAC-IUB Commission on Biochemical Nomenclature, *Biochemistry*, *13*, 1555 (1974).
13. IUPAC-IUB Commission on Biochemical Nomenclature, *Biochem. J.*, *147*, 1 (1975).
14. R. Bonnett, J. R. Cannon, A. W. Johnson, and A. R. Todd, *J. Chem. Soc.*, 1148 (1957).
15. M. J. Mahoney and L. E. Rosenberg, *J. Lab. Clin. Med.*, *78*, 302 (1971).
16. R. A. Firth, H. A. O. Hill, J. M. Pratt, R. G. Thorp, and R. J. P. Williams, *J. Chem. Soc.*, *A*, 381 (1969).
17. J. B. Armitage, J. R. Cannon, A. W. Johnson, L. F. J. Parker, E. L. Smith, W. H. Stafford, and A. R. Todd, *J. Chem. Soc.*, 3849 (1953).
18. W. Friedrich, and K. Bernhauer, *Z. Naturforsch.*, *9b*, 685 (1954).
19. D. Dolphin, *Methods Enzymol.*, *18*, 34 (1971).
20. J. L. Peel, *Biochem. J.*, *88*, 296 (1963).
21. G. N. Schrauzer, and J. W. Sibert, *Arch. Biochem. Biophys.*, *130*, 257 (1969).
22. R. O. Brady, and H. A. Barker, *Biochem. Biophys. Res. Commun.*, *4*, 373 (1961).
23. H. P. C. Hogenkamp, *J. Biol. Chem.*, *238*, 477 (1963).
24. H. P. C. Hogenkamp, J. N. Ladd, and H. A. Barker, *J. Biol. Chem.*, *237*, (1950) 1962.
25. J. N. Pratt, *J. Chem. Soc.*, 5154 (1964).
26. H. P. C. Hogenkamp, *Biochemistry*, *5*, 417 (1966).
27. A. W. Johnson, N. Shaw, and F. Wagner, *Biochim. Biophys. Acta. 72*, 107 (1963).
28. H. P. C. Hogenkamp, in *Cobalamin* (B. M. Babior, ed.), Wiley Interscience, New York, p. 21 (1975).
29. J. M. Wood, F. S. Kennedy, and C. G. Rosen, *Nature*, *220*, 173 (1968).
30. K. Bernhauer, P. Renz, and F. Wagner, *Biochem. Z.*, *335*, 443 (1962).
31. D. Dolphin, A. W. Johnson, and N. Shaw, *Nature*, *199*, 170 (1963).
32. J. A. Hill, J. M. Pratt, and R. J. P. Williams, *J. Chem. Soc.*, 5149 (1964).

33. H. C. Friedman in *Cobalamin* (B. M. Babior, ed.), Wiley Interscience, New York, p. 75 (1975).

34. H. C. Friedman, in *Vitamin B_{12}* (B. Zagalak and W. Friedrich, eds.), Walter de Gruyter, Berlin, p. 331 (1979).

35. A. R. Battersby and E. McDonald, in *B_{12}*, Vol. 1 (D. Dolphin, ed.), Wiley Interscience, New York, p. 107 (1982).

36. R. O. Brady, E. G. Castanera, and H. A. Barker, *J. Biol. Chem.*, *237*, 2325 (1962).

37. G. A. Walker, S. Murphy, and F. M. Huennekens, *Arch. Biochem. Biophys.*, *134*, 95 (1969).

38. J. Pawelkiewicz, M. Gorna, W. Fenrych, and S. Magar, *Ann. N.Y. Acad. Sci.*, *112*, 641 (1964).

39. G. S. Kerwar, G. Spears, B. McAnslan, and H. Weissbach, *Arch. Biochem. Biophys.*, *142*, 231 (1971).

40. R. T. Taylor, in *B_{12}*, Vol. 2 (D. Dolphin, ed.), Wiley Interscience, New York, p. 307 (1982).

41. B. M. Babior, in *Cobalamin* (B. M. Babior, ed.), Wiley Interscience, New York, p. 145 (1975).

42. G. Morrow, L. A. Barness, G. J. Cardinale, R. H. Abeles, and J. G. Flaks, *Proc. Natl. Acad. Sci. USA*, *63*, 191 (1969).

43. J. M. Poston, and T. C. Stadtman, in *Cobalamin* (B. M. Babior, ed.), Wiley Interscience, New York, p. 11 (1975).

44. L. G. J. Ljungdahl and H. G. Wood, in *B_{12}*, Vol. 2 (D. Dolphin, ed.), Wiley Interscience, New York, p. 165 (1982).

45. J. S. Levine, R. H. Allen, D. H. Alpers, and B. Seetharam, *J. Cell. Biol.*, *98*, 1111 (1984).

46. I. Chanarin, H. Muir, A. Hughes and A. V. Hoffbrand, *Br. Med. J.*, *i*, 1454 (1978).

47. J. Lindemans, Thesis, Erasmus University, Rotterdam (1979).

48. H. Olesen, B. L. Hom, and M. Schwartz, *Scand. J. Haematol.*, *5*, 5 (1968).

49. A. P. Skouby, E. Hippe, and H. Olesen, *Blood*, *38*, 769 (1971).

50. D. W. Bartholomew, M. L. Batshaw, R. H. Allen, C. R. Rae, D. Rosenblatt, D. L. Valle, and C. A. Francomano, *J. Pediatr.*, *112*, 32 (1988).

51. J. Pawelkiewicz, in *Vitamin B_{12} und Intrinsic Factor* (H. C. Heinrich, ed.), F. Enke Verlag, Stuttgart, p. 280 (1962).

52. W. Friedrich, *Vitamin B_{12} und verwandte corrinoide*, George Thieme Verlag, Stuttgart (1965).

53. G. Matsuda, *J. Vitaminol. 1*, 221 (1955).

54. H. Kubo, S. Fujita, and H. Ogino, *Chem. Abstr.*, *54*, 13153 (1960).

55. W. Friedrich and K. Bernhauer, *Z. Naturforsch.*, *9b*, 755 (1954).

56. M. W. Penley, D. G. Brown, and J. M. Wood, *Biochemistry*, *22*, 4302 (1970).

57. V. B. Koppenhagen, B. Elsenhaus, F. Wagner, and J. J. Pfiffner, *J. Biol.*

Chem., *249*, 6532 (1974).

58. E. V. Quadros, A. Hamilton, D. M. Matthews, and J. C. Linnell, *J. Chromatogr.*, *160*, 101 (1978).

59. S. H. Ford and H. C. Friedman, *Arch. Biochem. Biophys.*, *175*, 121 (1975).

60. W. A. Fenton and L. E. Rosenberg, *Anal. Biochem.*, *90*, 119 (1978).

61. P. Gimsing, E. Nexo, and E. Hippe, *Anal. Biochem.*, *129*, 296 (1983).

62. E. Stupperich, I. Steiner, and M. Rühlemann, *Anal. Biochem.*, *155*, 365 (1986).

63. D. W. Jacobsen, R. Green, E. V. Quadros, and Y. D. Montejano, *Anal. Biochem.*, *120*, 394 (1982).

64. E. P. Frenkel, R. Prough, and R. L. Kitchens, *Methods Enzymol.*, *67*, 31 (1980).

65. J. C. Linnell, H. M. Mackenzie, J. Wilson, and D. M. Matthews, *J. Clin. Pathol.*, *22*, 545 (1969).

66. J. C. Linnell, A. V. Hoffbrand, H. A.-A. Hussein, I. J. Wise, and D. M. Matthews, *Clin. Sci. Mol. Med.*, *46*, 163 (1974).

67. P. Gimsing, E. Hippe, and E. Nexo, in *Vitamin B$_{12}$* (W. Friedrich and B. Zagalak, eds.), Walter de Gruyter, Berlin, p. 665 (1979).

68. P. Gimsing, E. Hippe, I. Helleberg-Rasmusen, M. Moergaard, J. Lanng Nielson, P. Bastrup-Madsen, R. Berlin, and T. Hansen, *Scand. J. Haematol.*, *29*, 311 (1982).

69. M. C. Mahoney and L. E. Rosenberg, *Am. J. Med.*, *48*, 584 (1970).

70. P. Gimsing, E. Nexo, and E. Hippe, *Anal. Biochem.*, *129*, 288 (1983).

71. W. R. Bauriedel, J. C. Picken, Jr., and L. A. Underkofler, *Proc. Soc. Exp. Biol. Med.*, *91*, 377 (1956).

72. R. T. Taylor and M. L. Hanna, *Arch. Biochem. Biophys.*, *141*, 247 (1970).

73. E. L. Lien and J. M. Wood, *Biochim. Biophys. Acta.*, *264*, 530, (1972).

74. J. van Kapel, L. J. M. Spijkers, J. Lindemans, and J. Abels, *Clin. Chim. Acta*, *131*, 211 (1983).

75. G. Markus, and F. Karush, *J. Am. Chem. Soc.*, *79*, 134 (1957).

76. A. Lorber, C. C. Chang, D. Masuoka, and I. Meacham, *Biochem. Pharmacol.*, *19*, 1551 (1970).

77. R. B. Martin and J. T. Edsall, *J. Am. Chem. Soc.*, *81*, 4044 (1959).

78. J. Sedlak and R. H. Lindsay, *Anal. Biochem.*, *25*, 192 (1968).

79. R. H. Allen, and P. W. Majerus, *J. Biol. Chem.*, *247*, 7695 (1972).

80. J. F. Kolhouse and R. H. Allen, *J. Clin. Invest.*, *60*, 1381 (1977).

81. H. Kondo, J. F. Kolhouse, and R. H. Allen, *Proc. Natl. Acad. Sci. USA* 77, 817 (1980).

82. R. A. Firth, H. A. O. Hill, J. M. Pratt, and R. G. Thorp., *Anal. Biochem.*, *23*, 429 (1968).

83. T. M. Vickrey, R. N. Katz, and G. N. Schrauzer, *J. Am. Chem. Soc.*, *97*, 7248 (1975).

84. J. C. Linnell, H. A.-A. Hussein, and D. M. Matthews, *J. Clin. Pathol.*, *23*, 820 (1970).

85. J. C. Linnell, A. V. Hoffbrand, T. J. Peters, and D. M. Matthews, *Clin. Sci.*, *40*, 1 (1971).

86. E. Nexo and J. Andersen, *Scand. J. Clin. Lab. Invest.*, *37*, 723 (1977).

87. M. J. Dillon, J. M. England, D. Gompertz, P. A. Goodey, D. B. Grant, H. A.-A. Hussein, J. C. Linnell, D. M. Matthews, S. H. Mudd, G. H. Newns, J. W. T. Seakins, B. W. Uhlendorf, and I. J. Wisse, *Clin. Sci. Mol. Med.*, *47*, 43 (1974).

88. E.V. Quadros, D. M. Matthews, I. J. Wisse, and J. C. Linnell, *Biochim. Biophys. Acta.*, *421*, 141 (1976).

89. J. C. Linnell, M. J. Wilson, Y. B. Mikol, and L. A. Poirier, *J. Nutr.*, *113*, 124 (1983).

90. H. Vogelmann and F. Wagner, *J. Chromatogr.*, *76*, 359 (1973).

91. V. B. Koppenhagen, F. Wagner, and J. J. Pfiffner, *J. Biol. Chem.*, *248*, 7999 (1973).

92. G. Tortolani, P. Bianchini, and V. Mantovani, *Farm. Ed. Prat.*, *25*, 772 (1970).

93. G. Tortolani, P. Bianchini, and V. Mantovani, *J. Chromatogr.*, *53*, 577 (1970).

94. R. A. Gams, E. M. Ryel, and L. M. Meyer, *Proc. Soc. Exp. Biol. Med.*, *149*, 384 (1975).

95. R. A. Gams, E. M. Ryel, and F. Ostroy, *Blood*, *47*, 923 (1976).

96. P. Gimsing, and E. Hippe, *Scand. J. Haematol.*, *24*, 243 (1978).

97. J. A. Begley and C. A. Hall, *J. Chromatogr.*, *177*, 360 (1979).

98. S. L. Lee, *Methods Enzymol.*, *67*, 3 (1980).

99. M. Katada, S. Tyagi, A. Nath, R. L. Petersen, and R. K. Gupta, *Biochim. Biophys. Acta*, *584*, 149 (1979).

100. J. A. Schmit, R. A. Henry, R. C. Williams, and J. F. Dieckman, *J. Chromatogr. Sci.*, *9*, 645 (1971).

101. R. B. H. Wills, C. G. Shaw, and W. R. Day, *J. Chromatogr. Sci.*, *15*, 262 (1977).

102. Y. Maeda, M. Yamamoto, K. Owada, S. Sato, T. Masui, and H. Nakazowa, *J. Assoc. Off. Anal. Chem.*, *72*, 244 (1989).

103. E. Pellerin, J.-F. Letavernier, and N. Chanon, *Ann. Pharm. Fr.*, *9–10*, 413 (1977).

104. D. Mourot, B. Delepine, J. Boisseau, and G. Gayot, *Ann. Pharm. Fr.*, *5–6*, 235 (1979).

105. E. P. Frenkel, R. L. Kitchens, and R. Prough, *J. Chromatogr.*, *174*, 393 (1979).

106. D. W. Jacobsen and R. Green, in *Vitamin B$_{12}$* (W. Friedrich and B. Zagalak, eds.) Walter de Gruyter, Berlin, p. 663 (1979).

107. M. Binder, J. F. Kolhouse, K. C. van Horne, and R. H. Allen, *Anal. Biochem.*, *125*, 253 (1982).

108. E. Stupperich, H. J. Eisinger, and B. Kräutler, *Eur. J. Biochem.*, *172*, 459 (1988).

109. B. Kräutler, H.-P. E. Kohler and E. Stupperich, *Eur. J. Biochem.*, *176*, 461 (1988).
110. E. Nexo, *Scand. J. Haematol.*, *18*, 358 (1977).
111. W. Butte, H.-H. Riemann, and A. J. Walle, *Clin. Chem.*, *28*, 1778 (1982).
112. H. M. Schiebel and H.-R. Schulten, *Mass Spectrom. Rev.*, *5*, 249 (1986).
113. J. Seibl, *Adv. Mass Spectrom. 4*, 317 (1968).
114. M. von Ardenne, K. Steinfelder, and R. Tümmler, *Elektronenanlagerungs-Massenspektrographie organischer Substanzen*, Springer, Berlin (1971).
115. H.-R. Schulten and H. M. Schiebel, *Naturwissenschaften*, *65*, 223 (1978).
116. M. L. Vestal, *Science, 226*, 275 (1984).

13

PANTOTHENIC ACID

Jan Velíšek, Jiří Davídek, and Tomáš Davídek

Institute of Chemical Technology, Prague, Czechoslovakia

1. INTRODUCTION

The principal biologically active natural forms of pantothenic acid (vitamin B_5) are coenzyme A (CoA or CoASH) and acyl-carrier protein (ACP). In pharmaceuticals, because of simple handling and increased stability, the pantothenic acid sodium and calcium salt are used in solid preparations. Panthenol is usually used in liquid pharmaceutical preparations and in cosmetics.

A number of review articles and books on pantothenic acid and its natural and synthetic derivatives, their chemical, physical, and pharmaceutical properties, biological function, biosynthesis, nutritional aspects, and use have appeared during the last two decades (1–17).

1.1 History

The existence of pantothenic acid as a B-group vitamin, a dietary factor, whose absence caused a form of dermatitis in chicks, was anticipated around 1930 and discovered in 1931 by Williams (15,18,19). The name pantothenic acid, given to the active substance by Williams and his co-workers in 1933 (20), indicated its widespread occurrence in nature. The structure of pantothenic acid (Fig. 1) was established by Williams in 1938 (21) and the total synthesis was achieved by the Merck group in 1940 (22).

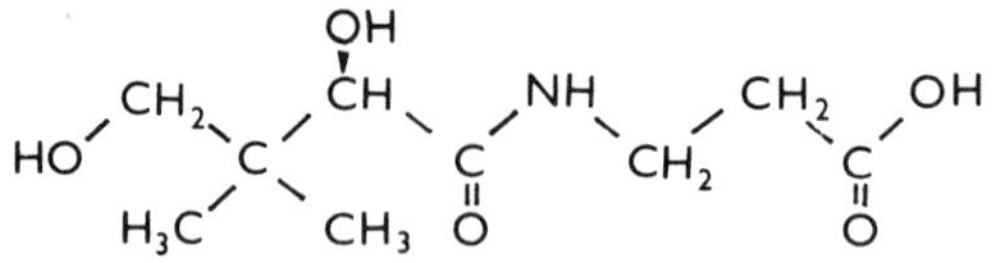

Figure 1 (R)-Pantothenic acid structure.

The first active form of pantothenic acid, coenzyme A (CoA, CoASH), was isolated and identified as the acyl transfer agent in two-carbon unit metabolism in 1946 (23,24). Its structure (Fig. 2) was elucidated in 1950 (25) and confirmed synthetically in 1961 (26,27).

The second active form of pantothenic acid is the acyl-carrier protein (ACP) involving the 4'-phosphopantetheine moiety linked with a serine residue in the respective molecule (Fig. 3). It was described by Pugh and Wakil in 1965 (28) and found to be a coenzyme of fatty acid synthetase, thyrocidine- and gramicidin-S-synthetase, and GTP-dependent acyl-CoA synthetase (6).

1.2 Chemistry

Pantothenic acid, still designated as D(+)-pantothenic acid, D(+)-α, γ-dihydroxy-β, β-dimethyl butyrylalanine, or N-(α, γ-dihydroxy-β, β-dimethylbutyryl)-β-alanine, is composed of D(+)-pantoic acid (2,4-dihydroxy-3,3-dimethylbutyric acid) linked by an amide bond to β-alanine (3-aminopropionic acid) (Fig. 1). Pantothenic acid occurs in nature only as the D(+) or the (R) enantiomer; the L(−) or (S) form has no vitamin activity, as biological effects of this group of compounds are specific and connected solely with the optically active dextrorotatory forms.

Pantothenic acid is a yellowish viscous oily liquid, which is readily soluble in water, alcohols, and dioxane, slightly soluble in diethyl ether and acetone, and virtually insoluble in benzene and chloroform. The stability of pantothenic acid in aqueous solutions is very pH dependent. It is most stable in slightly acidic medium (pH 4–5). Both in acidic and alkaline media it is hydrolytically cleaved to yield pantoic acid and its salts, respectively, and β-alanine. In acidic solutions, pantoic acid spontaneously dehydrates, forming (R)-2-hydroxy-3,3-dimethyl-4-butanolide (α-hydroxy-β, β-dimethyl-γ-butyrolactone), referred to as pantoyl lactone or pantolactone (Fig. 4).

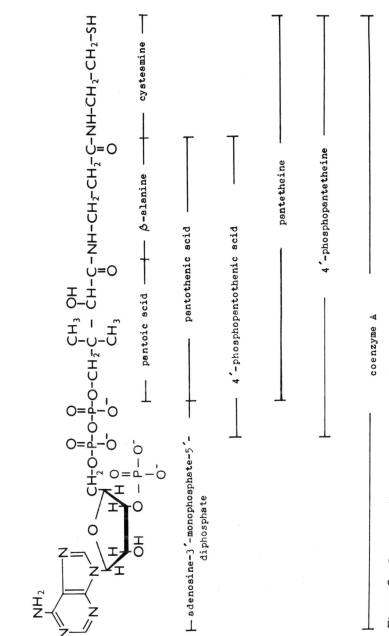

Figure 2 Coenzyme A structure.

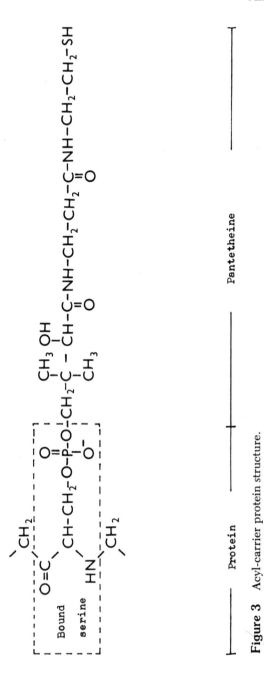

Figure 3   Acyl-carrier protein structure.

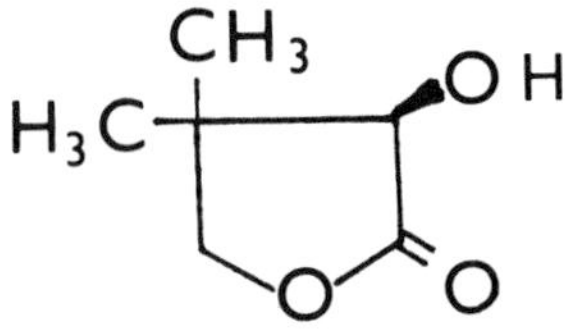

Figure 4   (R)-Pantolactone structure.

Pantothenic acid itself is not used as it is hygroscopic and unstable. Its more stable sodium salt and, especially, the calcium salt are synthesized chemically and used pharmaceutically, mainly in solid preparations and as an additive compound for domestic animal feeds. Calcium pantothenate is most stable at almost neutral pH (6–7). Salts of pantothenic acid are colorless crystals, less hygroscopic (especially the calcium salt) than pantothenic acid. The solubility of calcium pantothenate in water at 25°C is 0.356 g/ml, whereas the sodium salt also is very water soluble.

An alcohol related to pantothenic acid and referred to as D-panthenol or D-pantothenyl alcohol also possesses vitamin activity (Fig. 5). It is commonly used in liquid pharmaceutical and cosmetic preparations. Panthenol is a hygroscopic viscous oil that can be crystallized. Panthenol is very slightly soluble in water but very soluble in alcohol. The products of hydrolysis of panthenol are pantoic acid and 3-amino-1-propanol (β-alanol).

Pantetheine and coenzyme A are amorphous, colorless, water-soluble powders. Solutions of coenzyme A are relatively stable at pH 2–6. Both compounds form oxidation products, that is, pantethine and the coenzyme A disulfide form (15,18,29,30).

Some of the chemical and physical constants of pantothenic acid and the related compounds are summarized in Table 1.

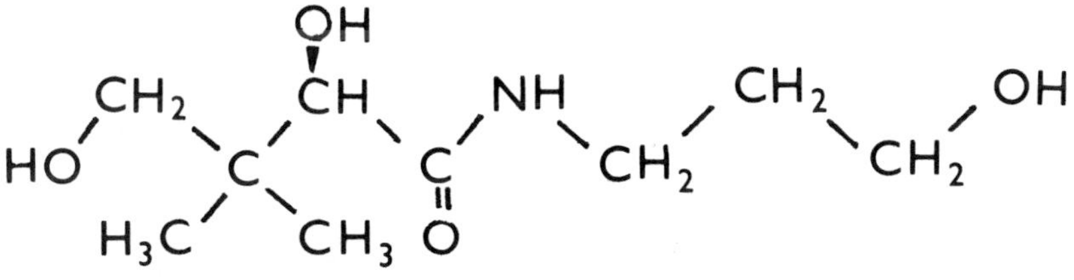

Figure 5   (R)-Panthenol structure.

Table 1 Some Constants of Pantothenic Acid and Related Compounds[a]

Compound	Molecular weight	Bruto formula	λ max (nm)	Optical rotation $[\alpha]_D^t$	Melting point (°C)	pK$_a$ at 25°C
Pantothenic acid	219.2	$C_9H_{17}O_5N$		+37.5°		4.41
Calcium pantothenate	476.5	$C_{18}H_{32}O_{10}N_2Ca$		+24.3° (+26 to +27.5°)	200 (dec.)	
Sodium pantothenate	241.2	$C_9H_{16}O_5NNa$		+26.5 to +28.5°	160–165 (122–124)	
Panthenol	205.3	$C_9H_{19}O_4N$		+29.5 to +31.5°		
Pantetheine	278.4	$C_{11}H_{23}O_4N_2S$				
4'-Phosphopantetheine	358.4	$C_{11}H_{23}O_7N_2SP$		+10.8°		
Pantethine	556.7	$C_{22}H_{44}O_8N_4S_2$		+13.5 to +17.7°		
Coenzyme A	767.6	$C_{21}H_{36}O_{16}N_7SP_3$	257			10.35
Pantolactone	130.1	$C_6H_{10}O_3$		+49.8°	92–93	

[a] From Refs. 15,18,29, and 30.

1.3 Biochemistry

Pantothenic acid is synthesized in plants and some microorganisms from pantoic acid and β-alanine. Pantoic acid is formed from 2-oxopantoic acid (4-hydroxy-3,3-dimethyl-2-oxobutyric acid) and 2-oxoisovaleric acid (3-methyl-2-oxobutyric acid), a precursor of valine. β-Alanine is formed by decarboxylation of L-aspartic acid. Enzymes involved include pantothenate synthetase (EC 6.3.2.1), oxopantoate reductase (EC 1.1.1.169), oxopantoate hydroxymethyltransferase (EC 4.1.2.12), and aspartate 1-decarboxylase (EC 4.1.1.12).

A degradative enzyme of some bacteria, pantothenase (EC 3.5.1.22) specifically splits pantothenic acid to pantoic acid and β-alanine.

Animals do not synthesize pantothenic acid. However, they, as do yeasts and bacteria, convert the exogenous vitamin derived from the diet to coenzyme A (CoA) and acyl-carrier protein (ACP), the two metabolically active forms. The reaction pathway is shown in Fig. 6.

The biosynthesis of CoA in animals requires five enzymes. The first three are found only in the cytosol, and the other two are also found in mitochondria. Reaction IV is reversible. Four moles of ATP are required for the biosynthesis of one mole CoA from one mole of pantothenic acid. Two additional enzymes in animal tissues are involved in the biosynthesis of holo-acyl-carrier protein (holo-ACP) and its hydrolysis of 4'-phosphopantetheine, respectively (15,31–34).

Ingested pantothenic acid is transported by the blood to the organs. The previously described five steps are required to re-form CoA from the pantothenic acid (35). The ingested CoA is first hydrolyzed in the intestinal lumen to pantothenic acid and pantetheine via 4'-phosphopantetheine. Panthenol is more easily absorbed than pantothenic acid and is converted to the latter (32). The excretion of pantothenic acid or its derivative occurs mainly via the urine, in which the free form of the vitamin predominates.

Coenzyme A can form high-energy bonds with acetic acid via its sulfhydryl group to yield acetyl-coenzyme A (acetyl-CoA), also referred to as activated acetate. Through a variety of biochemical sequences, CoA can also be converted to a number of other acyl-CoA derivatives such as malonyl-CoA, methylmalonyl-CoA, succinyl-CoA, etc. The energy required for the transformation of CoA to acetyl-CoA is derived either from the cleavage of ATP or from a thioclastic cleavage or oxidative decarboxylation. Acetyl-CoA is formed, for example, from fatty acids, amino acids, and carbohydrate metabolism or comes from its own metabolic pool. Acetyl-CoA and short-chain acyl-CoA esters subsequently enter various biochemical reactions that are of particular importance in the metabolism of carbohydrates, fats, and nitrogen-containing com-

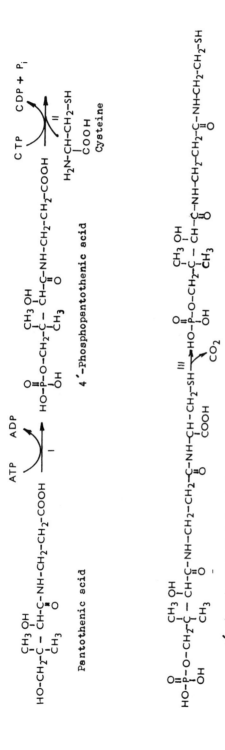
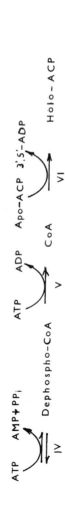

Figure 6 Biosynthesis of coenzyme A and acyl-carrier protein. I = pantothenate kinase (EC 2.7.1.33), II = phosphopantothenyl-cysteine synthetase (EC 6.3.2.5), III = phosphopantothenylcysteine decarboxylase (EC 4.1.1.36), IV = pantetheine phosphate adenylytransferase (EC 2.7.7.3), V = dephospho-CoA kinase (EC 2.7.1.24), VI = transferase.

pounds such as citrate cycle, fatty acid synthesis, phospholipid synthesis, steroid (cholesterol) synthesis, and heme synthesis. Acetyl-CoA facilitates the interchange of two-carbon units between donors such as pyruvate, acetoacetate, and acetyl phosphate, and acceptors such as acetoacetate, oxaloacetate, and choline. It is capable of "head condensation," carbon-carbonyl condensation, and "tail-condensation" such as the acetyl group of acetyl-CoA condensing through its methyl group with oxaloacetic acid forming citric acid; it is capable of acetylation of amines such as choline, aldol condensation of aldehydes, etc. The biosynthesis of the long-chain fatty acids takes place on the fatty acid-synthase complex. The growing chain of the fatty acid remains covalently bound to the enzyme, where the pantothenic acid serves as the binding agent. It is bound to a serine residue on the protein via a phosphate group forming the already-mentioned complex (Fig. 3) of pantetheine and protein called ACP (15,18,32,33).

The amount of about 6–8 mg per day has been established as the desirable pantothenic acid intake for adult human beings. Adolescent individuals (over 12 years) and pregnant and nursing women have a particularly high requirement for pantothenic acid. The normal diet contains 6–12 mg pantothenic acid per day (15). Although deficiency conditions are known, and although addition of pantothenic acid salts to food improves the nitrogen balance, so far few efforts have been made to supplement foods with this vitamin. Recent studies indicate that the increased use of processed foods has reduced the pantothenic acid levels in the diet of industrial countries, which suggests the need for pantothenic acid supplements (36).

The feed of domestic animals is currently supplemented to give an optimal level. For example, estimated minimum requirements for pantothenic acid for growing chicks and breeding hens are 10 mg/kg diet and for breeding turkeys 16 mg/kg diet (19).

Even small changes in (R)-pantothenic acid molecular structure reduce its biological activity very strongly or completely. Thus, (S)- or L(−)-pantothenic acid has no biological activity (37) and is an antimetabolite of (R)-pantothenic acid. Another effective antimetabolite of (R)-pantothenic acid is the so-called pantoyltaurine (sulfopantothenic acid) having a sulfhydryl group instead of carboxyl group in the β-alanine molecule. In animals, pantoyltaurine has no biological effect (15). The only universally effective antimetabolite of pantothenic acid is ω-methylpantothenic acid (with methyl group instead of hydroxymethyl group at the end of the molecule), which evokes symptoms of pantothenic acid deficiency even in human beings (37).

1.4 Occurrence and Stability in Foods

Pantothenic acid is found in practically all foods of plant and animal origin, but usually only in small quantities. It occurs rarely in free form as it is usually a component of coenzyme A, acyl-coenzymes A, and the acyl-carrier protein. The levels of pantothenic acid in individual foods vary greatly. Relatively large amounts are present in meats (especially in organs such as liver), fish, yeasts, several kinds of cheese, whole-grain products, and legumes. The lowest amounts have been found in milk, fruits, and vegetables (Table 2).

Pantothenic acid in foods has proven to be relatively labile during storage and, especially during thermal processing. The stability, even at elevated temperatures, is highest at pH 4–5 (40). The losses upon dissolution in water during operations such as washing and leaching into the cooking water during blanching and boiling often exceed losses due to the destruction of the vitamin by hydrolysis.

Losses of 12–50% were reported in various cooked meats, mainly caused by transfer to the drip or broth, depending on type of heat treatment, volume of water used, and other factors (41).

Pasteurization of milk apparently does not influence the vitamin content (31). During sterilization of milk (heating to 112°C for 10 min) the vitamin content reportedly decreases by 14% (42). The mean retention in UHT (ultra-high temperature) milk was approximately 96% (43).

Table 2 Pantothenic Acid Content of Some Foods[a]

Food	Content in mg/kg (edible portion)	Food	Content in mg/kg (edible portion)
Beef	3–20	Peas	2–6
Pork	4–30	Carrots	3
Liver (beef, pork, calf, chicken)	40–100	Cabbage	1–3
		Cauliflower	1–9
Eggs	16–55	Tomatoes	3–4
Milk	3–4	Apples	1
Cheese	55	Oranges	2
Wheat	8–13	Bananas	2
Bread	4–5	Mushrooms	20
Maize	5–9	Baker's yeasts	50–200
Potatoes	3		

[a] Modified from Refs. 15, 38, and 39.

After 6 weeks of storage at room temperature the losses increase to 30%, and the total pantothenic acid losses caused by UHT heat treatment and storage amount to 20–35% (44). In dried milk after storage for 8 weeks at 60°C the loss was 18% (45). The natural vitamin content in fermented milk products was affected only slightly by the fermentation (46).

In grains, the highest levels of pantothenic acid are present in the outer layer and the vitamin is mostly lost during milling (47). Relatively large amounts are present in whole-grain products including certain types of bread (48,49).

The losses of pantothenic acid in canned foods of animal origin ranged from 20 to 35%, in canned fruits and fruit juices the average loss was 50%, and in canned vegetables the losses varied from 46 to 78% (50).

1.5 Analysis

Biological, chemical, and physical methods used for the analysis of pantothenic acid and its derivatives have been reviewed in several excellent books and review articles (15,51–58).

The formerly frequently used animal tests have been gradually replaced by simpler, more rapid, and cheaper microbiological methods based on measurements of the growth of yeasts and bacteria. The microbiological methods are especially well suited for the determination of the vitamin in samples such as foods and feeds, where the vitamin is usually present in bound form. The detection limit of these methods is about 0.03–0.05 µg pantothenic acid/ml (55,57,59). The most commonly employed analytical assay is currently the assay procedure using *Lactobacillus plantarum*. This procedure can be extremely time-consuming, needs careful control of assay conditions, requires regular maintenance of cultures, and can be susceptible to interferences from unidentified compounds causing inhibition or stimulation of the microorganisms. Therefore numerous alternative biochemical, chemical, and physico-chemical methods have been developed.

Pantothenic acid and pantetheine may be assayed using several enzymatic tests with pantothenase (60–63). Immunoassays and, especially, radioimmunoassays have been used in the analysis of pantothenic acid in tissue fluids, because of their sensitivity, specificity, and high rates of sample throughput. The radioimmunoassay methods (RIA) have about the same sensitivity as microbiological tests (approximately 0.05 µg/ml). As an alternative to the radioimmunoassay, the enzyme-linked immunosorbent assay (ELISA) is particularly suitable for the routine analysis of foods (64–69).

Chemical methods are mainly based on analysis of pantothenic acid hydrolysis products by spectrophotometry or fluorometry. Although relatively rapid to perform, these methods lack the specificity and sensitivity needed to determine vitamin in foods or differentiate between D and L forms. Several spectrophotometric determinations of pantothenic acid and its salts have been developed. They are based on the reaction of pantolactone with hydroxylamine (70,71) and 2,7-naphthalenediol (62,72). Most published methods use the determination of β-alanine. Ninhydrin (73,74), 1,2-naphthoquinone (75,76), phthalaldehyde (77), acetylacetone (78,79), and some other reagents have been introduced for the spectrophotometric determination of pantothenates via β-alanine (80–82).

Some other chemical and physical methods such as thermal analysis (83), nuclear magnetic resonance analysis (84), and capillary isotachophoresis (85), have been occasionally used for the analysis of pantothenates in pharmaceutical preparations. Pure compounds can also be determined chelatometrically or using alkalimetric titration in nonaqueous solvents or can be analyzed after decomposition to ammonia (86,87).

Panthenol can be determined polarographically (88). A sensitive fluorometric determination in multivitamin preparations (hydrolysis, reaction with ninhydrin) has been described (89).

Because of the importance of coenzyme A and its acyl thioesters in metabolic control, several enzymatic assays in conjunction with spectroscopic or fluorometric monitoring have been developed to determine their total content in tissues (91–93).

2. PAPER AND THIN-LAYER CHROMATOGRAPHY AND CONVENTIONAL COLUMN CHROMATOGRAPHY

2.1 General Considerations

Paper chromatography (PC) and thin-layer chromatography (TLC) played a very important role in the beginning of the exploration of new chromatographic techniques for the separation of pantothenic acid and its derivatives. The reason for that was especially the simplicity of these methods, which allowed their application practically in any laboratory. With the development of HPLC and GLC techniques, PC and TLC lost their importance in the quantitative determination of pantothenic acid and its derivatives, but they are still of some value for the preliminary separation or cleanup of samples analyzed by other procedures. PC and TLC also play a very important role in qualitative determinations of pantothenic acid and its derivatives in pharmaceuticals as well as in biological materials. These methods are also very often used for controlling the purity of synthetic derivatives, especially on a laboratory scale. The main disadvantage of these methods is the rather poor sensitivity with the detection reagents used up to now. This disadvantage can be overcome by bioautographic methods, which are highly specific and sensitive (94,95).

2.2 Sample Handling

The handling and preparation of the sample prior to PC and TLC separation depend on the type of the sample. Pantothenic acid and its derivatives are relatively unstable compounds, and therefore all procedures during handling and analysis have to be done rapidly and with maximum care.

In most cases pantothenic acid and its derivatives in pharmaceutical samples are present as mixtures with other vitamins, especially with the vitamins of the B group. Liquid preparations can be directly used for PC and TLC analysis. Pantothenic acid in solid pharmaceutical samples has to be dissolved in a suitable solvent. Preference is given to organic solvents with a low boiling point, such as ethanol and acetone. Pantothenic acid and its derivatives for drug use are mostly incorporated tablets and hence are not chemically bound to the vehicle. Their isolation does not create any special problems. In the analysis of dragées, the coating materials might sometimes interfere and have to be removed either mechanically or from the aqueous extract. In cases where the vitamin concentration is below the detection limit, it is necessary to concentrate the samples prior to analysis using either evaporation under reduced pressure and at low temperature or ion-exchange chromatography.

In the analysis of foods and other biological samples, the sampling procedure is the most critical point. In all cases the pretreatment for conservation and transport to the laboratory is extremely important since the vitamin could easily be lost in the interval between sampling and performing the analysis. Unfortunately, no general procedure can be given because this matter has not been investigated thoroughly (94,95).

A practically applicable procedure for isolation of pantothenic acid and its derivatives including coenzyme A from animal tissues has been described by Lawrence et al. (96). Portions of 1–2 g of tissue are frozen in liquid nitrogen, pulverized, extracted with 5 volumes of perchloric acid (6% w/w), kept in ice for 10–15 min, and then centrifuged at 4°C. The supernatant fluid is titrated with $KHCO_3$ solution to pH 3.5 using dimethyl yellow as an indicator. After cooling in an ice bath for 10–15 min the precipitated potassium perchlorate is removed by centrifugation and the supernatant fluid is lyophilized. For chromatography, the lyophilized extracts are dissolved in water and amounts equivalent to 5–10 mg of the original tissue are subjected to PC or TLC.

2.3   Detection

For the detection of pantothenic acid and its derivatives, most often the ninhydrin reagent is used. The reaction is based on the interaction of the released β-alanine with ninhydrin. Besides ninhydrin, the reaction with potassium permanganate can be employed. Puech et al. (97) compared sensitivities of these two reagents. The detection sensitivity with $KMnO_4$ was as good as or better than that obtained with the ninhydrin reagent (Table 3). Iodoplatinate reagent, which is suitable for detection of alkaloids and various drugs, can also be used (94). Pantothenic acid and its derivatives can also be detected after conversion to pantolactone by acid hydrolysis. Pantolactone reacts with hydroxylamine to form hydroxamic acid. The latter reacts with Fe(III) ions, giving a typical red product (98).

For the detection of pantothenic acid derivatives, different reagents can be used. Phosphorous-containing compounds can be localized with the Hanes and Isherwood spray reagent (99), followed by UV irradiation. Thiols can be visualized by spraying with an aqueous ammonia solution after treatment with sodium nitroprusside, and disulfides can be localized with the nitroprusside spray reagent after reaction with potassium cyanide (100).

Lyle and Tehrani (101) developed a pyrolysis method for the visualization of calcium pantothenate. This procedure is not suitable for the detection itself, but can be applied for the GLC determination of volatile pyrolysis products.

Besides the mentioned chemical detection methods, bioautographic methods have been used (96). They are suitable for the detection of pantothenic acid and its derivatives, including coenzyme A and its short-chain acyl derivatives. The test microorganisms (*Torulopsis bovina* and *Gluconobacter oxydans*) allowed detection of nanomole amounts of compounds after separation by PC. *Torulopsis bovina* yeasts gave a bioautographic growth response to 1–2 ng of pantothenates and to 50 ng of β-alanine, but not to pantethine, coenzyme A, and its derivatives. To detect the latter compounds, it was necessary to hydrolyze them in situ before placing the chromatogram on the bioautographic plate. This can be achieved by spraying the sheets with an enzyme preparation containing alkaline phosphatase and enzymes isolated from avian liver. The sensitivity of this method depends upon the completeness of the hydrolysis. Amounts as low as 100 ng of pantethine, 50 ng of coenzyme A, and 50 ng of acetyl-coenzyme A can be detected. The bioautographic detection utilizing the bacterium *G. oxydans* can be improved by adding bromocresol green as an indicator to the medium and observing the acid production. This microorganism responded to pantothenate (50 ng), pan-

Table 3 Paper and Thin-Layer Chromatography Detection Reagents' Sensitivities[a]

	Detection reagent			
	KMnO$_4$		Ninhydrin	
Compound	Color	Sensitivity (μg)	Color	Sensitivity (μg)
Pantothenic acid	Yellow	1.00	Pinkish-violet	1.00
Calcium pantothenate	Yellow	0.50	Pinkish-violet	1.00
Sodium pantothenate	Yellow	0.50	Pinkish-violet	1.00
Panthenol	Yellow	0.50	Pink	1.00
Pantolactone	Yellow	0.05	—	—
β-Alanine	Yellow	0.10	Violet	0.10

[a] From Ref. 97.

529

toate (30 ng), and to coenzyme A and its short-chain acyl derivatives (2 ng) without the necessity of converting these compounds to pantothenate. Both described detection systems were also sufficiently sensitive to detect pantothenate-related compounds in extracts of rat tissues (96). The technique of bioautography takes advantage of the separation achieved by PC and the specificity provided by microorganisms with requirements for specific growth factors.

2.4 Paper Chromatography

Paper chromatography (PC) is a suitable method for qualitative and in some cases semi-quantitative determinations of pantothenic acid and its derivatives. Using two-dimensional PC, it was possible to separate all the vitamins in multivitamin preparations using a buffer saturated with phenol as the mobile phase (the buffer solution contained 6.3% w/w sodium citrate and 3.7% w/w KH_2PO_4) in the first direction and 1-butanol-propionic acid-water (fresh solution was prepared by mixing equal volumes of two solutions, the first of which was prepared from 1246 ml of 1-butanol and 84 ml of water, the second from 620 ml of propionic acid and 790 ml of water) in the second direction (102). Acetone-1-butanol-water (5:40:55, v/v/v) and 1-pentanol-acetone-water (6:3:3, v/v/v) mixtures have also been used (97). Panthenol in pharmaceutical products may be separated by using Amberlite ion-exchange paper WA-2 adjusted to pH 4.6 with an acetate buffer, with water as the mobile phase (103).

Mobilities of pantothenic acid and related compounds are given in Table 4; mobilities of CoA, its acyl analogues, and related compounds in several PC solvent systems are summarized in Table 5.

2.5 Thin-Layer Chromatography

Thin-layer chromatography is very often used for orientative determinations in multivitamin pharmaceutical preparations, premixes, and mixed feeds. Silica gel and cellulose were especially used as the sorbents. Gänshirt and Malzacher (108) separated pantothenic acid on silica gel G layers with acetic acid-acetone-menthol-benzene (5:5:20:70, v/v/v/v) as the mobile phase. Thielemann (109) used activated ready-prepared silica-gel sheets for the separation of pantothenic acid in multivitamin preparations. Blešová and Zahradníček (110) used Silufol UV_{254} sheets. Pharmaceutical preparations containing sodium and calcium pantothenates, pantolactone, and some other degradation products of pantothenic acid were separated on silica gel GF_{254} layers using chloroform-ethanol-acetic acid (10:7:3, v/v/v) as the mobile phase (111). The vitamins of the

Table 4 Mobilities of Pantothenic Acid and Related Compounds in Paper Chromatography Solvent Systems

Paper[a]	P1	P1	P1	P2	P2	P2	P2
Solvent[b]	S_1	S2	S3	S4	S5	S6	S7
Technique[c]	DE	AS	DE	AS	AS	AS	AS
Detection[d]	D1	D1	D2	D2-4	D2-4	D3-5	D3-5
Compound	R_{CoA}	R_F	R_F	R_F	R_F	R_F	R_F
Pantothenic acid			0.66	0.40			
Pantothenates	11.9	0.46					
Pantetheine				0.70	0.66		
Pantethine	11.9	0.96		0.65	0.35		
4'-Phosphopantetheine						0.55	0.26
4'-Phosphopantetheine						0.34	0.25
Homopantetheine				0.76	0.58		
Homopantethine				0.72	0.26		
α-Methylpantetheine				0.82	0.82		
α-Methylpantethine				0.81	0.48		
β-Methylpantetheine				0.75	0.76		
β-Methylpantethine				0.73	0.48		
Oxypantetheine				0.54	0.26		

[a] Paper: P1 = Whatman no. 1, P2 = Toyo no. 50.

[b] Solvent: S1 = 4 M ammonium acetate buffer (pH 4.7)-2-propanol (1:2, v/v); S2 = ethyl acetate-pyridine-water (1:1:1, v/v/v); S3 = phenol-buffer (100:25, v/v; buffer: 6.3% sodium citrate, 3.7% KH_2PO_4); S4 = 1-butanol saturated with water; S5 = methyl ethyl ketone saturated with water; S6 = 1-butanol-acetic acid-water (5:2:3, v/v/v); S7 = 1-propanol-ammonia (25%, w/w)-water (6:3:1, v/v/v).

[c] Technique: DE = descending, AS = ascending.

[d] Detection: D1 = bioautography, D2 = ninhydrin, D3 = sodium nitroprusside, D4 = potassium cyanide, sodium nitroprusside, D5 = Hanes-Isherwood reagent, UV irradiation.

Source: Modified from Refs. 96,99,100,102,104, and 105.

B complex, including pantothenic acid, can be separated on cellulose MN 300HR layers with 1-butanol-acetic acid-water (8:1:11, v/v/v) as the solvent system (112). For the separation of polyvitamin preparations in mixed feeds, silica gel GF$_{254}$ layers with different solvent systems have been successfully used (29).

The R_f values for various derivatives of pantothenic acid in various solvent systems used in TLC are given in Table 6.

Table 5 Mobilities of Coenzyme A and Related Compounds in Paper Chromatography Solvent Systems

Paper[a]	P1	P1	P1	P1	P2	P2	P2
Solvent[b]	S1	S2	S3	S4	S5	S6	S7
Technique[c]	DE	DE	AS	AS	AS	AS	AS
Detection[d]	D1	D1	D1	D1	D356	D356	D356
Compound	R_{CoA}	R_{CoA}	R_F	R_F	R_F	R_F	R_F
CoA	1.0	1.0	0.34	0.17	0.28	0.12	0.54
Acetyl-CoA	5.6	7.8	0.46	0.31			
Propionyl-CoA	6.4	10.3	0.38	0.27			
Isobutyryl-CoA		12.8	0.39	0.28			
α-(β-)Methyl-CoA					0.30	0.12	
α-Carboxy-CoA					0.26	0.05	
Homo-CoA					0.28	0.13	
Desulpho-CoA					0.30	0.13	
Inosino-CoA					0.24	0.09	0.38
Guanosino-CoA					0.21	0.07	0.36

[a] Paper: P1 = Whatman no. 1, P2 = Toyo no. 50.

[b] Solvent: S1 = 4 M ammonium acetate buffer (pH 4.7)-2-propanol (1:2, v/v); S2 = 0.1 M ammonium acetate buffer (pH 4.7)-2-propanol (1:4, v/v); S3 = 2-propanol-pyridine-water (1:1:1, v/v/v); S4 = ethyl acetate-pyridine-water (1:1:1, v/v/v); S5 = ethanol-0.5 M ammonium acetate buffer (pH 3.8) (5:2, v/v); S6 = ethanol-1 M ammonium acetate buffer (pH 4.7) (5:2, v/v); S7 = isobutyric acid-1M ammonia-0.1 M ethylenediamine tetraacetic acid disodium salt (100:60:1.6, v/v/v).

[c] Technique: DE = descendent, AS = ascendent.

[d] Detection: D1 = bioautography, D3 = sodium nitroprusside, D5 = Hanes-Isherwood reagent, UV irradiation, D6 = UV irradiation.

Source: Modified from Refs. 96,99,106, and 107.

A semiquantitative determination can be carried out by estimating the spot sizes and comparing them with those of a series of standards (113). Attempts have also been made to evaluate the ninhydrin spots quantitatively by reflectance spectrophotometry (114).

For quantitative purposes, the separation by TLC combined with GLC separation of the volatile pyrolysis products has been successfully used (101).

2.6 Ion-Exchange Chromatography

One of the first applications of chromatographic separations on strongly acidic cation exchange columns of Amberlite CG-400 (H^+) and similar

Table 6 Mobilities of Pantothenic Acid and Its Derivatives in Thin-Layer Chromatography Solvent Systems

Layer[a]	L1	L1	L1	L1	L2	L2	L3
Solvent[b]	S1	S2	S3	S4	S5	S6	S7
Detection[c]	D12	D12	D12	D12	D12	D12	D12
Compound	R_F	R_F	R_F	R_F	R_F	R_F	R_F
Pantothenic acid	0.89	0.57	0.56	0.80	0.89	0.40	
Calcium pantothenate				0.76		0.40	
Sodium pantothentate				0.77			
Panthenol	0.75	0.80	0.61	0.65	0.67		
Panthenol ethyl ester	0.95	0.68	0.02				
Pantetheine							0.63
Pantethine							0.72
Pantolactone				0.92			
β-Alanine				0.08	0.40		
3-Amino-1-propanol					0.65		

[a] Layer: L1 = silica gel GF_{254}, L2 = silica gel, L3 = cellulose MN300.

[b] Solvent: S1 = water (ref. 29); S2 = acetic acid-acetone-methanol-benzene (5:5:20:70, v/v/v/v) (ref. 115); S3 = ethanol (absolute); S4 = chloroform-ethanol-acetic acid (10:7:3, v/v/v); S5 = water (ref. 29); S6 = acetic acid-acetone-methanol-benzene (5:5:20:70, v/v/v/v) (ref. 115); S7 = 1-butanol-acetic acid-water (62:25:13, v/v/v).

[c] Detection: D1 = ninhydrin, D2 = potassium permanganate.

Source: Modified from Refs. 29 and 115.

resins was reported in connection with the preliminary purification of β-alanine and 3-amino-1-propanol in hydrolysates of calcium pantothenate and panthenol, respectively. The aim of this separation was to remove the interferences in the subsequent spectrophotometric determination of vitamins according to Wollish and Schmall (70) and Schmall and Wollish (75). Either ion-exchange chromatography or selective precipitation has been employed to separate panthenol from interfering substances such as riboflavin and pyridoxin in multivitamin preparations, followed by polarographic determination of panthenol (88). Ion-exchange sample cleanup on Dowex 50W × 4 (H^+) is useful to remove interferences (such as vitamins and minerals) in the HPLC determination of pantothenic acid in the form of β-alanine-fluorescamine complex (116). Amberlite IR-120 (H^+) was used for the conversion of calcium pantothenate to free acid to be directly determined in the eluate by alcalimetric titration (117). Dowex 1 (Cl^-) anion exchange resin has been used for the separation of adenosine 2′- and 3′-phosphate-5′-diphosphate in the course of studies on coenzyme A synthesis (118).

ECTEOLA-cellulose columns have been successfully employed for the separation of adenosine phosphates, intermediary products of coenzyme A synthesis; DEAE-cellulose proved to be a suitable sorbent for the separation of coenzyme A thiol and disulfide forms (119), as can be seen in Fig. 7. The same sorbent is useful for the separation of α-methyl-CoA (SH form) and α-methyl-CoA (disulfide form) from adenosine 3′, 5′-diphosphate, as well as α-carboxy-CoA (thiol) from its disulfide form and homo-CoA thiol from its disulfide form (107). Using the same sorbent and elution with water and a linear gradient of 0–0.075 M LiCl in 0.003 M HCl it was possible to separate the components of the fermentation medium (biosynthesis of CoA) into the following three fractions: (1) pantothenic acid and pantethine, (2) 4′-phosphopantothenate and 4′-phosphopantetheine, and (3) CoA and dephospho-CoA (120). Using a 120 × 10 mm DEAE-cellulose column equilibrated with 0.01 M TRIS buffer (pH 7.3) and elution with water and a linear gradient (0-0.075 M) of LiCl in 0.003 M HCl it was possible to separate CoA, free pantothenic acid, and 4′-phospho-5′-benzoylpantethein in rat liver extracts (121).

3. HIGH-PERFORMANCE LIQUID CHROMATOGRAPHY

3.1 General Considerations

In the last few years high-performance liquid chromatography (HPLC) has become a valuable method for the separation and quantitation of pantothenic acid and some of its derivatives. Several methods for the

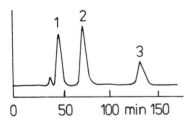

Figure 7 Chromatography of products involved in biosynthesis of coenzyme A. Column: DEAE-cellulose (Cl⁻), 290 × 30 mm; mobile phase: water (500 ml), a linear gradient with 0.003 M HCl (2250 ml) and 0.225 M LiCl in 0.003 M HCl (2250 ml); flow rate: 1.5 ml/min; detection: UV 257 nm; peak identification: (1) adenosine-3′, 5′-diphosphate, (2) coenzyme A (thiol), (3) coenzyme A (disulfide). (From Ref. 119.)

determination of pantothenic acid and its salts (mainly calcium pantothenate), or panthenol, in pharmaceutical preparations have been developed and are applied on a routine basis in a few research and control laboratories (122–128). However, none of these methods can be used for the analysis of complex matrices such as foods and feeds. Another limitation lies in the impossibility of separating optical isomers of the biologically active forms of compounds.

Of particular interest are the HPLC methods developed for the separation and quantitation of coenzyme A and its short-chain acyl analogues in biological materials (129–136).

HPLC techniques present several potential advantages over earlier spectrophotometric, fluorometric, and microbiological assay methods that are very tedious and often difficult to perform. These advantages include simple sample preparation, direct analysis of compounds without any derivatization, and potential simultaneous determination of several compounds in a single run, in addition to a reduction of analysis time, excellent precision, and relatively good sensitivity.

Only reversed-phase materials have been used, and most separations have been performed on octadecyl columns. Mixtures of polar organic solvents such as methanol or acetonitrile with water or appropriate buffers are the most common eluents. Only spectrophotometric and exceptionally refractometric detection are suitable for direct analysis. To facilitate the analysis and increase the sensitivity, suitable derivatives allowing fluorometric detection have been prepared.

Overviews of methods and applications are given in Tables 7 and 8.

3.2 Pantothenic Acid and Pantothenates

Pantothenic acid and its salts as well as its degradation products such as pantoic acid and β-alanine do not exhibit significant absorption above 220 nm. As a result, the limitation of the direct HPLC assays lies in the lack of a selective detection wavelength. Detection is mainly performed by UV absorption at low wavelength. Analysis using UV detection below 220 nm has inherent problems because of the limited number of common mobile phase solvents that have appropriate cutoff and because of dissolved oxygen that has to be removed via sonication under vacuum.

Pantothenic acid and pantothenates may also be analyzed following derivatization to extend the chromophore and hence allow UV detection at higher wavelengths or fluorometric detection. Hudson et al. (124) have attempted to analyze the vitamin as a β-alanine-fluorescamine complex. The derivatization procedure was lengthy and required extensive sample cleanup before the hydrolysis step due to the interference of riboflavin, niacinamide, and some minerals such as zinc, copper, man-

Table 7 HPLC Conditions for the Analysis of Calcium Pantothenate and Panthenol in Pharmaceutical Multivitamin Preparations

Compound separated	Sample preparation	Stationary phase	Mobile phase	Detection	Reference
Calcium pantothenate	Dissolve in mobile phase	Nucleosil 7 C18	Acetic acid-water (5:95, v/v)	RI	122
	Dissolve in methanol-water (25:75, v/v)	Zorbax C-8	Methanol-0.25 M NaH_2PO_4, pH 3.5 (12:88, v/v)	UV 214 nm	123
	Dissolve in 0.005 M KH_2PO_4, pH 5	LiChrosorb NH_2	Acetonitrile-0.005 M KH_2PO_4, pH 5 (87:13, v/v)	UV 210 nm	124,125
	Dissolve in 0.01 M NaH_2PO_4, pH 3	Nucleosil 5 C18	Acetonitrile-0.01 M NaH_2PO_4 pH 3 (3:97, v/v)	UV 208 nm	126
	Dissolve in water	Hypersil ODS C18	Acetonitrile-0.25 M NaH_2PO_4, pH 2.5 (3:97, v/v)	UV 205 nm	127
Panthenol	Dissolve in 0.5 M HCl, hydrolysis, derivatization with fluorescamine	Chromegabond C18	Methanol-sodium borate buffer, pH 8 (30:70, v/v)	Fluorescence: ex 390 nm, em 475–490 nm or UV 390 nm	128
	Dissolve in 0.5 M HCl, hydrolysis, derivatization with fluorescamine	μBondapak C18	Acetonitrile-0.1 M ammonium acetate (18:82, v/v)	Fluorescence: ex 390 nm, em 475–490 nm	125

Table 8 HPLC Conditions for the Analysis of CoA and Short-Chain Acyl-CoA Esters in Model Systems and Rat Liver Tissue

Sample preparation	Stationary phase	Mobile phase	Detection	Reference
Dissolve standards in mobile phase	LiChrosorb RP-8	0.01 M tetrabutylammonium hydroxide buffer, pH 5.5 in methanol-water (45:55, v/v)	UV 230 nm	135
Neutralized $HClO_4$ extract	Spherisorb 5 ODS	0.22 M KH_2PO_4 buffer, pH 4-methanol (88:12, v/v)	UV 254 nm	136
Neutralized $HClO_4$ extract	μBondapak C18	0.05 M KH_2PO_4 buffer, pH 5.3-methanol (90:10, v/v)	UV 254 nm	134
Neutralized $HClO_4$ extract	Spherisorb ODS II C18	(1) 0.22 M KH_2PO_4 buffer, pH 4; (2) chloroform-methanol (2:98, v/v)	UV 254 nm	129
Neutralized $HClO_4$ extract	ODS Ultrasphere C18	NaH_2PO_4 buffer-acetonitrile gradient	UV 254 nm	130
Neutralized $HClO_4$ extract, concentrated on a Sep-Pak C18 cartridge	Develosil ODS	Water-acetonitrile gradient	UV 260 nm	131

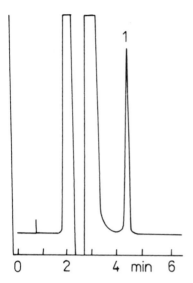

Figure 8 Determination of calcium pantothenate in multivitamin tablets. Chromatographic conditions: see Table 7. Peak identification: (1) pantothenate. (From Ref. 122.)

ganese, and molybdenum. Although these interferences were eliminated, the method did not yield reproducible results.

Technical notes of Hewlett-Packard (132) and DuPont (133) reported possibility to separate calcium pantothenate from other water-soluble vitamins by HPLC. The first successful separation of calcium pantothenate in multivitamin preparations that allowed the quantitative determination in less than 5 min was reported by Jonvel et al. (122). They used a 20-cm Nucleosil 7 C_{18} reversed-phase column, an acetic acid-water (5:95, v/v) mobile phase at a flow rate of 2 ml/min, and a refractometer as a detector. Samples were simply dissolved in the mobile phase and analyzed without any internal standard. Mean recoveries of the assays of commercially available calcium pantothenate tablets containing also thiamine, riboflavin, niacinamide, and pyridoxine ranged from 96.8 to 104.4%. The detection limit was 50 ng injected (Fig. 8).

Franks and Stodola (123) analyzed calcium panthothenate employing a 250×4.6 mm Zorbax C-8 column equipped with a guard MPLC 30-mm cartridge column packed with RP-18 Spheri-5 sorbent. Calcium pantothenate was extracted from tablets with a mixture of methanol-water (25:75, v/v) containing adipic acid as the internal standard. The mobile phase was a mixture of methanol-NaH_2PO_4 buffer (pH 3.5), and the effluent was monitored at 214 nm. A highly retained excipient peak eluted approximately 2 h after calcium pantothenate peak (retention time 8 min) and hence interfered with subsequent chromatograms. The use of a column-switching arrangement was employed to shorten the chromatography run time. Average recovery was 99.7%, and relative standard deviation ranged from 0.83 to 2.32%.

Pantothenic acid/calcium pantothenate in pharmaceutical products and vitamin premixes was also analyzed using low-wavelength ultraviolet (UV) detection (124,125). The vitamin was extracted from tablets or powdered premixes with 0.005 M KH_2PO_4 buffer (pH 4.5) and separated from other water-soluble vitamins on an aminopropyl-bonded silica column (LiChrosorb NH_2) eluted with an acetonitrile-0.005 M KH_2PO_4 buffer (pH 4.5) (87:13, v/v) and detected at 210 nm (Fig. 9). Quantitative recoveries (> 95%) and relative standard deviations 0.79–2.2% were obtained for multivitamin tablets, vitamin premixes, fortified yeasts, and raw materials. The limit of sensitivity was approximately 1 mg/g sample. The results were compared with those obtained by the standard microbiological procedure. Low levels of calcium pantothenate

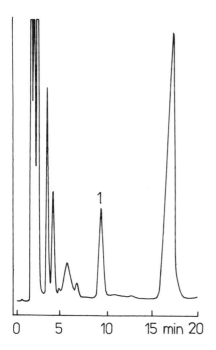

Figure 9 Determination of calcium pantothenate in multivitamin-multimineral tablets. Chromatographic conditions: see Table 7. Peak identification: (1) pantothenate. (From Ref. 125.)

(< 3 mg per tablet) were more precisely analyzed by the HPLC procedure than by the microbiological method.

A similar procedure employed for the determination of pantothenic acid in pharmaceuticals was described by Akeda (126). The vitamin was separated on a Nucleosil 5 C_{18} column with an acetonitrile-0.01 M phosphate buffer of pH 3 (3:97, v/v) and detected at 208 nm.

A fast, simple, and sensitive method was developed for the determination of calcium pantothenate in commercial multivitamin tablet formulations and raw materials (127). The chromatographic system included a 5-μm reversed-phase C18 column (150 × 4.6 mm) and a mobile phase consisting of acetonitrile and 0.25 M NaH$_2$PO$_4$ buffer of pH 2.5 (97:3, v/v). The column effluent was monitored by UV detection at 205 nm. The sample preparation involved only extraction in water followed by filtration of the extract. The method had the detection limit of approximately 50 ng/ml sample, with mean recovery ranging from 98.7 to 99.8%. The relative standard deviation ranged from 0.3 to 2.0% (Fig. 10).

3.3 Panthenol

Panthenol can be determined using the procedure developed by Umgat and Tscherne (128), which is useful for the analysis of panthenol in premixes and multivitamin preparations. The method is based on the acid hydrolysis of panthenol with 0.5 M HCl at 85°C and derivatization of the released 3-amino-1-propanol (β-alanol) with fluorescamine, a reagent that reacts specifically with primary amines. The condensation

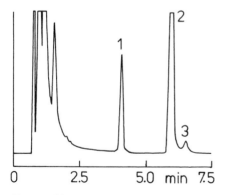

Figure 10   Determination of calcium pantothenate in chewable multivitamin tablets. Chromatographic conditions: see Table 7. Peak identification: (1) pantothenate, (2) saccharin, (3) 2-sulfamoylbenzoic acid. (From Ref. 127.)

product of aminopropanol and the corresponding derivative of 6-aminohexanoic acid (ϵ-aminocaproic acid) used as the internal standard were separated on a 300×4.6 mm Chromegabond C_{18} column and detected by using either a spectrofluorometer with the excitation wavelength at 390 nm and the emission wavelength of 475–490 nm or by measuring the absorbance of 390 nm (Fig. 11). The fluorometric measurement had to be used for trace analysis. The mobile phase was prepared by mixing methanol with 0.1 M borate buffer (adjusted to pH 8 with 2 M NaOH) in a ratio of 30:70, v/v (Table 7). In comparison to the earlier methods, the HPLC procedure was faster, more specific, and also suitable to monitor natural trace levels of aminopropanol in panthenol. The results obtained by the HPLC method were in close agreement with those obtained using nonaqueous titration with perchloric acid, spectrophotometric determination with 1,2-naphthoquinone 4-sulfonate, or microbiological assay. Recoveries found for pure D- and DL-panthenol were 99.6 and 100.5%, respectively, whereas for pharmaceutical preparations containing D-panthenol they ranged from 97.9 to 103.1%. In multivitamin preparations where large amounts of riboflavin were

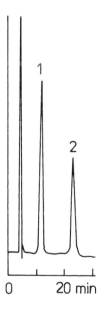

0   20 min

Figure 11   Determination of panthenol in multivitamin tablets. Chromatographic conditions: see Table 7. Peak identification: (1) 6-aminohexanoic acid (internal standard)-fluorescamine derivative, (2) 3-amino-1-propanol-fluorescamine derivative. (From Ref. 128.)

present, the peak of panthenol was not fully resolved from that of the internal standard, which elutes immediately after riboflavin. In that case, 2-aminoethanol had to be used as the internal standard.

A modification of this procedure was described by Hudson et al. (125) and used for the determination of panthenol in liquid multivitamin products. A sample aliquot containing approximately 1 mg panthenol was hydrolyzed for 30 min at 85°C in 0.5 M HCl, centrifuged, and the supernate was mixed with fluorescamine reagent and diluted with 1% (w/w) borate buffer. The aminopropanol-fluorescamine complex was chromatographed on a μBondapak C_{18} column with acetonitrile-0.1 M ammonium acetate (18:82, v/v) as mobile phase and using fluorescence detection (the excitation and emission wavelengths were set as mentioned above at 390 and between 475–490 nm, respectively) (Fig. 12). This procedure was limited to samples containing at least 100 μg/g panthenol. The average recovery was 99% and precision was 2.9% (relative standard deviation) at 1.03 mg/g panthenol. Excellent agreement was found when the HPLC method was compared with the microbiological assay procedure.

3.4   Coenzyme A and Related Compounds

Several HPLC methods have been developed to separate and determine coenzyme A and short-chain coenzyme A esters. The older methods pro-

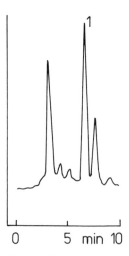

Figure 12   Determination of panthenol in multivitamin tablets. Chromatographic conditions: see Table 7. Peak identification: (1) 3-amino-1-propanol-fluorescamine derivative. (From Ref. 125.)

vided chromatographic separation of a few CoA esters only (135), employing corrosive ion-pairing reagents or a combination of three consecutive chromatographic systems (134). More recently, a reversed-phase chromatographic separation system suitable for the determination of CoA, dephospho-CoA, and acetyl-CoA has been developed (136), modified, and employed for the separation of CoA and various short-chain acyl CoA esters in rat tissues (129). Separation of the various compounds was accomplished by using a 250×4.6 nm Spherisorb ODS II, 5 μm C_{18} column fitted with a 45×4 mm guard column filled with reversed-phase Bio-Sil P1B-ODS beads. The mobile phase solvents were (1) 0.22 M KH_2PO_4 buffer of pH 4, containing 0.05% (v/v) thiodiglycol to prevent oxidation of CoA, and (2) chloroform-methanol (2:98, v/v). The effluent was monitored at 254 nm (at about the λ_{max} of adenosine), and nearly baseline separation was achieved for a standard mixture of free CoA, methylmalonyl-CoA, β-hydroxy-β-methylglutaryl-CoA, succinyl-CoA, acetoacetyl-CoA, acetyl-CoA, propionyl-CoA, β-methylcrotonyl-CoA, and isovaleryl-CoA. Profiles of metabolically accumulated CoA derivatives were determined in rat heart and liver and in isolated liver mitochondria. However, the method did not appear to be applicable to the direct determination of small amounts of these derivatives in tissues. The HPLC assay procedure gave results similar to the enzymatic assay of CoA.

The first quantitative determinations of HPLC of CoA compounds have been presented by King and Reiss (130). The authors developed a reversed-phase HPLC procedure to measure CoA and short-chain CoA compounds in rat liver tissue. Seventeen CoA-related standards in model experiments were separated and quantified in a 37-min run employing a 75×4.6 mm ODS Ultrasphere octadecylsilica column (Fig. 13). In rat liver CoA, acetyl-CoA and six minor CoA-related metabolites could be quantitated (Fig. 14). The separation was achieved using an Na_2HPO_4-acetonitrile gradient. The eluate was monitored at 254 nm. Recovery of CoA standards added in tissue extracts ranged from 83 to 107%. The procedure allowed measurement of as little as 12 pmol of CoA compounds injected.

More sensitive HPLC reversed-phase procedure for the determination of CoA and short-chain acyl-CoA esters in normal rat liver extracts have recently been developed by Hosokawa et al. (131). The acyl-CoA esters present in the neutralized $HClO_4$ extract were concentrated on a Sep-Pak C_{18} cartridge. The cartridge was washed with water and a series of organic solvents and subsequently the acyl-CoA esters were eluted with ethanol-water (65:35, v/v) containing 0.1 M ammonium acetate. The eluate was analyzed using 150×4.6 mm and 250×4.6 mm Develosil

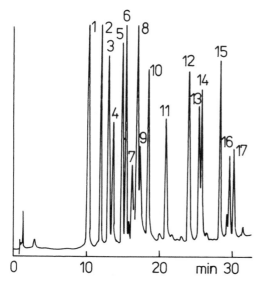

Figure 13 Separation of coenzyme A and its analogues (standards). Column: 3 μm, C18 (ODS Ultrasphere); 75×4.6 mm; temperature: 30°C; mobile phase: gradient elution from 0.6 to 18% acetonitrile with constant Na_2HPO_4 concentration of 0.2 M; flow rate: 1 ml/min; detection: UV at 254 nm; peak identification: (1) malonyl-CoA, (2) glutathione-CoA, (3) CoA (thiol), (4) methylmalonyl-CoA, (5) succinyl-CoA, (6) 3-hydroxy-3-methylglutaryl-CoA, (7) dephosphoCoA, (8) acetyl-CoA, (9) acetoacetyl-CoA, (10) CoA(disulfide), (11) propionyl-CoA, (12) crotonyl-CoA, (13) isobutyryl-CoA, (14) butyryl-CoA, (15) 3-methylcrotonyl-CoA, (16) isovaleryl-CoA, (17) valeryl-CoA. (From Ref. 130.)

ODS columns. The separation of eight CoA compounds was conducted with a linear gradient (from 1.75 to 10%) of acetonitrile in water (v/v). The elution was monitored at 260 nm. Isobutyryl-CoA was used as the internal standard. The lower detection limit of the individual acyl-CoA esters was about 50 pmol injected. Recoveries of authentic short-chain acyl-CoA esters ranged from 56 to 77%.

4. GAS-LIQUID CHROMATOGRAPHY

4.1 General Considerations

Pantothenic acid, its salts, and panthenol as such are not volatile enough for direct gas-liquid chromatography (GLC). However, it is possible to use this chromatographic technique after derivatization of the polar hydroxyl and carboxyl groups of the vitamin (58,137–155). The majority of the developed methods are, however, applicable only to relatively

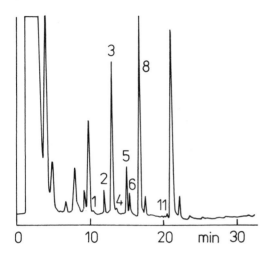

Figure 14 Determination of coenzyme A and its acyl derivatives in liver from a starved rat. Chromatographic conditions and peak identification: see Fig. 13. (From Ref. 130.)

pure and simple samples such as multivitamin preparations (137, 138,144,145,148) and certain biological samples, such as urine (149,150). Only a few methods are suitable for the determination of the vitamin in complex matrices such as foods (139,152,154).

Two approaches are currently used for the preparation of volatile derivatives of the vitamin. The first approach is mostly based on the conversion of pantothenic acid and/or panthenol to acetyl (137,138,153) or trimethylsilyl derivatives (137,145). A simpler and more convenient approach for most applications seems to be the procedure based on the hydrolysis of the vitamin in acidic medium and analysis of the hydrolysis products. Pantothenic acid, its salts, and coenzyme A as well as its analogues undergo acid hydrolysis with formation of β-alanine and pantolactone. Panthenol breaks down to 3-amino-1-propanol (β-alanol) and pantolactone. For instance, β-alanine can be analyzed as the corresponding N-trifluoroacetyl methyl ester or N-trifluoroacetyl butyl ester (142). Pantolactone is sufficiently volatile to be amenable to direct GLC (139,148,152), but it can also be analyzed as the corresponding trimethylsilyl ether (146), trifluoroacetyl or isopropylurethane derivative (140).

4.2 Pantothenic Acid and Pantothenates

The nature of the sample is indicative for the suitability for the determination of pantothenic acid or its salts. Most of the described methods are applicable to multivitamin and other pharmaceutical preparations, whereas only a few of them are also applicable to biological materials.

Pharmaceutical Preparations

Calcium and sodium pantothenate can be chromatographed following derivatization, degradation, or a combination of both. Derivatization is mostly based on the determination of the corresponding acetates or trimethylsilyl ethers. The determination of pantothenic acid and/or pantothenates as acetates (137,138,153) requires esterification of the carboxyl group prior to acetylation of the hydroxyl function.

Prosser and Sheppard (138) analyzed the vitamin as ethyl pantothenate diacetate. The pantothenate was first converted to ethyl pantothenate by using ethanolic HCl (2.5%) reaction (at room temperature, for 2h) and then to pantothenate diacetate using a mixture of acetic acid anhydride-pyridine (1:1, v/v; at room temperature, for 1 h). The product was chromatographed on a polar stationary phase (Table 9 and Fig. 15). Sensitivity of the determination was 5–8 ng of injected compound.

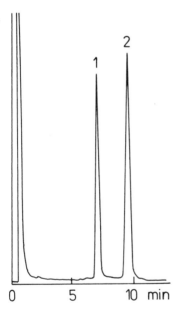

Figure 15 Determination of calcium pantothenate and panthenol as acetyl derivatives. Detector: FID; column: glass, 244 cm × 4 mm; stationary phase: 2% NPGS (neopentyl glycol sebacate); solid support: Anakrom ABS (110/120 mesh); temperatures: injector 280°C, column 230°C, detector 280°C; peak identification: (1) ethyl pantothenate diacetate, (2) panthenol triacetate. (From Ref. 138.)

Trifluoroacetyl derivatives of pantothenic acid and its salts have been prepared by Prosser and Sheppard (138).

A number of pharmaceutical preparations containing pantothenate have been analyzed after trimethylsilylation of the compound. The latter can be carried out using a 2:1:1 (v/v/v) mixture of bis(tri-methylsilyl)acetamide (BSA), -trimethylsilyl imidazole (TMSIM), or -tri-methylchlorosilane (TMCS) in dimethyl sulfoxide (at room temperature, for 10 min). The resulting product is analyzed on a nonpolar stationary phase (Fig. 16). The detection limit is 2–4 ng (137,145). Bis(trimethylsilyl)trifluoroacetamide (BSTFA) can be used instead of BSA (145). TMCS is required only in the derivatization of pantothenates, but pantothenic acid can be also derivatized using a simpler 4:1 (v/v) mixture of BSTFA with TMSIM (145).

A second group of analytical methods requires preliminary acid hydrolysis. This is conducted in 7 M HCl at 95–97°C for 4 h (145) or in 1 M HCl at 80°C for 3 h (148). The hydrolysis product β-alanine has been analyzed after its conversion to the corresponding N-trifluoroacetyl

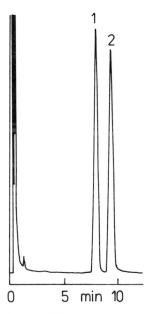

Figure 16 Determination of sodium pantothenate and panthenol as trimethyl-silyl derivatives. Detector: FID; column: glass, 2440 × 4 mm; stationary phase 5% SE-30; solid support: Gas Chrom Q (100/120 mesh); temperatures: injector 270°C, column 185°C, detector 270°C; peak identification: (1) trimethylsilyl derivative of panthenol, (2) trimethylsilyl derivative of pantothenic acid (sodium pantothenate). (From Ref. 145.)

Table 9 GLC Conditions for the Analysis of Pantothenic Acid, Pantothenates, and Panthenol with the Use of FID

Compound analyzed	Derivative	Column (length × ID in mm)	Stationary phase	Solid support (mesh)	Column temperature (°C)	Reference
Pantothenates, panthenol	Acetyl	Glass, 2440 × 4	2% Neopentyl-glycolsebacate	Anakrom ABS (110/120)	230	138
Pantothenates, panthenol	Trifluoro acetyl	Glass, 1830 × 4	3% OV-17	Diatomaceous earth (100/120)	135	138
Pantothenates, panthenol	Trimethyl-silyl	Glass, 2440 × 4	5% SE-30	Gas Chrom Q (100/120)	185	145
Pantothenates, panthenol	Trimethyl-silyl	Glass, 2440 × 4	3% OV-1	Anakrom ABS (110/120)	200	145
Pantothenates, panthenol	Pantolactone	Glass, 2100 × 4	1% Carbowax 20M	Gas-Chrom P (100/120 mesh)	115	148
Pantothenic acid, panthenol	Pantolactone	Glass, 3000 × 3	5% QF-1 or 4% XE-60	Gas-Chrom Q	Not specified	149
Pantothenates, panthenol, pantothein, pantolactone	Pantolactone	Glass, not specified	5% XE-60	Chromaton N-AW	Not specified	150,155
Coenzyme A, pantothenic acid	Pantolactone	Glass, 4300 × 3	LAC-2-R-446	Gas-Chrom Q (100/120)	140	139,144, 147,154
DL-Pantolactone	MTPA-panto-lactone	Glass, 2400 × 2.1	10% Carbowax 20M	Chromaton N-AW-DMCS (0.125-0.16 mm)	120–220 (5°C/min)	152

Compound	Derivative	Column	Stationary phase	Support	Temperature	Ref.
DL-Pantothenic acid	Trifluoroacetyl	Glass, 15,000 mm long capillary	XE-60-L-Val-(R)-α-phenylethylamide		From 130 (2°C/min)	140
Panthenol	Trimethylsilyl	Glass, 1800×3	3.8% SE-30	Diatoport S (80/100)	185	143
DL-Panthenol	Trifluoroacetyl	Fused silica, 15,000 mm long capillary	XE-60-L-Val-(S)-α-phenylethylamide		From 130 (1.5°C/min)	140
DL-Pantolactone	None	Fused silica, 50,000 m long capillary	XE-60-L-Val-(S)-α-phenylethylamide		160	140
DL-Pantolactone	Trifluoroacetyl	Glass, 40,000 m long capillary	XE-60-L-Val-(S)-α,α'-naphthylethylamide		80	140
DL-Pantolactone	Isopropylurethane	Glass, 15,000 m long capillary	XE-60-L-Val-(R)-α-phenylethylamide		From 145 (2°C/min)	140
Pantolactone	Trimethylsilyl	Glass, 1300×3.2	5% SE-30	Chromosorb G (AW-DMCS), (80/100)	170	146

methyl ester or *N*-trifluoroacetyl butyl ester. Derivatization of β-alanine is a two-step procedure. The compound is first converted to its methyl or butyl ester using ethanolic HCl and then to its *N*-trifluoroacetyl derivative by the use of trifluoroacetic acid anhydride. The resulting derivative is analyzed using a polar stationary phase (142).

More convenient are the methods based on degradation to pantolactone. This compound can be simply extracted in a suitable organic solvent, such as dichloromethane, chloroform, or ethyl acetate and chromatographed on polar stationary phases (Fig. 17) (148,149,154).

GLC is the only chromatographic method that enables the resolution of enantiomers of pantothenic acid and hence the specific determination of the biologically active form of pantothenic acid. Similarly to analysis of the other optically active compounds, the enantiomers of pantothenic acid and pantolactone can be separated either on optically active stationary phases (for instance, in the form of trifluoroacetates) or on common stationary phases (in the form of the corresponding diastereoisomers).

König and Sturm (140) separated DL-pantothenic acid in the form of methyl bis(trifluoroacetyl)pantothenate (MPTA) on a capillary column with a chiral polysiloxane phase XE-60-L-Val (R)-α-phenylethylamide

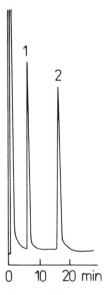

Figure 17 Determination of calcium pantothenate and panthenol as pantolactone. Detector: FID; column: glass, 2100×4 mm; stationary phase: 1% Carbowax 20M; solid support: Gas Chrom P (100/120 mesh); temperatures: injector (not stated), column 115°C, detector (not stated); peak identification: (1) *o*-toluidine (internal standard), (2) pantolactone. (From Ref. 148.)

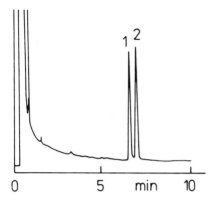

Figure 18 Separation of D- and L-pantothenic acid. Detector: FID; column: glass capillary (15m long); stationary phase: XE-60-L-Val-(R)-α-phenylethylamide (film thickness not stated); temperatures: injector (not stated), column from 130°C (2°C/min) detector (not stated): peak identification: (1) D-pantothenic acid (trifluoroacetyl derivative), (2) L-pantothenic acid (trifluoroacetyl derivative). (From Ref. 140.)

(Fig. 18). The volatile derivative was prepared by esterification of pantothenic acid with methanolic HC1 (20°C, for 14 h) and by acylation of methyl pantothenate formed with trifluoroacetanhydride in dichloromethane (20°C, for 20 min).

Optical purity of D-pantothenic acid can also be determined indirectly, for example, by analysis of pantolactone, as no racemization of pantothenic acid/pantolactone occurs in acidic or in alkaline aqueous media (141). The D- and L-pantolactone were analyzed on a chiral stationary phase, either as such or as trifluoroacetyl or isopropylurethane derivatives (Fig. 19) (140).

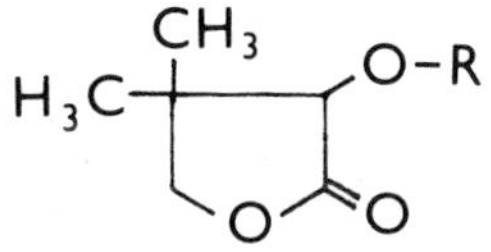

Isopropylamine: R= CO-NH-CH(CH$_3$)$_2$ (From Ref. 140)

MTPA derivative: R= CO-C(CF$_3$)(OCH$_3$)-C$_6$H$_5$ (From Ref. 141)

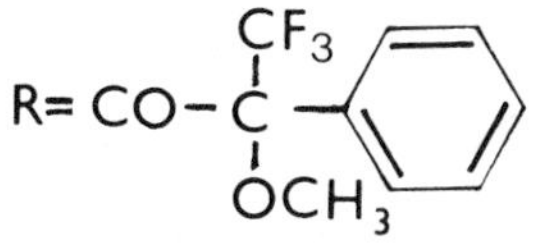

Figure 19 Some pantolactone derivatives structure.

The trifluoroacetate derivatives were prepared using a 4:1 (v/v) mixture of dichloromethane-trifluoroacetanhydride (at 20°C, for 20 min), and isopropylurethane derivatives using a 1:1 (v/v) mixture of dichloromethane-isopropyl isocyanate (at 100°C, for 30 min) (140).

Not only chiral phases but also common stationary phases have been used for the separation of DL-pantolactone isomers. Takase and Ohya (141) described the separation of MTPA derivatives of pantolactone isomers employing a packed column containing 2% OV-17 (Figs. 19 and 20). MTPA derivatives were prepared using a 5:5:2 (v/v/v) mixture of 1,2-dichloroethane- (−)-α-methoxy-α-(trifluoromethyl)-phenylacetyl chloride (MTPAC)-pyridine (at 80°C, for 30 min). N-Trifluoroacetyl-L-prolyl and some other derivatives were also tested but did not give adequate separation.

Biological Materials

Acetylation or trimethylsilylation is not suitable as a derivatization technique for the determination of pantothenic acid in biological materials. Only methods based upon the analysis of the hydrolysis products of pantothenic acid have been successfully employed. The determination of β-alanine is not applicable for the estimation of the pantothenic acid content, as β-alanine can arise not only from the pantothenic acid itself but also from some other substances such as aspartic acid or β-alanylhistidine dipeptides occurring in animal tissues (carnosine, anserine, etc.).

Schulze et al. (147) described a method useful for the analysis of pantothenic acid in urine. Samples were first purified by ion-exchange

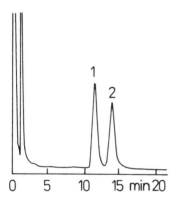

Figure 20 Separation of the MTPA derivatives of D- and L-pantolactone. Detector: FID; column: glass, 2000×3 mm; stationary phase: 2% OV-17; solid support: Gas Chrom Q (80/100 mesh); temperatures: injector 190°C, column 170°C, detector (not stated); peak identification: (1) MTPA derivative of L-pantolactone, (2) MTPA derivative of D-pantolactone. (From Ref. 141.)

chromatography and then hydrolyzed with HCl solutions; the generated pantothenic acid was extracted with dichloromethane and analyzed with methyl myristate as an internal standard on a polar stationary phase. The relative standard deviation of the method was 6–7%.

Determination of pantothenic acid in foods was described in detail by Davídek and Velíšek (58). This method is also based upon the acid hydrolysis of the vitamin and the separation of pantolactone. The hydrolysis is performed in 25% (w/w) HCl for 4–5 h at 95–100°C. Pantolactone can be extracted either directly from the hydrolysate or from the neutralized hydrolysate (at pH 5) into dichloromethane. The extract may be further purified by chromatography on a silica-gel column (139,154) or directly analyzed by GLC (152) using polar stationary phases such as polyethylene glycols (Fig. 21). Methyl myristate and ethyl laurate can be used as internal standards.

All of the described methods are suitable for the determination of the total content of the vitamin, that is, free pantothenic acid as well as its bound forms such as coenzyme A or pantetheine.

4.3 Panthenol

In pharmaceutical preparations, panthenol can be determined as a volatile derivative or as derivatives of its degradation products. Most commonly employed are acetyl and trimethylsilyl derivatives. The same

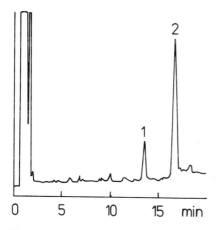

Figure 21 Gas chromatogram of fresh beef liver hydrolysate extract. Detector: FID; column: glass, 240 cm × 2.1 mm; stationary phase: 10% Carbowax 20M; solid support: Chromaton N-AW-DMCS (0.125/0.160 mm); temperatures: injector 220°C, column 120–220°C (5°C/min), detector 250°C; peak identification: (1) ethyl laurate (internal standard), (2) pantolactone. (From Ref. 152.)

derivatization procedures used for the acetylation of pantothenic acid can be employed for the conversion of panthenol into its triacetate, which can then be analyzed on polar stationary phases. Similarly, a tris(trimethylsilyl) ether of panthenol may be prepared using the derivatization procedures previously described. In addition, a 3:6:2 (v/v/v) mixture of TMCS-HMDS-dioxane (35°C, 100 min) has been used (143). Nonpolar polymethylsiloxanes are the stationary phases of choice.

The hydrolysis procedure leading to the formation of pantolactone, which can be analyzed as such, has been described above. The amount of residual pantolactone in panthenol can be estimated after conversion of both compounds to trimethylsilyl derivatives, which are chromatographed on nonpolar stationary phases with the trimethylsilyl ether of 2,6-dimethylphenol as the internal standard (146). For the derivatization, a 9:3:1 (v/v/v) pyridine-HMDS-TMCS mixture was used (room temperature, 30 s).

Enantiomers of panthenol can also be separated on chiral stationary phases. This separation can be performed either after conversion of panthenol isomers into their trifluoroacetates with a 4:1 (v/v) mixture of dichloromethane-trifluoroacetanhydride (20°C, 15 min) (140) or by analyzing free pantolactone formed in acidic medium (section 4.2).

4.4 Coenzyme A

Coenzyme A and its analogues have not yet been subjected to GLC separation. Only the indirect method based upon the analysis of pantolactone has been described and used for the evaluation of the degree of hydrolysis of CoA in HCl solutions (154). Pantolactone was extracted into dichloromethane and chromatographed on a polar stationary phase with methyl myristate as the internal standard. Recovery of the determination was 91% and the relative standard deviation was 3.6%.

Similarly to CoA, none of the other acyl-CoA analogues has been chromatographed using GLC. HPLC procedures and ion-exchange chromatographic methods are the only methods of choice.

Reported levels of pantothenic acid in biological samples obtained by the pantolactone GLC approach pertain not only to the free acid but always to all other active forms, such as CoA, acetyl-CoA, etc.

5. FUTURE TRENDS

The literature on chromatography of pantothenic acid and its derivatives that appeared during the last decade has shown that chromatographic techniques became useful analytical tools, especially for the quantitative determination of the vitamin in pharmaceuticals, for which they offer certain advantages over earlier analytical methods. The minor attention that has been paid to the analysis of naturally occurring pantothenic acid in foods can be, to a certain extent, ascribed to the fact that part of the vitamin is supplied by the intestinal microfloras of animals and humans. Together with the vitamin coming from the diet, the latter provides adequate quantities to cover nutritional requirements.

Modern chromatography of pantothenic acid and of the other compounds in pharmaceuticals that possess the vitamin activity is mainly restricted to HPLC and GLC techniques. The main reason is that HPLC allows simple sample preparation and fast determinations. Currently employed HPLC methods for pantothenic acid and/or pantothenates have been solely applied to pharmaceuticals, whereas assays of coenzyme A and its acyl analogues have also been successfully performed on animal tissues. However, the newly developed HPLC procedures require increased sensitivity to make them applicable to complex biological samples such as food. Appropriate GLC procedures have also been used for the analysis of pure vitamins, their optical isomers, pharmaceuticals and, rarely even foods. The main disadvantage of this group of chromatographic methods is the tedious and relatively time-consuming sample preparation (derivatization) prior to the GLC analysis. Currently used methods for quantitative estimation of the vitamin in foods and feeds still mainly rely on microbiological assay procedures. Bioautography of chromatograms appears to be a promising technique due to high sensitivity of the assays. Some other techniques, especially the sensitive radioimmunoassay procedures, also have been applied on a routine basis. Other chromatographic techniques, such as paper and thin-layer chromatography and ion-exchange chromatography, remain valuable particularly for qualitative analysis and preparative purposes.

REFERENCES

1. D. B. Coursin, *Prog. Food Nutr. Sci., 1*, 183 (1975).
2. W. A. Gauntt, *Proc. AFMA Nutr. Coun. 36*, 13 (1976).
3. R. H. Herman, F. B. Stifel, and H. L. Greene, *Sci. Pract. Clin. Med., 1*, 386 (1976).
4. A. Y. Rozanov, *Vitaminy, 9*, 34 (1976).
5. A. Fifanza, *Acta Vitaminol. Enzymol., 31*, 85 (1977).
6. M. Shimizu, *Method. Chim., 11*, 73 (1977).
7. A. G. Moiseenok, ed., in *Chemistry, Biochemical Function, and Use of a Pantothenic Acid*, Izd. Nauka Tekhnika, Minsk (1977).
8. O. Guillard, A. Pirou, and D. Reiss, *Gaz. Med. Fr., 86*, 1589 (1979).

9.   J. R. Morgan and H. L. Greene, *Am. J. Dis. Child.*, *133*, 308 (1979).
10. G. M. Browes and M. Williamson, *Adv. Enzymol. Related Areas Mol. Biol.*, *53*, 345 (1982).
11. A. G. Moiseenok, *Vopr. Pitan.*, 9 (1982).
12. I. Sharman, *Nutr. Food Sci.*, *78*, 12 (1982).
13. K. Imada, *New Food Ind.*, *25*, 10 (1983).
14. S. J. Gross, *Clin. Disord. Pediatr. Nutr.*, *3*, 185 (1985).
15. W. Friedrich, *Vitamins*, Walter de Gruyter, Berlin (1988).
16. V. M. Kopelevich and V. I. Gunar, *Khim. Prir. Soedin.*, 477 (1988).
17. N. Plesofsky-Vig and R. Brambl, *Annu. Rev. Nutr.*, *8*, 461 (1988).
18. A. F. Wagner and K. Folkers, *Vitamins and Coenzymes*, Wiley, New York, p. 98 (1964).
19. R. J. Williams and E. M. Bradway, *J. Am. Chem. Soc.*, *53*, 783 (1931).
20. R. J. Williams, C. M. Lyman, G. M. Goodyear, J. E. Truesdayl, and D. Holaday, *J. Am. Chem. Soc.*, *55*, 2912 (1933).
21. R. J. Williams, in *A Textbook of Chemistry*, Van Nostrand, New York (1938).
22. E. T. Stiller, S. A. Harris, J. Finkelstein, J. C. Keresztesy, and K. Folkers, *J. Am. Chem. Soc.*, *62*, 1785 (1940).
23. F. Lipman and M. O. Kaplan, *J. Biol. Chem.*, *162*, 743 (1946).
24. F. Lipman, M. O. Kaplan, G. D. Novelli, L. C. Tutte, and B. M. Guylard, *J. Biol. Chem.*, *167*, 869 (1947).
25. F. Lynen, E. Reichert, and L. Rueff, *Ann. Chem.*, *574*, 1 (1951).
26. J. G. Moffatt and H. G. Khorana, *J. Am. Chem. Soc.*, *83*, 663 (1961).
27. A. M. Michelson, *Biochim. Biophys. Acta*, *50*, 605 (1961).
28. E. L. Pugh and S. J. Wakil, *J. Biol. Chem.*, *240*, 4727 (1965).
29. E. Knobloch and J. Černá-Heyrovská, in *Fodder Biofactors. Their Methods of Determination*, Academia, Praha, p. 145 (1979).
30. J. Weichet, in *Vitamins, Their Chemistry and Biochemistry* (J. Fragner, ed.), NČSAV, Praha, p. 907 (1961).
31. K. Werkmeister, F. Wieland, and E. Schweizer, *Biochem. Biophys. Res. Commun.*, *96*, 483 (1980).
32. H. M. Fox, in *Handbook of Vitamins* (L. J. Machlin, ed.), Marcel Dekker, New York, p. 437 (1984).
33. P. Karlson, *Biochemie*, 12, Auflage, Thieme, Stuttgart, p. 373 (1984).
34. J. D. Robinshaw and J. R. Neely, *Am. J. Physiol.*, *246H*, 532 (1984).
35. K. Shibata, C. J. Gross, and L. M. Henderson, *J. Nutr.*, *118*, 2107 (1983).
36. J. V. Kathman and C. Kies, *Nutr. Res.*, *4*, 245 (1984).
37. S. Kimura, Y. Furukawa, J. Wakasugi, Y. Ishihara, and A. Nakayama, *J. Nutr. Sci. Vitaminol.*, *25*, 113 (1980).
38. L. L. Southern and D. H. Baker, *J. Anim. Sci.*, *53*, 403 (1981).
39. J. Davídek, G. Janíček, and J. Pokorný, in *Chemie potravin*, SNTL/ALFA, Praha, p. 149 (1983).
40. D. J. Robertson, *Food Flavour Ingred. Process.*, *1*, 79 (1979).
41. R. J. Priestley, in *Effect of Heating on Foodstuffs* (R. J. Priestley, ed.), Applied Science Publishers, London, p. 121 (1979).

42. L. P. Khrisanfova and V. P. Bubnova, *Doklady TSKhA*, *210*, 87 (1975).

43. R. Uherová and F. Görner, *Prumysl potravin*, *30*, 445 (1979).

44. F. Görner and R. Uherová, *Nahrung*, *24*, 373 (1980).

45. L. E. Ford, R. T. Hurrell, and P. A. Finot, *Br. J. Nutr.*, *49*, 355 (1983).

46. L. Alm, *Dairy Sci.*, *65*, 353 (1982).

47. R. K. Airas, *Anal. Biochem.*, *134*, 122 (1983).

48. J. Adrian, J. Boisselot-Lefevres, and A. Sitti, *Bull. Anc. Eleves Ecole Franc Meunerie*, *281*, 260 (1977).

49. J. Adrian, *Ann. Technol. Agric.*, *27*, 873 (1978).

50. H. A. Schroeder, *Am. J. Clin. Nutr.*, *24*, 562 (1971).

51. R. Strohecker and H. M. Henning, *Vitamin-Bestimmungen*, Verlag Chemie, Weinheim, p. 218 (1963).

52. M.-H. Hashmi, *Assay of Vitamins in Pharmaceutical Preparations*, Wiley, New York, p. 124 (1973).

53. R. J. Williams, *Lab. Equip. Drug.*, *14*, 67 (1976).

54. M. N. Voigt and R. R. Eitenmiller, *J. Food Prot.*, *41*, 730 (1978).

55. O. Solberg and I. K. Hegna, *Methods Enzymol.*, *62D*, 561 (1979).

56. H. M. Fox, *Food Sci. Technol.*, *13*, 437 (1984).

57. A. G. Moiseenoik, in *Metody Otsenki Kontrolya Vitam. Obespechennosti Naseleniya* (V. B. Spirichev, ed.), Nauka, Moscow, p. 111 (1984).

58. J. Davídek and J. Velíšek, *J. Micronutr. Anal.*, *2*, 25 (1986).

59. J. H. Walsh, *Diss. Abstr. Int.*, *B*, *41*, 900 (1980).

60. R. K. Airas, *Methods Enzymol.*, *122G*, 20 (1986).

61. S. Dupré, R. Chiaraluce, M. Nardini, C. Cannella, G. Ricci, and D. Cavallini, *Anal. Biochem.*, *142*, 175 (1984).

62. C. R. Szalkowski and J. H. Davidson, *Anal. Chem.*, *25*, 1192 (1953).

63. C. Wittwer, B. W. Wyse, and R. G. Hansen, *Anal. Biochem.*, *122*, 213 (1982).

64. B. W. Wyse, C. Wittwer, and R. G. Hansen, *Clin. Chem.*, *25*, 108 (1979).

65. J. H. Walsh, B. W. Wyse, and R. G. Hansen, *J. Food Biochem.*, *3*, 175 (1980).

66. K. M. Knights and R. Drew, *Anal. Biochem.*, *168*, 94 (1988).

67. G. Bertelsen, P. M. Finglas, J. Longhridge, J. M. Faulks, and M. R. A. Morgan, *Food Sci. Nutr.*, *42F*, 83 (1988).

68. H. C. Morris, P. M. Finglas, R. M. Faulks, and M. R. A. Morgan, *J. Micronutr. Anal.*, *4*, 33 (1988).

69. H. C. Morris, P. M. Finglas, R. M. Faulks, and M. R. A. Morgan, *J. Micronutr. Anal.*, *4*, 47 (1988).

70. E. G. Wollish and M. Schmall, *Anal. Chem.*, *22*, 1033 (1950).

71. E. Illner, *Pharmazie*, *35*, 186 (1980).

72. J. Wacheck, *Pharmazie*, *21*, 222 (1966).

73. M. Iamagishi and T. Yoshida, *J. Pharm. Soc. Jpn*, *74*, 1001 (1954).

74. M. S. Karawaya, M. G. Ghourab, and E. N. Ibralum, *J. Assoc. Off. Anal. Chem.*, *57*, 1357 (1974).

75. M. Schmal and E. G. Wollish, *Anal. Chem.*, *29*, 1509 (1957).

76. R. Crocaert and E. T. Bigwood, *Arch. Int. Physiol.*, *56*, 189 (1948).
77. R. B. Roy and A. Buccafuri, *J. Assoc. Off. Anal. Chem.*, *61*, 720 (1978).
78. P. Haefellinger and V. Bader-Beerli, *Z. Anal. Chem.*, *262*, 189 (1972).
79. R. Keeler, *Science*, *129*, 1617 (1959).
80. A. F. Zappala and C. A. Simpson, *J. Pharm. Sci.*, *50*, 845 (1961).
81. A. M. Diab, G. Bohn, and G. Ruecker, *Egypt. J. Pharm. Sci.*, *22*, 59 (1981).
82. T. Takeuchi, Y. Kabasawa, R. Horikawa, and T. Tanimura, *Analyst*, *113*, 1673 (1988).
83. M. Weselowski, *Microchem. J.*, *26*, 105 (1981).
84. J. V. Turezan, B. A. Goldwitz, and T. Medwick, *J. Agric. Food Chem.*, *25*, 594 (1977).
85. R. Röben and K. Rubach, *Proc. Int. Symp. Isotachophoresis*, 3rd, p. 345 (1982); *Chem. Abstr.*, *102*, 32367z (1985).
86. S. Tagami and S. Miyajima, *Buneski Kagaku*, *36*, T129 (1987); *Chem. Abstr.*, *108*, 82213g (1988).
87. C. Li, J. Zhong, J. Sun, J. Zhang, M. Xia, and X. Gao, *Yiyao Gongye*, *19*, 308 (1988); *Chem. Abstr.*, *109*, 176434c (1988).
88. G. Matta and E. S. Lopez, *Rev. Farm.*, *16*, 452 (1966).
89. R. G. Painier and J. A. Close, *J. Pharm. Sci.*, *53*, 108 (1964).
90. S. Skrede and J. Bremer, *Eur. J. Biochem.*, *14*, 465 (1970).
91. D. K. Reibel, B. W. Wyse, D. A. Berkich, and J. R. Neely, *J. Nutr.*, *112*, 1144 (1982).
92. P. K. Tubbs and P. B. Garland, *Methods Enzymol.*, *13*, 535 (1969).
93. G. Michael and H. U. Bergmeyer, in *Methods in Enzymatic Analysis* (H. U. Bermeyer, ed.), Vol. 4, Academic Press, New York, p. 1967 (1974).
94. G. Lapiczak, *Ann. Pharm. Fr.*, *36*, 191 (1978).
95. D. R. Osborne and P. Voogt, in *Analysis of Nutrients in Foods*, Academic Press, London, 1978.
96. L. M. Lewin, R. Golan, O. Wassercug, and S. Green, *J. Micronutr. Anal.*, *4*, 209 (1988).
97. A. Puech, J. Monleaud, M. Jacob, and G. Lapiczak, *Ann. Pharm. Fr.*, *36*, 191 (1978).
98. V. Šícho and B. Kakáč, *Cas. lék. čes.*, *92*, 1372 (1953).
99. C. S. Hanes and F. A. Isherwood, *Nature*, *164*, 1107 (1949).
100. O. Nagase, *Chem. Pharm. Bull.*, *15*, 648 (1967).
101. S. J. Lyle and M. S. Tehrani, *J. Chromatogr.*, *236*, 31 (1982).
102. E. L. Gadsten, C. H. Edwards, and G. A. Edwards, *Anal. Chem.*, *32*, 1415 (1960).
103. R. Hüttenrauch and L. Klotz, *Experientia*, *19*, 95 (1963).
104. M. Shimizu, G. Ochata, O. Nagase, S. Okada, and Y. Hosokawa, *Chem. Pharm. Bull.*, *13*, 180 (1965).
105. O. Nagase, H. Tagawa, and M. Shimizu, *Chem. Pharm. Bull.*, *16*, 977 (1968).
106. M. Shimizu, O. Nagase, S. Okada, and Y. Hosokawa, *Chem. Pharm. Bull.*, *18*, 313 (1970).

107. M. Shimizu, O. Nagase, Y. Hosokawa, and H. Tagawa, *Tetrahedron, 24,* 5241 (1968).

108. H. Gänshirt and A. Malzacher, *Naturwissenschaften, 47,* 279 (1960).

109. H. Thielemann, *Scientia Pharm., 42,* 145 (1974).

110. M. Blešová and M. Zahradník, *Čs. farmacie, 23,* 303 (1974).

111. A. Puech, J. Monleaud, M. Jacob, and G. Lapiczak, *Ann. Pharm. Fr., 36,* 191 (1978).

112. S. Boczyk and L. Szeczesniak, *Acta Pol. Pharm., 32,* 347 (1975).

113. G. Pataki, in *Technique of Thin-Layer Chromatography in Amino Acid and Peptide Chemistry,* Ann Arbor Science, Ann Arbor, MI (1968).

114. R. W. Frey and M. M. Frodyma, *Anal. Biochem., 9,* 310 (1964).

115. S. Ishikawa and G. Katsui, *Bitamin, 29,* 203 (1964).

116. T. S. Hudson, S. Subramanian, and R. J. Allen, *J. Assoc. Off. Anal. Chem., 67,* 994 (1984).

117. J. Jarzebinski, E. Lugowska, and M. Grabowska, *Acta. Pol. Pharm., 44,* 87 (1987).

118. Y. Hosokawa, Y. Yotsui, O. Nagase, and M. Shimizu, *Chem. Pharm. Bull., 18,* 1052 (1970).

119. M. Shimizu, O. Nagase, S. Okada, Y. Hosokawa, H. Tagawa, Y. Abiko, and T. Suzuki, *Chem. Pharm. Bull., 15,* 655 (1967).

120. A. G. Moiseenok, V. A. Gurinovich, and V. A. Lysenkova, *Khim. Prir. Soedin., 258* (1987).

121. V. A. Gurinovich, *Khim. Biokhim. Funkts. Primen. Pantotenovoi Kisloty,* Mater. Grodn. Simp., 4th, 36 (1977); *Chem. Abstr., 90,* 182532p (1979).

122. P. Jonvel, G. Andermann, and J. F. Barthelemy, *J. Chromatogr., 281,* 371 (1983).

123. T. J. Franks and J. D. Stodola, *J. Liq. Chromatogr., 7,* 823 (1984).

124. T. J. Hudson and R. J. Allen, *J. Pharm. Sci., 73,* 113 (1984).

125. T. J. Hudson, S. Subramanian, and R. J. Allen, *J. Assoc. Off. Anal. Chem., 67,* 994 (1984).

126. Y. Akada, *Bunseki Kagaku, 35,* 320 (1986); *Chem. Abstr., 104,* 230547d (1986).

127. J. A. Timmons, J. C. Meyer, D. J. Steible, and S. P. Assenza, *J. Assoc. Off. Anal. Chem., 70,* 510 (1987).

128. H. Umagat and R. Tscherne, *Anal. Chem., 52,* 1368 (1980).

129. M. S. DeBuysere and M. S. Olson, *Anal. Biochem., 133,* 373 (1983).

130. M. T. King and P. D. Reiss, *Anal. Biochem., 146,* 173 (1985).

131. Y. Hosokawa, Y. Shimomura, R. A. Harris, and T. Ozawa, *Anal. Biochem., 153,* 45 (1986).

132. R. Schuster, Hewlett-Packard Application Note, AN232-6, September 1978.

133. DuPont Liquid Chromatography Report E-25 475.

134. B. E. Corkey, M. Brandt, R. J. Williams, and J. R. Williamson, *Anal. Biochem., 118,* 30 (1981).

135. F. C. Baker and D. A. Schooley, *Anal. Biochem., 94,* 417 (1979).

136. O. C. Ingebretsen and M. Farstad, *J. Chromatogr., 202,* 439 (1980).

137. A. J. Sheppard and W. D. Hubbard, NBS Special Publication (U.S.), A New Frontier in Analytical Chemistry, *519*, 267 (1979).
138. A. R. Prosser and A. J. Sheppard, *J. Pharm. Sci.*, *58*, 718 (1969).
139. E. Tesmer, J. Leinert and D. Hötzel, *Nahrung*, *24*, 697 (1980).
140. W. A. Koenig and U. Sturm, *J. Chromatogr.*, *328*, 357 (1985).
141. A. Takasu and K. Ohya, *J. Chromatogr.*, *389*, 251 (1987).
142. P. Tarli, S. Benocci, and P. Nerli, *Farmaco, Ed. Prat.*, *25*, 504 (1970).
143. J. V. Wisniewski, *Facts Methods Sci. Res.*, *7*, 4 (1966).
144. E. Tesmer and D. Hötzel, *Z. Anal. Chem.*, *277*, 124 (1975).
145. A. R. Prosser and A. J. Sheppard, *J. Pharm. Sci.*, *60*, 909 (1971).
146. J. C. Stone and J. Wright, *J. Pharm. Sci.*, *60*, 163 (1971).
147. E. Schulze zur Wiesch, C. Hesse, and D. Hötzel, *Z. Klin. Chem. Klin. Biochem.*, *12*, 498 (1974).
148. P. Tarli, S. Benocci, and P. Nerli, *Anal. Biochem.*, *42*, 8 (1971).
149. C. Hesse, E. Schulze zur Wiesch, and D. Hötzel, *Klin. Wochenschr.*, *50*, 55 (1972).
150. A. G. Moisenok, V. S. Slyshenkov, E. V. Sanozova, and G. A. Gavrinovich, *Vop. Med. Khim.*, *30*, 126 (1984).
151. P. Jonvel, G. Andermann, and J. F. Barthelemy, *J. Chromatogr.*, *281*, 371 (1983).
152. J. Davídek, J. Velíšek, J. Černá, and T. Davídek, *J. Micronutr. Anal.*, *1*, 39 (1985).
153. A. J. Sheppard and A. R. Prosser, *Methods Enzymol.*, *18*, 311 (1970).
154. E. Tesmer, Dissertation, Reinischen Friedrich-Wilhelms-Universität, Bonn, 1978.
155. V. S. Slyshenkov and A. G. Moiseenok, *Khim.-Farm. Zh.*, *17*, 1513 (1983).

Index

Pyridoxal (−5′-phosphate)
  enzymatic determination, 425
  see vitamin B$_6$
Pyridoxamine (−5′-phosphate)
  see vitamin B$_6$
4-Pyridoxic acid
  in urine 430–431
  see vitamin B$_6$
Pyridoxine (−5′-phosphate)
  see vitamin B$_6$
Pyrovitamin D, 116–119,130,135

Quinolinic acid
  biosynthesis, 288
  determination in plasma, GC-MS,
    312
  determination in whole blood,
    GC-MS, 312
  GC, 311–312
  GC-MS, 312–313
  HPLC determination, 307–309
  selected ion monitoring, 312–313

RBP
  determination methods, 37–38
  size exclusion HPLC, 20
  transport of retinol, 5
Reduced NAD$^+$
  HPLC, 299,304–305
  stability, 287
Reduced NADP$^+$
  HPLC, 299,304–305
  stability, 287
Reductic acid
  internal standard in assays of vita-
    min C, 248–249
Retinal
  formation from carotenoids, 4,43
  GC of, 35
  geometric isomer separation by
    HPLC, 24–28
  HPLC separation from retinoic
    acid, 29
  HPLC separation from retinol, 24
  spectral properties, 14
  structure, 2

Retinal oximes
  HPLC separation, 25–28,33
Retinoic acid
  adsorption HPLC, 28,30
  biochemical function, 6
  detection, HPLC, 28
  determination in plasma, 30–31
  direct inlet mass spectrometry,
    30–31
  extraction from biological
    material, 7,28
  HPLC separation from retinol and
    retinal, 28
  HPLC separation from retinyl
    esters, 30–31
  protein binding, 5
  reversed phase HPLC, 28
  separation from 13-cis-retinoic, 28
  separation from metabolites,
    HPLC, 28,30–31
  spectrometric properties, 14
  structure, 2
Retinoids (natural)
  see Vitamin A
Retinoids (synthetic)
  GC, 35
  internal standard in assays of polar
    retinoids, 13
  internal standard in assays of
    retinoic acid, 13
  RP-HPLC separation, 32
  structures, 3
Retinol
  determination in buccal mucosa
    cells, 19
  determination in milk, 19
  determination in plasma/serum,
    18–19
  determination in tear fluid HPLC,
    19
  electrochemical detection HPLC,
    16
  fluorescence, 4,10,16
  fluorescence detection, HPLC, 16
  GC, 35–36
  GC-MS, 35